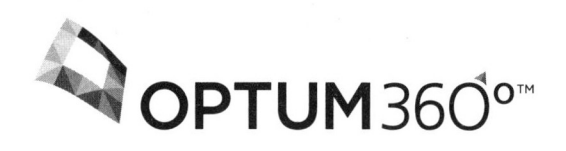

OPTUM360°™

REF

SAVE UP TO 25%*
when you renew your coding essentials.

>> Buy 1–2 items, save 15%
Buy 3–5 items, save 20%
Buy 6+ items, save 25%

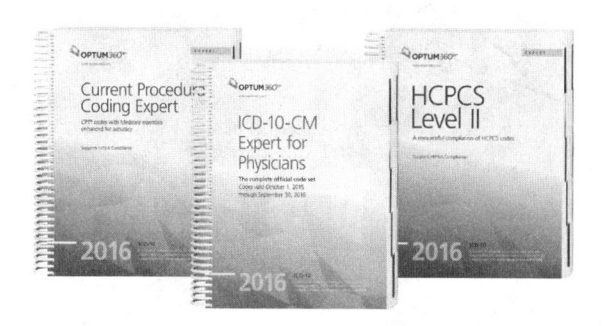

ITEM #	TITLE INDICATE THE ITEMS YOU WISH TO PURCHASE	QUANTITY	PRICE PER PRODUCT	TOTAL

Subtotal

(AK, DE, HI, MT, NH & OR are exempt)   Sales Tax

1 item $10.95 • 2–4 items $12.95 • 5+ CALL   Shipping & Handling

TOTAL AMOUNT ENCLOSED

Save up to 25% when you renew.

Visit **optumcoding.com** and enter the promo code below.

Call **1-800-464-3649, option 1,** and mention the promo code below.

Fax this order form with purchase order to **1-801-982-4033.** Optum360 no longer accepts credit cards by fax.

**PROMO CODE
FOBA16WA**

Mail this order form with payment and/or purchase order to:
Optum360, PO Box 88050, Chicago, IL 60680-9920.
Optum360 no longer accepts credit cards by mail.

Name

Address

Customer Number   Contact Number

○ CHECK ENCLOSED (PAYABLE TO OPTUM360)

○ BILL ME   ○ P.O.#

( )
Telephone
( )
Fax

@
E-mail

Optum360 respects your right to privacy. We will not sell or rent your email address or fax number to anyone outside Optum360 and its business partners. If you would like to remove your name from Optum360 promotions, please call 1-800-464-3649, option 1.

*Discount does not include digital coding solutions, workers' comp or bookstore products.
© 2015 Optum360, LLC. All rights reserved. OPTPRJ9368 SPRJ2351

OPTUM360°

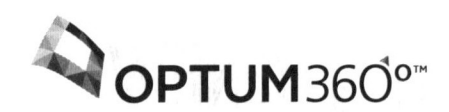

P1ONEER
THE NEW FRONTIER OF CODING

WITH A TRUSTED, INDUSTRY LEADER BY YOUR SIDE.

Navigate the changing landscape of coding and move forward with confidence.

With Optum360 tools and resources at your fingertips, you can open a world of opportunities and help build the foundation for greater efficiencies, financial gains, and competitive advantages. For over 30 years, our print resources have remained trusted tools for coding professionals, and our 2016 editions offer the same quality and reliability you have come to expect from us.

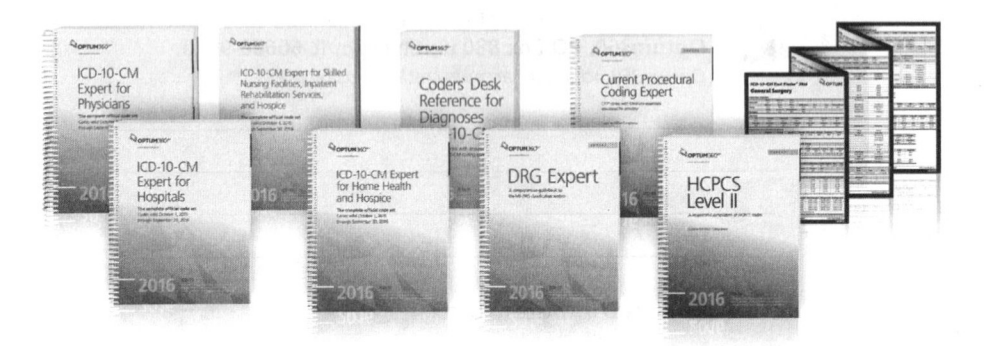

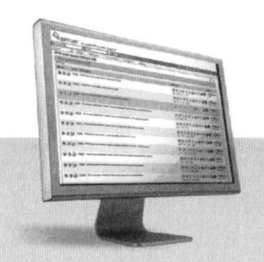

Eliminate roadblocks with web-based coding solutions.
ICD-10 will have 668 percent more codes than ICD-9. Web-based coding solutions can help you experience a smooth, successful transition with fast access to ICD-10 codes, data and mapping tools, and can easily be used in conjunction with our ICD-10 books. Learn more about EncoderPro.com and RevenueCyclePro.com today by visiting **optumcoding.com/transitions.**

The new frontier of coding awaits.
Save up to 25% on the ICD-10, CPT®, and HCPCS coding resources you need.

Visit OptumCoding.com and enter promo code **00000AD3** to save 25%

Call 1.800.464.3649, option 1 and mention promo code **00000AD3** to save 20%

© 2015 Optum360. LLC. All rights reserved.   OPTPRJ9371   SPRJ2353

ESSENTIALS CODING, BILLING & COMPLIANCE CONFERENCE

VISIT OPTUMCODING.COM/ESSENTIALS

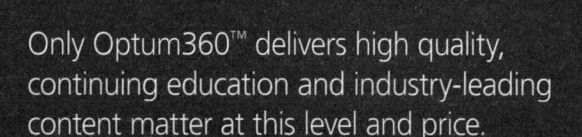

Only Optum360™ delivers high quality, continuing education and industry-leading content matter at this level and price.

Whether you're looking for daily tips to help make your job just a little easier, or you want to keep your skills current and relevant in this ever-changing world of coding, billing and compliance, Optum360 Essentials is truly, well, essential.

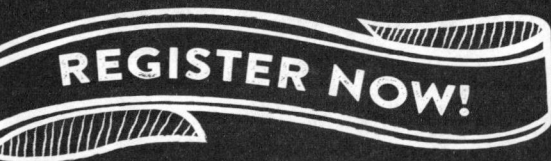

REGISTER NOW!

VISIT
optumcoding.com/essentials

CALL
1-510-463-6073

EMAIL
optumECBC@streamlinevents.com

WHY ATTEND?

- Choose from up to 40 educational sessions, all created to be timely and relevant with what's currently happening in the industry.
- Earn as many as 16 CEUs approved by both AAPC and AHIMA.
- Learn from nationally recognized experts on medical coding, billing and compliance.
- Learn about the CPT® code updates firsthand.
- Stay current with updates on ICD-10-CM/PCS, HCPCS, DRG codes, HCC, PQRS, IPPS and OPPS.
- Focus on ICD-10 with specialty sessions dedicated to your practice.
- Attend vetted presentations that are reviewed and approved by legal and clinical experts.
- Network with a wide spectrum of medical professionals, from entry-level to expert understanding.
- Join user group sessions to learn about the latest in Digital Coding solutions.

CPT is a registered trademark of the American Medical Association.

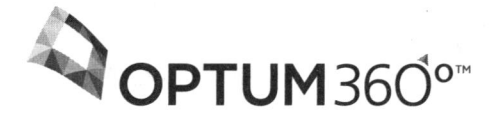

OPTUM360°™

Optum360™
ESSENTIALS
CODING, BILLING & COMPLIANCE CONFERENCE

© 2015 Optum360, LLC. All rights reserved. OPTPRJ9377 SPRJ2356

AMP IT UP

WHEN YOU TURN IT UP WITH DIGITAL CODING TOOLS.

Amp up your accuracy. Save time. Get more code sets and medical reference data and policies. Reduce denials.

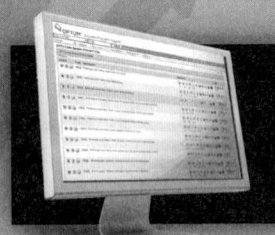

EncoderPro.com for physicians and payers
Quickly and easily access the content of 37 Optum360 code books in one place, with a few clicks of your mouse. Boost productivity and first-pass payment. Streamline coding and prep for ICD-10. **optumcoding.com/transition**

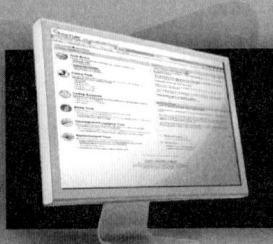

RevenueCyclePro.com for facilities
Simplify your research efforts with reference data compiled in one comprehensive, online problem-solving tool. Maximize your coding compliance efforts and minimize rejected and denied claims. Increase efficiency across the entire hospital revenue cycle. **optumcoding.com/transition**

Take Optum360 online digital coding tools for a spin the following ways at **optumcoding.com/transition**:

- Explore your options by market
- Sign up for a one-on-one customized demo
- Request a free 30-day trial
- Discover the digital coding webinar series

AMP UP YOUR CODING CAPABILITIES TODAY.

Call: 1-800-464-3649, option 1   **Visit:** optumcoding.com/transition

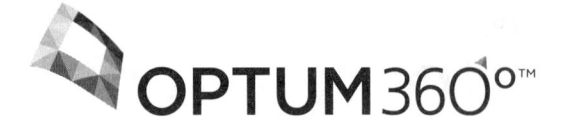

OPTUM 360°™

OPTPRJ9370 | SPRJ2352 | June 2015

OPTUM360°™

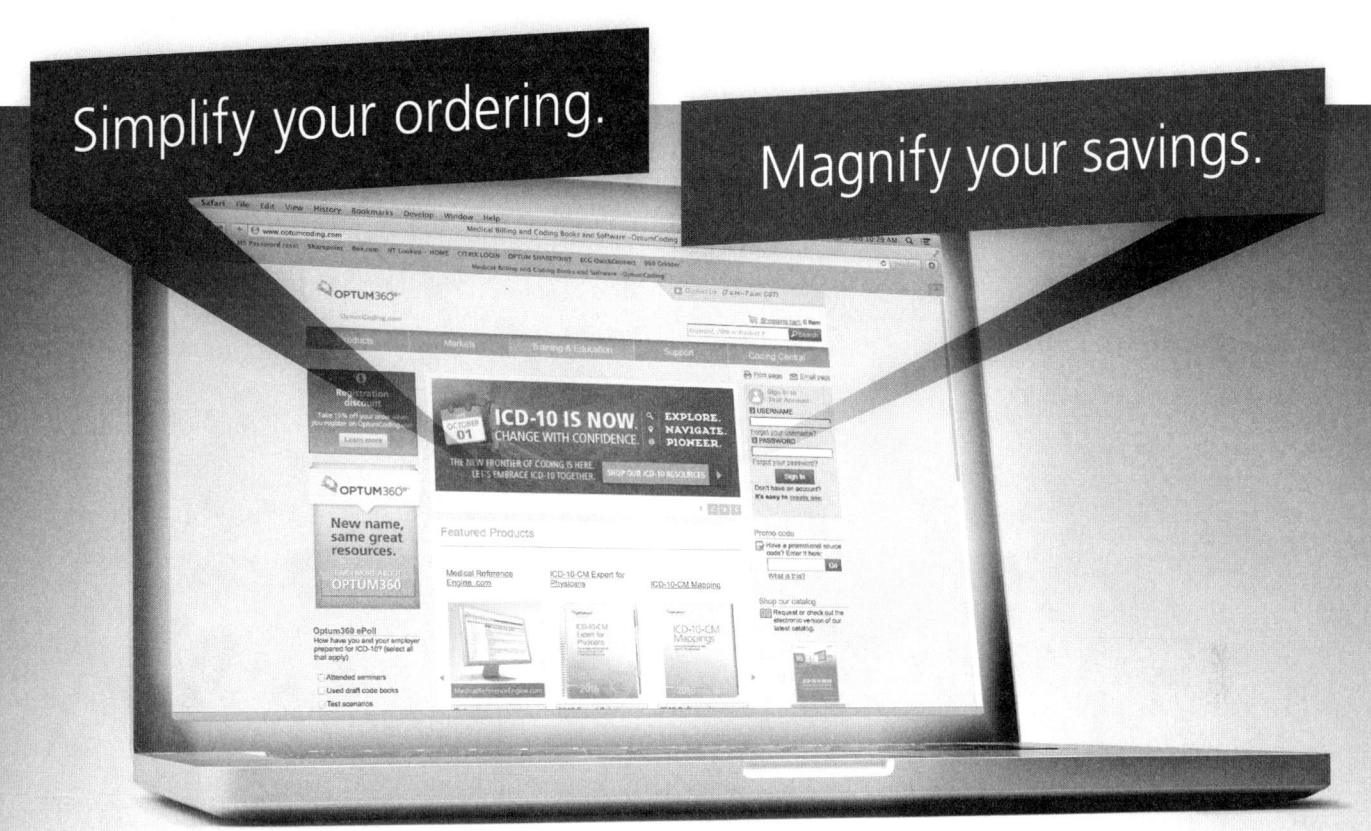

Simplify your ordering.

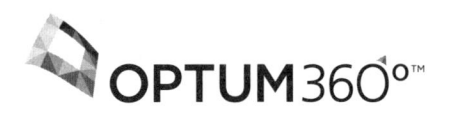

Magnify your savings.

❶ Click.

Visit optumcoding.com

- Find the products you need quickly and easily.
- View all available formats and edition years on the same page.
- Chat live with a customer service representative.
- Visit Coding Central for expert resources including articles, *Inside Track to ICD-10* and coding scenarios to test your knowledge.
- View our catalog online. Utilize our interactive online catalog features to view product information quickly and easily.

❷ Register.

By registering, you'll be able to:

- Enjoy special promotions, discounts and automatic rewards.
- Get recommendations based on your order history.
- Check on shipment status and tracking.
- View order and payment history.
- Pay invoices.
- Manage your address book and ship orders to multiple locations.
- Renew your order with a single click.
- Compile a wish list of the products you want and purchase when you're ready.

❸ Save.

Get 15% off your next order

Register for an account and receive a coupon via email for 15% off your next order.

Plus, save even more with our no-cost eRewards program.

OptumCoding.com
eRewards
program

Register for an account and you're automatically enrolled in our eRewards program, where you'll get a $50 coupon for every $500 you spend*. When logged in at optumcoding.com, the eRewards meter keeps track of purchases toward your next reward.

Visit us at optumcoding.com to register today!

*Offer valid only for customers who are NOT part of our Medallion or Partner Account programs. You must be registered at optumcoding.com to have your online purchases tracked for rewards purposes. Shipping charges and taxes still apply and cannot be used for rewards. Optum Coding eReward offers valid online only.
© 2015 Optum360, LLC. All rights reserved. OPTPRJ9371 SPRJ2354

2016

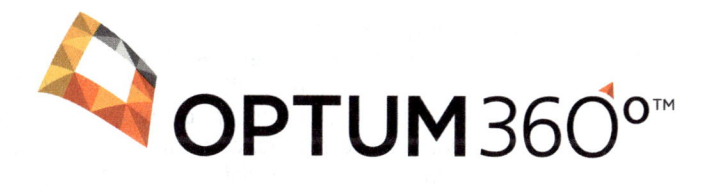

OPTUM360™

Optum360 Learning:
Comprehensive Anatomy and Physiology for ICD-10-CM and ICD-10-PCS Coding

Publisher's Notice

Optum360 Learning: Comprehensive Anatomy and Physiology for ICD-10-CM and ICD-10-PCS Coding is designed to be an accurate and authoritative source of information regarding coding, and every reasonable effort has been made to ensure accuracy and completeness of the content. However, Optum360 makes no guarantee, warranty, or representation that this publication is accurate, complete, or without errors. It is understood that Optum360 is not rendering any legal or other professional services or advice in this publication and that Optum360 bears no liability for any results or consequences that may arise from the use of this book. Please address all correspondence to:

Optum360
2525 Lake Park Blvd
West Valley City, UT 84120

Our Commitment To Accuracy

Optum360 is committed to producing accurate and reliable materials.

To report corrections, please visit www.optumcoding.com/accuracy or email accuracy@optum.com. You can also reach customer service by calling 1.800.464.3649, option 1.

Copyright

Copyright 2015 Optum360, LLC

All rights reserved. No part of this publication may be reproduced or transmitted in any form or by any means electronic or mechanical, including photocopy, recording, or storage in a database or retrieval system, without the prior written permission of the publisher.

Made in the USA

ISBN 978-1-60151-907-8

Acknowledgments

Gregory A. Kemp, MA, *Product Manager*
Karen Schmidt, BSN, *Technical Director*
Stacy Perry, *Manager, Desktop Publishing*
Lisa Singley, *Project Manager*
Karen Krawzik, RHIT, CCS, AHIMA-Approved ICD-10-CM/PCS Trainer, *Clinical/Technical Editor*
Anita Schmidt, BS, RHIT, AHIMA-Approved ICD-10-CM/PCS Trainer, *Clinical/Technical Editor*
Tracy Betzler, *Senior Desktop Publishing Specialist*
Hope M. Dunn, *Senior Desktop Publishing Specialist*
Katie Russell, *Desktop Publishing Specialist*
Kimberli Turner, *Editor*
Regina Heppes, *Editor*

Karen Krawzik, RHIT, CCS, AHIMA-approved ICD-10-CM/PCS Trainer

Ms. Krawzik has expertise in ICD-10-CM, ICD-9-CM, and CPT/HCPCS coding. Her coding experience includes inpatient, ambulatory surgery, and ancillary and emergency room records. She has served as a DRG analyst and auditor of commercial and government payer claims, and as a contract administrator. Most recently she was responsible for the conversion of the ICD-9-CM code set to ICD-10 and for analyzing audit results, identifying issues and trends, and developing remediation plans. Ms. Krawzik is credentialed by the American Health Information Management Association (AHIMA) as a Certified Coding Specialist (CCS) and is an AHIMA-approved ICD-10-CM/PCS trainer. She is an active member of AHIMA and the Missouri Health Information Management Association.

Anita Schmidt, BS, RHIT, AHIMA-approved ICD-10-CM/PCS Trainer

Ms. Schmidt has expertise in Level I Adult and Pediatric Trauma hospital coding, specializing in ICD-9-CM, DRG, and CPT coding. Her experience includes analysis of medical record documentation and assignment of ICD-9-CM codes and DRGs, and CPT code assignments for same-day surgery cases. She has conducted coding training and auditing inclusive of DRG validation, conducted electronic health record training, and worked with clinical documentation specialists to identify documentation needs and potential areas for physician education. Ms. Schmidt is an AHIMA-approved ICD-10-CM/PCS trainer, and is an active member of the American Health Information Management Association (AHIMA) and the Minnesota Health Information Management Association (MHIMA).

Contents

Introduction 1
    Welcome to Comprehensive Anatomy and Physiology for ICD-10-CM
        and ICD-10-PCS Coding 1
    Conventions, Guidelines and Coding Clinics 7
    Summary 8

Chapter 1. Introduction to the Human Body 9
    Anatomy Overview 9
        Figure 1.1: Tissue 10
        Figure 1.2: Anatomical Position 13
        Figure 1.3: Body Planes 14
        Figure 1.4: Motion 16
    Summary 16
    Knowledge Assessment Questions 17

Chapter 2. ICD-10-CM: Integumentary System 19
    Anatomic Overview 19
        Figure 2.1: Skin 19
        Figure 2.2: Hair and Glands 20
        Figure 2.3: Nail 20
        Figure 2.4: Female Breast 21
    Anatomy and Pathophysiology and the ICD-10-CM Code Set 22
        Figure 2.5: Surface and Solid Lesions 27
        Figure 2.6: Sac Lesions 32
        Figure 2.7: Four Stages of Pressure Ulcers 35
        Figure 2.8: Degrees of Burns 41
    Summary 41
    Knowledge Assessment Questions 43

Chapter 3. ICD-10-CM: Skeletal System and Articulations 45
    Anatomic Overview 45
        Figure 3.1: Cranium 46
        Figure 3.2: Facial Bones 47
        Figure 3.3: Vertebrae 48
        Figure 3.4: Spine 48
        Figure 3.5: Ribs and Sternum 49
        Figure 3.6: Shoulder/Upper Extremity 50
        Figure 3.7: Hand 51
        Figure 3.8: Right Coxal Bone 51
        Figure 3.9: Right Tibia and Fibula, Anterior View 52
        Figure 3.10: Right Foot, Dorsal 53
        Figure 3.11: Synovial Joint Structures 54
    Anatomy and Pathophysiology and the ICD-10-CM Code Set 55
        Figure 3.12: Tears of Meniscus 62
        Figure 3.13: Kyphosis and Lordosis 75
        Figure 3.14: Scoliosis and Kyphoscoliosis 75
    Summary 77
    Knowledge Assessment Questions 78

Chapter 4. ICD-10-CM: Muscular System 81
    Anatomic Overview 81
        Figure 4.1: Joint Structures 82
        Figure 4.2: Muscles of the Face 84

Figure 4.3: Eye Musculature 85
Figure 4.4: Associated Regions of Pain due to Neck Injuries 86
Figure 4.5: Muscles of Erector Spine 87
Figure 4.6: Diaphragm 88
Figure 4.7: Pectoralis Major 89
Figure 4.8: Posterior Thorax 90
Figure 4.9: Shoulder Muscles 90
Figure 4.10: Upper Arm 91
Figure 4.11: Forearm 92
Figure 4.12: Elbow 93
Figure 4.13: Thumb and Palm 93
Figure 4.14: Hand 94
Figure 4.15: Anatomy of Anterior Abdominal Wall 94
Figure 4.16: Male Pelvic Floor 95
Figure 4.17: Female Pelvic Floor 95
Figure 4.18: Anterior View of Hip 96
Figure 4.19: Gluteal Muscles 96
Figure 4.20: Anterior View of Thigh 97
Figure 4.21: Gluteus Maximus 97
Figure 4.22: Lower Leg 98
Figure 4.23: Foot 99
Figure 4.24: Foot 99
Anatomy and Pathophysiology and the ICD-10-CM Code Set 100
Summary 109
Knowledge Assessment Questions 110

Chapter 5. ICD-10-CM: Nervous System 113
Anatomic Overview 113
Figure 5.1: Brain 113
Figure 5.2: Spinal Column 114
Figure 5.3: Peripheral Nervous System 115
Figure 5.4: Adnexa 117
Figure 5.5: Eye Musculature 117
Figure 5.6: Ear Anatomy 118
Anatomy and Pathophysiology and the ICD-10-CM Code Set 119
Figure 5.7: Neuromuscular Junction 124
Figure 5.8: Parkinson's Disease 124
Figure 5.9: Pyramidal Pathways 126
Figure 5.10: Myelin and Nerve Structure 128
Figure 5.11: Circle of Willis 132
Figure 5.12: Cerebrovascular Arteries 133
Figure 5.13: Trigeminal and Facial Nerve Branches 134
Figure 5.14: Facial Nerves 135
Figure 5.15: Anterior Chamber 137
Figure 5.16: Posterior Segment of Eye 142
Figure 5.17: Glaucoma 144
Figure 5.18: Cataract 145
Figure 5.19: Arcus Senilis 147
Figure 5.20: External Ear 151
Figure 5.21: Middle and Inner Ear 152
Figure 5.22: Schematic of Labyrinth and Semicircular Ducts 154
Summary 157
Knowledge Assessment Questions 158

Chapter 6. ICD-10-CM: Endocrine System 161
Anatomic Overview 161
Figure 6.1: Endocrine System 163
Figure 6.2: Pancreas 163
Figure 6.3: Pituitary Gland 164

Figure 6.4: Thyroid 165
Figure 6.5: Dorsal View of Parathyroid Glands 166
Figure 6.6: Uterus and Ovaries 167
Figure 6.7: Male Pelvic Organs 168
Figure 6.8: Thymus Gland 168
Anatomy and Pathophysiology and the ICD-10-CM Code Set 169
Figure 6.9: Goiter 169
Figure 6.10: Cataract 175
Summary 188
Knowledge Assessment Questions 189

Chapter 7. ICD-10-CM: Cardiovascular System 191
Anatomic Overview 191
Figure 7.1: Sections of Heart Muscle 191
Figure 7.2: Anatomy 192
Figure 7.3: Blood Flow 192
Figure 7.4: Conduction System of the Heart 193
Figure 7.5: Arteries of the Heart 194
Figure 7.6: Capillary Bed 196
Figure 7.7: Cerebrovascular Arteries 197
Figure 7.8: Head Veins 197
Figure 7.9: Arterial System 198
Figure 7.10: Portal System 199
Anatomy and Pathophysiology and the ICD-10-CM Code Set 200
Figure 7.11: Valvular Function 200
Figure 7.12: Acute Myocardial Infarction 203
Figure 7.13: Thoracic and Abdominal Aortic Aneurysm 210
Figure 7.14: Venous System 211
Figure 7.15: Map of Major Veins 213
Figure 7.16: Veins of Lower Extremities 214
Summary 222
Knowledge Assessment Questions 223

Chapter 8. ICD-10-CM: Blood and Blood-Forming Organs 227
Anatomic Overview 227
Figure 8.1: Red Blood Cells 228
Figure 8.2: Blood Types 229
Figure 8.3: White Blood Cells 230
Figure 8.4: Platelets 231
Figure 8.5: Blood Coagulation 232
Anatomy and Pathophysiology and the ICD-10-CM Code Set 233
Figure 8.6: Thalassemia 234
Figure 8.7: Normal and Sickle Red Blood Cells 235
Summary 239
Knowledge Assessment Questions 240

Chapter 9. ICD-10-CM: Lymphatic System 243
Anatomic Overview 243
Figure 9.1: Lymphatic Capillaries 243
Figure 9.2: Lymphatic System 244
Figure 9.3: Thyroid Gland 245
Figure 9.4: Lymph Node 245
Figure 9.5: Axillary Lymph Nodes 246
Figure 9.6: Lymph Nodes of Trunk 246
Figure 9.7: Lymphatic Drainage 247
Figure 9.8: Tongue 248

Anatomy and Pathophysiology and the ICD-10-CM Code Set 248
Summary 258
Knowledge Assessment Questions 259

Chapter 10. ICD-10-CM: Respiratory System 261
Anatomic Overview 261
  Figure 10.1: Lower Respiratory System 262
  Figure 10.2: Larynx 263
  Figure 10.3: Lungs 264
  Figure 10.4: Upper Respiratory System 265
Anatomy and Pathophysiology and the ICD-10-CM Code Set 266
  Figure 10.5: Bronchoscopy 267
  Figure 10.6: Bronchioli and Alveoli 268
  Figure 10.7: Emphysema 271
  Figure 10.8: Alveoli, Asbestoses, Air Sacs 275
  Figure 10.9: Pleural Effusion 278
  Figure 10.10: Firearm Injury, X-ray 283
  Figure 10.11: Upper Respiratory System 285
Summary 286
Knowledge Assessment Questions 287

Chapter 11. ICD-10-CM: Digestive System 289
Anatomic Overview 289
  Figure 11.1: Digestive System 289
  Figure 11.2: Stomach and Pylorus 290
  Figure 11.3: Duodenum 291
Anatomy and Pathophysiology and the ICD-10-CM Code Set 292
  Figure 11.4: Teeth 292
  Figure 11.5: Saliva Glands 294
  Figure 11.6: Liver 295
  Figure 11.7: Pancreas 297
  Figure 11.8: Esophagus 298
  Figure 11.9: Stomach 300
  Figure 11.10: Volvulus and Diverticulitis 301
  Figure 11.11: Large Intestine 303
  Figure 11.12: Colostomy 307
Summary 310
Knowledge Assessment Questions 311

Chapter 12. ICD-10-CM: Urinary System 315
Anatomic Overview 315
  Figure 12.1: Urinary System 315
  Figure 12.2: Kidney 316
  Figure 12.3: Nephron 316
  Figure 12.4: Bladder 317
Anatomy and Pathophysiology and the ICD-10-CM Code Set 318
Summary 331
Knowledge Assessment Questions 332

Chapter 13. ICD-10-CM: Reproductive Systems 335
Anatomic Overview: Male Reproductive System 335
  Figure 13.1: Male Genitalia 335
  Figure 13.2: Glans Penis 336
  Figure 13.3: Testis and Sperm Generation 336
  Figure 13.4: Prostate and Seminal Vesicles 337
Anatomy and Pathophysiology and the ICD-10-CM Code Set: Male
  Reproductive System 338
  Figure 13.5: Male Urinary and Reproductive Systems 339

    Figure 13.6: Slitting of Prepuce 340
    Figure 13.7: Penis 343
Summary: Male Reproductive System 343
Anatomic Overview: Female Reproductive System 344
    Figure 13.8: Female External Genitalia 344
    Figure 13.9: Female Reproductive System 345
Anatomy and Pathophysiology and the ICD-10-CM Code Set: Female
    Reproductive System 347
    Figure 13.10: Ovary and Fallopian Tube 347
Summary: Female Reproductive System 350
Anatomic Overview: Pregnancy, Childbirth, and the Puerperium 350
Anatomy and Pathophysiology and the ICD-10-CM Code Set: Pregnancy,
    Childbirth, and the Puerperium 351
Summary: Pregnancy, Childbirth, and the Puerperium 356
Knowledge Assessment Questions 357

Chapter 14. ICD-10-PCS Introduction 361
Importance of Anatomy and Physiology in ICD-10-PCS 361
Overview 361
Character 1: Section 363
Character 2: Body System 363
Character 3: Root Operation 366
Character 4: Body Part 369
Character 5: Approach 374
Character 6: Device 376
Character 7: Qualifier 377
Summary 379
Knowledge Assessment Questions 380

Chapter 15. ICD-10-PCS:
Nervous and Circulatory Systems 383
Central Nervous System (Ø) 383
    Figure 15.1: Brain Sections 384
    Figure 15.2: Skull Layers 385
    Figure 15.3: Cranial Nerves 387
Peripheral Nervous System (1) 391
    Figure 15.4: Peripheral Nervous System 392
    Figure 15.5: Brachial Plexus 393
    Figure 15.6: Median and Ulnar Nerves 394
    Figure 15.7: Sympathetic Nervous System 396
Heart and Great Vessels (2) 399
    Figure 15.8: Coronary Arteries 400
    Figure 15.9: Heart Anatomy 400
Upper Arteries (3) 405
    Figure 15.10: Map of Upper Arteries 406
    Figure 15.11: Cerebrovascular Arteries 407
    Figure 15.12: Circle of Willis 408
    Figure 15.13: External Carotid 409
Lower Arteries (4) 411
    Figure 15.14: Lower Arteries 412
Upper Veins (5) 416
    Figure 15.15: Map of Upper Veins 417
    Figure 15.16: Head and Neck Veins 418
Lower Veins (6) 421
    Figure 15.17: Map of Lower Veins 422

Summary 425

Knowledge Assessment Questions 426

Chapter 16. ICD-10-PCS: Lymphatic, Sense Organ, and Respiratory Systems 429

Lymphatic and Hemic Systems (7) 429
  Figure 16.1: Lymphatic System 430
Eye (8) 434
  Figure 16.2: Eye 435
  Figure 16.3: Retina (E, F) 436
  Figure 16.4: Eye Musculature 436
  Figure 16.5: Lacrimal System 437
Ear, Nose, and Sinus (9)* 439
  Figure 16.6: Ear Anatomy 440
  Figure 16.7: Middle and Inner Ear 441
  Figure 16.8: Nasal Turbinates 442
  Figure 16.9: Paranasal/Accessory sinuses 443
Respiratory System (B) 444
  Figure 16.10: Bronchi 445
  Figure 16.11: Lungs 446
Summary 447
Knowledge Assessment Questions 448

Chapter 17. ICD-10-PCS: Digestive and Endocrine Systems 451

Mouth and Throat (C) 451
  Figure 17.1: Mouth Frontal View (Upper) 452
  Figure 17.2: Mouth Frontal View (Lower) 452
  Figure 17.3: Oral Anatomy 453
  Figure 17.4: Mandibular Glands 453
  Figure 17.5: Pharynx 454
Gastrointestinal System (D) 456
  Figure 17.6: Gastrointestinal System: Upper Intestinal Tract, Lower Intestinal Tract 457
  Figure 17.7: Stomach and Pylorus 458
  Figure 17.8: Lower GI 459
  Figure 17.9: Rectum and Anus 460
Hepatobiliary System and Pancreas (F) 462
  Figure 17.10: Liver 463
  Figure 17.11: Gallbladder and Ducts 464
  Figure 17.12: Pancreas 464
Endocrine System (G) 466
  Figure 17.13: Endocrine System 467
  Figure 17.14: Adrenal Glands 467
  Figure 17.15: Thyroid and Parathyroid Glands 468
  Figure 17.16: Thyroid (Frontal) 468
Summary 469
Knowledge Assessment Questions 470

Chapter 18. ICD-10-PCS: Skin, Subcutaneous Tissue, and Musculoskeletal Systems 473

Skin and Breast (H) 473
  Figure 18.1: Integumentary Anatomy (0-9, A-P) 474
  Figure 18.2: Nail Anatomy (Q, R) 475
  Figure 18.3: Breast (T-X) 475
Subcutaneous Tissue and Fascia (J) 477
Muscles (K) 480
  Figure 18.4: Muscles 481

Tendons (L)	485
Figure 18.5: Wrist and Forearm Cross-section	486
Figure 18.6: Tendons of the Wrist and Hand	486
Figure 18.7: Shoulder Tendons	487
Figure 18.8: Leg Muscles and Tendons	487
Figure 18.9: Lower Leg Tendons	488
Bursae and Ligaments (M)	489
Figure 18.10: Shoulder Anatomy	490
Figure 18.11: Wrist Ligaments	491
Figure 18.12: Knee Bursae	492
Figure 18.13: Knee Ligaments	493
Head and Facial Bones (N)	494
Figure 18.14: Head and Facial Bones	495
Figure 18.15: Skull Bones	496
Upper Bones (P)	498
Figure 18.16: Humerus and Scapula	499
Figure 18.17: Radius and Ulna	500
Figure 18.18: Hand Bones	501
Lower Bones (Q)	502
Figure 18.19: Hip Bone Anatomy	503
Figure 18.20: Pelvic and Lower Bones	504
Figure 18.21: Foot Bones	505
Upper Joints (R)	507
Figure 18.22: Vertebral Joint	508
Figure 18.23: Shoulder Joint	509
Figure 18.24: Hand Joints	510
Lower Joints (S)	512
Figure 18.25: Hip Joint	514
Figure 18.26: Knee Joint (C, D)	514
Figure 18.27: Lateral View, Knee (C, D)	515
Figure 18.28: Foot	516
Summary	517
Knowledge Assessment Questions	518
Chapter 19. ICD-10-PCS: Genitourinary Systems	**521**
Urinary System (T)	521
Figure 19.1: Genitourinary System	522
Figure 19.2: Kidney	522
Figure 19.3: Bladder	523
Female Reproductive System (U)	525
Figure 19.4: Female Reproductive System	526
Figure 19.5: Female External Structures	527
Male Reproductive System (V)	528
Figure 19.6: Male Reproductive System	529
Figure 19.7: Penis	530
Summary	530
Knowledge Assessment Questions	531
Chapter 20. ICD-10-PCS: Anatomical Regions Systems	**533**
Anatomical Regions	533
Summary	534
Knowledge Assessment Questions	535
Appendix A. Knowledge Assessment Answers	**537**
Chapter 1. Introduction to the Human Body	537
Chapter 2. ICD-10-CM: Integumentary System	539
Chapter 3. ICD-10-CM: Skeletal Systems and Articulations	541

Chapter 4. ICD-10-CM: Muscular System 544
Chapter 5. ICD-10-CM: Nervous System 547
Chapter 6. ICD-10-CM: Endocrine System 550
Chapter 7. ICD-10-CM: Cardiovascular System 552
Chapter 8. ICD-10-CM: Blood and Blood-Forming Organs 557
Chapter 9. ICD-10-CM: Lymphatic System 560
Chapter 10. ICD-10-CM: Respiratory System 563
Chapter 11. ICD-10-CM: Digestive System 567
Chapter 12. ICD-10-CM: Urinary System 571
Chapter 13. ICD-10-CM: Reproductive Systems 573
Chapter 14. ICD-10-PCS Introduction 579
Chapter 15. ICD-10-PCS: Nervous and Circulatory Systems 582
Chapter 16. ICD-10-PCS: Lymphatic, Sense Organ, and Respiratory Systems 584
Chapter 17. ICD-10-PCS: Digestive and Endocrine Systems 586
Chapter 18. ICD-10-PCS: Skin, Subcutaneous Tissue, and Musculoskeletal Systems 588
Chapter 19. ICD-10-PCS: Genitourinary Systems 591
Chapter 20. ICD-10-PCS: Anatomical Regions Systems 593

Appendix B. Body Part Key 595

Appendix C. Body Part Definitions 615

Appendix D. Root Operation Definitions 629

Appendix E. Root Operation Conversion Table 637

Introduction

Welcome to Comprehensive Anatomy and Physiology for ICD-10-CM and ICD-10-PCS Coding

The transition from ICD-9-CM to ICD-10-CM and ICD-10-PCS marks a transformation in coding in the United States. Not only have code choices increased five-fold, but the code descriptions themselves are much more specific. The greater level of detail in ICD-10 demands that coders have an in-depth knowledge of anatomy, physiology, and pathophysiology if they are to select the most appropriate code in the new system. Optum360's *Comprehensive Anatomy and Physiology for ICD-10-CM and ICD-10-PCS Coding* is a great initial step in that education.

Before delving into the details of anatomy and physiology, however, it is important to understand the transition from ICD-9 to ICD-10 and the differences between the code sets.

ICD-9-CM to ICD-10 Transition

The codes within ICD-9-CM fall woefully short of today's medical reporting needs. ICD-9-CM was created more than 25 years ago as a modern and expandable system that was then only partially filled. Thousands of codes have been added to ICD-9-CM over the years to classify new procedures and diseases, and today the remaining space in ICD-9-CM procedure and diagnosis coding systems cannot accommodate new technologies or new understanding of diseases.

In response to ICD-9-CM's shortcomings, new coding systems were developed and soon will be implemented in the United States. The World Health Organization (**WHO**) created and adopted ICD-10 in 1994 and it has been used in much of the world since then. This system is the basis for the new U.S. diagnosis coding system, International Classification of Diseases, 10th Revision, Clinical Modification (ICD-10-CM).

Concurrent to the clinical modification of ICD-10 by the National Center for Health Statistics (**NCHS**), the Centers for Medicare and Medicaid Services (**CMS**) commissioned 3M Health Information Management to develop a new procedure coding system to replace volume 3 of ICD-9-CM, used for inpatient procedure coding. Now that the coding systems have been designed and written, they need only be implemented, but progress is slow. The government is moving cautiously toward implementation, partly because the scope of change is massive and will profoundly affect all care providers, payers, and government agencies, but also because the change is massive and costly enough to carry considerable political impact.

On January 16, 2009, the Department of Health and Human Services (HHS) published a final rule in the *Federal Register*, 45 CFR part 162, "HIPAA Administrative Simplification: Modifications to Medical Data Code Set Standards to Adopt ICD-10-CM and ICD-10-PCS" (downloadable at http://edocket.access.gpo.gov/2009/pdf/E9-743.pdf). This final rule adopts modifications to standard medical data code sets for coding diagnoses and inpatient hospital procedures by adopting ICD-10-CM for diagnosis coding, including the *Official ICD-10-CM Guidelines for Coding and Reporting*, and ICD-10-PCS for inpatient hospital procedure coding, effective October 1, 2013. The most current 2016 update release is available for public viewing, and additional updates are expected before implementation. On September 5, 2012, HHS announced a final rule that would delay the implementation of the ICD-10-CM code sets from October 2013 to October 2014. This delay gives the health care community additional time to prepare and test systems appropriately.

> **DEFINITIONS**
>
> **CMS.** Centers for Medicare and Medicaid Services. Federal agency that provides health insurance for more than 74 million Americans through Medicare, Medicaid, and Children's Health Insurance Program. CMS contracted with 3M HIS to develop a new procedure coding system (ICD-10-PCS). Find CMS at http://www.cms.gov/.
>
> **NCHS.** National Center for Health Statistics. U.S. government agency that, jointly with CMS, refines the diagnostic portion of ICD-9-CM and is responsible for the clinical modification of ICD-10. NCHS holds several hearings a year to consider changes or additions to diagnosis coding. Find NCHS at http://www.cdc.gov/nchs.
>
> **WHO.** World Health Organization. International agency that maintains an international nomenclature of diseases, causes of death, and public health practices. WHO, with advice from participating countries, developed ICD-9 to track morbidity and mortality statistics worldwide. It recently updated diagnosis coding with ICD-10. Find WHO at http://www.who.int/en.

On April 2, 2014, Congress enacted the Protecting Access to Medicare Act of 2014, which contained a provision to delay the implementation of ICD-10 CM/PCS by at least a year. The act prohibits HHS from adopting the ICD-10 CM/PCS code sets as the mandatory standard until at least October 1, 2015.

HHS issued an interim final rule on August 4, 2014, finalizing October 1, 2015, as the new ICD-10 compliance date. This rule will also require HIPAA-covered entities to continue to use ICD-9-CM through September 30, 2015. This interim final rule may be viewed at http://www.gpo.gov/fdsys/pkg/FR-2014-08-04/pdf/2014-18347.pdf.

Everyone in facilities will be affected: coders, human resources staff, accountants, information systems staff, physicians—just to name a few. The proposed codes provide tremendous opportunities for disease and procedure tracking but also create enormous challenges. Computer hardware and software, medical documentation, and the revenue cycle are just three elements of medical reimbursement that will be shaken when implementation occurs.

Understanding the changes the World Health Organization made in moving from ICD-9 to ICD-10 is a good basis for learning about the clinical modifications to ICD-10. The first clue to the revisions is in the full title: International Statistical Classification of Diseases and Related Health Problems. WHO felt this change would not only clarify the classification's content and purpose, but show how the scope of the system has moved beyond the classification of disease and injuries to the coding of ambulatory care conditions and risk factors frequently encountered in primary care.

Overall, the 10th revision goes into greater clinical detail than does ICD-9-CM and addresses information about previously classified diseases, as well as those diseases discovered since the last revision. Conditions are grouped with general epidemiological purposes and the evaluation of health care in mind. New features have been added, and conditions have been reorganized, although the format and conventions of the classification remain unchanged for the most part.

Other adaptations of the ICD include:

- International Classification of Diseases for Oncology, third edition (ICD-O-3)
- International Classification of External Causes of Injury (ICECI)
- International Classification of Primary Care, second edition (ICPC-2)
- The ICD-10 for Mental and Behavioral Disorders Diagnostic Criteria for Research
- The ICD-10 for Mental and Behavioral Disorders Clinical Descriptions and Diagnostic Guidelines

In the United States, the clinical modification of ICD-10, ICD-10-CM, will replace the clinical modification of ICD-9, ICD-9-CM. The parent classification system, the International Classification of Disease (ICD), is owned and copyrighted by WHO, which publishes the classification. As with ICD-9-CM, WHO authorized the development of an adaptation of ICD-10 for use in the United States. This adaptation, the clinical modification (CM), must conform to WHO conventions for the ICD.

If many of the codes considered new in ICD-10 seem familiar to users of ICD-9-CM, it is because ICD-10 is a further evolution of the ICD-9 classification, as ICD-10-CM is a further evolution of ICD-9-CM. The underlying basic structure, conventions, and philosophy remain the same. The clinical modification in use in the United States (ICD-9-CM) has been maintained and updated annually since 1985. The following example using angina pectoris classifications illustrates the evolution from the preclinical modification ICD-9 version to the current 2016 version of ICD-10-CM:

ICD-9:

413   Angina pectoris

ICD-9-CM:

411.1	Intermediate coronary syndrome (includes unstable angina)
413.0	Angina decubitus
413.1	Prinzmetal angina
413.9	Other and unspecified angina pectoris

ICD-10 and ICD-10-CM:

All diseases of the circulatory system appear under the letter "I" in ICD-10.

I20.0	Unstable angina
I20.1	Angina pectoris with documented spasm — (includes Prinzmetal angina)
I20.8	Other forms of angina pectoris — (includes angina of effort and stenocardia)
I20.9	Angina pectoris, unspecified

ICD Structure

WHO published ICD-10 in three volumes: an index, an instructional manual, and a tabular list. ICD-10-CM will be published in two volumes: an index and a tabular list.

The index is an alphabetical list of terms with the corresponding code, and the tabular list is a chronological list of alphanumeric codes divided into chapters based on body system or condition. The index consists of the following parts: the Index to Diseases and Injuries, the Neoplasm Table, the Table of Drugs and Chemicals, and the Index to External Causes.

Tabular List

Volume 1 of ICD-9-CM contains the tabular listing of alphanumeric codes. The same hierarchical organization of ICD-9 applies to ICD-10: All codes with the same first three characters have common traits.

Each character beyond three adds more specificity. In ICD-10, valid codes can contain anywhere from three to five characters. However, ICD-10-CM for use in the United States has been expanded with valid codes containing anywhere from three to seven characters. In some instances, the final character may be an alphabetic character, known as an alpha extension, and not a number. In some cases, the use of a "reserve" subclassification (identified as an "X") has been incorporated into codes that continue with greater specificity beyond a fourth or fifth character to allow for built-in expansion within that established level of specificity. For example:

H83.3 Noise effects on inner ear
    Acoustic trauma of inner ear
    Noise-induced hearing loss of inner ear

H83.3X Noise effects on inner ear

H83.3X1	Noise effects on right inner ear
H83.3X2	Noise effects on left inner ear
H83.3X3	Noise effects on inner ear, bilateral
H83.3X9	Noise effects on inner ear, unspecified ear

This reserve subclassification, and simply the additional characters themselves, allow for more specific codes. This additional specificity can present a hurdle for some coders who may have not had a great deal of training in anatomy and physiology in the past. New terms are being used in the ICD-10-CM system, and they may be different from what the physician is using in his or her documentation. For this reason, coders need to be well educated about anatomy and physiology at a deeper level than was previously required for ICD-9-CM coding.

Alphabetic Index

In ICD-9-CM, the alphabetic index is a reference for the tabular list. As in the ICD-9-CM index, terms in the ICD-10 index are arranged alphabetically by diagnosis. This is no different for ICD-10-CM. Therefore, a code for a supernumerary nipple would be accessed by looking under "Supernumerary," then "nipple."

Alphabetical Index to Diseases and Nature of Injury in ICD-10-CM

Supernumerary (congenital)
- aortic cusps Q23.8
- auditory ossicles Q16.3
- bone Q79.8
- breast Q83.1
- carpal bones Q74.0
- cusps, heart valve NEC Q24.8
    - aortic Q23.8
    - mitral Q23.2
    - pulmonary Q22.3
- digit(s) Q69.9
- ear (lobule) Q17.0
- fallopian tube Q50.6
- finger Q69.0
- hymen Q52.4
- kidney Q63.0
- lacrimonasal duct Q10.6
- lobule (ear) Q17.0
- mitral cusps Q23.2
- muscle Q79.8
- nipple(s) Q83.3
- organ or site not listed — *see* Accessory
- ossicles, auditory Q16.3
- ovary Q50.31
- oviduct Q50.6
- pulmonary, pulmonary cusps Q22.3
- rib Q76.6
    - cervical or first (syndrome) Q76.5
- roots (of teeth) K00.2
- spleen Q89.09
- tarsal bones Q74.2
- teeth K00.1
- testis Q55.29
- thumb Q69.1
- toe Q69.2
- uterus Q51.2
- vagina Q52.1
- vertebra Q76.49

Code Structure

All codes in ICD-10 and ICD-10-CM are alphanumeric as opposed to the strictly numeric characters in the main classification of ICD-9-CM. Of the 26 available letters, all but the letter U is used, which is reserved for additions and changes that may need to be incorporated in the future or to resolve classification difficulties that may arise between revisions.

Codes for terrorism were created after September 11, 2001, within the framework of ICD-10 and ICD-9-CM. They have been incorporated into ICD-9-CM since 2002 and proposed for implementation in ICD-10 as U codes for terrorism and have not officially been adopted by WHO. If the codes are adopted, they will be identified as U.S. codes by an asterisk to distinguish them from official ICD codes.

In ICD-10-CM, external causes due to acts of terrorism are classified to code category Y38. This category includes seven-character codes that identify injuries resulting from acts of terrorism, defined as "the unlawful use of force or violence against persons or property to intimidate or coerce a government, the civilian population, or any segment thereof, in furtherance of political or social objective." An additional

> **KEY POINT**
>
> The alphabetic index in ICD-10-CM is arranged alphabetically by diagnosis, much like the ICD-9-CM index.

code from category Y92 should be assigned to specify place of occurrence. The seventh character reports the encounter as A (initial encounter), D (subsequent encounter), or S (sequela).

The code structures of ICD-9-CM and ICD-10-CM are similar in that each classification system is maintained to be as congruent to the other as possible, pending transition. As ICD-9-CM expanded its classification and code structure, ICD-10-CM was similarly expanded and maintained.

Though the use of alphabetic characters I and O may be confused with the numbers 1 and 0, coders should remember that the first character in ICD-10-CM is always a letter. The second character is a numeral, followed by a numeral or alphabetic character in the third character space. Codes may also contain an alphabetic extension in the final character position or a reserve subclassification, denoted as "X."

> ✓ **QUICK TIP**
>
> Be careful of alphabetic characters I and O versus numbers 1 and 0. They look similar, but remember that the first character in any ICD-10-CM code is always a letter and the second is always a number. Others could vary, so be cautious with code assignment.

ICD-9-CM:

Diseases of Arteries, Arterioles, and Capillaries (440–449)

440	Atherosclerosis
441	Aortic aneurysm and dissection
442	Other aneurysm
443	Other peripheral vascular disease
444	Arterial embolism and thrombosis
445	Atheroembolism
446	Polyarteritis nodosa and allied conditions
447	Other disorders of arteries and arterioles
448	Disease of capillaries
449	Septic arterial embolism

ICD-10-CM:

Diseases of Arteries, Arterioles and Capillaries (I70–I79)

I70	Atherosclerosis
I71	Aortic aneurysm and dissection
I72	Other aneurysm
I73	Other peripheral vascular diseases
I74	Arterial embolism and thrombosis
I75	Atheroembolism
I76	Septic arterial embolism
I77	Other disorders of arteries and arterioles
I78	Diseases of capillaries
I79	Disorders of arteries, arterioles and capillaries in diseases classified elsewhere

Importance of Anatomy and Physiology to ICD-10-CM

Throughout the many years they have used the ICD-9-CM system, providers have become used to the system's terminology, and many document cases based on that terminology. ICD-9-CM also has many codes that are fairly general; for instance, there are many unspecified or unlisted codes that must be used because more specific codes are not available for the conditions the patient is presenting with. In ICD-10-CM, this lack of specificity is diminished significantly.

ICD-10-CM will require coders to have a greater understanding of human anatomy, physiology, and disease pathology for multiple reasons. First, the code set itself is in many cases much more specific. For example:

Coding for Unspecified Cellulitis and Abscess of Finger

ICD-9-CM		ICD-10-CM	
681.00	Unspecified cellulitis and abscess of finger	L02.511	Cutaneous abscess of right hand
		L02.512	Cutaneous abscess of left hand
		L02.519	Cutaneous abscess of unspecified hand
		L03.011	Cellulitis of right finger
		L03.012	Cellulitis of left finger
		L03.019	Cellulitis of unspecified finger
		L03.021	Acute lymphangitis of right finger
		L03.022	Acute lymphangitis of left finger
		L03.029	Acute lymphangitis of unspecified finger

What was described as an "unspecified" cellulitis or abscess of the finger in ICD-9-CM will now require that the coder review the documentation and determine whether the patient was seen for a cutaneous abscess, cellulitis, or acute lymphangitis. Also, notice that the code set specifies laterality, another level of detail provided by ICD-10-CM.

This greater level of detail will demand that providers augment the clinical information in their documentation. Previously, a push for a higher level of documentation tended to focus on a few areas—particularly evaluation and management coding in the outpatient realm in addition to various items on the inpatient side. With ICD-10-CM, there will be a big push for documentation improvement across all services for diagnostic information, but much of that push will need to come from the coders. Coders well trained in human anatomy, physiology, and pathophysiology will be able to help providers document accurately what is going on clinically with the patient.

ICD-9-CM to ICD-10-PCS Transition

As discussed previously, the current ICD-9-CM coding system was never intended to be used for anywhere near 30 years. This same principle applies to the procedural coding system, as the ICD-9-CM Volume 3 code set was never developed to represent the highly complex and technically advanced procedures performed in hospitals today. The following table highlights the basic differences between ICD-9-CM Volume 3 procedure codes and ICD-10-PCS codes. A detailed explanation of the importance of anatomy and physiology as it relates to the ICD-10-PCS coding system is provided in chapter 14.

ICD-9-CM Volume 3	ICD-10-PCS
Uses ICD structure (developed for diagnosis codes)	Designed specifically for procedures, with all characters representing procedural concepts
Codes are maintained as a fixed/finite set in list format, using a "look-up" process	Codes are constructed from specifically defined character value components using tables
Codes are numeric	Codes are alphanumeric
Codes are three or four digits	Codes are seven characters, without exception
There are a finite number of potential codes; chapters easily fill up	Character values may be added or deleted, with an exponential amount of codes available

Conventions, Guidelines and *Coding Clinics*

Conventions and Guidelines: New detailed coding conventions and guidelines have been developed specifically for ICD-10-CM and PCS. Coders must carefully review these before applying codes for either of these code sets. Some of the guidelines pertaining to the human body are highlighted throughout this book. The complete and most recent guidelines for ICD-10-CM and ICD-10-PCS can be found at http://www.cms.gov/Medicare/Coding/ICD10/2016-ICD-10-CM-and-GEMs.html and http://www.cms.gov/Medicare/Coding/ICD10/2016-ICD-10-PCS-and-GEMs.html.

Coding Clinic: Published by the AHA Central Office (American Hospital Association), AHA *Coding Clinic* is the only official publication for ICD-10-CM and ICD-10-PCS coding guidelines and advice as designated by the four cooperating parties—American Hospital Association (AHA), American Health Information Management Association (AHIMA), Centers for Medicare and Medicaid Services (CMS), and National Center for Health Statistics (NCHS) plus the Editorial Advisory Board. Beginning in the fourth quarter of 2012, information has been published relating to codes, guidelines, and conventions for ICD-10-CM and ICD-10-PCS. This question and answer format is published by AHA on a quarterly basis and is available by subscription. *Coding Clinics* are not a substitute for physician documentation and should only be considered as guidance. The references used from AHA *Coding Clinics* in this book are taken from information published through the second quarter of 2015. When referenced in this book, it will be noted with the quarter, year, and page of the publication.

How to Use the *Comprehensive Anatomy and Physiology for ICD-10-CM and ICD-10-PCS Coding*

The **Comprehensive Anatomy and Physiology for ICD-10-CM and ICD-10-PCS Coding** has been set up to allow coders to study a single body area or organ system at a time if they wish or to review the entire body if that suits their study needs. The body has been broken down into 13 different areas and systems under ICD-10-CM, and arranged in body system order in the ICD-10-PCS section.

- Introduction to the Human Body
- Integumentary System
- Skeletal System and Articulations
- Muscular System
- Nervous System
- Endocrine System
- Cardiovascular System
- Blood and Blood-Forming Organs
- Lymphatic System
- Respiratory System
- Digestive System
- Urinary System
- Reproductive System
- Introduction to ICD-10-PCS
- ICD-10-PCS: Nervous and Circulatory Systems
- ICD-10-PCS: Lymphatic, Sense Organ, and Respiratory Systems
- ICD-10-PCS: Digestive and Endocrine Systems
- ICD-10-PCS: Skin, Subcutaneous Tissue, and Musculoskeletal Systems
- ICD-10-PCS: Genitourinary Systems
- ICD-10-PCS: Anatomical Region Systems

Within each ICD-10-CM chapter is an anatomic overview, providing the coder with a basic knowledge of the anatomy and physiology of the particular body area or organ system. Following the overview is a detailed comparison of the ICD-9-CM and ICD-10-CM codes affecting that section, and how anatomy, physiology, and pathophysiology differ between the two code sets. For example, what is the difference between a cutaneous abscess, cellulitis, and acute lymphangitis? Detailed illustrations are provided for both the basic anatomy and the comparison sections.

Tables are used to illustrate some of the differences between the ICD-9-CM and ICD-10-CM coding systems. These tables are provided to demonstrate the level of specificity and knowledge required by the coder in order to select the appropriate ICD-10-CM code. The tables are not meant to indicate any potential mapping as the examples provided may not include all of the available code choices for a given situation.

Chapters 14 through 20 feature the anatomy and physiology of ICD-10-PCS medical and surgical sections, detailing the importance of these topics in the procedural side of ICD-10 coding. These chapters include tables similar to those found in the ICD-10-PCS manual, in a more condensed format, detailing all valid character values for each body system. Information about the root operation characters, body part characters, and approach characters is provided, such as the types of procedures included in extirpation and what might fall into the body part character value of intracranial vein.

In some instances, it will be necessary to reference the basic anatomy information found in the first 13 chapters, as it may impact ICD-10-PCS coding as well. Detailed illustrations are provided in the ICD-10-PCS chapters, indicating the various body part characters. In addition, appendixes have been added to supplement chapters 14 through 20. Appendix B, Body Part Key and Appendix C, Body Part Definitions are two mapping tools in which anatomical terms are linked to their ICD-10-PCS character value or vice versa; both of which can be useful tools in ICD-10-PCS coding. Appendix D provides ICD-10-PCS official definitions for the root operations assigned in the medical and surgical section.

Also included in the **Comprehensive Anatomy and Physiology for ICD-10-CM and ICD-10-PCS Coding** are knowledge review questions for each of the chapters to enable the coder to test himself or herself on information in the chapter. Answers as well as rationales are included for the knowledge review questions.

To assist in the overall learning experience, key information has been included in the margins of the book, including interesting anatomy and physiology facts, key points, quick tips, clinical points, definitions, and more. Although much of the medical terminology used in the ICD-10-CM and ICD-10-PCS manuals are defined within the text itself, there are times when the text doesn't lend itself to this information. In these cases, the terms are placed in bold and italicized font, and the definition can be found in the margin.

Summary

The **Comprehensive Anatomy and Physiology for ICD-10-CM and ICD-10-PCS Coding** is a great start to learning about ICD-10-CM and ICD-10-PCS. Although it is not meant to teach coders how to code under these new code sets, it does help them understand the anatomy and physiology differences, as well as provide a ready reference to use side by side with their books when they are learning ICD-10-CM and ICD-10-PCS. The new coding systems are a much-needed change, and although this is just one part of the training needed, it is an important—and essential—step in coder education.

Chapter 1.
Introduction to the Human Body

Anatomy Overview

The human body is a complex organization of body areas and organ systems. Although coders often look at one particular disease process or a group of injuries at a time, it is also important to be aware of certain aspects of the overall function of the human body, as well as the layout of its anatomy. This chapter discusses structural organization of the human body, basic life processes, and anatomical positions and briefly outlines organ systems and body areas.

Structural Organization of the Human Body

Although people tend to think of themselves as simply human beings, the human body really exists on several different levels of organization. From smallest to broadest, these levels include:

- Chemical
- Cellular
- Tissue
- Organ
- System
- Organismal

The most basic level, the **chemical** level, breaks the body down into its most minute parts. Humans are made up of chemicals, atoms, and molecules, which make up the body's cells. Oxygen, carbon, nitrogen, and hydrogen are all important building blocks for genetic material, organs, and everything needed to keep the body functioning on a daily basis.

The **cellular** level of organization includes cells, the smallest living units in the body and the building blocks for all organs, muscles, blood, and more. Cells serve many roles throughout the body, ranging from helping preserve *homeostasis*, to serving as structural support and helping fight off infections. The principal parts of a cell are the plasma membrane, the cytoplasm, and the nucleus, where *DNA* is housed. A *chromosome*, which is a single molecule of DNA, contains thousands of genes that direct the aspects of cellular structure and function.

The **tissue** level of structural organization is next; it is at this point that items more regularly recognizable in the coding world appear. There are four basic types of tissue found in the human body:

- Epithelial tissue
- Connective tissue
- Muscle tissue
- Nervous tissue

> **DEFINITIONS**
>
> **chromosome.** Single thread of genetic material, or DNA, that controls the aspects of cellular function and structure, as well as the inheritance of certain traits.
>
> **DNA.** Deoxyribonucleic acid. Molecule of genetic information that is found in the nucleus of a cell.
>
> **homeostasis.** State of relative constancy within the internal environment of the human body.

Figure 1.1: Tissue

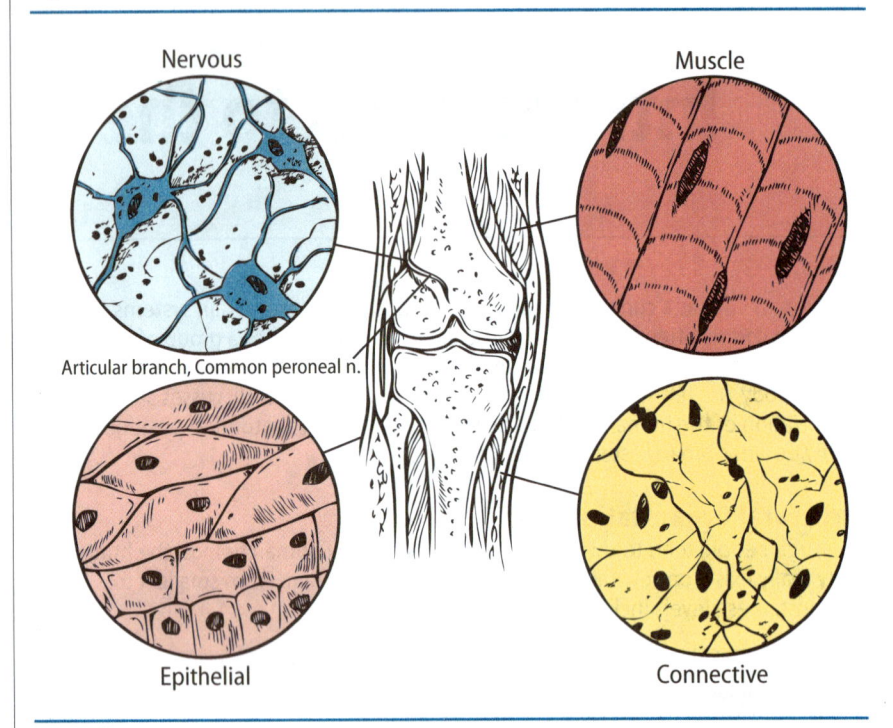

Nervous | Muscle
Articular branch, Common peroneal n.
Epithelial | Connective

Epithelial tissue covers the surfaces of the body, lines body cavities, ducts, and hollow organs, and forms glands in the body. It consists of cells arranged in continuous sheets, in single layers or multiple layers, depending on the thickness of the tissue in that area. Some examples of epithelial tissue are the skin, the lining of the peritoneum, and the thyroid gland.

Connective tissue is found distributed throughout several different areas of the body, making it one of the most abundant tissues found in the human body. Like epithelial tissue, it serves several functions within the body. Connective tissue protects and insulates internal organs, serves as the major transport system throughout the body, supports and strengthens other body tissue, and is the main site of stored energy reserves as well as immune responses. The five main types of connective tissue found in the body are:

- **Loose connective tissue:** Fat tissue, subcutaneous layer of the skin
- **Dense connective tissue:** Tendons, ligaments, fascia
- **Cartilage:** Ends of long bones, larynx, trachea
- **Osseous tissue:** Bones *(turns into bones)*
- **Blood:** Within blood vessels and heart

Muscle tissue is made up of elongated cells that are often referred to as muscle fiber. This muscle fiber serves many purposes within the body, such as maintaining posture, generating body heat, and producing the many different movements of the body. There are three types of muscle tissue: skeletal, cardiac, and smooth. Skeletal muscle tissue is found in various places throughout the body and is usually attached to bones. It is commonly referred to as voluntary muscle because its activity, either contraction or relaxation, is under conscious control. Cardiac muscle forms the walls of the heart. It is an involuntary muscle fiber, meaning that its contractions are not consciously controlled. Smooth muscle tissue is also an involuntary type of muscle fiber that is found in the walls of hollow internal structures of the body. For example, smooth muscle can be found in the blood vessels, the intestines, and the urinary bladder. These fibers work involuntarily to move and process food through the

---

INTERESTING A & P FACT

Connective tissue binds organs together, stores energy reserves as fat, and helps provide immunity.

gastrointestinal tract, move fluids through the body, and eliminate wastes, among other functions.

Nervous tissue is made up of two main types of cells: neurons and neuroglia. The neurons are the main nerve cells and are sensitive to various stimuli. They take that stimuli and convert it into an electrical impulse, to be sent off to various other parts of the body such as another neuron, muscle tissue, glands, or the brain. Neuroglia cells nourish and protect the neurons, which are very fragile cells.

Organs make up the next level of body structure. Each organ consists of various types of tissue and has a specific function to perform to help the body operate properly. Some examples of organs in the human body include the stomach, the lungs, the skin, and the brain. Proper function of these organs is vital to maintaining good health.

The **system** level of body structure groups related organs together that have some commonality in function. There are 11 commonly accepted systems of the human body, which are described throughout this book in various chapters.

- Integumentary system
- Skeletal system
- Muscular system
- Nervous system
- Endocrine system
- Cardiovascular system
- Lymphatic system
- Respiratory system
- Digestive system
- Urinary system
- Reproductive system

> **CLINICAL NOTE**
>
> Each organ is made up of several layers of tissue and membrane, each with its own function.

The *integumentary system* includes skin as well as the structures contained in the skin, such as the hair, the nails, and the sweat and oil glands. One of its main purposes is to protect the body. The *skeletal system* consists of the bones and joints. It supports and protects the body and aids in movement. The *muscular system* includes the skeletal muscle tissue throughout the body and produces movement through voluntary muscle control.

The *nervous system* consists of the brain, spinal cord, and nerves, as well as the special sensory organs such as the eyes and the ears. This system plays many important roles for the body, mainly involving monitoring outside activity and communicating that activity to the brain to regulate body activities. The *endocrine system* includes all of the hormone-producing glands throughout the body, such as the hypothalamus and the pituitary gland, as well as any hormone-producing cells that reside in another part of the body. These glands and cells release hormones that help regulate various body activities.

The *cardiovascular system* includes the blood, the heart, and all of the blood vessels. Its main function is to pump the blood throughout the body to carry oxygen and nutrients to the cells and to carry wastes away from the cells. The *lymphatic system* includes lymph nodes and vessels, as well as the lymphatic vessels. It also contains the spleen, the thymus, and the tonsils. One of the lymphatic system's main functions is to return fluid and protein to the bloodstream. The *respiratory system* consists of the lungs and the air passageways. Its main function is to transfer the oxygen from the inhaled air into something that is usable by the bloodstream, as well as transfer the waste carbon dioxide from the bloodstream into the exhaled air.

> ✓ **QUICK TIP**
>
> Sometimes organs are part of more than one system, as they may serve several functions. For example, the pancreas is typically included in both the digestive and endocrine systems.

The *digestive system* includes all of the organs and accessory structures of the gastrointestinal tract, which include the mouth, the pharynx, the esophagus, the stomach, the small and large intestines, the anus, the salivary glands, the liver, the gallbladder, and the pancreas. The main purpose of the digestive system is to break down food both physically and chemically so that the body can absorb it. The *urinary system* consists of the kidneys, ureters, urinary bladder, and the urethra. Its main function is to produce, store, and eliminate urine. The main function of the *reproductive system*, which contains the reproductive organs, is to produce gametes (oocytes or sperm) in order to reproduce and create a new organism. In males, the testes, epididymis, vas deferens, and penis make up the reproductive organs. In females, the reproductive organs consist of the ovaries, fallopian tubes, uterus, and vagina.

The final and highest level of structural organization of the body is the **organismal level.** The organism is a living, breathing creature. Each of these previous levels rolls up into the organism, a single living person.

Basic Life Processes

Some basic life processes within humans separate us from nonliving things. Problems with these processes are the roots of many of the diseases and disorders that coders deal with each day in their health care organizations. Below is a discussion of six of these basic life processes: metabolism, responsiveness, movement, growth, differentiation, and reproduction.

Metabolism is really an aggregate (collection) of all of the various chemical processes that take place within the body. It has two aspects: catabolism and anabolism. Catabolism is the process of breaking down a very complex chemical substance into a simpler one, such as breaking down a protein in food into its component parts such as amino acids. Anabolism is the opposite. It takes those smaller component parts and creates complex chemical substances. In anabolism, the body may take those amino acids it broke down before and build them into new proteins for building muscles and bones throughout the body. The metabolism is a comprehensive bodily function that is necessary for growth, generation of energy, distribution of nutrients, and elimination of wastes throughout the body.

Responsiveness denotes the body's ability to respond to stimuli, be they internal or external. If the body's ability to respond to internal and external environments is diminished, its ability to survive is also diminished. In many instances nerve cells respond to stimuli by telling muscle cells to contract or relax, causing movement, or by raising or lowering body temperature in response to the environment. There are many ways the body can respond to different circumstances, all helping it to survive and maintain health.

Movement is a basic life process that is often associated simply with the external movements of appendages (accessories). However, movement also occurs within the body, such as blood moving through the vessels, food moving through the digestive tract, or white blood cells traveling to damaged tissue to speed healing.

Growth is the body's ability to grow from its initial size at birth to its adult size. The body can grow by adding additional cells, by having existing cells grow larger, or by having the material that surrounds the cells expand, such as in the case of bone growth.

Differentiation is a process whereby unspecialized cells become specialized. Most of the cells in the body are highly specialized in structure and function, with one exception, the *stem cell*. Stem cells, found in the red bone marrow, are considered unspecialized and can undergo differentiation to become one of several types of cells, such as a red blood cell or a white blood cell.

Reproduction is the final basic life process this section examines. This process refers not only to creating a new human being, but also to producing new cells and new tissues for repair. Because cells and tissues constantly die, the body must continually reproduce those cells and tissues. The body also reproduces cells and tissues to repair wounds from traumatic injury.

☞ INTERESTING A & P FACT

There are more than 100 entries in the ICD-10-CM index under Disorders, Metabolism. That is more than twice as many as were listed in ICD-9-CM. Many of the listed entries are inherited or genetic, some caused by organ dysfunction, and others by nutritional disorders. New disorders continue to be discovered so it is a benefit that ICD-10-CM has the capability to expand.

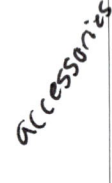

Body Positions

There are various terms that describe the body in different positions, as well as references that describe imaginary planes that transect the body. These terms are crucial to coders, especially in ICD-10-CM. With the higher level of specificity found in the new coding system, providers often use these terms to describe specific areas of the body affected by a condition. It is important for all coders to be very familiar with these terms and understand their use.

When a body is in the *anatomical position,* the patient is in the forward-facing position, with the head level, and eyes facing forward. His or her feet are flat on the floor, and the palms are turned forward. A patient who is face down in a reclining position is in the *prone* position. In the *supine* position, the patient is face up in a reclining position.

Figure 1.2: Anatomical Position

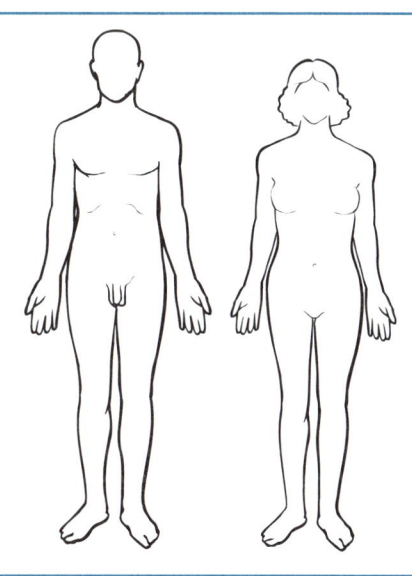

The anatomical position can be divided into imaginary planes and sections and can also be used to demonstrate various directional terms describing parts of the body in relation to one another.

Directional Terms

There are several important directional terms to be aware of, used in various ways. Some describe a body part relative to the anatomical position. Some compare positions of various anatomical structures. It is important to be accurate in descriptions regardless of the type of use.

- **Superior:** Toward the top of the body, or toward the head. The esophagus is superior to the stomach, to which it is attached. (Also referred to as cranial, cephalic)
- **Inferior:** Toward the lower part of the body, or toward the feet. Immediately inferior to the diaphragm lies the abdominal cavity. (Also referred to as caudal)
- **Anterior:** To the front of, or nearer to the front. The nose is on the anterior surface of the head. The anterior surface of the hand is the palm. (Also, ventral)
- **Posterior:** To the back of, or nearer to the back. The heel occupies the posterior part of the foot. (Also, dorsal)

- **Medial:** Toward the middle or toward the medial plane. The external auditory canal extends medially to the tympanic membrane, or eardrum.
- **Lateral:** Farther away from the middle or away from the medial plane. The heart lies in the left lateral compartment of the mediastinum.
- **Intermediate:** Between two structures. The transverse colon is intermediate between the ascending and descending colons.
- **Ipsilateral:** On the same side of the body as another structure. The left lung and the heart are ipsilateral.
- **Contralateral:** On the opposite side of the body from another structure. The ascending colon and the heart are contralateral.
- **Proximal:** Nearest to the point of origin, or nearest to the trunk. The thoracic portion of the aorta is proximal to its passage through the diaphragm.
- **Distal:** Farthest from the point of origin, or farthest from the trunk. The patella, or kneecap, partially overlies the most distal portion of the femur.
- **Superficial:** Closest to the surface. The epidermal layer is superficial to the dermis.
- **Interior:** Nearer the center. Two chambers divided by a septum occupy the interior of the heart.
- **Exterior:** Farther from the center. The muscular exterior of the esophagus works to facilitate swallowing.

Figure 1.3: Body Planes

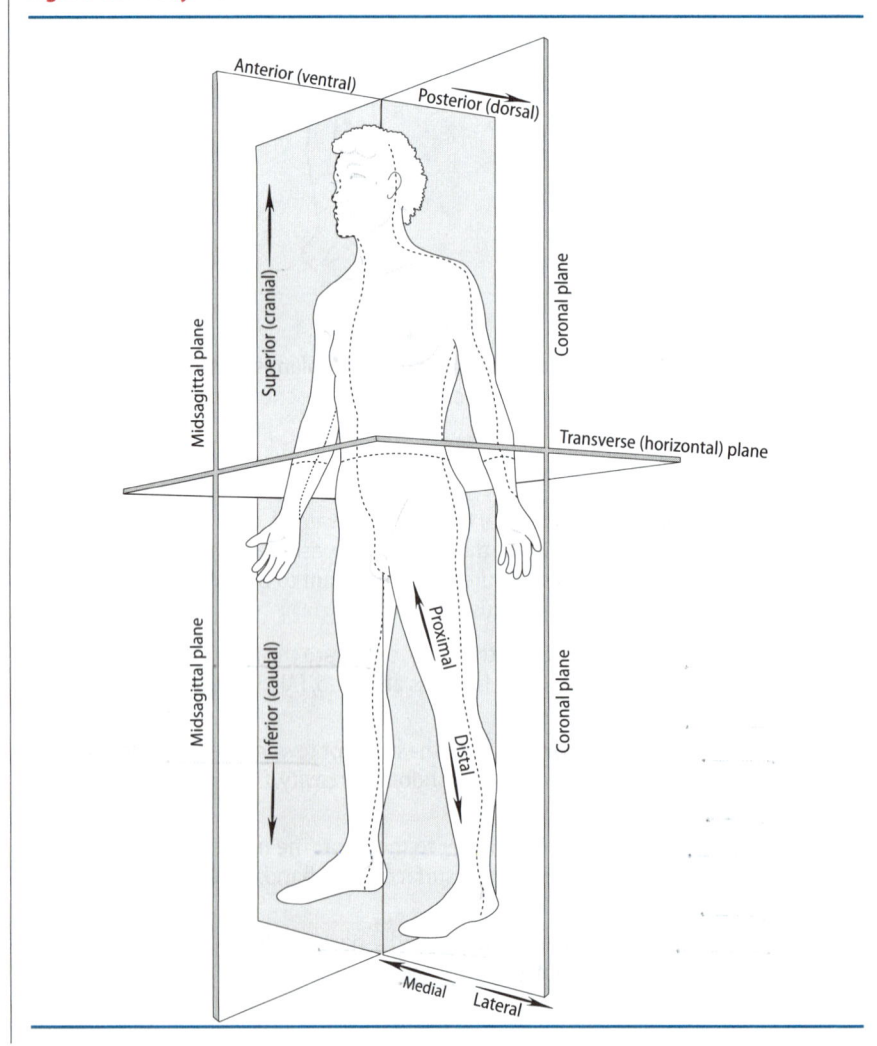

Planes

References to body sites often mention imaginary planes that pass through the body. The median or midsagittal plane runs vertically through the center of the body, dividing it exactly into the right side and the left side. There are any number of sagittal planes that run parallel to the median plane. Frontal or coronal planes run at right angles to the median plane to divide the body into front and back portions. Horizontal planes run at right angles to both the median plane and the coronal planes and may also be called transverse planes or cross-sectional planes. You can see some of these planes denoted in the above illustration.

Types of Movement

Some basic terms describe types of movement, specifically directions of movement usually of the extremities. This information is important for coding purposes, as these terms can often be the difference between one code and another, especially in the more detailed ICD-10-CM code set. Below are definitions of terms used to describe types of movement:

- **Flexion:** The movement causing decreased angle of a joint.
- **Extension:** The movement causing increased angle, or straightening, of a joint.
- **Abduction:** The movement away from the median plane.
- **Adduction:** The movement toward the median plane.
- **Eversion:** The movement, usually of the foot at the ankle, away from the medial plane.
- **Inversion:** The movement, usually of the foot at the ankle, toward the medial plane.
- **Afferent:** Conveying toward a center. For example, afferent nerves carry impulses to the central nervous system.
- **Efferent:** Conveying away from the center. For example, efferent nerves carry information away from the central nervous system to muscles and glands.
- **Supination:** The movement of the lower arm that rotates the palm and forearm anteriorly (as in the anatomical position).
- **Pronation:** The movement of the lower arm that rotates the palm and forearm posteriorly (opposite position of supination).

> ✓ **QUICK TIP**
>
> Internal rotation, also known as medial rotation, is rotation toward the center of the body. External rotation, also known as lateral rotation, is rotation away from the center of the body.

Figure 1.4: Motion

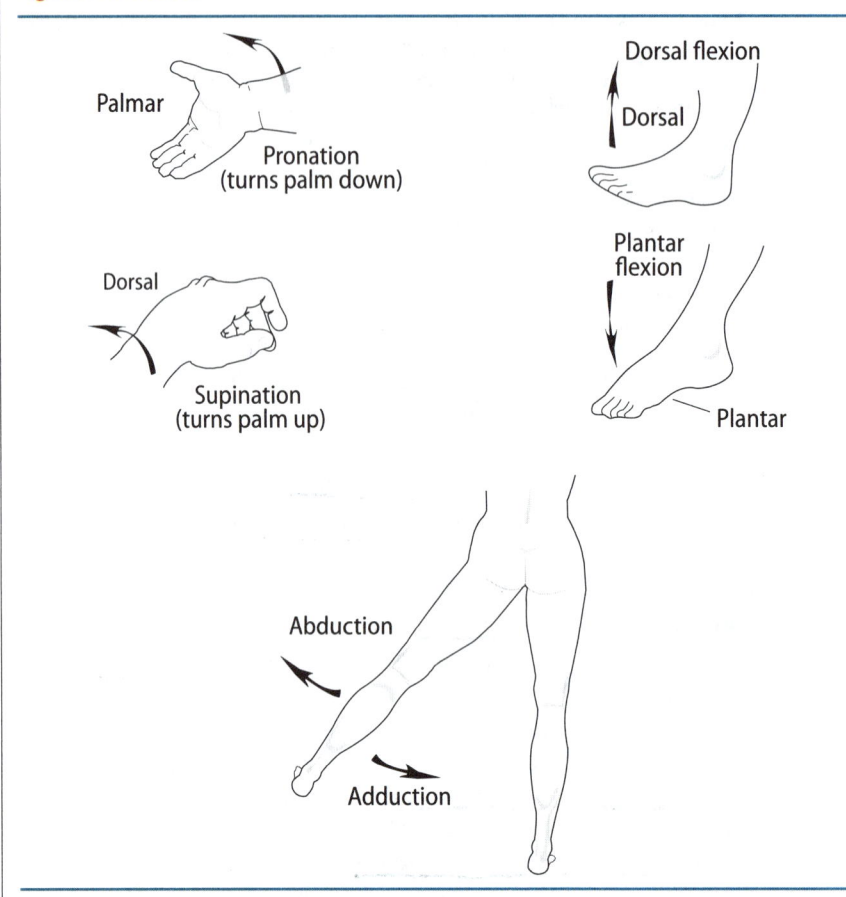

Summary

This chapter has reviewed the basics of the human body and some of the important terminology related to its anatomy and functions. The following chapters go into each of the organ systems and body areas in detail. They also discuss how the transition from ICD-9-CM to ICD-10-CM and ICD-10-PCS will require coders to learn more about anatomy and pathophysiology in certain areas.

Chapter 2. ICD-10-CM: Integumentary System

Anatomic Overview

Skin

The skin is the largest organ system, covering the entire external surface of the body. Known as the integumentary system, the skin serves many purposes. It protects tissue layers from damage and provides waterproofing and cushioning. It also helps the body excrete wastes properly and regulate temperature, and provides the nerves with a surface for originating sensory receptors.

The top layer of the skin is known as the epidermis. This thinner portion of the skin mainly exists to absorb nutrients and to protect deeper tissue layers. The deeper and thicker layer of the skin is the dermis. The dermis is the connective tissue layer and contains the sweat glands, hair roots and follicles, blood vessels, sensory receptors, and other important structures of the integumentary system. Beneath the dermis is the hypodermis, or subcutaneous layer. This layer is not part of the skin itself, but the tie between the integumentary system and the fascia below.

> **INTERESTING A & P FACT**
>
> The skin accounts for approximately 16 percent of the body's total weight.

Figure 2.1: Skin

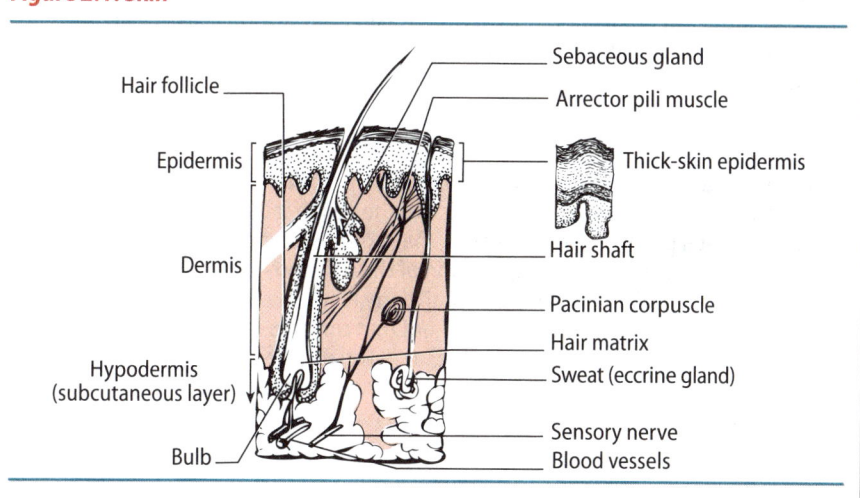

[Diagram of skin cross-section with labels: Hair follicle, Epidermis, Dermis, Hypodermis (subcutaneous layer), Bulb, Sebaceous gland, Arrector pili muscle, Thick-skin epidermis, Hair shaft, Pacinian corpuscle, Hair matrix, Sweat (eccrine gland), Sensory nerve, Blood vessels]

As indicated above, the dermal layer contains many different blood vessels, as well as glands, hair follicles, nerves, and sensory receptors. It is made up mainly of connective tissue, and all of these elements are embedded into that connective tissue.

The sweat glands, also known as sudoriferous glands, are found throughout the body. There are 3 to 4 million of these glands, which release perspiration onto the surface of the skin through small holes known as pores. This process helps regulate body temperature by releasing the perspiration and allowing it to evaporate.

The dermal layer also contains sebaceous glands, which are oil glands. These glands secrete sebum, an oily substance that keeps the skin and hair from drying out. The sebaceous glands are attached to a portion of the hair follicles. The hair and follicles are quite a complex system, allowing for continuous growth and regeneration. Hair,

> **INTERESTING A & P FACT**
>
> There are two types of sweat glands in the body: eccrine and apocrine. Eccrine glands are found over most of the body and they secrete sweat to cool body temperature in response to temperature increase. Apocrine glands, concentrated in the armpits, groin, and scalp, secrete a different type of sweat triggered by stress or intense emotions. This sweat is comprised of a thicker, fattier substance and is generally considered to be the cause of unpleasant body odor.

Comprehensive Anatomy and Physiology for ICD-10-CM and ICD-10-PCS Coding

DEFINITIONS
keratin. Tough fibrous protein commonly found in the hair and nails.

itself, can be thought of as a recycling system, using dead, **keratinized** epidermal cells to bond with proteins to create the hair within the follicle. The hair shaft grows out from the follicle, through the epidermis, and out of the skin entirely. The hair's purpose depends on its location—some helps avoid heat loss, while some protects from foreign bodies.

Figure 2.2: Hair and Glands

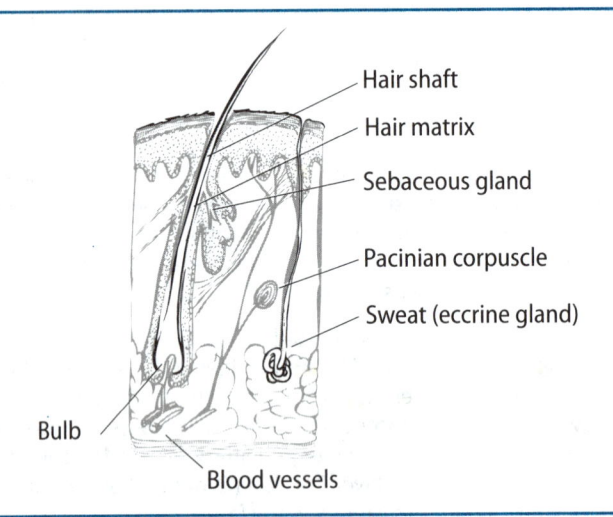

- Hair shaft
- Hair matrix
- Sebaceous gland
- Pacinian corpuscle
- Sweat (eccrine gland)
- Bulb
- Blood vessels

Nails

The nails, although not technically part of the skin itself, are typically considered part of the integumentary system. Nails are keratinized epidermal cells that form a solid covering over the surface of the end of the finger or toe. Outside of their aesthetic function, nails provide a protective covering helping to shield from traumatic injuries. They also assist in the gripping and maneuvering of small objects.

While the anatomy of the nail system is detailed, there are only a few important terms to be aware of. The nail body is the portion of the nail that can be seen, and the free edge is the distal portion of the nail body that extends beyond the end of the finger or toe. The nail root is the proximal portion of the nail body buried in a fold of skin. The nail bed is the skin upon which the nail body rests. The nail matrix is a portion of the nail bed found deep beneath the nail root that contains nerves and vessels. This is the portion of the nail system responsible for new nail growth. Nails typically grow at a rate of three to four millimeters per month, although there are several factors that can affect nail growth. Complete regrowth of a nail plate takes approximately six months.

Figure 2.3: Nail

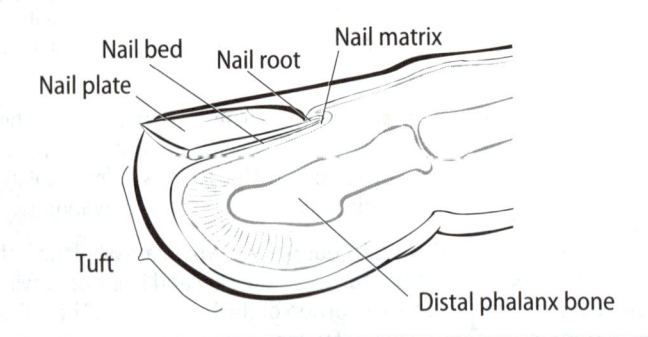

- Nail bed
- Nail root
- Nail matrix
- Nail plate
- Tuft
- Distal phalanx bone

Breast

Commonly seen as part of the integumentary system, as well as the reproductive system, breasts are found on the anterior aspect of the surface of the chest in men and women. The breasts contain the mammary glands, responsible for lactation in women associated with pregnancy and childbirth. The breast itself is connected to pectoralis major and serratus anterior muscles of the chest wall via a layer of fascia.

Each breast contains one pigmented projection, the nipple. In women, the nipple contains a series of small openings called the lactiferous ducts, which are closely spaced openings where milk emerges. There is also a circular pigmented area that surrounds the nipple known as the areola. This area contains a series of sebaceous glands, which create a rough looking appearance. The suspensory ligaments of the breast run between the skin and fascia to support the breast.

Within each female breast is a mammary gland, which is a modified sudoriferous or sweat gland that produces milk. Each gland is made up of 15 to 20 lobes, which are separated by adipose tissue. The lobes contain smaller lobules containing milk-secreting glands called alveoli. From the alveoli, milk drains to various tubules and ducts to be stored in the lactiferous sinuses until it is needed. Additional detail regarding the breast and its function in the reproductive system is found in chapter 13.

> **CODING AXIOM**
>
> ICD-10-CM Official Coding Guideline I.C.2. states, "A primary malignant neoplasm that overlaps two or more contiguous (next to each other) sites should be classified to the subcategory/code .8 ('overlapping lesion'), unless the combination is specifically indexed elsewhere. For multiple neoplasms of the same site that are not contiguous such as tumors in different quadrants of the same breast, codes for each site should be assigned."

Figure 2.4: Female Breast

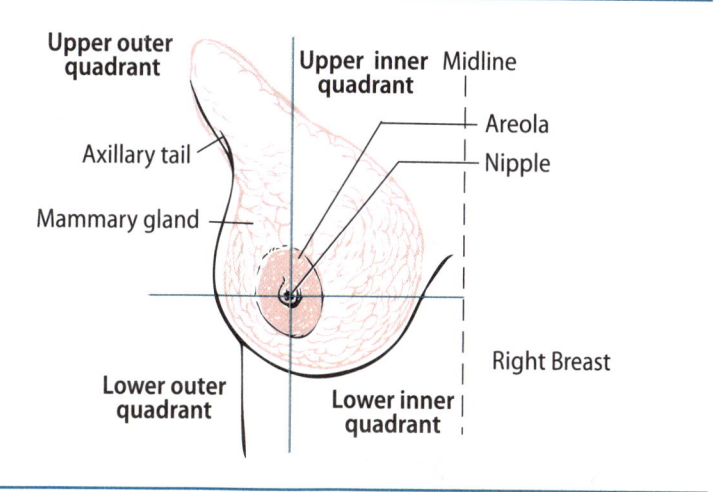

The male breast develops from the same tissue as the female breast. However, at puberty the hormones in the female develop the breast tissue in a different way than the hormones in the male, creating a different end result. Men can deal with several types of breast disorders, such as gynecomastia and male breast cancer.

Anatomy and Pathophysiology and the ICD-10-CM Code Set

The integumentary system can be affected by many different disease states. It is also the main site for traumatic injury, such as open wounds and burns. It is important to understand the terminology surrounding many of these disease states and injuries, as the ICD-10-CM code set is intricately detailed.

Skin Infections and Inflammation of Connective Tissue

There are many types of skin infections and inflammations, a few of which are discussed here.

An abscess is an infection in a cavity under the skin that contains pus, surrounded by inflamed tissue. Abscesses can occur nearly anywhere in the body. Those occurring in the integumentary system are known as **cutaneous abscesses**. Often a cutaneous abscess requires incision and drainage to heal appropriately.

A *furuncle*, more commonly known as a boil, is a localized skin infection typically caused by the *Staphylococcus aureus* bacterium. A furuncle is a specific type of abscess that usually begins in a gland or hair follicle, where a core of dead tissue is formed, causing pain, redness, and swelling. The dead tissue may simply reabsorb into the system, which resolves the problem, or it may spontaneously extrude itself. In some instances, surgical removal of the necrotic tissue may be required.

A *carbuncle* is larger than a furuncle and typically consists of several interconnected sites of infection that eventually discharge pus to the skin's surface. Carbuncles are also often caused by the *Staphylococcus aureus* bacterium and can vary greatly in size. Some carbuncles can be small, similar to the size of a pea, but others can grow to be quite large, greater than the size of a golf ball. Much like furuncles, some carbuncles heal on their own by reabsorption into the system or spontaneous extrusion. However, sometimes surgical treatment and antibiotics are required.

Coding for these three types of skin infections is more complex under the ICD-10-CM code set than in ICD-9-CM, and coders need to understand more about the anatomy, physiology, and pathology of the areas in question to code accurately. In ICD-9-CM, carbuncle and furuncle were grouped together under category 680. In ICD-10-CM, carbuncle and furuncle are separate codes, as indicated in the following table.

Coding for Carbuncles and Furuncles

ICD-9-CM		ICD-10-CM	
680.0	Carbuncle and furuncle of face	L02.02	Furuncle of face
		L02.03	Carbuncle of face
680.1	Carbuncle and furuncle of neck	L02.12	Furuncle of neck
		L02.13	Carbuncle of neck
680.2	Carbuncle and furuncle of trunk	L02.221	Furuncle of abdominal wall
		L02.222	Furuncle of back [any part, except buttock]
		L02.223	Furuncle of chest wall
		L02.224	Furuncle of groin
		L02.225	Furuncle of perineum
		L02.226	Furuncle of umbilicus
		L02.229	Furuncle of trunk, unspecified
		L02.231	Carbuncle of abdominal wall
		L02.232	Carbuncle of back [any part, except buttock]
		L02.233	Carbuncle of chest wall
		L02.234	Carbuncle of groin
		L02.235	Carbuncle of perineum
		L02.236	Carbuncle of umbilicus
		L02.239	Carbuncle of trunk, unspecified

DEFINITIONS

carbuncle. Several interconnected skin infection sites.

cutaneous abscess. Infection in a cavity under the skin that contains pus, surrounded by inflamed tissue.

furuncle. Also known as a boil, a localized skin infection in a gland or hair follicle.

Chapter 2. ICD-10-CM: Integumentary System

ICD-9-CM		ICD-10-CM	
680.3	Carbuncle and furuncle of upper arm and forearm	L02.421	Furuncle of right axilla
		L02.422	Furuncle of left axilla
		L02.423	Furuncle of right upper limb
		L02.424	Furuncle of left upper limb
		L02.429	Furuncle of limb, unspecified
		L02.431	Carbuncle of right axilla
		L02.432	Carbuncle of left axilla
		L02.433	Carbuncle of right upper limb
		L02.434	Carbuncle of left upper limb
		L02.439	Carbuncle of limb, unspecified
680.4	Carbuncle and furuncle of hand	L02.521	Furuncle right hand
		L02.522	Furuncle left hand
		L02.529	Furuncle unspecified hand
		L02.531	Carbuncle of right hand
		L02.532	Carbuncle of left hand
		L02.539	Carbuncle of unspecified hand

To report skin infections correctly in ICD-10-CM, the type of infection must be known. Did the patient present with a cutaneous abscess, a furuncle, or a carbuncle? Was it **cellulitis** or **lymphangitis**, which is a separate code set within ICD-10-CM. Additionally, the organism causing the infection should be coded, if known.

Once the type of infection has been determined, the location of the skin infection must be identified.

Coding for Cellulitis and Cutaneous Abscesses

ICD-9-CM		ICD-10-CM	
682.0	Cellulitis and abscess of face	K12.2	Cellulitis and abscess of mouth
		L02.01	Cutaneous abscess of face
		L03.211	Cellulitis of face
		L03.212	Acute lymphangitis of face
682.1	Cellulitis and abscess of neck	L02.11	Cutaneous abscess of neck
		L03.221	Cellulitis of neck
		L03.222	Acute lymphangitis of neck
682.2	Cellulitis and abscess of trunk	L02.211	Cutaneous abscess of abdominal wall
		L02.212	Cutaneous abscess of back [any part, except buttock]
		L02.213	Cutaneous abscess of chest wall
		L02.214	Cutaneous abscess of groin
		L02.215	Cutaneous abscess of perineum
		L02.216	Cutaneous abscess of umbilicus
		L02.219	Cutaneous abscess of trunk, unspecified
		L03.311	Cellulitis of abdominal wall
		L03.312	Cellulitis of back [any part, except buttock]
		L03.313	Cellulitis of chest wall
		L03.314	Cellulitis of groin
		L03.315	Cellulitis of perineum
		L03.316	Cellulitis of umbilicus
		L03.319	Cellulitis of trunk, unspecified
		L03.321	Acute lymphangitis of abdominal wall
		L03.322	Acute lymphangitis of back [any part, except buttock]
		L03.323	Acute lymphangitis of chest wall
		L03.324	Acute lymphangitis of groin

(Continued on next page)

> **DEFINITIONS**
>
> **cellulitis.** Sudden, severe, suppurative inflammation and edema in subcutaneous tissue or muscle, most often caused by bacterial infection secondary to a cutaneous lesion. *affecting the skin*
>
> **lymphangitis.** Inflammation of the lymph glands.

Comprehensive Anatomy and Physiology for ICD-10-CM and ICD-10-PCS Coding

ICD-9-CM		ICD-10-CM	
682.2	Cellulitis and abscess of trunk *(Continued)*	L03.324	Acute lymphangitis of groin
		L03.325	Acute lymphangitis of perineum
		L03.326	Acute lymphangitis of umbilicus
		L03.329	Acute lymphangitis of trunk, unspecified
682.3	Cellulitis and abscess of upper arm and forearm	L02.411	Cutaneous abscess of right axilla
		L02.412	Cutaneous abscess of left axilla
		L02.413	Cutaneous abscess of right upper limb
		L02.414	Cutaneous abscess of left upper limb
		L02.419	Cutaneous abscess of limb, unspecified
		L03.111	Cellulitis of right axilla
		L03.112	Cellulitis of left axilla
		L03.113	Cellulitis of right upper limb
		L03.114	Cellulitis of left upper limb
		L03.119	Cellulitis of unspecified part of limb
		L03.121	Acute lymphangitis of right axilla
		L03.122	Acute lymphangitis of left axilla
		L03.123	Acute lymphangitis of right upper limb
		L03.124	Acute lymphangitis of left upper limb
		L03.129	Acute lymphangitis of unspecified part of limb

In the table above, there are multiple ICD-10-CM codes for cellulitis and cutaneous abscesses. Code selection depends on the type and location of skin infection or inflammation. The detail in these code descriptions is much greater than that provided in ICD-9-CM. For example, look at ICD-9-CM code 680.2 Carbuncle and Furuncle of Trunk. In ICD-10-CM, 14 codes are used in its place, seven specific to furuncles and seven specific to carbuncles. The sixth character indicates the infection site:

- 1 Abdominal wall
- 2 Any part of back except buttock
- 3 Chest wall
- 4 Groin
- 5 Perineum
- 6 Umbilicus
- 9 Trunk, unspecified

Sixth-character specifications are added not only to carbuncle and furuncle codes, but also to cutaneous abscess, cellulitis, and acute lymphangitis codes. Similar anatomical breakdowns occur in the other sections as well, such as right side versus left side, upper limbs versus lower limbs, or upper arm versus *axillae*. There is also an unspecified code option in many of these code sets. However, it is not known how payers will handle unspecified codes under the ICD-10-CM code set, so it is important to always code to the highest level of specificity. This may mean querying the provider for additional information. Providers must document any additional information via a query form or an addendum to the medical record.

Dermatitis and Eczema

Simply stated, *dermatitis* is inflammation of the skin. *Eczema* is one form of dermatitis. ICD-10-CM uses these terms interchangeably. Contact dermatitis, a fairly common form of the condition, is inflammation that results from an allergic reaction (allergic contact dermatitis) or exposure to some type of skin irritant (irritant contact dermatitis).

Dermatitis and eczema can be something as simple as redness of the skin or a bumpy rash, to something more serious such as blisters. Generally, the treatment for

---

DEFINITIONS

axilla. Area under the arm.

dermatitis. Inflammation of the skin.

eczema. Inflammatory form of dermatitis with red, itchy breakouts of exudative vesicles that lead to crusting and scaling.

dermatitis depends on the cause and includes medications such as corticosteroids. In most cases, the use of an antihistamine cream helps control itchiness of the affected area.

Once again, ICD-10-CM coding for dermatitis and eczema requires more detail in documentation than its ICD-9-CM counterpart. One of the major differences is the breakdown of allergic- and irritant-related contact dermatitis codes.

Coding for Contact Dermatitis and Eczema

ICD-9-CM		ICD-10-CM	
692.3	Contact dermatitis and other eczema due to drugs and medicines in contact with skin	L23.3	Allergic contact dermatitis due to drugs in contact with skin
		L24.4	Irritant contact dermatitis due to drugs in contact with skin
		L25.1	Unspecified contact dermatitis due to drugs in contact with skin
692.4	Contact dermatitis and other eczema due to other chemical products	L23.1	Allergic contact dermatitis due to adhesives
		L23.5	Allergic contact dermatitis due to other chemical products
		L24.5	Irritant contact dermatitis due to chemical products
		L25.3	Unspecified contact dermatitis due to other chemical products

ICD-10-CM codes differentiate between the various types of skin responses to solar radiation. These more detailed ICD-10-CM codes provide additional granularity in coding but also require that the coder be more knowledgeable about these types of conditions.

A phototoxic response to a drug is different clinically from a photoallergic response, and they are coded differently in ICD-10-CM. A phototoxic response is a rapidly appearing, sunburn-like response generated by exposure to light and a photosensitizing substance. A photoallergic response is a delayed skin reaction of some sort, due to hypersensitivity to light caused by a photosensitizing substance. Photocontact dermatitis is yet another type of dermatitis that involves an interaction between UV radiation and certain substances, fruits, or vegetables. Finally, solar *urticaria* is a condition classified as hives or wheals caused specifically by exposure to the sun or UV radiation. In ICD-9-CM, these services are classified to general acute dermatitis code 692.72, but now all have specific diagnosis codes in ICD-10-CM.

> **DEFINITIONS**
>
> **excoriated.** Condition resulting from abrading the skin or otherwise scratching off the surface of the skin.
>
> **urticaria.** Well circumscribed areas of redness and edema of the skin, commonly referred to as hives.

Coding for Acute Dermatitis Due to Solar Radiation

ICD-9-CM		ICD-10-CM	
692.72	Acute dermatitis due to solar radiation	L56.0	Drug phototoxic response
		L56.1	Drug photoallergic response
		L56.2	Photocontact dermatitis [berloque dermatitis]
		L56.3	Solar urticaria

ICD-9-CM code 691.8 Other atopic dermatitis and related conditions, includes a list of less common types of dermatitis that can be reported with this code. However, in ICD-10-CM, many of these conditions have their own codes, making it imperative that providers adequately document the different types of dermatitis in medical record documentation.

Besnier's prurigo is a form of atopic dermatitis associated with pregnancy. Also known as prurigo gestationis, it is a dermatological condition of pregnancy typically affecting women between the 20th and 34th week of gestation. It normally consists of an eruption of itchy, red papules that can be *excoriated* as well. There are several treatments that can make the patient more comfortable, although given the pregnancy, not all prescription treatments are an option.

Flexural eczema is a form of atopic dermatitis found in the flexures of the body, such as the elbows, wrists, and knees. This type of dermatitis often affects children, although it isn't exclusive to youth. It typically results in **lichenification,** as well as cracking and weeping of the area.

There are various other conditions that fall within this section. It is important to review documentation and determine whether the information best fits within a detailed diagnosis, or whether the diagnosis is still a more general atopic dermatitis diagnosis. Coders unable to identify the diagnosis based on incomplete documentation should query the provider.

> **DEFINITIONS**
>
> **lichenification.** Thickening and hardening of the epidermis, which often results in an exaggeration of its normal markings.

Coding for Other Atopic Dermatitis

ICD-9-CM		ICD-10-CM	
691.8	Other atopic dermatitis and related conditions	L20.0	Besnier's prurigo
		L20.81	Atopic neurodermatitis
		L20.82	Flexural eczema
		L20.84	Intrinsic (allergic) eczema
		L20.89	Other atopic dermatitis
		L20.9	Atopic dermatitis, unspecified

ICD-9-CM code 692.9 Contact dermatitis and other eczema due to an unspecified cause, maps to several ICD-10-CM codes, some unspecified codes, but others more specific.

Nummular dermatitis is typically characterized by itchy, oval lesions. In ICD-9-CM, nummular dermatitis is reported with 692.9. In ICD-10 CM, it has its own code (L30.0).

Cutaneous autosensitization is a secondary dermatitis caused by an inflammatory response somewhere else in the body. This autosensitization dermatitis is also coded to 692.9 in ICD-9-CM but has its own code (L30.2) in ICD-10-CM. Although there are several code options for unspecified dermatitis diagnoses, it is important to note that there is a great deal of uncertainty as to how payers will react to unspecified codes in the ICD-10-CM environment. There are many specific dermatitis codes as well, and it could be a good idea to query the provider for additional detail on the specific type of dermatitis.

Coding for Contact Dermatitis

ICD-9-CM		ICD-10-CM	
692.9	Contact dermatitis and other eczema due to unspecified cause	L23.9	Allergic contact dermatitis, unspecified cause
		L24.9	Irritant contact dermatitis, unspecified cause
		L25.9	Unspecified contact dermatitis, unspecified cause
		L30.0	Nummular dermatitis
		L30.2	Cutaneous autosensitization
		L30.8	Other specified dermatitis
		L30.9	Dermatitis, unspecified

ICD-9-CM code 692.73 Actinic reticuloid and actinic granuloma, is separated into two codes in ICD-10-CM: L57.1 Actinic reticuloid, and L57.5 Actinic granuloma. Actinic reticuloid is a form of chronic photosensitivity dermatitis in which the patient's skin becomes inflamed due to sunlight exposure or other artificial light sources, often of the face and neck. Treatment includes a prescription for oral steroids and avoidance of light sources.

Actinic granuloma typically manifests itself as ring-shaped lesions on the skin. It is thought that these are the result of sun damage. Although the lesions tend to generally be asymptomatic, they can cause the patient problems when exposed to the sun. There is some confusion about whether actinic granuloma is related to another skin condition, granuloma annulare. However, there is no proof of a definitive link between the two conditions, although they are similar.

[handwritten: showing no symptoms]

Figure 2.5: Surface and Solid Lesions

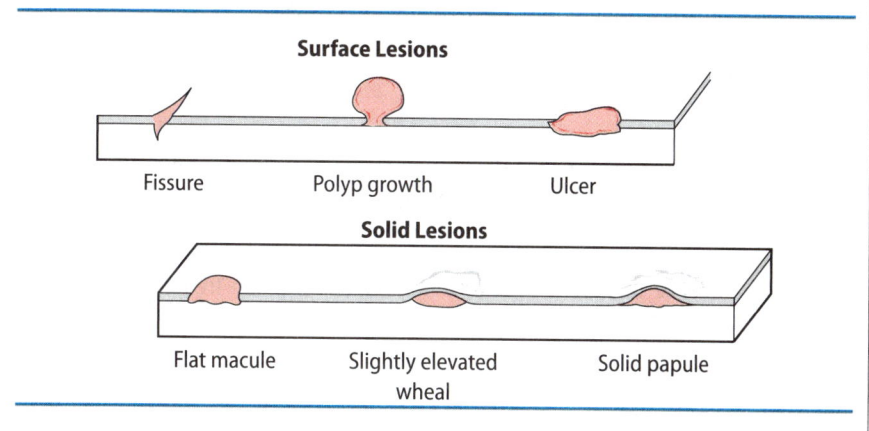

Surface Lesions

Fissure   Polyp growth   Ulcer

Solid Lesions

Flat macule   Slightly elevated wheal   Solid papule

Psoriasis and Other Similar Disorders

In ICD-9-CM, psoriasis and other similar disorders group to category 696 without a great deal of detail. In ICD-10-CM, there are more than 25 codes representing these conditions, providing much more detail in the code description than in ICD-9-CM.

Arthropathic Psoriasis

Arthropathic psoriasis is a form of inflammatory arthritis that affects patients with psoriasis. It causes joint inflammation but can also cause tendinitis, issues with the nails, and swelling of the digits. There are various forms of this condition, described by distinctive names. Many of these forms have been assigned different codes in the ICD-10-CM code set.

Distal interphalangeal psoriatic arthropathy is arthropathic psoriasis characterized by inflammation in the distal portions of the fingers and toes. In this particular type of arthropathy, there are often changes noted in the nails as well, including pitting, discoloration, ridging, and thickening.

Psoriatic arthritis mutilans is a severe, deforming form of arthritis. It gets progressively worse over months or even years, causing resorption of bones and severe joint damage. It is not a common condition, affecting less than 5 percent of patients with arthropathic psoriasis.

Psoriatic spondylitis is a type of arthropathic psoriasis that results in pain and stiffness of the spine and neck. This occurs predominantly in male patients. These patients may show unusual radiological features, such as paravertebral ossification.

Psoriatic juvenile arthropathy is arthropathic psoriasis with an onset in childhood. The average age of onset is 9 to 10 years, and it occurs predominantly in female patients. Luckily, the disease tends to be mild in children. Psoriatic juvenile arthropathy accounts for 8 to 20 percent of all childhood arthritis.

Other Psoriasis and Similar Disorders

Psoriasis vulgaris is the most common form of psoriasis, affecting 80 to 90 percent of all psoriasis diagnoses. Also known as plaque psoriasis, it presents as raised and inflamed red areas covered with silvery/white scaly skin. These areas are known as plaques and can be itchy and painful. Treatment for psoriasis varies based on the severity, but ranges from topical agents to oral pharmaceuticals to various types of phototherapies.

Acrodermatitis continua is a form of pustular psoriasis that results in skin lesions on the ends of the fingers and toes. It is quite rare and is referred to by many different names, such as acropustulosis, acrodermatitis continua of Hallopeau, dermatitis repens, and pustular acrodermatitis. This condition tends to be resistant to common psoriasis treatment, so it can require more aggressive treatment even for what seems like a less serious form of psoriasis.

Pustulosis palmaris et plantaris, or palmoplantar pustulosis (PPP), causes pustules specifically on the hands and feet, hence its name. It is a persistent condition, typically recurring over and over. Interestingly, it is suggested that patients with PPP refrain from smoking, as nicotine has been known to cause flare-ups.

Guttate psoriasis is characterized by small red spots on the skin, as opposed to the large, scaly regions of other types of psoriasis. They are usually found on the upper body, specifically the trunk and upper limbs. It is predominantly found in adolescents and young adults and can be precipitated by many different types of illnesses, such as an upper respiratory infection, strep throat, tonsillitis, or even simply stress or the administration of certain drugs. It is important this condition be treated so it does not become a more serious form of psoriasis in the future.

Parapsoriasis

Pityriasis lichenoides et varioliformis acuta (PLEVA) is a serious disease involving the immune system. It is characterized mainly by rashes and small lesions on the skin, caused by the immune system inappropriately "fighting" the skin cells and causing damage. It is often misdiagnosed as various similar looking conditions, such as chicken pox or rosacea. Common treatment for the condition is a combination of pharmaceuticals and phototherapy. Localized wound care may be required for large ulcerations or infections.

Pityriasis lichenoides chronica is the milder, chronic form of PLEVA. This condition is characterized by the gradual development of symptomless, small, scaling papules that spontaneously flatten and regress over a period of weeks or months. The patient may have lesions at various stages present at any one time. Patients with this condition often have exacerbations and relapses of the condition, which can last for months or years.

Lymphomatoid papulosis is a chronic skin disease with histological features consistent with malignant lymphoma. It is characterized by pruritic papules on the trunk and limbs that heal over time but leave scarring. What is interesting about this condition is that it is histologically malignant, exhibiting the clinical features of a lymphoma. However, because of its benign clinical course and fairly spontaneous resolution, many clinicians were reluctant to classify this as a malignancy and as such, it was classified in ICD-9-CM to code 709.8 Other specified disorders of skin. This has changed in ICD-10-CM, however, with lymphomatoid papulosis being reclassified to category C86 Other specified types of T/NK-cell lymphoma, and reported with code C86.6 Primary cutaneous CD30-positive T-cell proliferations.

Small plaque parapsoriasis is a mild version of parapsoriasis, resulting in small skin lesions typically on the trunk. This condition often resolves on its own and rarely, if ever, progresses.

Large plaque parapsoriasis is a serious chronic inflammatory disorder that results in large skin lesions. This condition can be concerning, not because of the skin issues themselves, which are quite treatable, but because approximately 10 percent of patients with large plaque parapsoriasis progress to cutaneous T-cell lymphoma or mycosis fungoides, both serious conditions. Treatments include topical pharmaceuticals in conjunction with phototherapy.

Retiform parapsoriasis is a form of large plaque parapsoriasis. It causes large skin lesions that result in a netlike pattern on the body and can also cause the skin to atrophy. As is the case with all large plaque parapsoriasis, treatment is important in avoiding disease progression.

> **INTERESTING A & P FACT**
>
> Many skin conditions, including many of the psoriasis and parapsoriasis conditions, have no identifiable cause. Many researchers hypothesize, but in most cases have not been able to agree on, a solid cause for most of these conditions.

Poikiloderma vasculare atrophicans (PVA) is a condition characterized by hypopigmentation or hyperpigmentation of the skin, atrophy of the skin, and telangiectasia (dilated blood vessels) near the surface of the skin. These issues are often related to another condition, such as mycosis fungoides, other parapsoriasis, and other conditions that might cause the skin issues. Treatment for PVA is typically geared toward the underlying condition. The classification of poikiloderma vasculare atrophicans (PVA) has been changed in ICD-10-CM to a localized connective tissue disorder, reported with code L94.5 Poikiloderma vasculare atrophicans, rather than parapsoriasis as in ICD-9-CM.

Other Psoriasis and Similar Disorders, Other

Pityriasis rubra pilaris is a chronic skin condition resulting in reddish orange scaly plaques and keratotic papules of the follicles. It can also cause palmoplantar keratoderma, which is a thickening of the skin on the palms of the hands and the soles of the feet. Treatment for this condition can include topical and/or oral medications and possibly phototherapy.

Infantile papular acrodermatitis, also known as Gianotti-Crosti syndrome, is a skin condition in children caused by the body's reaction to a viral infection. It is typically characterized by pink to pale flesh-colored papules covering the buttocks, the extremities, and the face. Rarely are other areas of the body involved. Hepatitis B was one of the initial viruses thought to cause this condition, although it is now just one of many seen as the root cause. In general, medications treat the symptoms but do not lessen the course of the condition. Topical agents can be used to soothe the itching, as can oral antihistamines.

Coding for Psoriasis and Other Similar Disorders

ICD-9-CM		ICD-10-CM	
696.0	Psoriatic arthropathy	L40.50	Arthropathic psoriasis, unspecified
		L40.51	Distal interphalangeal psoriatic arthropathy
		L40.52	Psoriatic arthritis mutilans
		L40.53	Psoriatic spondylitis
		L40.54	Psoriatic juvenile arthropathy
		L40.59	Other psoriatic arthropathy
696.1	Other psoriasis and similar disorders	L40.0	Psoriasis vulgaris
		L40.1	Generalized pustular psoriasis
		L40.2	Acrodermatitis continua
		L40.3	Pustulosis *palmaris* et *plantaris*
		L40.4	Guttate psoriasis
		L40.8	Other psoriasis
		L40.9	Psoriasis, unspecified
696.2	Parapsoriasis	L41.0	Pityriasis lichenoides et varioliformis acuta
		L41.1	Pityriasis lichenoides chronica
		L41.3	Small plaque parapsoriasis
		L41.4	Large plaque parapsoriasis
		L41.5	Retiform parapsoriasis
		L41.8	Other parapsoriasis
		L41.9	Parapsoriasis, unspecified
		L94.5	Poikiloderma vasculare atrophicans
696.8	Other psoriasis and similar disorders, other	L44.0	Pityriasis rubra pilaris
		L44.8	Other specified papulosquamous disorders
		L45	Papulosquamous disorders in diseases classified elsewhere

---

DEFINITIONS

infantile. Having to do with infants or children. When this term is used in conjunction with a condition or disease state, it usually indicates onset at a young age.

palmar. Pertaining to the palm. The root term is "palmo-."

plantar. Pertaining to the foot.

Pemphigoid

Pemphigoid is another skin condition in which there is a notable difference between the ICD-9-CM and ICD-10-CM code sets, with the ICD-10-CM code set requiring that the coder have a greater understanding of the different types of pemphigoid to code accurately.

Pemphigoid is an autoimmune disease that results in the body's own immune system attacking the cells of the integumentary system. It is important not to confuse it with pemphigus, which is a somewhat similar condition but is coded differently (L10.9 Pemphigus unspecified).

Bullous pemphigoid presents with blistering at the site of the attack and is accompanied by itching and pain. Treatment includes corticosteroids and/or immunosuppressants, as well as wound care to make sure the site stays clean and uninfected.

Other types of pemphigoid, such as gestationis pemphigoid, are reported with L12.8 Other pemphigoid, as more specific codes are not available.

Coding for Pemphigoid

ICD-9-CM		ICD-10-CM	
694.5	Pemphigoid	L12.0	Bullous pemphigoid
		L12.8	Other pemphigoid
		L12.9	Pemphigoid, unspecified

Rosacea

Rosacea is a common skin condition coded to a single ICD-9-CM code, 695.3. In ICD-10-CM, however, there are four separate codes with more specific terminology.

Perioral dermatitis is not exclusively related to rosacea but is a condition afflicting many with rosacea. Perioral refers to the area around the mouth. This form of dermatitis typically results in redness of the skin, small bumps that can be pus-filled, and peeling of the skin on the chin, the sides of the mouth, and around the nose. There is usually a band of skin around the mouth that is spared. There are various treatments for this condition, but the most common is the use of oral antibiotics, such as tetracycline. Corticosteroid creams are used in some cases but have been known to cause additional flare-ups.

Rhinophyma is the most recognizable condition related to rosacea. Although this condition isn't exclusive to rosacea, in most instances rosacea is involved. Rhinophyma results in the nose taking on a large, bulbous, distorted appearance, typically red in color. This distortion is caused over time by the hypertrophy of the sebaceous glands of the nose. It is often thought to be related to alcoholism, although there is no direct link. Heavy alcohol use, however, can aggravate the condition in patients with existing disease. Treatment for rhinophyma can include dermabrasion, laser resurfacing procedures, or other plastic surgery techniques to remove the damaged skin.

Coding for Rosacea and Related Conditions

ICD-9-CM		ICD-10-CM	
695.3	Rosacea	L71.0	Perioral dermatitis
		L71.1	Rhinophyma
		L71.8	Other rosacea
		L71.9	Rosacea, unspecified

Acne

In ICD-9-CM, acne codes are fairly generic, with most types of acne mapping to one of two codes. In ICD-10-CM, there are several codes for acne, all of which require that the coder have extensive knowledge about the specific form.

Acne vulgaris, also known as common acne, is a skin disorder faced by many adolescents who may deal with the disorder into adulthood. It is typically characterized by outbreaks of pimples, cysts, comedones, and inflammation. In youth, acne can have psychological effects as well, such as reduced self-esteem. Treatment for acne vulgaris can be as simple as over-the-counter benzoyl peroxide creams, or as complex as dermabrasion and surgical treatments, depending on severity.

Acne conglobata is a severe but somewhat rare form of acne that causes nodules on the skin, typically the trunk, upper arms, buttocks, thighs, and face. Also called cystic acne, these nodules create abscesses that become interconnected under the skin, creating a network of abscesses. This can cause significant scarring, to the point of disfigurement. It is typically treated with pharmaceuticals, but surgical excision may be required as well.

Acne tropica, or tropical acne, is seen in tropical climates. The warm air and humidity cause this condition, especially when the body is not used to higher temperatures. Acne tropica is caused by a significant build-up of oil, dead skin cells, and bacteria in the pores, which causes a heat rash-like reaction. Perspiration from the hot and humid weather exacerbates the condition, causing a vicious cycle. Treatment for acne tropica is much like that for acne vulgaris. Most patients are advised to use an over-the-counter benzoyl peroxide or salicylic acid treatment.

It is important that medical documentation differentiate between acne vulgaris and acne tropica, as well as between acne tropica and a heat rash, as each is coded differently under the ICD-10-CM system.

Infantile acne affects infants, typically starting around 2 to 3 months of age. There is no specific explanation for this form of acne, although there is a hypothesis that it is genetic in nature. It typically affects the nose and cheeks of the infant, but can spread to the chin and forehead. It usually dissipates by 6 months of age, but some cases have lasted up to age 3. Depending on the severity and the age of the patient, treatment may consist of nothing or may be similar to other acne treatments outlined above.

Acne excoriée des jeunes filles, also known as excoriated acne or picker's acne, is characterized by **comedones** or **pustules** that have been excoriated, or "picked," leaving open wounds or scratch marks. In most instances, much of the acne resolves, but scarring and sores remain. Treatment for this condition varies, based on severity and the root cause of excoriation [scratch or abrasion of skin]. In some cases, the excoriation can be caused by an underlying psychological condition, for which the patient may need to seek treatment. The acne itself can be treated with oral pharmaceuticals. In some cases, aggressive treatment to resolve the acne can curtail the patient's habitual picking, thus breaking the cycle.

Acne keloids are a form of **keloid** scarring that typically occurs at the base of the neck. It is associated with the occlusion of hair follicles in that area and is most often encountered in black and Asian men. The skin in the area becomes inflamed and bumpy, and it can be quite painful. Treatment varies, based on the severity of the condition. The use of antibiotics and steroid gels is common and, in more advanced cases, intralesional steroid injections may be required. Larger keloids may require surgical removal.

DEFINITIONS

comedones. Accumulation of sebum in the opening of a hair follicle. An open comedone is a blackhead, and a closed comedone is a whitehead.

keloid. Progressive overgrowth of cutaneous scar tissue that is raised and irregular in shape, caused by excessive formation of collagen during connective tissue repair.

pustule. Small skin elevation typically containing a purulent fluid, or pus.

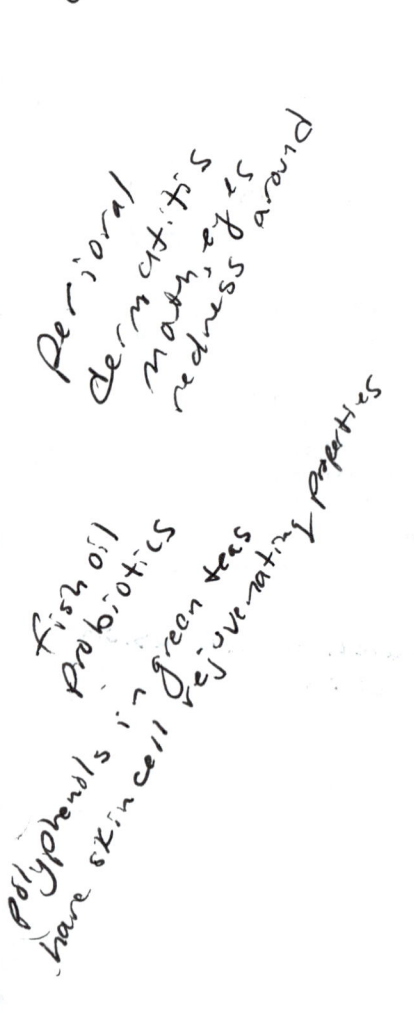

Coding for Acne

ICD-9-CM		ICD-10-CM	
706.1	Other acne	L70.0	Acne vulgaris
		L70.1	Acne conglobata
		L70.3	Acne tropica
		L70.4	Infantile acne
		L70.5	Acne excoriee des jeunes filles
		L70.8	Other acne
		L70.9	Acne, unspecified
		L73.0	Acne keloid

Heat-Related Skin Conditions

Prickly heat, or heat rash, uses significantly different terminology in ICD-9-CM from that used in ICD-10-CM. ICD-9-CM uses a more "layman" approach to the condition, whereas ICD-10-CM has taken a more clinical approach.

Miliaria rubra is the second most serious heat rash condition. It tends to affect adults in hot and humid conditions or neonates aged 1 to 3 weeks. It occurs deep within the epidermis and can cause pruritic papules across the body. The lesions tend to resolve quickly after the patients leave hot and humid climates.

Miliaria profunda is the most serious form of heat rash, caused by repeated episodes of miliaria rubra. This condition causes deep pustules to form at the dermal/epidermal junction. These pustules block the sweat glands and can make it impossible for the body to cool itself properly if widespread. In warm climates, patients with this condition are more likely to be predisposed to heat exhaustion.

Miliaria crystallina is the mildest form of heat rash. It tends to affect adults with other conditions that may be causing a fever or neonates younger than 2 weeks. Some adults who have relocated to a significantly warmer climate may be affected by this condition as well. This form affects the most superficial layer of the skin, causing what almost looks like tiny beads of liquid on the skin. It tends to be asymptomatic and often disappears on its own within a few days.

Coding for Prickly Heat/Heat Rash

ICD-9-CM		ICD-10-CM	
705.1	Prickly heat	L74.0	Miliaria rubra
		L74.1	Miliaria crystallina
		L74.2	Miliaria profunda
		L74.3	Miliaria, unspecified

Other Skin Conditions, Cysts

Sebaceous cysts are another type of skin condition difficult to code in ICD-10-CM without extensive knowledge. In ICD-9-CM, sebaceous cysts are grouped to a single code, 706.2. In ICD-10-CM, codes are assigned based on location and depth.

Figure 2.6: Sac Lesions

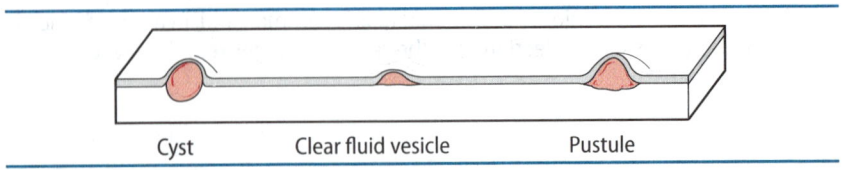

Cyst   Clear fluid vesicle   Pustule

Epidermal cysts, L72.0, are benign cysts of the skin resulting from any number of things, including a blocked pore or a traumatic injury. Such a cyst can be filled with pus or other purulent material and most likely needs to be removed surgically.

Trichodermal cysts, L72.12, are benign, fluid-filled cysts found at the hair follicle. They are often found on the scalp, although not exclusively. These cysts can grow together and form groups or channels, which can become problematic. Surgical excision is usually required.

Steatocystoma multiplex, L72.2, is a condition typically described as congenital, causing multiple cysts over the body. These cysts, typically small and fluid filled, are usually found in areas with the highest concentration of sebaceous glands (chest, arms, axillae, and neck). Treatment includes excision of particularly large or disfiguring lesions and pharmaceuticals to help prevent complications.

Nail Conditions

In ICD-9-CM, diseases of the nail are classified to one of three codes, two of which are generic. In ICD-10-CM, more specificity has been added, requiring that the coder be more knowledgeable about the various conditions that affect the nail.

Onychocryptosis, or an ingrown nail, is a painful condition that results in the nail plate growing and penetrating the skin, frequently causing infection. Although similar in appearance, this condition is different from onychia, which is an infection of the nail bed that can result in nail loss, or paronychia, which is an infection of the soft tissue surrounding the nail.

In onycholysis, the nail separates from the nail bed, typically starting at the distal free margin and separating proximally. It can occur for many reasons, including traumatic injuries, systemic diseases, and infections. Patients may be placed on medication to avoid a potential fungal infection related to this nail separation.

Onychogryphosis is a nail condition also known as "ram's horn nails." It is a hypertrophy of the nail that causes the nail to grow in a claw or a horn shape. It can be caused by various disease states or trauma, or it can be caused by neglect of the nail over a long period of time. Treatment often involves surgical avulsion of the nail plate.

Nail dystrophy is a general term relating to malformation of the nail. It can be a congenital malformation, but, in many cases, it is a deformity caused by some other condition or a drug or substance the patient has taken or been exposed to.

Beau's lines are horizontal depressions or lines across the nail bed. These lines grow out as the nail continues to grow. They can be caused by infections or trauma, or potentially even medication use.

Yellow nail syndrome is a rare condition characterized by yellow-tinted nails. The nails lack cuticles and can grow quite slowly. These patients are also typically affected by onycholysis.

Coding for Other Specified Diseases of the Nail

ICD-9-CM		ICD-10-CM	
703.8	Other specified disease of nail	L60.1	Onycholysis
		L60.2	Onychogryphosis
		L60.3	Nail dystrophy
		L60.4	Beau's lines
		L60.5	Yellow nail syndrome
		L60.8	Other nail disorders
		L62	Nail disorders in diseases classified elsewhere

Hair Conditions

Conditions related to the hair are more detailed in ICD-10-CM than in ICD-9-CM, requiring more knowledge to assign codes accurately. Various conditions affecting the hair and hair follicles, grouped to nonspecific codes in ICD-9-CM, have their own code descriptor.

In ICD-9-CM, unspecified alopecia is reported with 704.00. In ICD-10-CM, this condition maps to four codes.

Drug-induced androgenic alopecia, L64.0, is a hair loss condition in males and females caused by the ingestion of or exposure to some drug or substance. In many cases, this hair loss can be stopped by preventing exposure, and there is potential that the patient will have hair regrowth as well.

Androgenic alopecia, L64.8 and L64.9, is a general term for the most common form of hair loss. It is often referred to as male or female pattern baldness. There are various causes of hair loss, including stress, abnormal hormone levels, and disease states. In most instances, people are genetically predisposed to certain types of hair loss. Treatments available for androgenic alopecia include topical pharmaceuticals to attempt to generate hair growth, as well as surgical hair transplant techniques. However, most of these treatments are considered cosmetic in nature.

Alopecia areata (AA) is another type of hair loss affecting a smaller population than androgenic alopecia. Several researchers believe alopecia areata is an autoimmune disorder in which the immune system attacks the hair follicles causing the hair to fall out. In ICD-9-CM, alopecia areata is coded to 704.01. In ICD-10-CM, coding for AA isn't terribly complex, but there is one variant of the condition mentioned separately—ophiasis, L63.2. Patients with ophiasis typically have hair loss on the back of their head in the shape of a wave, near the nape of the neck. Outside of this specific pattern, there is no difference between ophiasis and other types of alopecia areata.

Other alopecia, previously coded as 704.09 in ICD-9-CM, has been separated into several components in ICD-10-CM.

Alopecia capitis totalis is total, typically permanent, hair loss on the scalp. Alopecia universalis is a total hair loss on the body, including eyebrows and eyelashes. Unlike alopecia totalis, however, the hair can grow back in some cases. Interestingly, there is no known cause for these conditions, as is the case for most forms of alopecia. Some researchers consider these conditions to be autoimmune disorders.

Anagen effluvium is hair loss that affects hair follicles specifically in the anagen stage of hair development. This hair loss most commonly occurs in patients undergoing radiation therapy or systemic chemotherapy treatments but can be caused by exposure to other pharmaceuticals or chemicals. Unfortunately, there is no treatment for the hair loss, but hair does typically regrow following conclusion of the therapies.

Alopecia mucinosa is characterized by patches of hair loss, as well as purulent papules and plaques. There is no known cause for this condition. Treatments can include topical medications and phototherapies, although these help with the papules and plaques more than they do hair loss. There is no standard treatment protocol for this condition, and it seems that in many cases the issue resolves on its own.

Pseudopelade is a form of cicatricial alopecia. It is characterized by irregularly shaped, slightly depressed lesions of the scalp. Sometimes there are a few hairs remaining in the lesion; otherwise it is typically hypopigmented in appearance. Once these lesions have occurred, there is unfortunately no medical treatment available. However, the patient may take pharmaceuticals to avoid other lesions from occurring. In serious cases, skin grafts and hair transplants may be used to replace hair loss if the disease has stabilized.

Folliculitis decalvans is another form of scarring alopecia. This condition is characterized by recurrent waves of follicular pustules that cause the hair to fall out.

> **INTERESTING A & P FACT**
>
> The name of the ophiasis pattern of alopecia areata comes from the Greek word for snake, ophis. A patient with the opposite hair loss pattern from the ophiasis pattern (hair loss everywhere except for the wave on the back of the head) is said to have sisaipho (the inverse of ophiasis, slightly altered for the sake of pronunciation).

Treatment for this condition is typically a combination of topical corticosteroids and oral tetracycline to control the infection and thus the hair loss.

Coding for Other Types of Alopecia

ICD-9-CM	ICD-10-CM	
704.09 Other alopecia	L63.0	Alopecia (capitis) totalis
	L63.1	Alopecia universalis
	L64.0	Drug-induced androgenic alopecia
	L64.8	Other androgenic alopecia
	L65.1	Anagen effluvium
	L65.2	Alopecia mucinosa
	L65.8	Other specified nonscarring hair loss
	L66.0	Pseudopelade
	L66.2	Folliculitis decalvans
	L66.8	Other cicatricial alopecia
	L66.9	Cicatricial alopecia, unspecified

Skin Ulcers

In ICD-9-CM, pressure and other types of ulcers are reported with multiple codes, although they are not specific to anatomical location. In ICD-10-CM, coders can pinpoint with a single code the ulcer site, type of ulcer, and whether it is related to a disease process. The coding of ulcers will not be reviewed in this publication; however, some anatomy and physiology concepts will be discussed to aid with coding accuracy.

Pressure Ulcer Stages

Pressure ulcer stages play an important role in ICD-9-CM and ICD-10-CM coding. Unfortunately, providers do not always document the specific stage of the ulcer, so wound descriptors may need to be scrutinized. Carefully review the many guidelines pertaining to the coding of pressure ulcers. These guidelines can be found in the front section of Optum360's *ICD-10-CM Complete Official Code Set* book or online at the Centers for Medicare and Medicaid Services (CMS) website.

> **CODING AXIOM**
>
> ICD-10-CM Official Coding Guideline I.C.12.a.3. states, "Assignment of the pressure ulcer stage code should be guided by clinical documentation of the stage or documentation of the terms found in the Alphabetic Index. For clinical terms describing the stage that are not found in the Alphabetic Index, and there is no documentation of the stage, the provider should be queried."
>
> The stage descriptions in figure 2.7 use the terms found in the alphabetic index.

Figure 2.7: Four Stages of Pressure Ulcers

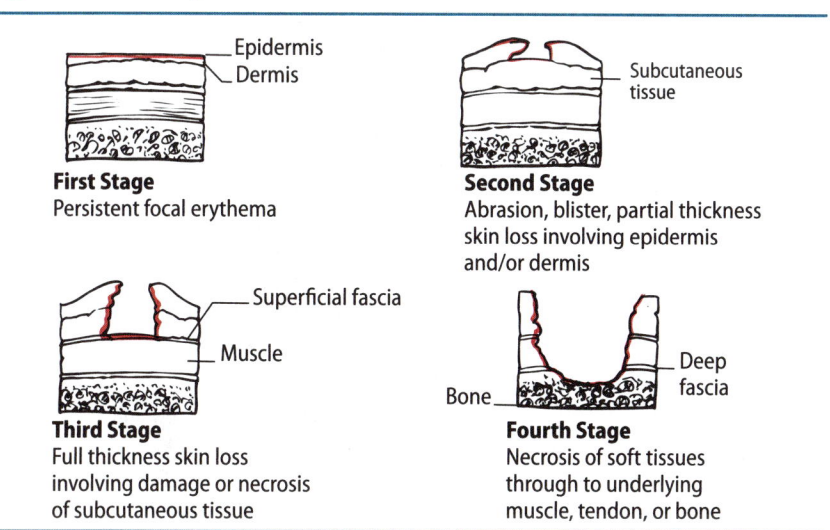

First Stage
Persistent focal erythema

Second Stage
Abrasion, blister, partial thickness skin loss involving epidermis and/or dermis

Third Stage
Full thickness skin loss involving damage or necrosis of subcutaneous tissue

Fourth Stage
Necrosis of soft tissues through to underlying muscle, tendon, or bone

Anatomy

When reporting skin ulcers in ICD-10-CM, the anatomical site must be identified. For example, in ICD-9-CM, pressure ulcer of the lower back is reported with 707.03. In ICD-10-CM, documentation needs to specify whether the ulcer is on the right or left lower back, the sacral region, or the buttock or hip. If the site is not specified, the coder must query the provider.

Conditions Involving the Breast

The most prominent difference between the classification of conditions of the breast in ICD-9-CM and ICD-10-CM is related to laterality. In ICD-9-CM, coding was limited to a description of the diagnosis itself.

> 610.0   Solitary cyst of breast

However, in ICD-10-CM, that coding becomes much more specific, requiring more detailed documentation from the physician.

> N60.01   Solitary cyst of right breast
>
> N60.02   Solitary cyst of left breast
>
> N60.09   Solitary cyst of unspecified breast

The clinical documentation needs to state in which breast the cyst is found, or the unspecified code needs to be assigned. Laterality is also used to code diffuse cystic mastopathy, fibroadenosis of breast, fibrosclerosis of breast, mammary duct ectasia, other specified benign mammary dysplasias, and benign mammary dysplasia, unspecified. There are some disorders of the breast found in categories N60–N65 of ICD-10-CM that do not indicate laterality, though many have added that additional detail.

Regarding conditions of the male breast, there is also a greater level of detail required in the documentation for ICD-10-CM than was required in ICD-9-CM.

Coding for Malignant Neoplasm of Other or Unspecified Sites of the Male Breast

> **DEFINITIONS**
>
> **quadrant of the breast.** Breasts are divided into four quadrants by drawing straight vertical and horizontal lines, intersecting at the nipple.

ICD-9-CM		ICD-10-CM	
175.9	Malignant neoplasm of other and unspecified sites of male breast	C50.121	Malignant neoplasm of central portion of right male breast
		C50.122	Malignant neoplasm of central portion of left male breast
		C50.129	Malignant neoplasm of central portion of unspecified male breast
		C50.221	Malignant neoplasm of upper-inner **quadrant** of right male breast
		C50.222	Malignant neoplasm of upper-inner quadrant of left male breast
		C50.229	Malignant neoplasm of upper-inner quadrant of unspecified male breast
		C50.321	Malignant neoplasm of lower-inner quadrant of right male breast
		C50.322	Malignant neoplasm of lower-inner quadrant of left male breast
		C50.329	Malignant neoplasm of lower-inner quadrant of unspecified male breast
		C50.421	Malignant neoplasm of upper-outer quadrant of right male breast
		C50.422	Malignant neoplasm of upper-outer quadrant of left male breast
		C50.429	Malignant neoplasm of upper-outer quadrant of unspecified male breast
(Continued on next page)		C50.521	Malignant neoplasm of lower-outer quadrant of right male breast

ICD-9-CM		ICD-10-CM	
175.9	Malignant neoplasm of other and unspecified sites of male breast *(Continued)*	C50.522	Malignant neoplasm of lower-outer quadrant of left male breast
		C50.529	Malignant neoplasm of lower-outer quadrant of unspecified male breast
		C50.621	Malignant neoplasm of **axillary tail** of right male breast
		C50.622	Malignant neoplasm of axillary tail of left male breast
		C50.629	Malignant neoplasm of axillary tail of unspecified male breast
		C50.821	Malignant neoplasm of overlapping sites of right male breast
		C50.822	Malignant neoplasm of overlapping sites of left male breast
		C50.829	Malignant neoplasm of overlapping sites of unspecified male breast
		C50.921	Malignant neoplasm of unspecified site of right male breast
		C50.922	Malignant neoplasm of unspecified site of left male breast
		C50.929	Malignant neoplasm of unspecified site of unspecified male breast

> **DEFINITIONS**
>
> **axillary tail.** Breast tissue that extends into the axilla or armpit area.

As demonstrated in the above table, additional clinical information about the exact location of the neoplasm within the male breast is required for ICD-10-CM. This level of detail was required in ICD-9-CM for malignant neoplasms of the female breast. However, this is a new requirement in ICD-10-CM for the male breast, as well as the addition of the laterality component. If a situation arises where the exact site of the neoplasm is not specified, query the provider for more information. Provider queries allow coders to collect detailed clinical information in order to assign the most accurate code for the patient's diagnosis.

Conditions Involving the Skin and Subcutaneous Tissue in Other Areas of ICD-10-CM

Diseases involving the skin and subcutaneous tissue are generally found in chapter 12 of ICD-10-CM (L00–L99). However, these conditions are not limited to this chapter and can be found throughout the ICD-10-CM manual.

Neoplasms

According to the most widely accepted definition, a neoplasm is an abnormal mass of tissue, the growth of which exceeds and is uncoordinated with that of normal tissues. It persists in the same excessive manner after cessation of the stimulus that evoked the cell changes.

For coding classification purposes, neoplasms are described in the following four ways:

- Behavior
- Functional activity
- Morphology
- Site

The behavior of a neoplasm refers to its biological behavior. The ICD-10-CM coding system recognizes the following behavioral types:

- **Malignant:** Tumors that behave in a life-threatening manner. The behavior that makes certain neoplasms malignant is their ability to invade surrounding tissues, as well as to metastasize. Malignant tumors can be further subdivided as:
  - **malignant primary:** Originating site of the tumor.
  - **malignant secondary:** Site to which a primary tumor has metastasized.
  - **carcinoma in situ:** Tumors confined to their point of origin that have not invaded surrounding tissue.
- **Benign:** Tumors in which the dividing cells adhere to each other, with the resulting neoplastic mass remaining as a circumscribed lesion.
- **Uncertain:** Neoplasm whose behavior cannot be determined at the time of discovery and that require continued study to accurately classify the neoplasm by behavior.
- **Unspecified:** Assigned when medical documentation does not specify the neoplasm behavior.

Functional activity refers to the effects certain neoplasms have on tissues that are functionally active and is reported with a secondary code from another chapter of ICD-10-CM.

A *basal cell* carcinoma is a malignant tumor found in the lowest layer of the epidermis, usually in areas exposed to sunlight, such as the head or neck. This is the most common form of carcinoma in the United States. These tumors are slow growing and rarely spread.

A *squamous cell* carcinoma originates in the squamous cells of the epidermis. Like basal cell, these lesions most frequently develop in areas exposed to the sun. However, unlike basal cell carcinoma, squamous cell carcinoma may spread to distant parts of the body and can be fatal.

Malignant *melanoma* begins in the melanocytes, the pigment-producing skin cells. Melanomas vary in size, shape, and color. Melanomas may grow deep into the skin and subcutaneous tissues, with the deepest ones having an increased risk of spreading through the lymphatic and blood system and metastasizing elsewhere in the body. Melanomas that spread are often fatal.

There are also a number of benign neoplasms that affect the skin. Examples include:

- Papilloma
- Acquired keratoderma
- Seborrheic keratosis
- Hemangioma

Site refers to the anatomic location of the neoplasm and is used as a subdivision for the four types of behaviors. ICD-9-CM codes do not differentiate greatly between neoplasm sites. In ICD-10-CM, however, there is greater differentiation in laterality, as well as upper versus lower. The following table illustrates the difference in anatomical terminology used in ICD-9-CM versus ICD-10-CM for neoplasms of the ear.

Coding for Other Malignant Neoplasm of the Skin of the Ear and External Canal

ICD-9-CM		ICD-10-CM	
173.29	Other specified malignant neoplasm of skin of ear and external auditory canal	C44.291	Other specified malignant neoplasm of skin of unspecified ear and external auricular canal
		C44.292	Other specified malignant neoplasm of skin of right ear and external auricular canal
		C44.299	Other specified malignant neoplasm of skin of left ear and external auricular canal

---

DEFINITIONS

basal cell. Malignant epithelial cell tumor that begins as a papule, but enlarges peripherally. They tend to develop a central crater that erodes, crusts, and then bleeds.

melanoma. Highly metastatic malignant neoplasm composed of melanocytes that occur most often on the skin from a preexisting mole or nevus but may also occur in the mouth, esophagus, anal canal, or vagina. Melanoma has four stages. Stage 0: cells are found only in the outer layer of skin cells and have not invaded deeper tissues. Stage I: Tumor is no more than 1 mm thick and the outer layer of skin may appear scraped or ulcerated; or the tumor is between 1 and 2 mm thick with no ulceration and no spread to nearby lymph nodes. Stage II: Tumor is at least 1 mm thick with ulceration or the lesion is more than 2 mm thick without ulceration and no spread to lymph nodes. Stage III: Cells have spread to one or more nearby lymph nodes or to tissues just outside the original lesion. Stage IV: Malignant cells have spread to other organs, lymph nodes, or areas of the skin distant from the original tumor.

squamous cell. Slow-growing malignant tumor of the squamous epithelium, found in the skin as well as the lungs, anus, cervix, larynx, nose, and bladder.

Note that in ICD-9-CM, the term auditory canal describes the external portion of the ear canal. However, in ICD-10-CM that term has been changed to auricular canal.

ICD-10-CM provides a few options for coding benign neoplasms. It is important that the coder have as much detail as possible before selecting the appropriate code.

Coding for Benign Neoplasm of Skin of Other and Unspecified Parts of the Face

ICD-9-CM		ICD-10-CM	
216.3	Benign neoplasm of skin of other and unspecified parts of face	D22.30	Melanocytic nevi of unspecified part of face
		D22.39	Melanocytic nevi of other parts of face
		D23.30	Other benign neoplasm of skin of unspecified part of face
		D23.39	Other benign neoplasm of skin of other parts of face

Melanocytic nevi do not have their own code in ICD-9-CM, although they are included in morphology coding scenarios. These benign neoplasms are made of melanocytes, which are pigment-producing cells, typically giving them a dark color varying from tan to black. These nevi can be surgically removed for cosmetic purposes or if the provider is concerned that they may progress into something more serious.

Symptoms, Signs, and Ill-Defined Conditions Involving the Skin and Subcutaneous Tissue

In ICD-9-CM, chapter 16 is reserved for signs and symptoms that cross over many body and organ systems. ICD-10-CM chapter 18 is similar, and some of the conditions listed involve the integumentary system.

From an anatomy and physiology perspective, most of the signs and symptoms involving the skin and subcutaneous tissues are similar between the two manuals. However, in ICD-10-CM, special attention needs to be paid to anatomical site. For example, in ICD-9-CM, localized superficial swelling, mass, or lump is assigned to a single code, 782.2. In ICD-10-CM, there are 12 distinct codes, differentiated by anatomical site, including:

R22.0	Localized swelling, mass and lump, head
R22.1	Localized swelling, mass and lump, neck
R22.2	Localized swelling, mass and lump, trunk
R22.30	Localized swelling, mass and lump, upper limb, unspecified side
R22.31	Localized swelling, mass and lump, right upper limb
R22.32	Localized swelling, mass and lump, left upper limb
R22.33	Localized swelling, mass and lump, upper limb, bilateral
R22.40	Localized swelling, mass and lump, lower limb, unspecified side
R22.41	Localized swelling, mass and lump, right lower limb
R22.42	Localized swelling, mass and lump, left lower limb
R22.43	Localized swelling, mass and lump, lower limb, bilateral
R22.9	Localized swelling, mass and lump, unspecified

There is also some additional specificity added to ICD-10-CM for some skin conditions. For example, in ICD-9-CM, disturbance of skin sensation is reported with a single code, 782.0. In ICD-10-CM, there is a series of codes representing various levels of the disturbance.

Comprehensive Anatomy and Physiology for ICD-10-CM and ICD-10-PCS Coding

Anesthesia of skin is a disturbance of skin sensation resulting in a complete loss of sensation to a particular area of the skin. In most instances, anesthesia refers to induction of an anesthetic for a surgical procedure or pain control; however, this is not the case for this diagnosis.

Hypoesthesia of the skin is a reduced sense of touch or feeling in the skin. It is not a complete anesthesia, but is a noticed decrease in sensation in the affected area. Hyperesthesia is the opposite, an increased sensitivity in the skin.

Paraesthesia is a combination of hypoesthesia with a tingling or prickling feeling in the affected area. It is commonly referred to as "pins and needles" or the area "falling asleep." Patients often complain of paraesthesias in the extremities, which can be secondary to various conditions or pharmaceutical therapies. Treatment depends on the root cause.

Coding for Disturbance of Skin Sensation

ICD-9-CM		ICD-10-CM	
782.0	Disturbance of skin sensation	R20.0	Anesthesia of skin
		R20.1	Hypoesthesia of skin
		R20.2	Paraesthesia of skin
		R20.3	Hyperesthesia
		R20.8	Other disturbances of skin sensation
		R20.9	Unspecified disturbances of skin sensation

Injuries Involving the Skin and Subcutaneous Tissue

In the ICD-10-CM code set, lacerations and open wounds with and without complications are no longer the "norm." Close attention must be paid to the injury site, the mechanism of the injury, the patient encounter, and whether foreign bodies are involved.

Coding for Open Wounds of Scalp

ICD-9-CM		ICD-10-CM	
873.0	Open wound of scalp without mention of complication	S01.00XA	Unspecified open wound of scalp, initial encounter
		S01.01XA	Laceration without foreign body of scalp, initial encounter
		S01.03XA	Puncture wound without foreign body of scalp, initial encounter
		S01.05XA	Open bite of scalp, initial encounter
		S08.0XXA	Avulsion of scalp, initial encounter
873.1	Open wound of scalp, complicated	S01.02XA	Laceration with foreign body of scalp, initial encounter
		S01.04XA	Puncture wound with foreign body of scalp, initial encounter

As illustrated in the table above, what was previously an open wound in ICD-9-CM is now a *laceration,* a *puncture wound,* an *open bite,* or an *avulsion* in ICD-10-CM. [handwritten: pulling/tearing away]

In ICD-9-CM, codes for lacerations and open wounds include descriptors "with or without complications." In ICD-10-CM, this terminology is no longer used, but code descriptions focus instead on whether the wound includes a foreign body.

Burns

Burns are the result of an injury or destruction to the tissue and can be due to the effects of thermal energy, chemicals, electricity, or radiation. Many complications arise in burn patients, including hypovolemic shock, inhalation injury, inability to regulate temperature, infection, scarring, and contractures.

CODING AXIOM

Examples for injuries involving the skin and subcutaneous tissue include only initial encounters in this publication. However, codes are also differentiated between subsequent encounters and sequelae in ICD-10-CM.

DEFINITIONS

avulsion. Traumatic injury caused by the forcible tearing away of a part.

laceration. Tearing injury, or a torn, ragged-edged wound.

open bite. Traumatic injury caused by an animal or another human.

puncture wound. Traumatic injury caused by an object, such as a knife, nail, or fragment of a solid substance like glass or wood.

There are three degrees of burn depending on the level of skin lost:

- **First-degree burns:** Also known as erythema, first-degree burns are limited to tissue damage to the outer layer of the epidermis.
- **Second-degree burns:** Blistering with extension beyond the epidermis to partial thickness of the dermis.
- **Third-degree burns:** Full-thickness skin loss. Third-degree burns with presence of necrotic tissue is termed deep necrosis.

Figure 2.8: Degrees of Burns

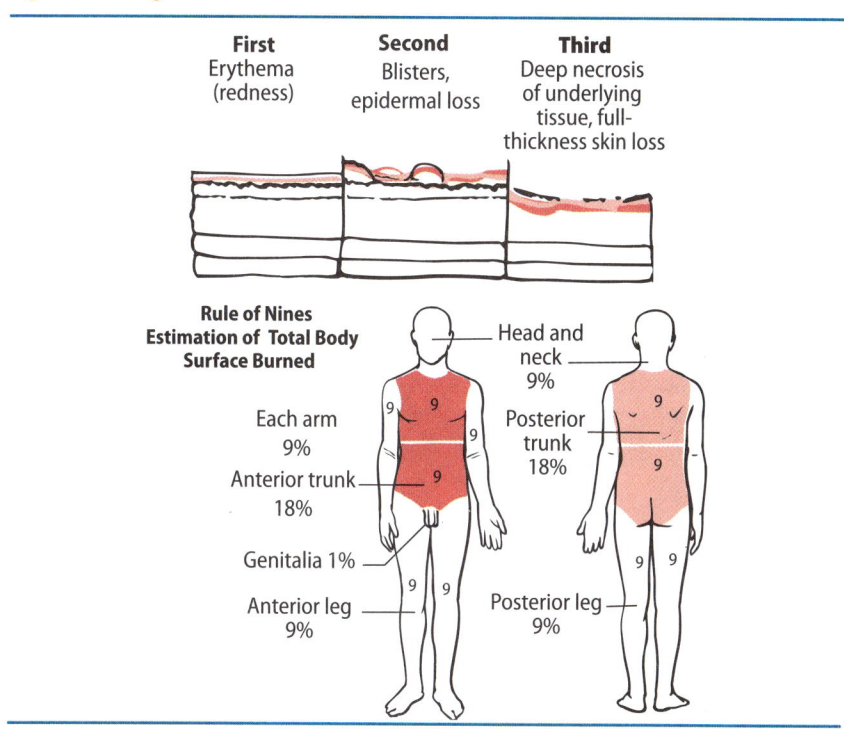

First — Erythema (redness)
Second — Blisters, epidermal loss
Third — Deep necrosis of underlying tissue, full-thickness skin loss

Rule of Nines Estimation of Total Body Surface Burned:
- Head and neck 9%
- Each arm 9%
- Anterior trunk 18%
- Posterior trunk 18%
- Genitalia 1%
- Anterior leg 9%
- Posterior leg 9%

The terminology used for burns varies between ICD-9-CM and ICD-10-CM. Common terminology includes first-, second-, and third-degree burns, as well as the "rule of nines" for calculating the total body surface area (TBSA) burned. However, ICD-10-CM also differentiates between burn types.

There are separate ICD-10-CM codes for burns and corrosions. Burns are traditional thermal burns, and corrosions are chemical burns.

Coding for Burns of Chin

ICD-9-CM		ICD-10-CM	
941.14	Erythema due to burn of chin	T20.13XA	Burn of first degree of chin, initial encounter
		T20.53XA	Corrosion of first degree of chin, initial encounter

> **CODING AXIOM**
>
> ICD-10-CM Official Coding Guideline I.C.19.d. states, "ICD-10-CM makes a distinction between burns and corrosions. The burn codes are for thermal burns, except sunburns that come from a heat source, such as a fire or hot appliance. The burn codes are also for burns resulting from electricity and radiation. Corrosions are burns due to chemicals. The guidelines are the same for burns and corrosions."
>
> All guidelines associated with the coding of burns and corrosions can be found in the front section of Optum360's *ICD-10-CM Complete Official Code Set* book or online at the Centers for Medicare and Medicaid Services (CMS) website.

Summary

The integumentary system is truly a diverse system, literally covering the human body from head to toe. In this chapter, the basics of the integumentary system were covered, as well as some of the coding differences between ICD-9-CM and ICD-10-CM. Pay close attention to detail when coding anatomical sites, as a simple left versus right or upper versus lower makes a major difference in ICD-10-CM coding.

Also note that because new terminology is used in ICD-10-CM, the coder may have to ask the physician for clarification. Physicians and other providers will be learning about this new code set as well, and many will likely be willing to assist coders in learning more about the clinical side of medicine.

Chapter 3. ICD-10-CM: Skeletal System and Articulations

Anatomic Overview

The skeletal system is comprised of bones, cartilage, articulations, and ligaments. It is responsible for shaping and supporting the body, providing protection for internal organs, and aiding in and restricting movement. It also plays a role in blood cell production and mineral storage.

Bones

Bones provide the support for and shape of the body. They are the structural foundation for the rest of the body, as well as protection for many vital organs. For instance, the ribs, sternum, scapula, and clavicle protect the heart and lungs, while the bony spine protects the spinal cord and blood vessels within the vertebrae.

A bone consists of two tissue types, the difference between which is seen only microscopically. Compact bone, also known as cortical bone, is tightly packed tissue with minimal gaps and spaces. Spongy or cancellous bone looks disorganized with what appears to be random gaps and holes in the tissue.

The bones also produce and house a highly specialized connective tissue called bone marrow. There are two types of bone marrow: yellow and red. Yellow bone marrow stores fat for the body and is found mainly in the hollow spaces in the long bones of adults. Blood cell formation occurs in red bone marrow, which is primarily stored in spongy bone.

Bones can be classified into five major categories: long, short, flat, irregular, and sesamoid.

Long bones, such as the femur (the thigh bone), are longer than they are wide. They are made up of a shaft, or **diaphysis**, and two bulbous ends, or **epiphyses**. The epiphyses form a joint with another bone and are covered in **articular cartilage** where bones meet to lessen friction during movement. The rest of a long bone is covered in a hard, vascular shell called the periosteum. Within the shaft of a long bone is compact tissue surrounding a space called the medullary cavity; this is where yellow marrow is stored. The epiphyses are covered in an outer layer of compact bone but are mostly composed of spongy bone.

The composition of short, flat, and irregular bones is different from that of a long bone, but similar to each other. They each consist of thin plates of compact bone covering the spongy bone in the middle. Red marrow is found within the spongy tissue of these bones, but there is no actual hollow cavity present. These bone types are classified according to their individual shapes. Short bones are cubelike, such as the bones in the wrist or ankle. Flat bones are platelike; most bones in the skull are flat bones. Irregular bones are those that have complicated shapes, such as the pelvic bones, vertebrae, and some facial bones.

Sesamoid bones are a unique type of bone that forms within **tendons**. They are small and round (some classify these as a type of short bone) and vary in size and number in different individuals. The function of most sesamoid bones is to direct the pull of a tendon. The kneecap, or patella, is the most commonly recognized bone associated with this classification.

The external surfaces of all bone types have visible bulges, depressions, and holes for various physiological purposes, including providing sites for muscle, ligament, and

---

> **INTERESTING A & P FACT**
>
> The skeleton accounts for approximately 30 to 40 percent of the body's total weight.

> **CLINICAL NOTE**
>
> Red marrow is primarily found in the spongy bone of the ribs, skull, sternum, clavicles, vertebrae, and pelvis of adults.

> **DEFINITIONS**
>
> **articular cartilage.** Smooth living tissue that covers and protects moving surfaces, resulting in the reduction of friction.
>
> **diaphysis.** Central shaft of a long bone.
>
> **epiphysis.** Enlarged proximal and distal ends of a long bone.
>
> **tendon.** Dense fibrous connective tissue that connects muscle to bone.

> **INTERESTING A & P FACT**
>
> Extra sesamoid bones can form throughout life within tendons as a response to friction where the tendon passes over bony protrusions.

© 2015 Optum360, LLC

tendon attachment to passageways for blood vessels and nerves. Some of the more commonly referred to markings for the purposes of coding are:

- **Condyle:** Rounded process that articulates with another bone.
- **Epicondyle:** Raised area on or above a condyle.
- **Facet:** Smooth surface that articulates with another bone.
- **Foramen:** Round opening through a bone.
- **Process:** Prominent projection.
- **Trochanter:** Very large, blunt process (found only on the femurs).
- **Tubercle:** Small rounded process.
- **Tuberosity:** Large rounded process.

The Axial Skeleton

The 206 bones that make up the adult skeleton can be divided into two classifications: the axial skeleton and appendicular skeleton. The axial, or "center," skeleton is formed by the bones and cartilaginous tissue in the skull, vertebral column, and thoracic cage. It supports and protects the organs of the head, neck, and trunk.

The skull consists of eight cranial bones, 14 facial bones, and the hyoid bone. The cranial bones form the cranium, which protects the brain and provides attachments for the muscles of the head and neck. The bones that form the cranium are:

- Two parietal
- Two temporal
- Frontal
- Occipital
- Sphenoid
- Ethmoid

Figure 3.1: Cranium

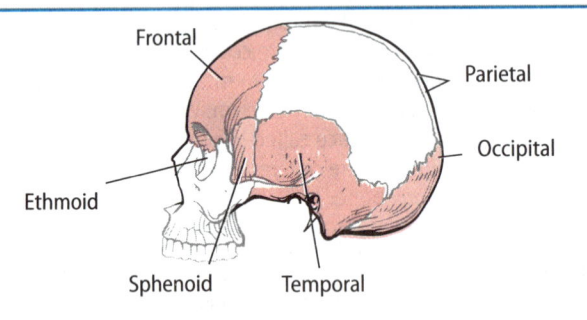

The facial bones provide the facial structure and provide attachments for the muscles that control facial and jaw movement. The face consists of 13 stationary bones and one mobile bone. The mandible (jawbone) is the only facial bone that moves and is also the largest and strongest bone of the face. The remaining bones of the face are:

- Two maxilla
- Two palatine
- Two zygomatic (cheekbones)
- Two lacrimal
- Two nasal
- Two inferior nasal concha (thin, curved bones that form the lateral walls of the nasal cavity)
- Vomer (located along the midline of the nasal cavity forming part of the nasal septum)

Figure 3.2: Facial Bones

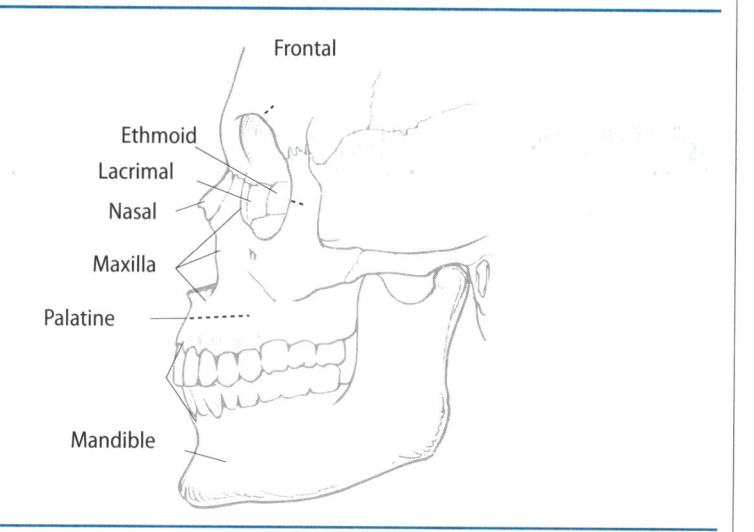

The hyoid bone is not really a part of the skull, as it does not articulate with any bones of the head. It is located in the neck just below the mandible. It supports the tongue and provides attachments for the muscles that move the larynx during speech and swallowing.

Also found in the head but outside of the skull are the bones that make up the middle ear. There are three bones found in each ear: the malleus, incus, and stapes. These bones are the smallest in the human body.

Attaching the skull to the body is the vertebral column, or bony spine. The vertebral column supports the head and trunk of the body and protects the spinal cord. It is composed of 26 individual bones. Of these bones, 24 are vertebrae that are separated by cartilage called intervertebral discs. Vertebrae have a common structure consisting of a body, *pedicles*, and *lamina* that form the vertebral arch. The body and arch come together and form an opening called the vertebral foramen, through which the *spinal cord* passes. Extending laterally off the vertebral arch are three processes: the two on each side are transverse processes, and the one in the middle is the spinous process. There are also processes that extend above and below the vertebral arch, known respectively as the inferior and superior articular processes.

> **DEFINITIONS**
>
> **lamina.** Thin plate of membrane or other tissue.
>
> **pedicle.** Narrow bony spike coming off a larger bone.
>
> **spinal cord.** Portion of the central nervous system that extends from the brain through the vertebral canal.

Figure 3.3: Vertebrae

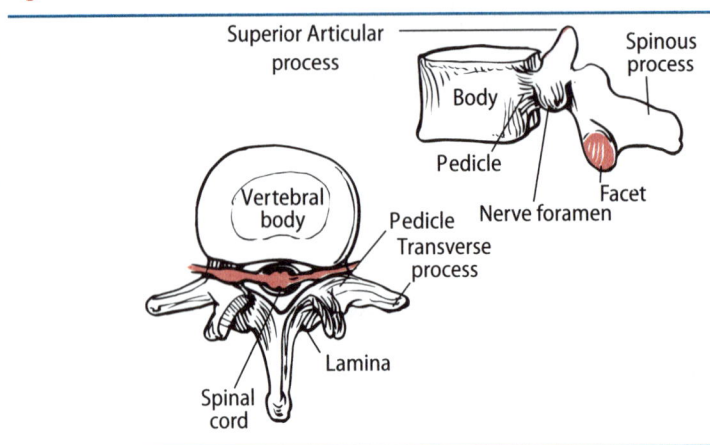

The vertebrae can be divided into three groups:

- Seven cervical (C1-C7; C1 is also known as atlas, C2 as axis)
- Twelve thoracic (T1-T12)
- Five lumbar (L1-L5)

Figure 3.4: Spine

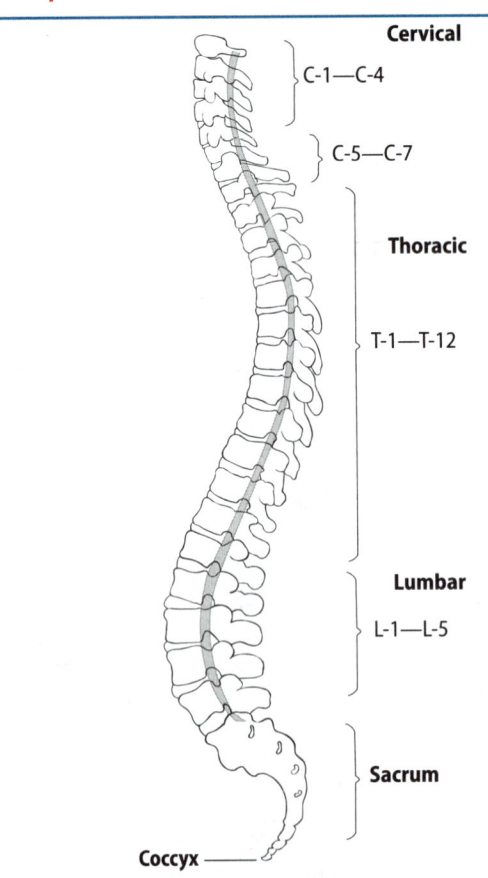

Below the lumbar vertebrae is the sacrum, which articulates with the pelvic bones of the appendicular skeleton. The last bone at the end of the vertebral column is the coccyx, or tail bone.

The spine has naturally occurring curves in it to increase its resilience. These curves allow it to function as a spring, bending and flexing with movement and impact. The names of the curves correspond with the vertebrae associated with it: the cervical, thoracic, and lumbar curvatures.

Articulating with the thoracic vertebrae are 12 pairs of flat bones known as the ribs. The first seven pairs of ribs meet up with the sternum directly via costal cartilage. The cartilage for the next three pairs of ribs joins with the costal cartilage of the seventh rib. The last two rib pairs do not join the sternum at all. The combination of these bones and cartilage form the thoracic cage, or bony thorax. This structure protects the lungs, heart, and great blood vessels. It also supports the shoulders and upper limbs and provides attachments for the muscles of the neck, back, chest, and shoulders.

Figure 3.5: Ribs and Sternum

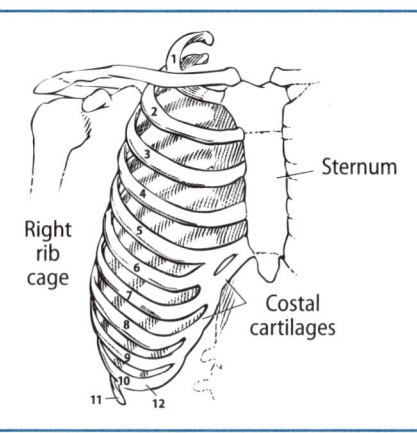

The Appendicular Skeleton

The bones that attach to the axial skeleton are referred to as the appendicular skeleton, which consists of the extremities and their respective girdles. This part of the skeleton enables the body to move.

The shoulder girdle consists of two bones on each side: the clavicle, or collar bone, and the scapula, or shoulder blade. It supports the upper limbs and provides the greatest range of movement found in the human body. The clavicle is found on the anterior side of the shoulder and the scapula on the posterior. The clavicles act as braces for the scapulas and arms by holding them outward.

The upper extremities are formed by 30 bones each and can be distinguished regionally as the upper arm, forearm, wrist, and hand. The bone in the upper arm is the humerus. Its superior epiphysis, or the humeral head, articulates with the glenoid cavity of the scapula to form the shoulder joint. At its inferior end, it articulates with the radius and ulna, the two bones that form the forearm. The radius is the long bone on the thumb side of the arm, and the ulna is located on the side of the little finger.

Figure 3.6: Shoulder/Upper Extremity

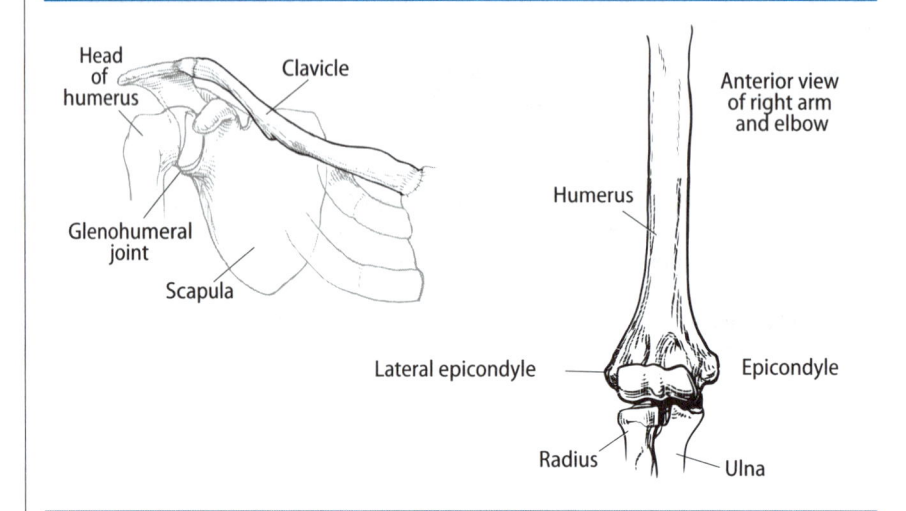

The wrist is composed of eight short bones called carpals that meet with the radius and ulna. These eight bones are:

- Scaphoid
- Capitate
- Trapezium
- Trapezoid
- Hamate
- Pisiform
- Triquetral
- Lunate

The carpals articulate with the metacarpals, which are the five bones that form the palm of the hand. The heads of the metacarpals are commonly referred to as knuckles, where the metacarpals join with the phalanges. Phalanges are the bones that form the fingers. There are three phalanges in all fingers, except for thumbs, which have only two. The phalanges that meet with the metacarpal heads are known as the proximal phalanges, then the middle phalanges, and, last, the distal phalanges.

Figure 3.7: Hand

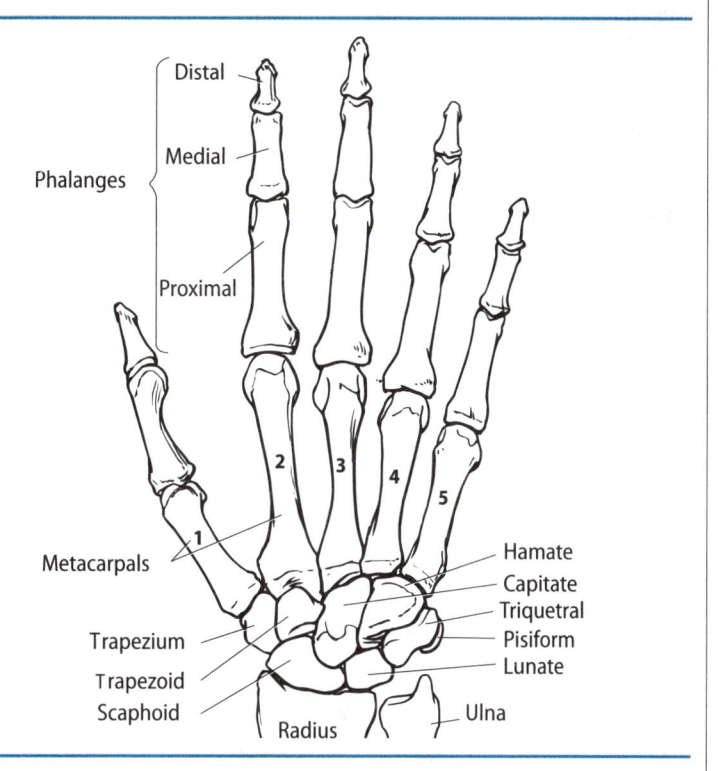

Similar to the upper extremity, the lower extremity follows the same basic structure with the pelvic girdles to attach the lower limbs to the axial skeleton. The pelvic or hip girdle distributes the weight of the body to the legs. It is composed of a coxal bone on each side that joins with the sacrum of the spine at the sacroiliac joint. The coxal bones can be divided into three parts:

- Ilium
- Ischium
- Pubis

Figure 3.8: Right Coxal Bone

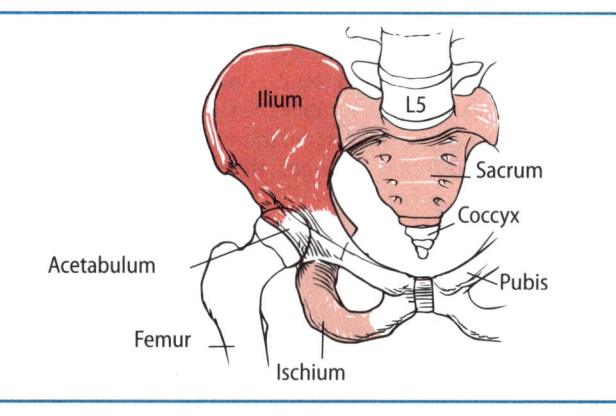

Where the three parts of the pelvic bone fuse is referred to as the acetabulum. It is a deep-seated pocket that accepts the rounded upper epiphysis of the thigh bone, or femoral head, to form the hip joint.

> **INTERESTING A & P FACT**
>
> The coxal bones are three separate bones at birth. By adulthood, they are fused together as a single bone. However, the names of the three original bones are retained to identify the different regions of the bone: ilium, ischium, and pubis.

The femur is the only bone in the thigh and is the largest and strongest bone in the body. It joins the tibia (shin bone) distally to form the knee joint. The knee joint is protected by a sesamoid bone called the patella, or the knee cap. The tibia also articulates with a second bone found alongside it within the lower leg known as the fibula. The fibula is the lateral bulge, or lateral malleolus, of the ankle; the tibia is the medial bulge, or medial malleolus.

Figure 3.9: Right Tibia and Fibula, Anterior View

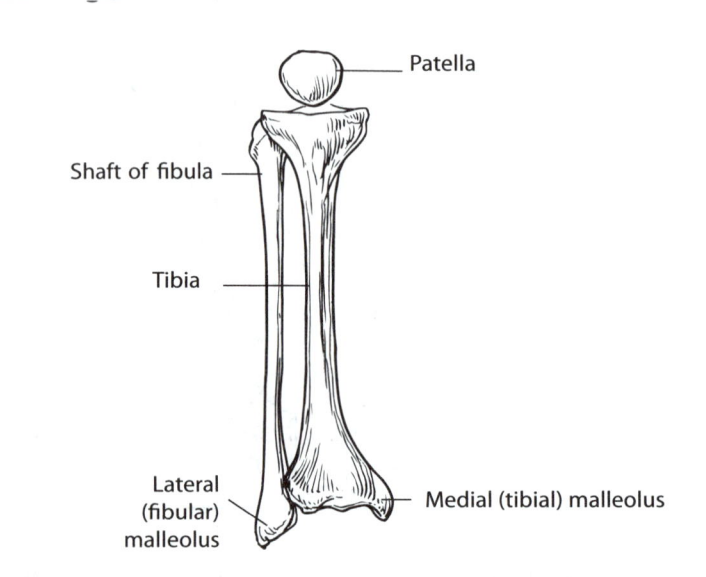

> **CODING AXIOM**
>
> ICD-10-CM Official Coding Guideline I.C.13.a.1. identifies the importance of knowing whether the condition being coded is affecting a bone near a joint or the joint structure itself. It states, "For certain conditions, the bone may be affected at the upper or lower end (e.g., avascular necrosis of bone, M87, Osteoporosis M80, M81). Though the portion of the bone affected may be at the joint, the site designation will be the bone, not the joint."

The tibia and fibula meet with the talus, the most superior of the seven tarsal bones, to form the ankle. The talus sits upon the calcaneus, or heel bone. Between the calcaneus and the metatarsals are the remaining five tarsals, known as:

- Cuboid
- Navicular
- Medial cuneiform
- Intermediate cuneiform
- Lateral cuneiform

Much the same as the bones in the wrist and hand, the tarsals meet with five small long bones in the foot called the metatarsals. The metatarsals meet up with phalanges. The toe phalanges are generally the same in structure and arrangement as the finger phalanges but are smaller and therefore less agile. Again, similar to the fingers, all of the toes have three phalanges, proximal, middle, and distal, with the exception of the great toe, or hallux.

Figure 3.10: Right Foot, Dorsal

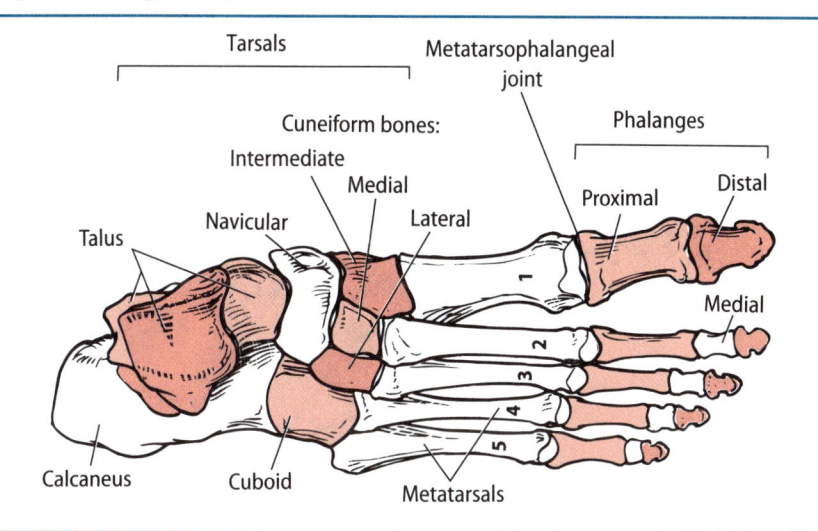

Articulations

Articulations, or joints, join two bones together and allow for movement in response to muscle contractions. There are three classifications of joints based on the structure or type of tissue the joint is composed of, including:

- Fibrous
- Cartilaginous
- Synovial

Fibrous joints are held together by dense tissue and are limited in movement by the length of that tissue. Most of these types of articulations are immovable or slightly moveable at best. There are three types of fibrous joints: sutures, or seams, between bones held together by connective tissue, such as those found in the cranium; gomphosis, a second type of fibrous joint, is found only as a tooth in its socket; and syndesmoses are bones joined by a **ligament**. The articulation between the tibia and fibula is an example of syndesmoses.

Cartilaginous joints are joined by cartilage. The first rib to the sternum is a cartilaginous articulation, as are the intervertebral joints and pubic symphysis. These types of joints do provide for some movement, albeit extremely minimal.

The majority of joints in the human body are synovial. These are free moving and therefore structurally more complex than the preceding two types. Synovial articulations all have a fluid-filled cavity separating the bones it joins. This cavity is called the synovial cavity, and the fluid is synovial fluid. The joint cavity is surrounded by a two-layer capsule called the articular capsule. The external layer of the capsule is a dense connective tissue that is contiguous with the periosteum of the related bones. The internal layer is a synovial membrane that covers all surfaces within the joint cavity except for the opposing bone surfaces. Articular cartilage covers those surfaces. Synovial joints are also unique in that they are reinforced by ligaments.

> **DEFINITIONS**
>
> **ligament.** Fibrous tissue binding joints together connecting bone to bone or bone to cartilage.

Figure 3.11: Synovial Joint Structures

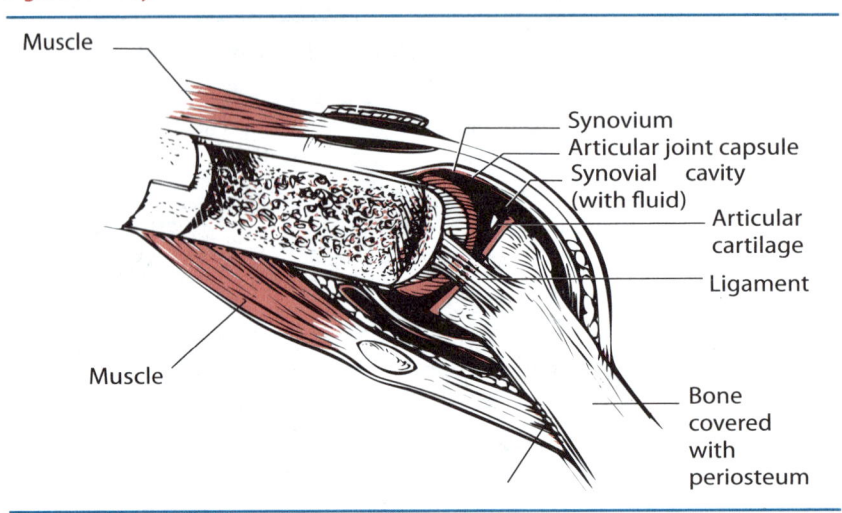

Synovial joints can be further classified by the movements they allow, including:

- **Ball-and-socket:** Head of a long bone ("ball") and depression of another bone ("socket') joint. The shoulder (humeral head and glenoid depression of the scapula) and hip joints (femoral head and acetabulum of a coxa bone) are ball-and-socket articulations.
- **Condyloid:** Protrusion of one bone meets a depression of another to form this type of joint. Examples are the wrist (radius and carpals) and knuckles (metacarpal and proximal phalange).
- **Hinge:** Convex portion of a bone meets with the concave part of another to form a hinge joint. The elbow and knee are large hinge joints.
- **Pivot:** Rounded or pointed protrusion of one bone fits into a ring composed of bone or bone and ligaments of another bone. The articulation between the C1 and C2 vertebrae that allows the head to move back and forth is a pivot joint.
- **Planar:** Flat surfaces of two bones glide against one another. The joints between the short carpals (intercarpal joint) and tarsals (intertarsal joint) are planar.
- **Saddle:** One bone has a depression shaped somewhat like an equestrian saddle; the joint is formed by a second bone straddling that depression. An example of this type of articulation is where the trapezium meets the metacarpal of the thumb. This joint allows the unique *opposition* of the human thumb.

DEFINITIONS

opposition. Act of touching the thumb to the tips of each finger on the same hand.

Anatomy and Pathophysiology and the ICD-10-CM Code Set

It is important to recognize the many differences between ICD-9-CM and ICD-10-CM when it comes to the skeletal system and its articulations. To assign the appropriate ICD-10-CM code, the coder needs advanced knowledge of the anatomy and physiology of the skeletal system and its articulations, as well as the ability to identify what additional information is needed.

Injuries

Injuries to the skeletal system are quite common as it is a rigid structure. The joints are also fairly susceptible to injury because part of their purpose is to maintain alignment, regardless of extraneous external forces.

Fractures, or breaks in the bone, are a common injury. There are roughly 6.8 million fractures reported in the United States annually.

In ICD-9-CM, the appropriate fracture code depends on the bone fractured, whether the fracture was *pathological* or traumatic, and whether it was considered open or closed. ICD-10-CM requires much more information than does ICD-9-CM.

For discussion purposes, ICD-9-CM and ICD-10-CM coding of a closed fracture of the greater tuberosity of the humerus will be compared. A difference in coding can be spotted immediately just by looking at the ICD-10-CM and ICD-9-CM alphabetic index. In ICD-10-CM, the fracture must be identified as traumatic or pathological before proceeding any further in code selection. In ICD-9-CM, the site of the fracture may be selected first, followed by whether it is pathological in nature. In ICD-9-CM, an injury is assumed to be traumatic unless further clarified. With the information provided, code 812.03 Fracture of humerus, upper end, closed, greater tuberosity, may be assigned in ICD-9-CM.

In ICD-10-CM, the above information is not sufficient for code assignment—there are two more considerations. First, is the fracture traumatic or pathological? Second, does the patient also have a diagnosis of *osteoporosis*? If the patient does have osteoporosis, according to ICD-10-CM coding guidelines, the fracture should be reported as a pathological fracture of the humerus, even if the patient had a minor fall or trauma, if that fall or trauma would not usually break a normal, healthy bone. For demonstration purposes, assume the fracture is specified as traumatic, which leads us to S42.25 Fracture of greater tuberosity of humerus.

Traumatic fractures must be further clarified with the following information:

- Is the bone *displaced*? If this is unspecified, ICD-10-CM Coding Guidelines direct the coder to assume the fracture is displaced.
- On which side of the body did the injury occur?

These two answers determine the sixth character of the ICD-10-CM code. However, since fracture codes require a seventh character, even more information is needed. This alphabetic character is based on multiple factors as listed below:

- Is this the initial encounter for the fracture? If yes, is the fracture:
  - *open*
  - *closed*
- Is this a subsequent encounter? If yes:
  - Is the healing of the fracture routine or delayed?
  - Is there a *nonunion* or *malunion*?
  - Is there a sequela or late effects of the fracture?

Due to the extensive nature of code selection for a fracture in ICD-10-CM, there is a "one-to-many" match between the two coding classification systems as demonstrated in the following table.

CODING AXIOM

ICD-10-CM Official Coding Guideline section I.C.19.c.1. states, "A code from category M80 Osteoporosis with current pathological fracture, not a traumatic fracture code, should be used for any patient with known osteoporosis who suffers a fracture, even if the patient had a minor fall or trauma, if that fall or trauma would not usually break a normal, healthy bone."

CODING AXIOM

ICD-10-CM Official Coding Guideline section I.C.19.c. states, "A fracture not indicated as open or closed should be coded to closed. A fracture not indicated whether displaced or not displaced should be coded to displaced."

DEFINITIONS

closed fracture. Bone fracture not accompanied by a break in skin.

displaced. Bone break in which the two broken ends are separated.

fracture. Break in bone or cartilage.

malunion. Fractured bone that has healed or is healing in an incorrect position.

nonunion. Fractured bone that has failed to heal.

open fracture. Fracture in which the broken end or ends of the bone have pierced the skin.

osteoporosis. Disorder characterized by bone degeneration. Osteoporosis is caused by the breakdown of the bony matrix without equivalent regeneration, resulting in a weak, porous, fragile bone structure.

pathological. Relating to a condition that is caused by or involves a disease process.

Comprehensive Anatomy and Physiology for ICD-10-CM and ICD-10-PCS Coding

> **CODING AXIOM**
>
> If the provider's documentation only identifies that a fracture is present but does not provide the specific location of the fracture, an x-ray report can be used to ascertain the needed specificity.
>
> *Coding Clinic,* 1Q, 13, 28

Coding for Closed Fracture of Greater Tuberosity of the Humerus

ICD-9-CM		ICD-10-CM	
812.03	Fracture of greater tuberosity of humerus, closed	S42.251A	Displaced fracture of greater tuberosity of right humerus, initial encounter for closed fracture
		S42.252A	Displaced fracture of greater tuberosity of left humerus, initial encounter for closed fracture
		S42.253A	Displaced fracture of greater tuberosity of unspecified humerus, initial encounter for closed fracture
		S42.254A	Nondisplaced fracture of greater tuberosity of right humerus, initial encounter for closed fracture
		S42.255A	Nondisplaced fracture of greater tuberosity of left humerus, initial encounter for closed fracture
		S42.256A	Nondisplaced fracture of greater tuberosity of unspecified humerus, initial encounter for closed fracture

Note that in ICD-9-CM, if a fracture is specified as complicated by a malunion or nonunion, the fracture site is irrelevant as there are only two applicable codes: 733.81 Malunion of fracture, and 733.82 Nonunion of fracture. However, documentation of the site, laterality, and type of complication is imperative in ICD-10-CM, as the same traumatic fracture codes are used but with a seventh character identifying malunion or nonunion.

Additionally, to appropriately assign a seventh character for malunion or nonunion of an open fracture, a coder must be aware of the differences between the types of open fractures as described below:

- Type I: The wound is less than 1 cm in length and clean.
- Type II: The wound is greater than 1 cm in length, clean, and there is minimal to no soft tissue injury.
- Type III: The wound is greater than 1 cm in length, and there is significant soft tissue injury. Type III fractures can be further classified as:
    - IIIA: There is enough local soft tissue to cover the wound and bone without the need for skin grafting.
    - IIIB: The injury to the soft tissue is significant enough that skin grafting is necessary to cover the bone.
    - IIIC: The injury is associated with an arterial injury that requires repair.

The differences in coding for malunion and nonunion are captured in the following table. Please note that due to extensive mapping, the table is a sample of the ICD-10-CM codes that represent the various concepts.

Coding for Malunion and Nonunion of Traumatic Fractures

ICD-9-CM		ICD-10-CM	
733.81	Malunion of fracture	S42.021P	Displaced fracture of shaft of right clavicle, subsequent encounter with malunion
		S42.022P	Displaced fracture of shaft of left clavicle, subsequent encounter with malunion
		S42.023P	Displaced fracture of shaft of unspecified clavicle, subsequent encounter with malunion
		S42.024P	Nondisplaced fracture of shaft of right clavicle, subsequent encounter with malunion
		S42.025P	Nondisplaced fracture of shaft of left clavicle, subsequent encounter with malunion
		S42.026P	Nondisplaced fracture of shaft of unspecified clavicle, subsequent encounter with malunion
		S52.011P	*Torus fracture* of upper end of right ulna, subsequent encounter with malunion
		S52.024Q	Nondisplaced fracture of olecranon process without intraarticular extension of right ulna, subsequent encounter for open fracture type I or II with malunion
		S52.032P	Displaced fracture of olecranon process with intraarticular extension of left ulna, subsequent encounter for closed fracture with malunion
733.82	Nonunion of fracture	S32.82XK	Multiple fractures of pelvis without disruption of pelvic ring, subsequent encounter with nonunion
		S42.021K	Displaced fracture of shaft of right clavicle, subsequent encounter with nonunion
		S42.022K	Displaced fracture of shaft of left clavicle, subsequent encounter with nonunion
		S42.023K	Displaced fracture of shaft of unspecified clavicle, subsequent encounter with nonunion
		S42.024K	Nondisplaced fracture of shaft of right clavicle, subsequent encounter with nonunion
		S42.025K	Nondisplaced fracture of shaft of left clavicle, subsequent encounter with nonunion
		S42.026K	Nondisplaced fracture of shaft of unspecified clavicle, subsequent encounter with nonunion
		S52.011K	Torus fracture of upper end of right ulna, subsequent encounter with malunion
		S52.033M	Displaced fracture of olecranon process with intraarticular extension of unspecified ulna, subsequent encounter for open fracture type I or II with nonunion
		S52.044K	Nondisplaced fracture of coronoid process of right ulna, subsequent encounter for closed fracture with nonunion

> **DEFINITIONS**
>
> **torus fracture.** Buckling or bowing of the bone with little or no displacement at the end and no breakage, usually occurring in children due to softer bone tissue.

In addition to expanding the traumatic fracture categories to include malunion and nonunion, ICD-10-CM expands the same traumatic fracture codes to capture sequelae or the late effects of fractures. In ICD-9-CM, codes 905.0 through 905.5 report any abnormal condition arising as a reaction to a fracture. In ICD-10-CM, the same codes for the initial fracture are reported but with a seventh character of S as demonstrated in the following table. Please note that due to extensive mapping, the table is a sample of the ICD-10-CM codes that represent the various concepts.

Comprehensive Anatomy and Physiology for ICD-10-CM and ICD-10-PCS Coding

> **DEFINITIONS**
>
> **apophyseal fracture.** Avulsion fracture in which a bony prominence, such as a process or tuberosity, is removed from its bone.
>
> **comminuted fracture.** Any type of fracture in which the bone is splintered or crushed, resulting in multiple bone fragments.
>
> **greenstick fracture.** Incomplete fracture in which the bone is bent but fractured only on the outer arc of the bend.
>
> **Monteggia's fracture.** Break in the proximal half of the ulnar shaft accompanied by a dislocation of the radial head.
>
> **neoplastic.** Relating to any abnormal growth of new tissue, benign or malignant; in this case, usually a malignancy.
>
> **osteomyelitis.** Inflammation of bone that may remain localized or spread to the marrow, cortex, or periosteum, in response to an infecting organism.
>
> **Salter-Harris fracture.** Fractures through a growth plate.
>
> **spiral fracture.** Bone break in which the disruption of the bone is spiral to the shaft of the bone.

Coding Late Effects of Traumatic Fractures

ICD-9-CM		ICD-10-CM	
905.0	Late effect of fracture of skull and face bones	S02.0XXS	Fracture of vault of skull, sequela
		S02.110S	Type I occipital condyle fracture, sequela
		S02.111S	Type II occipital condyle fracture, sequela
		S02.112S	Type III occipital condyle fracture, sequela
		S02.2XXS	Fracture of nasal bones, sequela
		S02.3XXS	Fracture of orbital floor, sequela
905.1	Late effect of fracture of spine and trunk without mention of spinal cord lesion	S12.030S	Displaced posterior arch fracture of first cervical vertebra, sequela
		S12.031S	Nondisplaced posterior arch fracture of first cervical vertebra, sequela
		S12.040S	Displaced lateral mass fracture of first cervical vertebra, sequela
		S12.041S	Nondisplaced lateral mass fracture of first cervical vertebra, sequela
905.2	Late effect of fracture of upper extremities	S42.011S	Anterior displaced fracture of sternal end of right clavicle, sequela
		S42.015S	Posterior displaced fracture of sternal end of left clavicle, sequela
		S52.271S	*Monteggia's fracture* of right ulna, sequela
		S52.311S	*Greenstick fracture* of shaft of right radius, right arm, sequela
905.3	Late effect of fracture of neck of femur	S72.111S	Displaced fracture of greater trochanter of right femur, sequela
		S72.134S	Nondisplaced *apophyseal fracture* of right femur, sequela
905.4	Late effect of fracture of lower extremities	S72.341S	Displaced *spiral fracture* of shaft of right femur, sequela
		S72.354S	Nondisplaced *comminuted fracture* of shaft of right femur, sequela
		S79.011S	*Salter-Harris* Type I physeal fracture of upper end of right femur, sequela
		S82.035S	Nondisplaced transverse fracture of left patella, sequela

Just as with traumatic fractures, the coding of pathological fractures is also extremely different in ICD-10-CM. In ICD-9-CM, the only documentation needed to assign a code from subcategory 733.1 Pathological fracture, is the location of the fracture and confirmation that it is pathological in nature. However, in ICD-10-CM, much more information is needed.

The most obvious difference is the division of the pathological codes by the disease process responsible for the fracture. Because these types of fractures are caused by underlying disease processes, ICD-10-CM has split the code sets to reflect the most common causes of pathological fractures. There are categories for fractures due to **neoplastic** disease, age-related and other osteoporosis, and other specified diseases to capture the not-so-common contributing factors, such as **osteomyelitis**.

After identifying the disease process, the coder must also specify site and laterality, whether the encounter is initial or subsequent, and any healing issues.

Coding for Initial Visit for Pathological Fracture of Neck of Femur

ICD-9-CM		ICD-10-CM	
733.14	Pathologic fracture of neck of femur	M80.051A	Age related osteoporosis with current pathological fracture, right femur, initial encounter
		M80.052A	Age related osteoporosis with current pathological fracture, left femur, initial encounter
		M80.059A	Age related osteoporosis with current pathological fracture, unspecified femur, initial encounter
		M80.851A	Other osteoporosis with current pathological fracture, right femur, initial encounter
		M80.852A	Other osteoporosis with current pathological fracture, left femur, initial encounter
		M80.859A	Other osteoporosis with current pathological fracture, unspecified femur, initial encounter
		M84.451A	Pathological fracture, right femur, initial encounter
		M84.452A	Pathological fracture, left femur, initial encounter
		M84.459A	Pathological fracture, unspecified femur, initial encounter
		M84.551A	Pathologic fracture in neoplastic disease, right femur, initial encounter
		M84.552A	Pathologic fracture in neoplastic disease, left femur, initial encounter
		M84.553A	Pathologic fracture in neoplastic disease, unspecified femur, initial encounter
		M84.559A	Pathologic fracture in neoplastic disease, hip, unspecified, initial encounter
		M84.651A	Pathologic fracture in other disease, right femur, initial encounter
		M84.652A	Pathologic fracture in other disease, left femur, initial encounter
		M84.653A	Pathologic fracture in other disease, unspecified femur, initial encounter
		M84.659A	Pathologic fracture in other disease, hip, unspecified, initial encounter

Note that in ICD-9-CM, the verbiage "collapsed vertebra" is synonymous with a pathological fracture and, therefore, 733.13 is reported for this condition. ICD-10-CM, however, differentiates between a vertebral collapse and pathological fracture. There is an entire category for collapsed vertebrae that are not specified as being due to a pathological fracture.

> **DEFINITIONS**
>
> **acromioclavicular joint.** Joint between the acromion of the scapula and the clavicle.
>
> **dislocation.** Displacement of a bone from its normal position within an articulation.
>
> **subluxation.** Incomplete dislocation.

Coding for Collapsed Vertebra

ICD-9-CM		ICD-10-CM	
733.13	Pathological fracture of vertebrae	M48.50XA	Collapsed vertebra, not elsewhere classified, site unspecified, initial encounter
		M48.51XA	Collapsed vertebra, not elsewhere classified, occipito-atlanto-axial region, initial encounter
		M48.52XA	Collapsed vertebra, not elsewhere classified, cervical region, initial encounter
		M48.53XA	Collapsed vertebra, not elsewhere classified, cervicothoracic region, initial encounter
		M48.54XA	Collapsed vertebra, not elsewhere classified, thoracic region, initial encounter
		M48.55XA	Collapsed vertebra, not elsewhere classified, thoracolumbar region, initial encounter
		M48.56XA	Collapsed vertebra, not elsewhere classified, lumbar region, initial encounter
		M48.57XA	Collapsed vertebra, not elsewhere classified, lumbosacral region, initial encounter
		M48.58XA	Collapsed vertebra, not elsewhere classified, sacral and sacrococcygeal region, initial encounter

Another fairly common acute injury affecting the skeletal system is dislocation of a joint. ICD-9-CM coding for this condition is straightforward; the code system classifies *subluxation* and *dislocation* together, and the code is based on the articulation that has been disrupted and whether that disruption is open or closed. For most body sites in ICD-10-CM, code selection is also basic, being determined by site and laterality, but it is further divided by whether the injury is a subluxation or true dislocation. For certain sites of dislocation or subluxation, code selection is further divided by degree or direction of separation. There is no subdivision in ICD-10-CM for open and closed joint dislocation or subluxation. ICD-10-CM codes for dislocation and subluxation include an instructional note indicating a separate code is assigned for any associated open wound. Please note that due to extensive mapping, the table below is a sample of the ICD-10-CM codes that represent the various concepts discussed.

Coding for Dislocation and Subluxation

ICD-9-CM		ICD-10-CM	
831.04	Closed dislocation of the *acromioclavicular (joint)*	S43.101A	Unspecified dislocation of right acromioclavicular joint, initial encounter
		S43.102A	Unspecified dislocation of left acromioclavicular joint, initial encounter
		S43.109A	Unspecified dislocation of unspecified acromioclavicular joint, initial encounter
		S43.111A	Subluxation of right acromioclavicular joint, initial encounter
		S43.121A	Dislocation of right acromioclavicular joint, 100%-200% displacement, initial encounter
		S43.131A	Dislocation of right acromioclavicular joint, greater than 200% displacement, initial encounter
		S43.141A	Inferior dislocation of right acromioclavicular joint, initial encounter
		S43.151A	Posterior dislocation of right acromioclavicular joint, initial encounter

ICD-9-CM		ICD-10-CM	
839.61	Closed dislocation of sternum (*sternoclavicular joint*)	S43.201A	Unspecified subluxation of right sternoclavicular joint, initial encounter
		S43.202A	Unspecified subluxation of left sternoclavicular joint, initial encounter
		S43.203A	Unspecified subluxation of unspecified sternoclavicular joint, initial encounter
		S43.204A	Unspecified dislocation of right sternoclavicular joint, initial encounter
		S43.205A	Unspecified dislocation of left sternoclavicular joint, initial encounter
		S43.206A	Unspecified dislocation of unspecified sternoclavicular joint, initial encounter
		S43.211A	Anterior subluxation of right sternoclavicular joint, initial encounter
		S43.221A	Posterior subluxation of right sternoclavicular joint, initial encounter

> **DEFINITIONS**
>
> **sternoclavicular joint.** Joint between the sternum and the clavicle.

Another common affliction impacting certain joints of the skeletal system is a torn meniscus. This is most commonly seen in the knee joint where two C shaped, cartilage-based cushions are found. They are sandwiched between the lateral and medial condyles of each femur where they articulate with the condyles of the tibia; one on the inside of the knee (the medial meniscus) and one on the outside (lateral meniscus). There are two usual causes of a meniscus tear: trauma and degeneration. A traumatic tear is usually acute and repairable; a tear caused by degeneration is usually chronic or old and irreparable. Only a physician can determine the acuity of the injury. ICD-10-CM guidelines help coders distinguish between acute versus old or chronic musculoskeletal conditions by stating that recurrent conditions or conditions that are the result of a healed injury are considered old.

Coding old, chronic, or recurrent meniscus tears is relatively the same in both classification systems, with the exception that ICD-10-CM differentiates laterality of the injury. On the other hand, acute meniscus tears are different. In ICD-9-CM, the site of the tear, lateral or medial meniscus, is the only consideration. The newer classification, however, expands that information to also include the laterality and type of tear. The different types of meniscus tears included in ICD-10-CM code selection are:

- **Bucket handle:** Tear in which the inner portion of the meniscus displaces into the joint causing the meniscus to resemble a bucket and its handle. These are always traumatic injuries.
- **Complex:** Describes more than one type of tear or a tear that goes in more than one direction.
- **Peripheral:** Indicates tears located in the peripheral or outer third of the meniscus. This area is susceptible to healing as it has access to a rich blood supply.

Figure 3.12: Tears of Meniscus

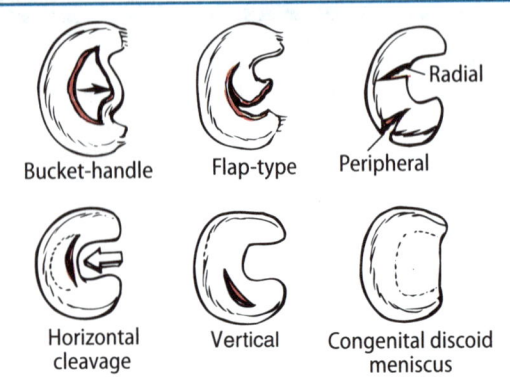

- Bucket-handle
- Flap-type
- Peripheral (Radial)
- Horizontal cleavage
- Vertical
- Congenital discoid meniscus

It is important to note, that like fractures and dislocations, acute meniscus tears also require a seventh character distinguishing the encounter as initial (A), subsequent (D), or a sequela of the injury (S). For discussion purposes, only the initial encounter is highlighted below.

Coding for Meniscus Tears

ICD-9-CM		ICD-10-CM	
836.0	Tear medial cartilage or meniscus of knee, current	S83.211A	Bucket handle tear of medial meniscus, current injury, right knee, initial encounter
		S83.212A	Bucket handle tear of medial meniscus, current injury, left knee, initial encounter
		S83.219A	Bucket handle tear of medial meniscus, current injury, unspecified knee, initial encounter
		S83.221A	Peripheral tear of medial meniscus, current injury, right knee, initial encounter
		S83.222A	Peripheral tear of medial meniscus, current injury, left knee, initial encounter
		S83.229A	Peripheral tear of medial meniscus, current injury, unspecified knee, initial encounter
		S83.231A	Complex tear of medial meniscus, current injury, right knee, initial encounter
		S83.232A	Complex tear of medial meniscus, current injury, left knee, initial encounter
		S83.239A	Complex tear of medial meniscus, current injury, unspecified knee, initial encounter
		S83.241A	Other tear of medial meniscus, current injury, right knee, initial encounter
		S83.242A	Other tear of medial meniscus, current injury, left knee, initial encounter
		S83.249A	Other tear of medial meniscus, current injury, unspecified knee, initial encounter

ICD-9-CM		ICD-10-CM	
836.1	Tear lateral cartilage or meniscus of knee, current	S83.251A	Bucket handle tear of lateral meniscus, current injury, right knee, initial encounter
		S83.252A	Bucket handle tear of lateral meniscus, current injury, left knee, initial encounter
		S83.259A	Bucket handle tear of lateral meniscus, current injury, unspecified knee, initial encounter
		S83.261A	Peripheral tear of lateral meniscus, current injury, right knee, initial encounter
		S83.262A	Peripheral tear of lateral meniscus, current injury, left knee, initial encounter
		S83.269A	Peripheral tear of lateral meniscus, current injury, unspecified knee, initial encounter
		S83.271A	Complex tear of lateral meniscus, current injury, right knee, initial encounter
		S83.272A	Complex tear of lateral meniscus, current injury, left knee, initial encounter
		S83.279A	Complex tear of lateral meniscus, current injury, unspecified knee, initial encounter
		S83.281A	Other tear of lateral meniscus, current injury, right knee, initial encounter
		S83.282A	Other tear of lateral meniscus, current injury, left knee, initial encounter
		S83.289A	Other tear of lateral meniscus, current injury, unspecified knee, initial encounter

Infections

Like any other system in the body, the skeletal system and its joints are susceptible to infection. An infection of the bone is known as osteomyelitis. Bacteria, most commonly *Staphylococcal aureus,* are usually the infecting agent, but occasionally fungi are responsible. Infection can be caused by direct exposure to the organism via open fracture or bone surgery and can occur at the site of internal orthopedic devices or adjacent soft tissue infections. Osteomyelitis can be acute or chronic in nature. Chronic osteomyelitis persists over time and can cause many complications, such as bone deformity and pathological fractures. ICD-9-CM categorizes osteomyelitis by acuity and site, as does ICD-10-CM. However, that is just the beginning of code selection for ICD-10-CM. In addition to distinguishing laterality, the coder must also determine whether the osteomyelitis is:

- Acute:
    - Is the infection **hematogenous**?
    - Is the infection actually acute or is it **subacute**?
- Chronic
    - Is there a draining **sinus**?
    - Is the infection hematogenous?
    - Is the infection **multifocal**?

Coding for Osteomyelitis of the Sternum

ICD-9-CM		ICD-10-CM	
730.08	Acute osteomyelitis, other specified site	M86.08	Acute hematogenous osteomyelitis, other sites
		M86.18	Other acute osteomyelitis, other site
		M86.28	Subacute osteomyelitis, other site

> **CLINICAL NOTE**
>
> Chronic osteomyelitis occurs in 5 to 25 percent of patients that have had acute osteomyelitis.

> **DEFINITIONS**
>
> **hematogenous.** Originating or transported in blood.
>
> **multifocal.** Having many points of origin.
>
> **sinus.** Cavity or channel leading to a pocket of purulent material.
>
> **subacute.** Being present as a disease or other abnormal condition in a person who appears to be clinically well.

ICD-9-CM		ICD-10-CM	
730.18	Chronic osteomyelitis, other specified site	M86.38	Chronic multifocal osteomyelitis, other site
		M86.48	Chronic osteomyelitis with draining sinus, other site
		M86.58	Other chronic hematogenous osteomyelitis, other site
		M86.68	Other chronic osteomyelitis, other site
		M86.8x8	Other osteomyelitis, other site

An infection of the fluid and tissues of a joint is referred to as septic or pyogenic arthritis. These infections are caused mainly by bacteria but can also be caused by fungi. ICD-10-CM has divided the classification for septic arthritis by bacterial organism in addition to the site and side affected.

Coding for Septic Arthritis of the Hip

ICD-9-CM		ICD-10-CM	
711.05	Pyogenic arthritis pelvic region and thigh	M00.051	Staphylococcal arthritis, right hip
		M00.052	Staphylococcal arthritis, left hip
		M00.059	Staphylococcal arthritis, unspecified hip
		M00.151	Pneumococcal arthritis, right hip
		M00.152	Pneumococcal arthritis, left hip
		M00.159	Pneumococcal arthritis, unspecified hip
		M00.251	Other streptococcal arthritis, right hip
		M00.252	Other streptococcal arthritis, left hip
		M00.259	Other streptococcal arthritis, unspecified hip
		M00.851	Arthritis due to other bacteria, right hip
		M00.852	Arthritis due to other bacteria, left hip
		M00.859	Arthritis due to other bacteria, unspecified hip

Occasionally, a joint is affected by an infection elsewhere. Inflammation of a joint as a reaction to another disease is referred to as reactive arthropathy. A secondary infection can also arise within a joint, referred to as direct infection. Although the two conditions are very different, ICD-9-CM classifies both under the same categories, 711.4 to 711.6, distinguished by site of the affliction and type of organism: bacterial, viral, or fungal (mycosis). On the other hand, ICD-10-CM has distinguished between reactive arthropathy and a direct infection, giving each its own category, but it has lost some of the detail of ICD-9-CM by not distinguishing the type of organism afflicting the joint. Both code sets require a code be assigned first for the underlying disease, such as leprosy, mycoses, or paratyphoid fever.

Coding for Arthropathy of the Right Shoulder Associated with Other Infectious Diseases

ICD-9-CM		ICD-10-CM	
711.41	Arthropathy associated with other bacterial disease, shoulder region	M01.X11	Direct infection of right shoulder in infectious and parasitic diseases classified elsewhere
		M02.811	Other reactive arthropathies, right shoulder
711.51	Arthropathy associated with other viral diseases, shoulder region	M01.X11	Direct infection of right shoulder in infectious and parasitic diseases classified elsewhere
		M02.811	Other reactive arthropathies, right shoulder

ICD-9-CM	ICD-10-CM	
711.61 Arthropathy associated with mycoses, shoulder region	M01.X11	Direct infection of right shoulder in infectious and parasitic diseases classified elsewhere
	M01.X12	Direct infection of left shoulder in infectious and parasitic diseases classified elsewhere
	M01.X19	Direct infection of unspecified shoulder in infectious and parasitic diseases classified elsewhere

Inflammatory and Degenerative Conditions

As the human body ages, the cartilage of the joints begins to degenerate and lose its elasticity from wear and tear and the natural aging process. This degeneration is referred to as primary osteoarthritis. The same type of disorder can also be caused by other disease processes, such as trauma, obesity, and some metabolic disorders. Osteoarthritis caused by something other than aging is called secondary osteoarthritis.

ICD-9-CM and ICD-10-CM osteoarthritis codes are similar in that there are categories for generalized, primary, secondary, localized, and unspecified osteoarthritis, further divided by site. In fact, localized and unspecified osteoarthritis codes are direct, one-to-one matches between the two classification systems. However, in many instances ICD-10-CM requires more detail, including laterality and cause in the case of secondary osteoarthritis. When the osteoarthritis site is the hand, ICD-10-CM also distinguishes between the first carpometacarpal joint and all other joints. The following table is not a complete mapping of all of the types of osteoarthritis that may occur, but gives the coder an idea of what may be seen in ICD-10-CM. For detailed information on ICD-9-CM to ICD-10-CM mapping, see Optum360's *ICD-10-CM Mappings*.

Coding for Secondary Osteoarthritis

ICD-9-CM	ICD-10-CM	
715.21 Secondary localized osteoarthrosis, shoulder region	M19.111	Post-traumatic osteoarthritis, right shoulder
	M19.112	Post-traumatic osteoarthritis, left shoulder
	M19.119	Post-traumatic osteoarthritis, unspecified shoulder
	M19.211	Secondary osteoarthritis, right shoulder
	M19.212	Secondary osteoarthritis, left shoulder
	M19.219	Secondary osteoarthritis, unspecified shoulder
715.22 Secondary localized osteoarthrosis, upper arm	M19.121	Post-traumatic osteoarthritis, right elbow
	M19.122	Post-traumatic osteoarthritis, left elbow
	M19.129	Post-traumatic osteoarthritis, unspecified elbow
	M19.221	Secondary osteoarthritis, right elbow
	M19.222	Secondary osteoarthritis, left elbow
	M19.229	Secondary osteoarthritis, unspecified elbow
715.23 Secondary localized osteoarthrosis, forearm	M19.131	Post-traumatic osteoarthritis, right wrist
	M19.132	Post-traumatic osteoarthritis, left wrist
	M19.139	Post-traumatic osteoarthritis, unspecified wrist
	M19.231	Secondary osteoarthritis, right wrist
	M19.232	Secondary osteoarthritis, left wrist
	M19.239	Secondary osteoarthritis, unspecified wrist

ICD-9-CM		ICD-10-CM	
715.25	Secondary localized osteoarthritis, pelvic region and thigh	M16.2	Bilateral osteoarthritis resulting from hip dysplasia
		M16.30	Unilateral osteoarthritis resulting from hip dysplasia, unspecified hip
		M16.31	Unilateral osteoarthritis resulting from hip dysplasia, right hip
		M16.32	Unilateral osteoarthritis resulting from hip dysplasia, left hip
		M16.4	Bilateral post-traumatic osteoarthritis of hip
		M16.50	Unilateral post-traumatic osteoarthritis, unspecified hip
		M16.51	Unilateral post-traumatic osteoarthritis, right hip
		M16.52	Unilateral post-traumatic osteoarthritis, left hip
		M16.6	Other bilateral secondary osteoarthritis of hip
		M16.7	Other unilateral secondary osteoarthritis of hip
715.26	Secondary localized osteoarthritis, lower leg	M17.2	Bilateral post-traumatic osteoarthritis of knee
		M17.30	Unilateral post-traumatic osteoarthritis, unspecified knee
		M17.31	Unilateral post-traumatic osteoarthritis, right knee
		M17.32	Unilateral post-traumatic osteoarthritis, left knee
		M17.4	Other bilateral secondary osteoarthritis of knee
		M17.5	Other unilateral secondary osteoarthritis of knee

Definitions

paresthesia. Sensation of tingling, pricking, or numbness of skin.

spastic paresis. Condition in which the muscles are affected by persistent spasms and exaggerated tendon reflexes.

Degenerative osteoarthritis occurring in the spine is called spondylosis. Spondylosis can cause compression on nerves and blood vessels that are affiliated with or near the spine. Compression that disturbs spinal cord function is referred to as myelopathy. Myelopathy manifests itself in various ways, including **paresthesia** and **spastic paresis**. Another manifestation, radiculopathy, also known as a pinched nerve, can occur, causing pain, weakness, and numbness. In severe cases of spondylosis, the anterior spinal artery and/or the vertebral artery may be compressed, called compression syndrome.

ICD-9-CM divides the spondylosis codes by spinal region and whether myelopathy was present. ICD-10-CM also uses these distinct identifiers to assign codes but increases detail by further specifying the spinal region and differentiating between myelopathy and radiculopathy. New codes identify when the spondylosis has progressed to include blood vessel compression.

Coding for Spondylosis

ICD-9-CM		ICD-10-CM	
721.0	Cervical spondylosis without myelopathy	M47.21	Other spondylosis with radiculopathy, occipito-atlanto-axial region
		M47.22	Other spondylosis with radiculopathy, cervical region
		M47.23	Other spondylosis with radiculopathy, cervicothoracic region
		M47.811	Spondylosis without myelopathy or radiculopathy, occipito-atlanto-axial region
		M47.812	Spondylosis without myelopathy or radiculopathy, cervical region
		M47.813	Spondylosis without myelopathy or radiculopathy, cervicothoracic region
		M47.891	Other spondylosis, occipito-atlanto-axial region
		M47.892	Other spondylosis, cervical region
		M47.893	Other spondylosis, cervicothoracic region
721.1	Cervical spondylosis with myelopathy	M47.011	Anterior spinal artery compression syndromes, occipito-atlanto-axial region
		M47.012	Anterior spinal artery compression syndromes, cervical region
		M47.013	Anterior spinal artery compression syndromes, cervicothoracic region
		M47.021	Vertebral artery compression syndromes, occipito-atlanto-axial region
		M47.022	Vertebral artery compression syndromes, cervical region
		M47.029	Vertebral artery compression syndromes, site unspecified
		M47.11	Other spondylosis with myelopathy, occipito-atlanto-axial region
		M47.12	Other spondylosis with myelopathy, cervical region
		M47.13	Other spondylosis with myelopathy, cervicothoracic region
721.2	Thoracic spondylosis without myelopathy	M47.24	Other spondylosis with radiculopathy, thoracic region
		M47.25	Other spondylosis with radiculopathy, thoracolumbar region
		M47.814	Spondylosis without myelopathy or radiculopathy, thoracic region
		M47.815	Spondylosis without myelopathy or radiculopathy, thoracolumbar region
		M47.894	Other spondylosis, thoracic region
		M47.895	Other spondylosis, thoracolumbar region

ICD-9-CM		ICD-10-CM	
721.3	Lumbosacral spondylosis without myelopathy	M47.26	Other spondylosis with radiculopathy, lumbar region
		M47.27	Other spondylosis with radiculopathy, lumbosacral region
		M47.28	Other spondylosis with radiculopathy, sacral and sacrococcygeal region
		M47.816	Spondylosis without myelopathy or radiculopathy, lumbar region
		M47.817	Spondylosis without myelopathy or radiculopathy, lumbosacral region
		M47.818	Spondylosis without myelopathy or radiculopathy, sacral and sacrococcygeal region
		M47.896	Other spondylosis, lumbar region
		M47.897	Other spondylosis, lumbosacral region
		M47.898	Other spondylosis, sacral and sacrococcygeal region
721.41	Spondylosis with myelopathy, thoracic region	M47.14	Other spondylosis with myelopathy, thoracic region
		M47.15	Other spondylosis with myelopathy, thoracolumbar region
721.42	Spondylosis with myelopathy, lumbar region	M47.16	Other spondylosis with myelopathy, lumbar region

Definitions

gout. Metabolic condition causing painful and inflamed joints.

idiopathic. Having no known cause.

As mentioned earlier, secondary arthritis can also be caused by certain disorders, such as *gout*. In gout, uric acid crystals can collect around the joint structures, causing inflammation. ICD-9-CM and ICD-10-CM give gouty arthropathy its own categories arranged first by acute versus chronic diagnosis. ICD-10-CM further clarifies acute gouty arthropathy by anatomical site and laterality (where applicable), as well as whether the gout is *idiopathic* or drug-induced.

Coding for Acute and Unspecified Gouty Arthropathy

ICD-9-CM		ICD-10-CM	
274.00	Gouty arthropathy, unspecified	M10.00	Idiopathic gout, unspecified site
		M10.01[1,2,9]	Idiopathic gout, shoulder
		M10.02[1,2,9]	Idiopathic gout, elbow
		M10.03[1,2,9]	Idiopathic gout, wrist
		M10.04[1,2,9]	Idiopathic gout, hand
		M10.05[1,2,9]	Idiopathic gout, hip
		M10.06[1,2,9]	Idiopathic gout, knee
		M10.07[1,2,9]	Idiopathic gout, ankle and foot
		M10.08	Idiopathic gout, vertebrae
		M10.09	Idiopathic gout, multiple sites
		M10.20	Drug-induced gout, unspecified site
		M10.21[1,2,9]	Drug-induced gout, shoulder
		M10.22[1,2,9]	Drug-induced gout, elbow
		M10.23[1,2,9]	Drug-induced gout, wrist
		M10.24[1,2,9]	Drug-induced gout, hand
		M10.25[1,2,9]	Drug-induced gout, hip
		M10.26[1,2,9]	Drug-induced gout, knee
		M10.27[1,2,9]	Drug-induced gout, ankle and foot
		M10.28	Drug-induced gout, vertebrae
		M10.29	Drug-induced gout, multiple sites

6th Character meanings for codes as indicated
1 right   2 left   9 unspecified

Chapter 3. ICD-10-CM: Skeletal System and Articulations

ICD-9-CM	ICD-10-CM	
274.01 Acute gouty arthropathy	M10.00	Idiopathic gout, unspecified site
	M10.01[1,2,9]	Idiopathic gout, shoulder
	M10.02[1,2,9]	Idiopathic gout, elbow
	M10.03[1,2,9]	Idiopathic gout, wrist
	M10.04[1,2,9]	Idiopathic gout, hand
	M10.05[1,2,9]	Idiopathic gout, hip
	M10.06[1,2,9]	Idiopathic gout, knee
	M10.07[1,2,9]	Idiopathic gout, ankle and foot
	M10.08	Idiopathic gout, vertebrae
	M10.09	Idiopathic gout, multiple sites
	M10.20	Drug-induced gout, unspecified site
	M10.21[1,2,9]	Drug-induced gout, shoulder
	M10.22[1,2,9]	Drug-induced gout, elbow
	M10.23[1,2,9]	Drug-induced gout, wrist
	M10.24[1,2,9]	Drug-induced gout, hand
	M10.25[1,2,9]	Drug-induced gout, hip
	M10.26[1,2,9]	Drug-induced gout, knee
	M10.27[1,2,9]	Drug-induced gout, ankle and foot
	M10.28	Drug-induced gout, vertebrae
	M10.29	Drug-induced gout, multiple sites

6th Character meanings for codes as indicated
1 right   2 left   9 unspecified

Just as in ICD-9-CM, ICD-10-CM classifies chronic gouty arthropathy by whether a **tophus** is present and further divides the classifications by anatomical site, laterality (where applicable), and cause. The following table is not a complete mapping of all of the types of chronic gouty arthropathy that may occur, but gives the coder an idea of what may be seen in ICD-10-CM. For detailed information on ICD-9-CM to ICD-10-CM mapping, see Optum360's *ICD-10-CM Mappings*.

DEFINITIONS

tophus. Calculus that forms in fibrous tissue.

Coding for Chronic Gouty Arthropathy

ICD-9-CM	ICD-10-CM	
274.02 Chronic gouty arthropathy without mention of tophus	M1A.00X0	Idiopathic chronic gout, unspecified site without tophus (tophi)
	M1A.01[1,2,9]0	Idiopathic chronic gout, shoulder without tophus (tophi)
	M1A.02[1,2,9]0	Idiopathic chronic gout, elbow without tophus (tophi)
	M1A.03[1,2,9]0	Idiopathic chronic gout, wrist without tophus (tophi)
	M1A.04[1,2,9]0	Idiopathic chronic gout, hand without tophus (tophi)
	M1A.05[1,2,9]0	Idiopathic chronic gout, hip without tophus (tophi)
	M1A.20X0	Drug-induced chronic gout, unspecified site without tophus (tophi)
	M1A.21[1,2,9]0	Drug-induced chronic gout, shoulder without tophus (tophi)
	M1A.22[1,2,9]0	Drug-induced chronic gout, elbow without tophus (tophi)

6th Character meanings for codes as indicated
1 right   2 left   9 unspecified

© 2015 Optum360, LLC

ICD-9-CM		ICD-10-CM	
274.03	Chronic gouty arthropathy with tophus	M1A.09X1	Idiopathic chronic gout, multiple sites with tophus (tophi)
		M1A.20X1	Drug-induced chronic gout, unspecified site with tophus (tophi)
		M1A.21[1,2,9]1	Drug-induced chronic gout, shoulder with tophus (tophi)
		M1A.22[1,2,9]1	Drug-induced chronic gout, elbow with tophus (tophi)
		M1A.30X1	Chronic gout due to renal impairment, unspecified site with tophus (tophi)
		M1A.31[1,2,9]1	Chronic gout due to renal impairment, shoulder with tophus (tophi)
		M1A.32[1,2,9]1	Chronic gout due to renal impairment, elbow with tophus (tophi))

6th Character meanings for codes as indicated
1 right   2 left   9 unspecified

Another common type of arthritis is rheumatoid arthritis (RA). RA is inflammation and destruction of the joint tissues due to an autoimmune disorder. RA can also affect other body systems and organs and is, therefore, sometimes considered a systemic disease.

In ICD-10-CM, it is important to understand the different musculoskeletal manifestations of RA. In ICD-9-CM, a code for RA (714.0) is reported first, followed by a code for any manifestations. The newer classification system expands the categories for RA by anatomical site and common manifestation. Complications identified in ICD-10-CM are myopathy, neuropathy, bursitis, and nodules. Myopathy is any abnormal condition affecting the muscles due to RA; this could be in the form of atrophy, weakness, myalgia, or similar symptoms. Neuropathy can be caused by inflammation and disfigurement of the joints, causing compression and entrapment of nerves. Bursitis, an inflammation of the connective tissue surrounding a joint, in RA is a result of the increased pressure put on joints. And lastly, rheumatoid nodules are firm, rounded masses occurring subcutaneously at areas of pressure, such as the elbows. These occur in approximately 25 percent of patients and are usually associated with more complicated extensions of the disease process.

If there is no manifestation mentioned, documentation specifying whether the patient has an abnormal antibody, called the rheumatoid factor, present in the blood can help in assigning a more detailed code. Rheumatoid factor is present in 80 percent of patients diagnosed with RA. The following table is not a complete mapping of all of the types of rheumatoid arthritis that may occur, but gives the coder an idea of what may be seen in ICD-10-CM. For detailed information on ICD-9-CM to ICD-10-CM mapping, see Optum360's *ICD-10-CM Mappings*.

Chapter 3. ICD-10-CM: Skeletal System and Articulations

Coding for Rheumatoid Arthritis

ICD-9-CM	ICD-10-CM	
714.0 Rheumatoid Arthritis	M05.41[1,2,9]	Rheumatoid myopathy with rheumatoid arthritis of shoulder
	M05.42[1,2,9]	Rheumatoid myopathy with rheumatoid arthritis of elbow
	M05.53[1,2,9]	Rheumatoid polyneuropathy with rheumatoid arthritis of wrist
	M05.54[1,2,9]	Rheumatoid polyneuropathy with rheumatoid arthritis of hand
	M05.75[1,2,9]	Rheumatoid arthritis with rheumatoid factor of hip without organ or systems involvement
	M05.76[1,2,9]	Rheumatoid arthritis with rheumatoid factor of knee without organ or systems involvement
	M05.77[1,2,9]	Rheumatoid arthritis with rheumatoid factor of ankle and foot without organ or systems involvement
	M06.07[1,2,9]	Rheumatoid arthritis without rheumatoid factor, ankle and foot
	M06.08	Rheumatoid arthritis without rheumatoid factor, vertebrae
	M06.26[1,2,9]	Rheumatoid bursitis, knee
	M06.27[1,2,9]	Rheumatoid bursitis, ankle and foot
	M06.28	Rheumatoid bursitis, vertebrae
	M06.38	Rheumatoid nodule, vertebrae
	M06.39	Rheumatoid nodule, multiple sites

6th Character meanings for codes as indicated
1 right   2 left   9 unspecified

Additional problems can arise when any type of arthritis affects the spine. One of the most common conditions is spinal stenosis, narrowing of a foramen of the spine that puts pressure on the nerves and causes pain, numbness, and weakness of limbs. Stenosis can also be a part of the normal aging process, as the cartilage loses its elasticity and the bones can form spurs, also decreasing the space for the nerves. There are multiple causes of spinal stenosis and ICD-10-CM puts this into perspective by providing categories for narrowing caused by subluxation, bony deformity, connective tissue disorders, intervertebral disc disorders, or any combination of these conditions. It also specifies whether the narrowing is of the vertebral foramen ("neural canal") or the ***intervertebral foramen***.

> **DEFINITIONS**
>
> **intervertebral foramen.** Opening between vertebrae where the nerves of the spinal cord extend to sites outside of the spine, such as the extremities.

Coding for Spinal Stenosis

ICD-9-CM		ICD-10-CM	
723.0	Spinal stenosis in cervical region	M48.01	Spinal stenosis, occipito-atlanto-axial region
		M48.02	Spinal stenosis, cervical region
		M48.03	Spinal stenosis, cervicothoracic region
		M99.20	Subluxation stenosis of neural canal of head region
		M99.21	Subluxation stenosis of neural canal of cervical region
		M99.30	Osseous stenosis of neural canal of head region
		M99.31	Osseous stenosis of neural canal of cervical region
		M99.40	Connective tissue stenosis of neural canal of head region
		M99.41	Connective tissue stenosis of neural canal of cervical region
		M99.50	Intervertebral disc stenosis of neural canal of head region
		M99.51	Intervertebral disc stenosis of neural canal of cervical region
		M99.60	Osseous and subluxation stenosis of intervertebral foramina of head region
		M99.61	Osseous and subluxation stenosis of intervertebral foramina of cervical region
		M99.70	Connective tissue and disc stenosis of intervertebral foramina of head region
		M99.71	Connective tissue and disc stenosis of intervertebral foramina of cervical region
724.01	Spinal stenosis of thoracic region	M48.04	Spinal stenosis, thoracic region
		M48.05	Spinal stenosis, thoracolumbar region
		M99.22	Subluxation stenosis of neural canal of thoracic region
		M99.32	Osseous stenosis of neural canal of thoracic region
		M99.42	Connective tissue stenosis of neural canal of thoracic region
		M99.52	Intervertebral disc stenosis of neural canal of thoracic region
		M99.62	Osseous and subluxation stenosis of intervertebral foramina of thoracic region
		M99.72	Connective tissue and disc stenosis of intervertebral foramina of thoracic region
724.02	Spinal stenosis of lumbar region without neurogenic claudication	M48.06	Spinal stenosis, lumbar region
		M48.07	Spinal stenosis, lumbosacral region
		M99.23	Subluxation stenosis of neural canal of lumbar region
		M99.33	Osseous stenosis of neural canal of lumbar region
		M99.43	Connective tissue stenosis of neural canal of lumbar region
		M99.53	Intervertebral disc stenosis of neural canal of lumbar region
		M99.63	Osseous and subluxation stenosis of intervertebral foramina of lumbar region
		M99.73	Connective tissue and disc stenosis of intervertebral foramina of lumbar region

Deficiencies and Anomalies

Occasionally, bones become soft due to a phosphate or calcium deficiency, known as osteomalacia in adults and rickets in children. Multiple factors can contribute to the insufficient minerals required for normal bone strength, including:

- Vitamin D deficiency due to nutritional deficits or malfunctioning metabolization—vitamin D is imperative to calcium absorption
- Malabsorption possibly due to digestive surgery or disease
- Malnutrition
- Pregnancy
- Pharmaceuticals, such as certain long-term anticonvulsants
- Kidney or liver disorders, which may impact the body's ability to process vitamins and minerals
- Aluminum bone disease—aluminum in high quantities prevents phosphate absorption

There are a couple of differences between ICD-9-CM and ICD-10-CM coding for this condition, most notably the reclassification of osteomalacia from the endocrine, nutritional, and metabolic immunity chapter to the musculoskeletal chapter. ICD-10-CM also differentiates code assignment by the documented cause of the bone softening.

Coding for Osteomalacia

ICD-9-CM		ICD-10-CM	
268.2	Osteomalacia, unspecified	M83.0	**Puerperal** osteomalacia
		M83.1	Senile osteomalacia
		M83.2	Adult osteomalacia due to malabsorption
		M83.3	Adult osteomalacia due to malnutrition
		M83.4	Aluminum bone disease
		M83.5	Other drug-induced osteomalacia in adults
		M83.8	Other adult osteomalacia
		M83.9	Adult osteomalacia, unspecified

Another disease that can impact the integrity of the skeletal structure is aseptic necrosis, also known as osteonecrosis and avascular necrosis (AVN). In this condition, the bone lacks a blood supply and the tissue then dies, leaving weakened bones that have the potential to fracture or collapse. There are multiple etiologies for aseptic necrosis, including trauma to blood vessels supplying the area, disease such as sickle cell or lupus, pharmaceuticals, and poor circulation. ICD-10-CM takes into consideration the documented etiology of the aseptic necrosis, as well as anatomical site and laterality. Please note that due to extensive mapping, the table is a sample of the ICD-10-CM codes that represent the various concepts.

> **DEFINITIONS**
>
> **puerperal.** Pertaining to the time from the end of the third stage of labor until the uterus and other reproductive organs return to their normal state, which is approximately three to six weeks following childbirth.

Coding for Aseptic Necrosis

ICD-9-CM		ICD-10-CM	
733.41	Aseptic necrosis of head of humerus	M87.011	Idiopathic aseptic necrosis of right shoulder
		M87.012	Idiopathic aseptic necrosis of left shoulder
		M87.019	Idiopathic aseptic necrosis of unspecified shoulder
		M87.021	Idiopathic aseptic necrosis of right humerus
		M87.022	Idiopathic aseptic necrosis of left humerus
		M87.029	Idiopathic aseptic necrosis of unspecified humerus
		M87.121	Osteonecrosis due to drugs, right humerus
		M87.122	Osteonecrosis due to drugs, left humerus
		M87.129	Osteonecrosis due to drugs, unspecified humerus
		M87.221	Osteonecrosis due to previous trauma, right humerus
		M87.222	Osteonecrosis due to previous trauma, left humerus
		M87.229	Osteonecrosis due to previous trauma, unspecified humerus
		M87.321	Other secondary osteonecrosis, right humerus
		M87.322	Other secondary osteonecrosis, left humerus
		M87.329	Other secondary osteonecrosis, unspecified humerus
		M87.821	Other osteonecrosis, right humerus
		M87.822	Other osteonecrosis, left humerus
		M87.829	Other osteonecrosis, unspecified humerus
733.44	Aseptic necrosis of talus	M87.074	Idiopathic aseptic necrosis of right foot
		M87.075	Idiopathic aseptic necrosis of left foot
		M87.076	Idiopathic aseptic necrosis of unspecified foot
		M87.174	Osteonecrosis due to drugs, right foot
		M87.175	Osteonecrosis due to drugs, left foot
		M87.176	Osteonecrosis due to drugs, unspecified foot
		M87.274	Osteonecrosis due to previous trauma, right foot
		M87.275	Osteonecrosis due to previous trauma, left foot
		M87.276	Osteonecrosis due to previous trauma, unspecified foot
		M87.374	Other secondary osteonecrosis, right foot
		M87.375	Other secondary osteonecrosis, left foot
		M87.376	Other secondary osteonecrosis, unspecified foot
		M87.874	Other osteonecrosis, right foot
		M87.875	Other osteonecrosis, left foot
		M87.876	Other osteonecrosis, unspecified foot

Sometimes the normal curvatures in the spine become deformed. There are three types of these deformities:

- **Scoliosis**, a lateral curvature of the spine
- **Kyphosis**, an abnormal posterior convex curvature of the spine
- **Lordosis**, an exaggerated inward curvature of the lower back

Figure 3.13: Kyphosis and Lordosis

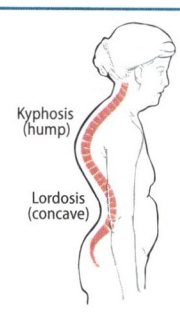

Figure 3.14: Scoliosis and Kyphoscoliosis

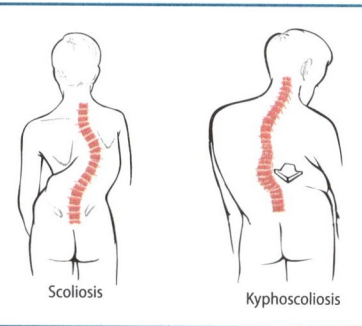

For the most part, ICD-10-CM mimics ICD-9-CM when it comes to coding kyphosis and lordosis, having equivalent one-to-one mapping or, if there is a one-to-many match, the classification is simply divided by spinal region (i.e., cervical, thoracic, or lumbar). However, there are a few distinct differences surrounding the crosswalk for scoliosis and kyphoscoliosis, subcategory 737.3 in ICD-9-CM. In order to appropriately assign a code for (kypho-) scoliosis in ICD-10-CM, the coder must understand the different physiologies of the disease.

There are four major types of scoliosis:

- Congenital
- Neuromuscular, which is due to spinal muscle weakness or nerve damage
- Degenerative
- Idiopathic, which has an unknown cause and is the most common form of the disease. It can be divided by the age of the patient:
    - infantile: birth to 3 months
    - juvenile: 3 months to 9 years
    - adolescent: 10 to 18 years

ICD-9-CM does distinguish between infantile and other types of idiopathic scoliosis, as well as whether the infantile disease is progressive or resolving. In ICD-10-CM, however, the distinction between the age classifications is further specified, and juvenile and adolescent idiopathic scoliosis are also given their own categories, but the detail of whether the disease is progressing or resolving is lost in ICD-10-CM.

In addition to codes clarifying idiopathic scoliosis, codes have been added in ICD-10-CM for neuromuscular and other secondary forms of scoliosis, such as that caused by disc herniation.

Coding for (Kypho-) Scoliosis

ICD-9-CM		ICD-10-CM	
737.30	Scoliosis, idiopathic	M41.112	Juvenile idiopathic scoliosis, cervical region
		M41.113	Juvenile idiopathic scoliosis, cervicothoracic region
		M41.114	Juvenile idiopathic scoliosis, thoracic region
		M41.115	Juvenile idiopathic scoliosis, thoracolumbar region
		M41.116	Juvenile idiopathic scoliosis, lumbar region
		M41.117	Juvenile idiopathic scoliosis, lumbosacral region
		M41.119	Juvenile idiopathic scoliosis, site unspecified
		M41.122	Adolescent idiopathic scoliosis, cervical region
		M41.123	Adolescent idiopathic scoliosis, cervicothoracic region
		M41.124	Adolescent idiopathic scoliosis, thoracic region
		M41.125	Adolescent idiopathic scoliosis, thoracolumbar region
		M41.126	Adolescent idiopathic scoliosis, lumbar region
		M41.127	Adolescent idiopathic scoliosis, lumbosacral region
		M41.129	Adolescent idiopathic scoliosis, site unspecified
		M41.20	Other idiopathic scoliosis, site unspecified
		M41.22	Other idiopathic scoliosis, cervical region
		M41.23	Other idiopathic scoliosis, cervicothoracic region
		M41.24	Other idiopathic scoliosis, thoracic region
		M41.25	Other idiopathic scoliosis, thoracolumbar region
		M41.26	Other idiopathic scoliosis, lumbar region
		M41.27	Other idiopathic scoliosis, lumbosacral region
737.31	Resolving infantile idiopathic scoliosis	M41.00	Infantile idiopathic scoliosis, site unspecified
		M41.02	Infantile idiopathic scoliosis, cervical region
		M41.03	Infantile idiopathic scoliosis, cervicothoracic region
		M41.04	Infantile idiopathic scoliosis, thoracic region
		M41.05	Infantile idiopathic scoliosis, thoracolumbar region
		M41.06	Infantile idiopathic scoliosis, lumbar region
		M41.07	Infantile idiopathic scoliosis, lumbosacral region
		M41.08	Infantile idiopathic scoliosis, sacral and sacrococcygeal region
737.32	Progressive infantile idiopathic scoliosis	M41.00	Infantile idiopathic scoliosis, site unspecified
		M41.02	Infantile idiopathic scoliosis, cervical region
		M41.03	Infantile idiopathic scoliosis, cervicothoracic region
		M41.04	Infantile idiopathic scoliosis, thoracic region
		M41.05	Infantile idiopathic scoliosis, thoracolumbar region
		M41.06	Infantile idiopathic scoliosis, lumbar region
		M41.07	Infantile idiopathic scoliosis, lumbosacral region
		M41.08	Infantile idiopathic scoliosis, sacral and sacrococcygeal region

Chapter 4. ICD-10-CM: Muscular System

Anatomic Overview

The muscles and muscle tissue perform five major functions for the human body. This system produces movement (within organs and organ systems as well as external movements), stabilizes posture, reinforces the articulations of the skeleton, helps with storage and regulation of substances within the body, and generates heat.

There are three types of muscle tissue: cardiac, smooth, and skeletal (or striated). Each type shares one or more of the four functional characteristics below that distinguish it as muscle tissue:

- **Excitability:** Ability to receive and react to irritation or stimulation.
- **Contractility:** Ability to reduce in size.
- **Extensibility:** Ability to lengthen or stretch.
- **Elasticity:** Ability to regain its original size and shape after contraction or extension.

Although all three types of tissue have specific attributes that differentiate between them, their general function—providing movement—is the same.

Cardiac Muscle

Cardiac muscle is found only in the heart. It forms the heart walls and performs the contractions that push blood through the vessels of the body. This type of muscle consists of linked fibers (similar to a skeletal muscle) that involuntarily contract (like a smooth muscle) in unison, producing the heartbeat. The movement of this muscle is controlled by electrical impulses sent by the heart's pacemaker. The cardiac muscle is unique because it is **striated** as a skeletal muscle is but involuntarily contracts like a smooth muscle. Because cardiac muscle is found only in the heart, the physiology of this type of muscle will be discussed in detail in the cardiac chapter.

Smooth Muscle

Smooth muscle is involuntary in its movements but is not striated, hence the name "smooth" muscle. This type of muscle lines the hollow organs of the body and contracts to force fluids and other bodily substances through the proper channels. It is found in organs such as the gastrointestinal tract, the uterus, urinary bladder, and blood vessels. Smooth muscle is also responsible for closing these channels to store contents or prevent "backflow" via ring-like bands of muscle called sphincters. Because of the various sites and functions of smooth muscle, the physiology of smooth muscle diseases will be discussed in more detail in the chapters coinciding with the location of the organ in which the muscle is found. For example, discussion of the smooth muscle lining the urinary bladder is found in the urinary chapter.

Skeletal Muscle

Skeletal muscle, as its name implies, moves the skeleton. It is responsible for the bumps and bulges under the skin associated with body builders and athletes. Skeletal muscle is striated and moves voluntarily, or consciously. In some cases, such as the movement of the diaphragm for breathing or the muscles that maintain posture, the movement is subconscious but still considered voluntary because a person can consciously cease or change the movement. Each muscle is attached at both ends: the origin (where the muscle is anchored to the bone) and the insertion (the point where the muscle attaches to the bone it moves). Generally, the origin

---

DEFINITIONS

striated. Something that is striped, marked by parallel lines, or has structural lines.

INTERESTING A & P FACT

Skeletal muscles make up approximately 40 percent of the body's mass.

bone does not move but forms an anchor so that when the muscle contracts, the insertion bone is moved toward the origin bone. This will be discussed in more detail later in this chapter. The fleshy contractile part is called the muscle belly.

Due to the various movements skeletal muscles perform depending on their location and function in the body, the structure of each may differ just as with the bones of the skeletal system. However, their basic components are the same. All skeletal muscles are composed of muscle tissue, nerves, blood vessels, and substantial amounts of connective tissue.

There are three kinds of connective tissue associated with muscle structure. Enclosing the entire muscle is a fibrous tissue called the epimysium, which may be commonly referred to as the muscle sheath. This tissue surrounds the outside of the muscle, holding it together. Within the epimysium lies many perimysium, tissue that groups individual muscle fibers together to form bundles called fascicles. Fascicles are the "grain" of the muscle and can be seen with the naked eye, such as in a piece of beef. Surrounding each individual muscle fiber found within these bundles is the endomysium. This complex and layered design allows for each fiber to move somewhat individually.

Also covering the muscle and providing further protection is a dense tissue called fascia. The fascia's main purpose is to hold muscles in place and separate them from surrounding organs or other muscles. It is also important to note that the fascia allows free movement, fills the spaces between muscles, and provides a mechanism for nerves, blood, and lymph vessels to reach the muscles. The space that contains the muscle within the fascia is known as a compartment.

In some cases, the fascia extends past the muscle it surrounds, forming a cord-like structure that attaches to the periosteum of a bone; this cord is referred to as a tendon. Certain tendons are further reinforced by an additional layer of connective tissue referred to as a tendon sheath. In other cases, the fascia extends past its muscle to form broad, thick sheets of connective tissue, called aponeurosis, that connect the muscle to an adjacent muscle.

In certain instances, mainly where muscles and tendons make contact with bone, there are fluid-filled sacs called bursae. A bursa reduces the friction between the muscle or tendon and the bone it moves across.

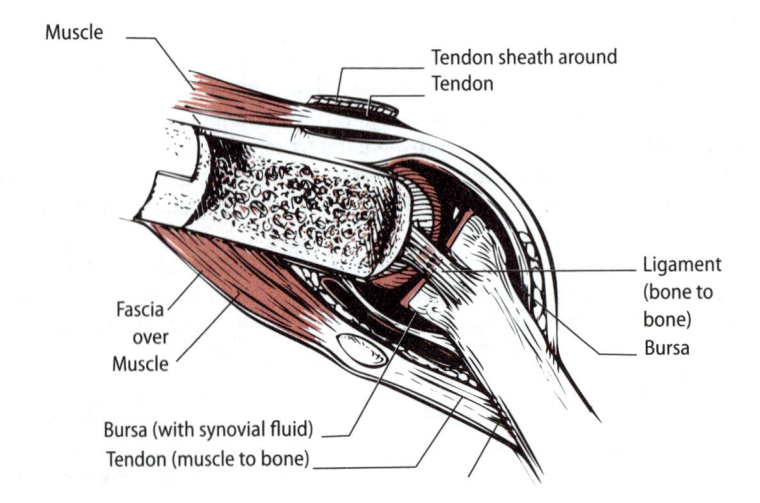

Figure 4.1: Joint Structures

The muscles' movement depends on the origin and insertion of the associated tendons. The origin of a muscle is where the tendon attaches to a stationary bone. For example, when flexing the muscle in the front of the upper arm (bicep), the upper arm/shoulder does not move, making this the origin of the muscle of the upper arm. The bones of the lower arm come closer to the body to cause the contraction in the bicep, making the lower arm the "moveable" attachment, or the insertion. In other words, when a muscle contracts, the insertion is pulled toward the origin.

Also influencing muscle movement is the arrangement of the individual muscle's fascicles. There are five basic shapes the fascicles form:

- **Parallel:** Fascicles follow the long axis of the muscle, forming a strap-like shape.
- **Fusiform:** Fascicles follow the long axis of the muscle but form a belly or bulge in the middle, forming a spindle-like shape.
- **Pennate:** Fascicles are short and feather out from a tendon.
    - **unipennate:** Fascicles attach only to one side of a tendon.
    - **bipennate:** Fascicles attach to both sides of a tendon.
    - **multipennate:** Fascicles attach to all parts of a tendon or both sides of multiple tendons in the same muscle.
- **Convergent:** Fascicles start out broad and end narrow, forming a triangular shape.
- **Circular:** Fascicles are arranged in concentric rings.

Skeletal muscles cause various movements based not only on their origins, insertions, and shape but also coordination with other muscles. Many muscles are in groups that define their actions—when one contracts, another relaxes. The muscle that contracts is called the agonist, and the relaxing muscle is the antagonist. Using the upper arm muscles as an example again, when the bicep contracts, the muscle on the posterior side of the arm (the tricep) relaxes and vice versa. In addition to these obvious muscles, there are also stabilizing muscles that interact with the agonist/antagonist relationship. Known as synergists, these muscles help coordinate the motion or stop unwanted movement. Those that stop unwanted movement are called fixators.

The multiple groups of muscles within the body provide many types of movement. The following terms describe the general body movements:

- **Flexion:** Bending of a joint so that its angle decreases (bending the elbow).
- **Extension:** Straightening of the angle of the joint (straightening at the elbow).
- **Hyperextension:** Extension of the joint beyond its normal anatomical position (bending the head back to look straight up).
- **Abduction:** Movement away from midline (reaching out with the arm).
- **Adduction:** Movement closer to midline (pulling the arm close to the body).
- **Rotation:** Movement around an axis (shaking head "no").
- **Circumduction:** Movement of a part so that the end moves (swinging the arms in circles).
- **Protraction:** Moving forward of a body part (pushing chin out).
- **Retraction:** Movement backward (pulling chin in).
- **Elevation:** Raising of a body part (shrugging the shoulders).
- **Depression:** Lowering of a body part (drooping the shoulders).

It is important to point out that the names of skeletal muscles are based on their basic characteristics: size, shape, action, location, and/or attachments. Many muscle names are formed by using combinations of the basic word roots in medical terminology to describe a distinct attribute of that muscle. Therefore understanding the meaning of a muscle's name gives a clue to that muscle's specific attributes.

Major Skeletal Muscle Groups

There are nearly 700 individual muscles in the body. For ICD-10-CM purposes, only the major muscle groups need to be discussed.

Muscles of the Head

The muscles in the head have three main functions: facial expression, **mastication**, and movement of the eyes.

There are four pairs of major muscles in addition to two single muscles that control facial expression. These muscles are unique in that their insertion points are attached to the skin or muscles of the face and scalp rather than the bones of the skull, making these muscles the most visible in the body.

Starting at the top of the head is the epicranius muscle, which is formed by the two frontalis muscles (over the frontal bone) and two occipitalis muscles (over the occipital bone). These two bundles of muscle tissue are connected by the epicranial aponeurosis. When contracted, this wrinkles the skin of the forehead. Below the bilateral frontalis muscles are two ring-like muscles that circle each of the eyes. The orbicularis oculi causes the eyelids to close or blink. Contracting this muscle causes the skin at the outer edge of the eyes to wrinkle, commonly called "crow's feet." Below the eyes is a pair of zygomaticus muscles, which attach to the cheekbones and lift the corners of the mouth to form a smile or laugh. Beneath the zygomaticus are the buccinators, which form the meaty part of the cheeks; when this muscle contracts, the cheeks "suck" in. Medial to these is the "kissing muscle" encircling the lips. This muscle is known as the orbicularis oris and as its nickname suggests, it is responsible for closing and puckering the lips. At the bottom of the face, covering the chin and front of the neck, is a thin, sheet-like muscle called the platysma. Its main functions are to pull the corners of the lips down to form a frown and help in lowering the mandible to open the mouth.

Figure 4.2: Muscles of the Face

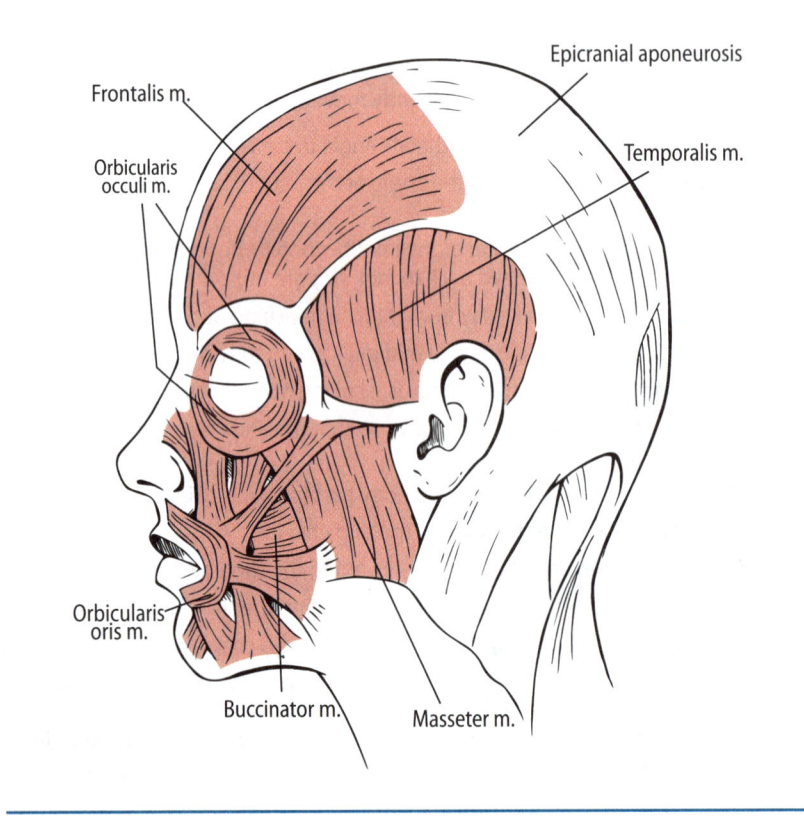

> **DEFINITIONS**
>
> **mastication.** Process of chewing food to ready it for the digestive system.

Four pairs of muscles in the face control the chewing process. The three pairs that aid in closing the jaw are the masseter, temporalis, and medial pterygoid. The masseter sits in front of the ear and clenches the jaw by contracting. Sitting just above the ear is the temporalis (covering the temporal bone). The medial pterygoid is found underneath the masseter and aids not only in closing the mouth but also moving the mandible from side to side. The fourth pair of muscles sits adjacent to the medial pterygoid beneath the masseter, attaching the mandible to the sphenoid bone. This muscle is called the lateral pterygoid, and its main purpose is to open the mouth. It also aids in pushing the chin outward and moving the jaw from side to side.

Last, six muscles move each eyeball. These are usually called "extrinsic" eye muscles because they are outside of the eye. They are unique in that their insertion points are on the eyeball itself. The first four muscles, the superior, inferior, lateral, and medial rectus, are aptly named for the direction in which they move the eyeball when contracted. For example, when a person goes cross-eyed, this is the contraction of both medial rectus muscles. The other two muscles, the superior and inferior obliques, move the eyeballs in the "in between" directions missed by the recti.

> **INTERESTING A & P FACT**
>
> The extrinsic eye muscles are some of the most exact and fastest reacting muscles in the body.

Figure 4.3: Eye Musculature

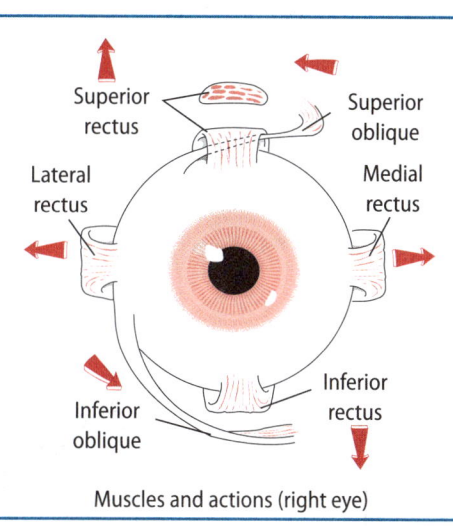

Muscles and actions (right eye)

Muscles of the Neck and Spine

On each side of the neck, running from behind the ear to the top of the sternum, are the sternocleidomastoid muscles. These muscles turn the head and pull the chin toward the chest. They also aid in lifting the sternum during deep breathing. In the back of the neck, there are multiple paired muscle groups. Starting toward midline and working outward are the spinalis capitis, the semispinalis capitis, and the longissimus capitis, which connect various lower cervical and upper thoracic vertebrae to the base of the skull. Lying on top of these muscles is the splenius capitis, a long muscle that extends from the skull to vertebrae in the head and neck. All of these muscles combined act to rotate the head and move the head, as well as hold it upright. Most superior in the back of the neck and connecting to the tops of the shoulders, forming the "crook" of the neck, is the trapezius muscle. This muscle stabilizes and controls movements of the shoulder. Although its superior location is the neck, it extends into the posterior thorax musculature.

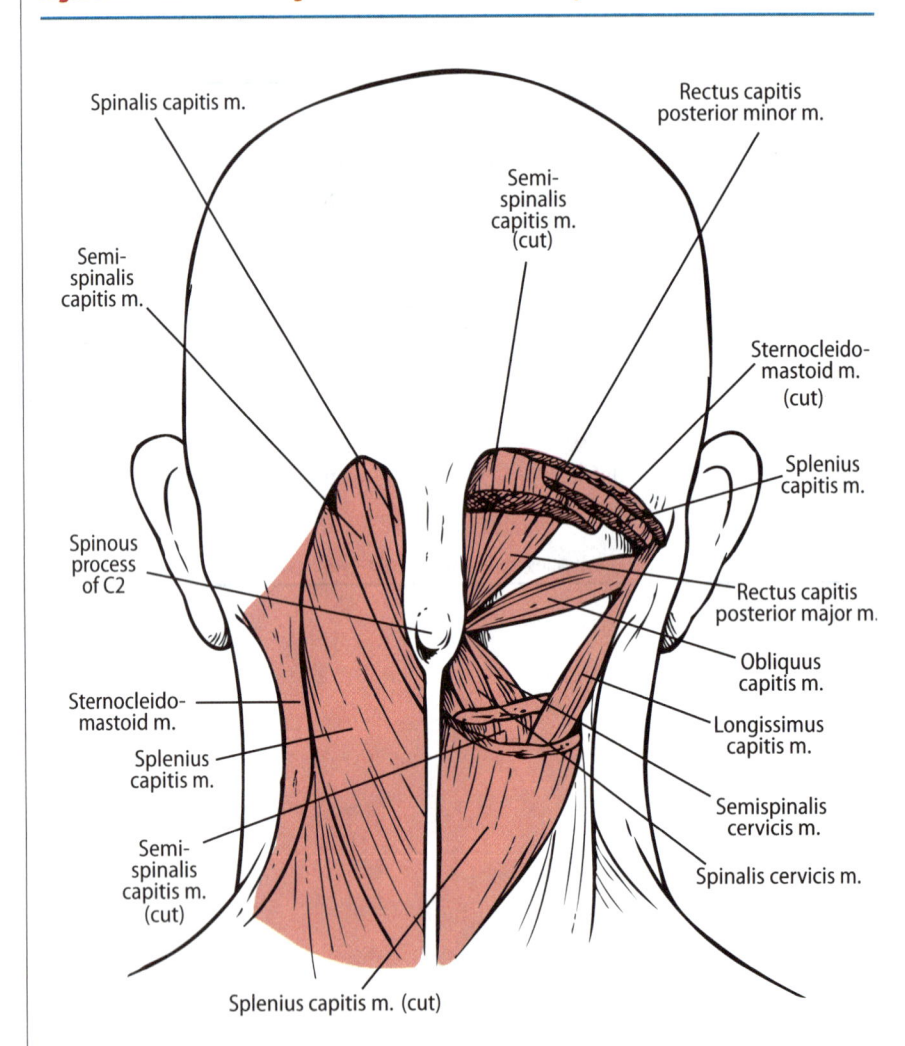

Figure 4.4: Associated Regions of Pain due to Neck Injuries

Further down the vertebrae, the erector spinae muscles run along the bony spine, connecting it to various bones in the axial skeleton. These muscles maintain upright posture and assist in movements. The erector spinae can be divided into three major groups of muscles depending on their proximity to the spine, and then they are divided by their insertion points on the vertebrae. Listed from closest (medial) to the spine to the furthest (lateral), the muscle groups of the erector spinae are:

- **Spinalis:** Spinalis cervicis, spinalis thoracis
- **Longissimus:** Longissimus cervicis, longissimus thoracis
- **Iliocostalis:** Iliocostalis cervicis, iliocostalis thoracis, iliocostalis lumborum

Figure 4.5: Muscles of Erector Spine

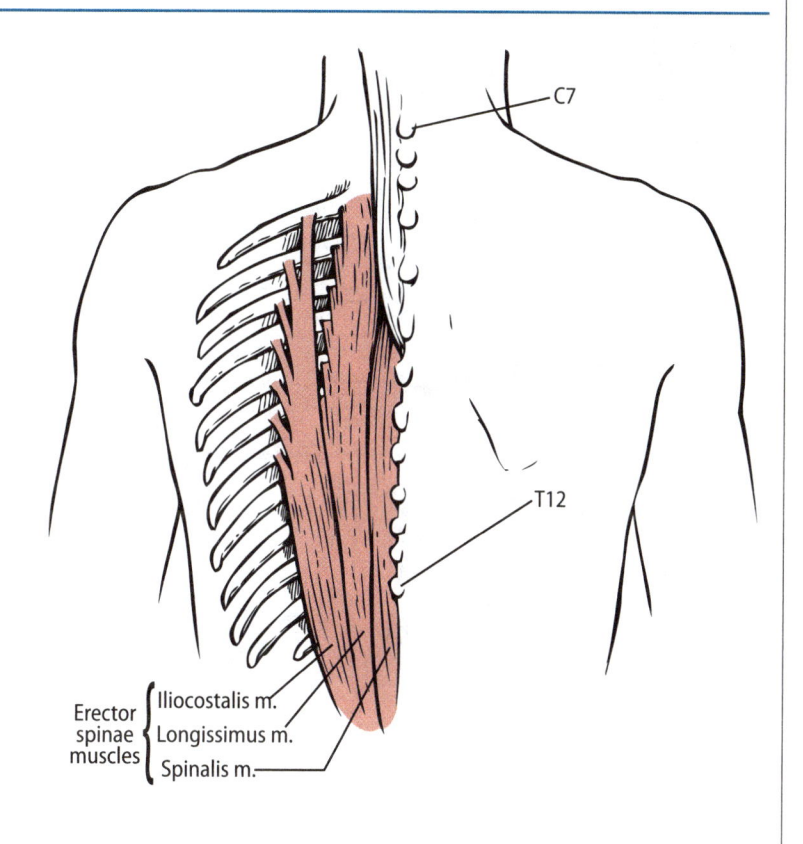

Muscles of the Thorax

There are two main functions of the muscle groups in the thorax. The first group of muscles aid in respiration, and the second aid in the movement and stabilization of the thoracic area. Those that aid in breathing control the expansion and contraction of the thoracic cavity, where the lungs are located. The cavity must expand on inhalation and contract during exhalation. The most significant of these muscles is the diaphragm. Serving as a dome-shaped divider between the thoracic and abdominal cavities, this muscle flattens when it contracts, making more space available to the lungs. Also helping to make more space on inspiration, the 11 pairs of external intercostal muscles running between the ribs lift and expand the rib cage. Sitting further inside the rib cage are the internal intercostal muscles, which counteract the external intercostals by compressing the rib cage on expiration.

Figure 4.6: Diaphragm

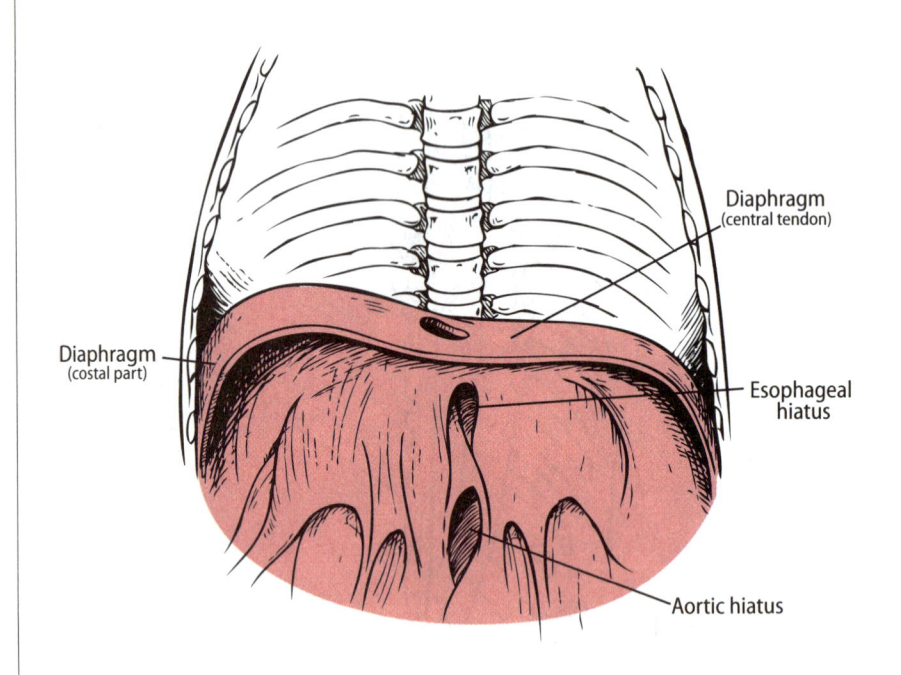

Anterior to the costal muscles are those muscles that aid in the movement and aesthetics of the chest. The most superficial and exposed muscle in the chest is the pectoralis major, forming bulges on both sides of the sternum. Although this muscle is predominantly seen on the chest, its function is to flex, adduct, and rotate the arm. Lying deep to this muscle is the pectoralis minor, running from the scapula to the second or third to fourth or fifth ribs. This muscle abducts the scapula, pulling the shoulder back, and also contributes to forceful inhalation when needed. Superior to the pectoralis minor, attaching the mid-distal clavicle to the first rib, is the subclavius, whose main function is stabilizing the thorax and shoulder. Wrapping around the sides of the thorax, sitting on top of the superior eight or nine ribs, is the serratus anterior. This muscle acts as an anterior stabilizer for the scapula and pushes the shoulder forward.

Figure 4.7: Pectoralis Major

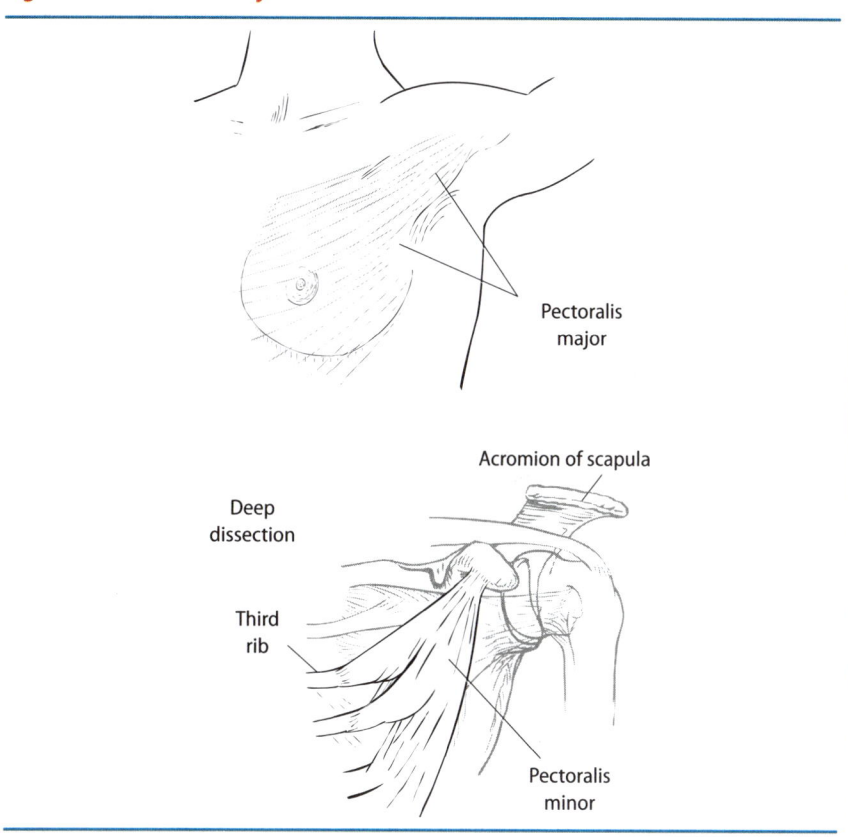

The most superficial muscle in the posterior thorax is also found in the neck, the trapezius. This muscle has origins on the occipital bone and also on the lower cervical and all thoracic vertebrae. The trapezius gets its name from the trapezoid shape of this paired muscle group in the back. Just inferior to the lowest-most portion of the trapezius is the latissimus dorsi. Attached to the lower vertebrae and extending up underneath the arm, this large muscle extends, adducts, and rotates the arm medially. Also lying deep to the trapezius is the rhomboid major and rhomboid minor, which aid in adding force to downward movements of the arms, as well as further stabilizing the scapula.

Figure 4.8: Posterior Thorax

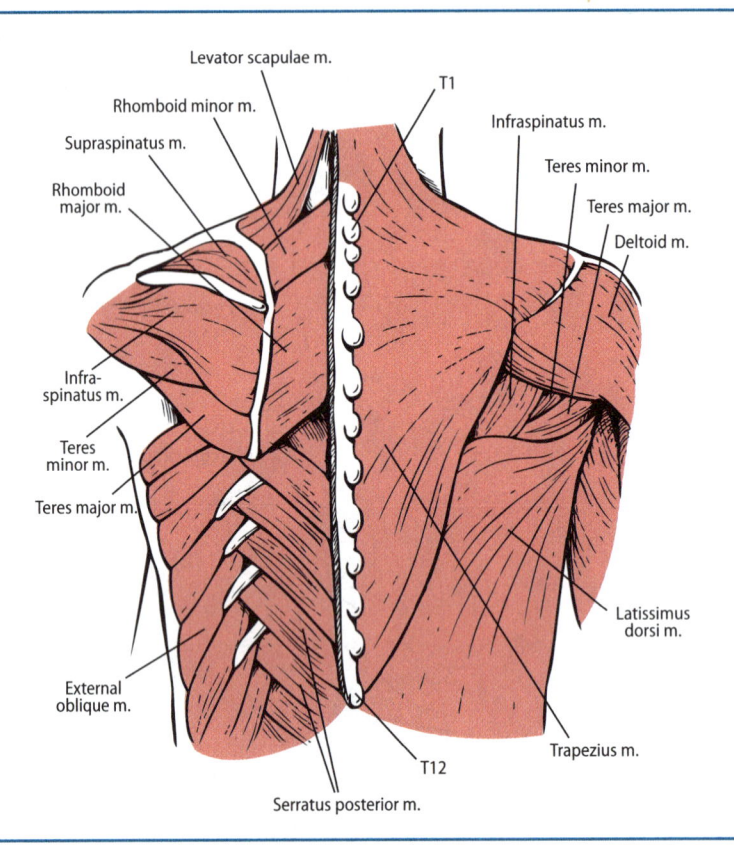

Muscles of the Shoulder and Upper Extremity

Lateral to the rhomboid muscles is the infraspinatus, connecting the scapula to the upper head of the humerus. The infraspinatus muscle connects to the scapula below the spinous process. On the opposite side of the scapula's spinous process is the supraspinatus. Inferior to these muscles are the teres minor and teres major, forming the lower area of the armpit where the back and the arm come together. Sitting on top of these muscles, capping the shoulder, is the deltoid. These muscles all work together to choreograph the various movements of the shoulder joint.

Figure 4.9: Shoulder Muscles

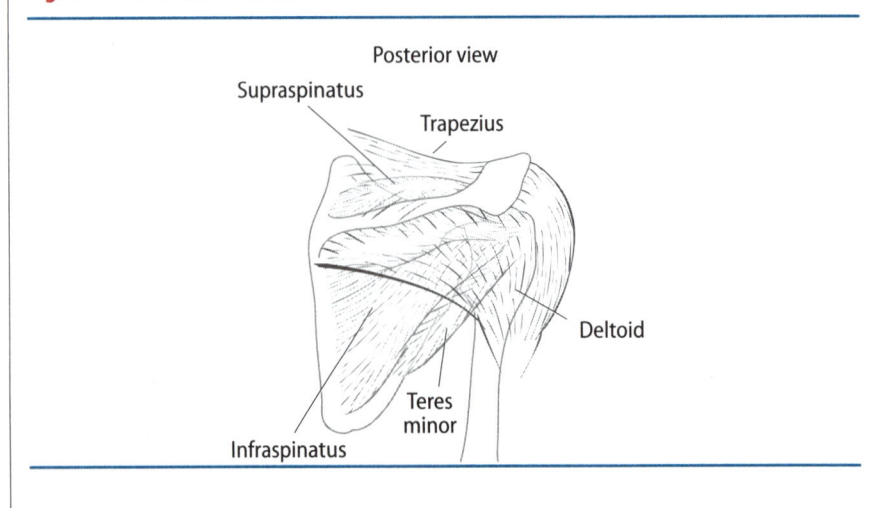

The upper arm has three major muscles. The anterior-most muscle associated with strong arms is called the biceps brachii. This muscle flexes the arm at the shoulder and the elbow. Just deep to the biceps is the brachialis, the most powerful *flexor* at the elbow joint. And last, there is one large muscle on the posterior side of the upper arm known as the triceps brachii. It is the most powerful *extensor* at the elbow joint.

Figure 4.10: Upper Arm

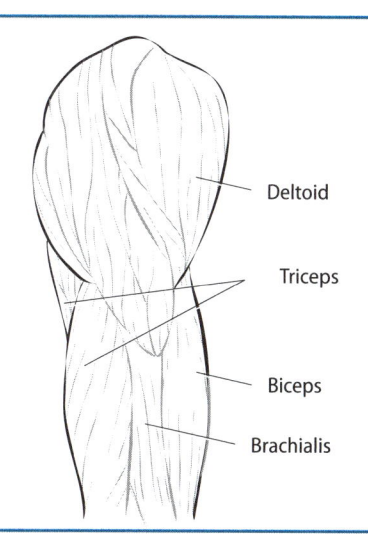

> **DEFINITIONS**
>
> **extensor.** Any muscle or tendon that extends a joint.
>
> **flexor.** Muscle or tendon that bends or flexes a limb or part as opposed to extending it.

Crossing over the elbow joint, connecting the humerus and ulna to the radius, is a short muscle called the pronator teres. Its main function is to rotate the lower arm medially or to face the palm of the hand down. Performing the opposite action of rotating the forearm laterally and also crossing the elbow joint is the supinator. Also aiding the rotation of the forearm, wrist, and hand is the pronator quadratus, which connects the radius and ulna at the anterior wrist.

Figure 4.11: Forearm

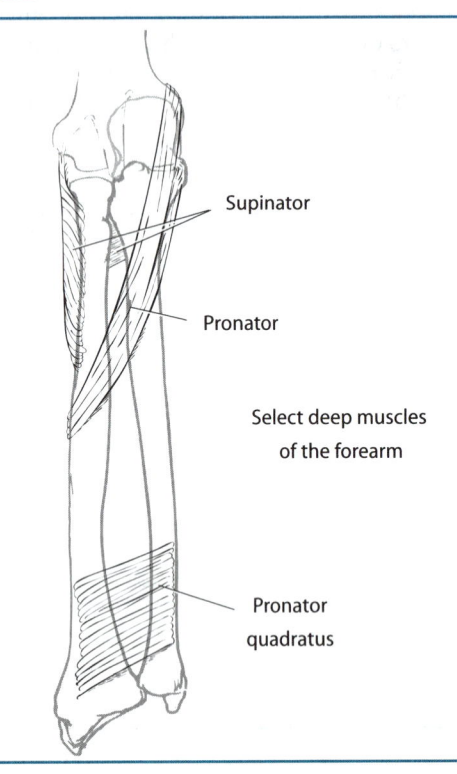

Supinator

Pronator

Select deep muscles of the forearm

Pronator quadratus

The rest of the muscles in the forearm can be classified as a flexor or extensor, depending upon the hand movements the muscles are responsible for. The flexors of the lower arm are:

- **Flexor carpi radius:** Located in the anterior medial part of the forearm; it flexes and abducts the hand.
- **Flexor carpi ulnaris:** Located along the pinkie finger side of the lower arm; it flexes and adducts the hand.
- **Palmaris longus:** Between the flexor carpi radius and flexor carpi ulnaris; it flexes the hand at the wrist.
- **Flexor digitorum:** Centrally located and posterior to flexor carpi ulnaris; it flexes the distal phalange joints.
- **Flexor digitorum superficialis:** Centrally located beneath the flexor carpi ulnaris; it flexes fingers and hand.

There are four extensors:

- **Extensor carpi radialis longus:** Located on the thumb side of the forearm; it extends and abducts the hand at the wrist.
- **Extensor carpi radialis brevis:** Medial to the extensor carpi radialis; it extends and abducts the hand at the wrist.
- **Extensor carpi ulnaris:** Located in the medial posterior part of the forearm; it extends and adducts the hand at the wrist.
- **Extensor digitorum:** Located alongside the extensor carpi ulnaris; it extends the fingers.

Figure 4.12: Elbow

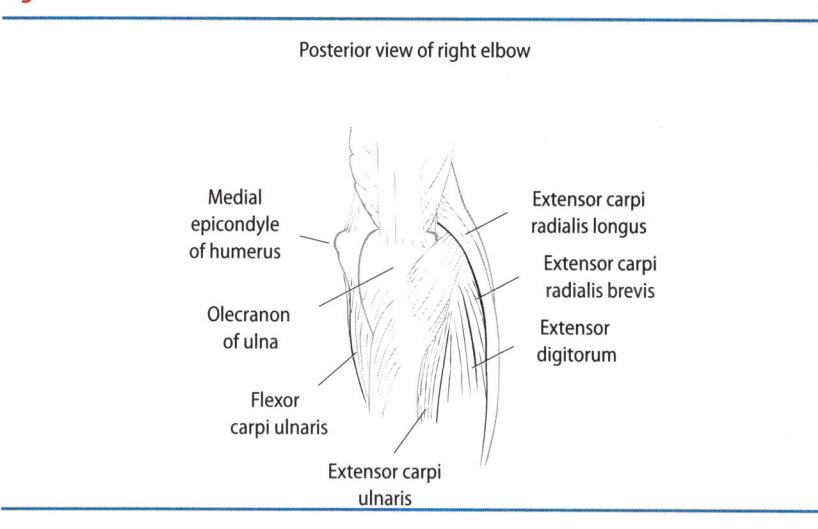

Posterior view of right elbow

- Medial epicondyle of humerus
- Olecranon of ulna
- Flexor carpi ulnaris
- Extensor carpi radialis longus
- Extensor carpi radialis brevis
- Extensor digitorum
- Extensor carpi ulnaris

The muscles in the forearm tend to control the less delicate hand movements; the intrinsic muscles in the hands perform the precise and fluid movements of the fingers. There are four muscles that move the thumb: the abductor pollicis brevis, opponens pollicis, flexor pollicis brevis, and the adductor pollicis. These muscles come together to form the bulge at the bottom of the hand on the palm below the thumb, called the thenar eminence.

Figure 4.13: Thumb and Palm

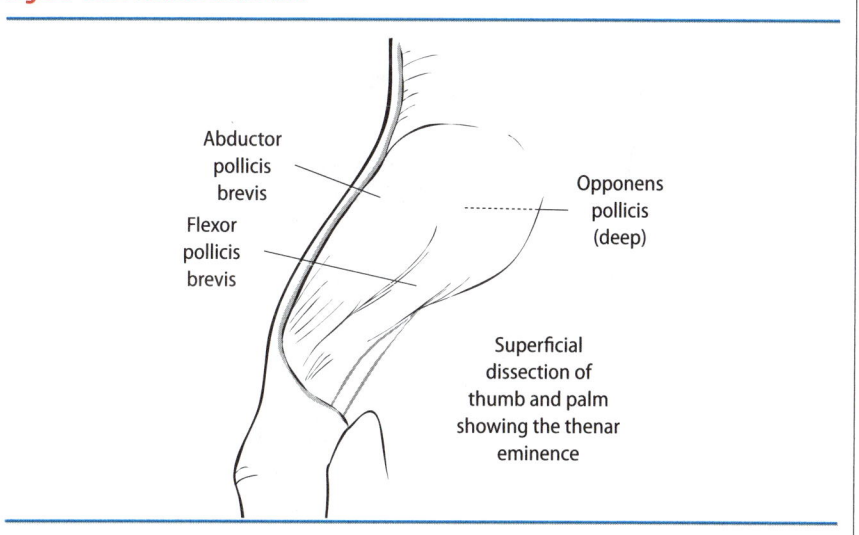

- Abductor pollicis brevis
- Flexor pollicis brevis
- Opponens pollicis (deep)

Superficial dissection of thumb and palm showing the thenar eminence

Moving the little finger (or fifth digit) are three unique muscles as well: the abductor digiti minimi, flexor digiti minimi brevis, and the opponens digiti minimi. The other fingers are controlled by four lumbricals (one laterally flanking the tendons of each finger), three palmar interossei (beside the metacarpal shafts), and four dorsal interossei (on the opposite side of the metacarpal shafts from the palmar interossei).

Figure 4.14: Hand

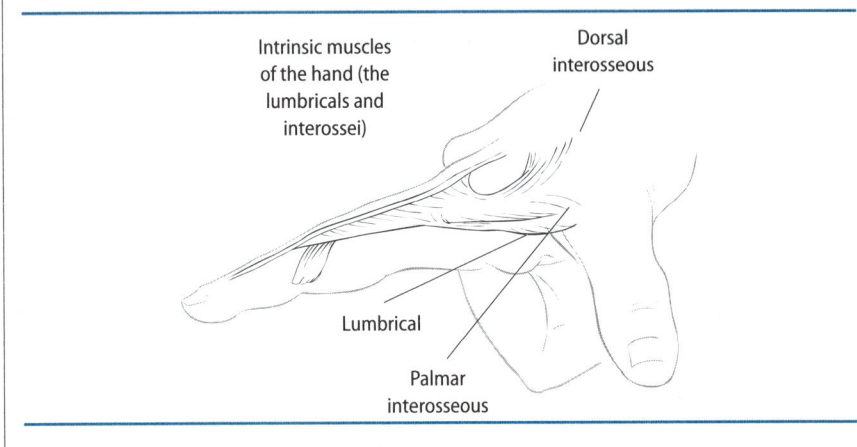

Muscles of the Abdominal Wall

Looking at the abdominal wall, the image of "six-pack" abdominal muscles comes to mind. Those individual definitions are all parts of one large muscle, called the rectus abdominus, covering the entire abdominal area from the ribs and sternum down to the pubis. This large muscle is covered by aponeuroses. There are three pairs of muscles that form the lateral sides of the abdomen. The most superficial of these is the external obliques, followed by the internal oblique and the transversus abdominus, the deepest.

Figure 4.15: Anatomy of Anterior Abdominal Wall

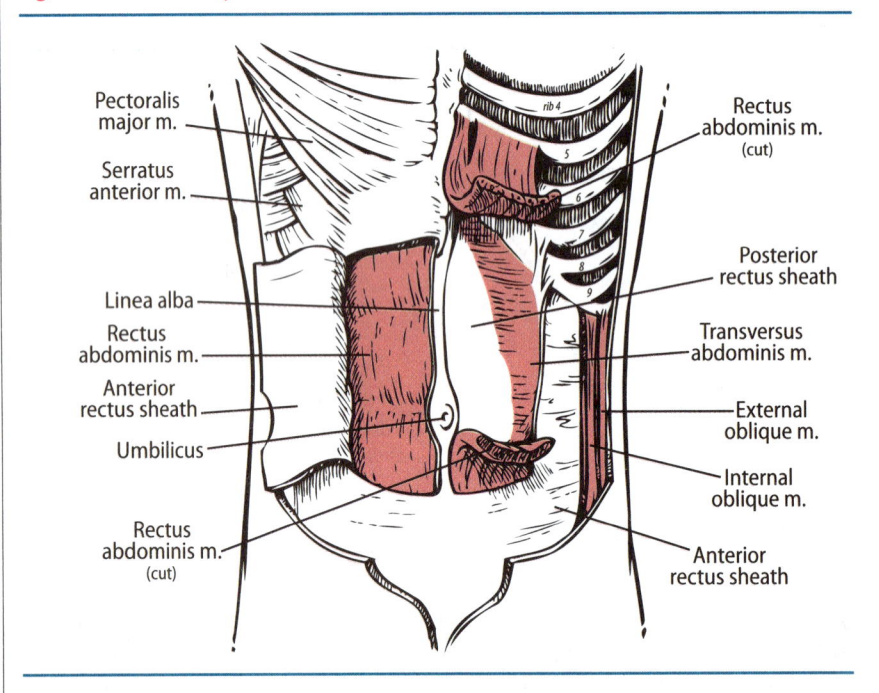

Muscles of the Pelvis

Although male and female anatomy varies significantly in the pelvic area, the muscular structure is surprisingly similar. The muscles in the pelvis can be divided into two distinct classifications based on location. Those that form the pelvic floor are considered part of the deeper pelvic diaphragm, and those that fill the space between the coxal bones are part of the urogenital diaphragm.

There are only two muscles that form the pelvic diaphragm: the levator ani and coccygeus. These muscles come together to support the pelvic floor and assist with the sphincter-like actions of the anus and vagina.

Also helping to support the pelvis is the superficial transversus perinea, a pair of muscles located along the posterior of the urogenital diaphragm. Anterior to these structures is the bulbospongiosus. This muscle is located at the bottom of the penis in men and surrounds the posterior part of the vaginal opening in women. In women, it is the muscle used to contract the vagina. It also aids in urination. To each side of the bulbospongiosus is an ischiocavernosus muscle that assists it with its functions. Both males and females also have a muscle called the sphincter urethrae that encircles the opening of the urethra to restrict or promote urinary flow.

Figure 4.16: Male Pelvic Floor

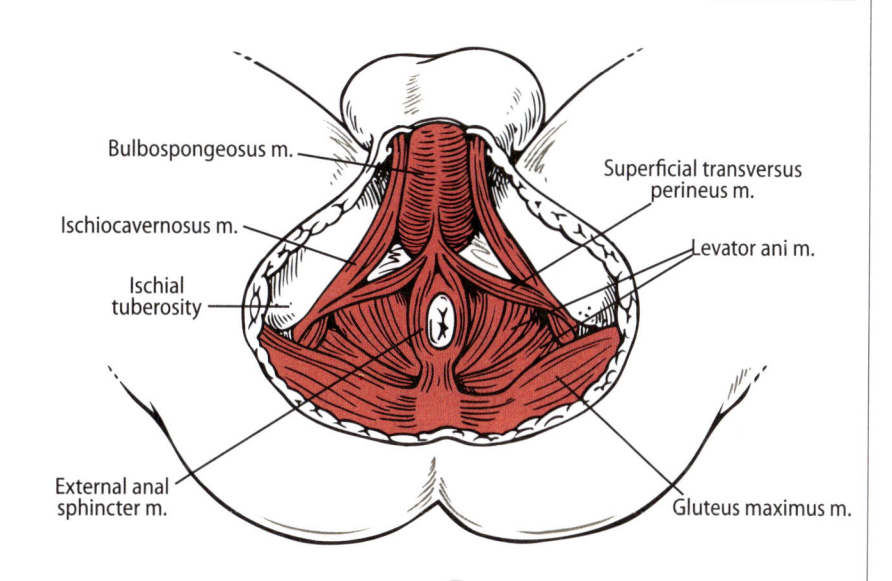

Figure 4.17: Female Pelvic Floor

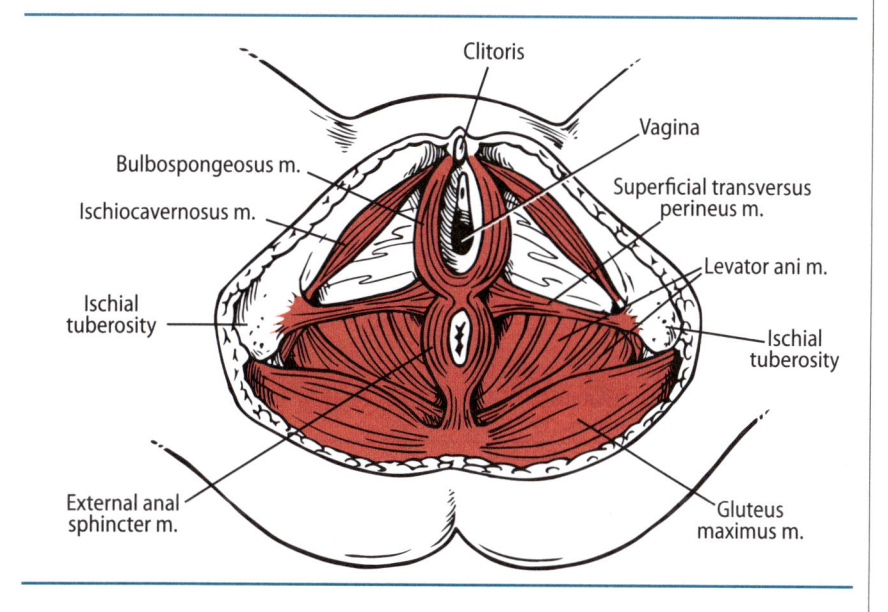

Muscles of the Hips and Lower Extremities

Within the anterior part of the hip region are psoas major and the iliacus. The psoas major is a straplike muscle that connects the lumbar spine to the femur and flexes the upper thigh. The iliacus is a larger, fan-shaped muscle that covers the ilium portion of the pelvic bones. Its main purpose is to assist the psoas major in moving the upper leg in the action of walking. Moving laterally on the hip is the tensor fasciae latae, which sits on the lateral anterior part of the hip.

Figure 4.18: Anterior View of Hip

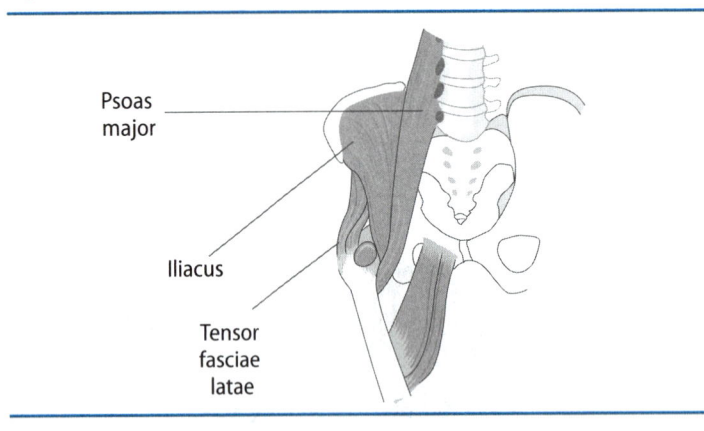

The next muscle moving toward the back of the hip is the gluteus medius, which also covers the gluteus minimus. These two muscles together abduct the thigh and rotate it medially. Partially covering the gluteus medius and forming the buttock is the gluteus maximus; its main functions are to straighten the lower limb and provide the force to stand from a sitting position.

Figure 4.19: Gluteal Muscles

> **INTERESTING A & P FACT**
> The gluteus maximus is the largest muscle in the body.

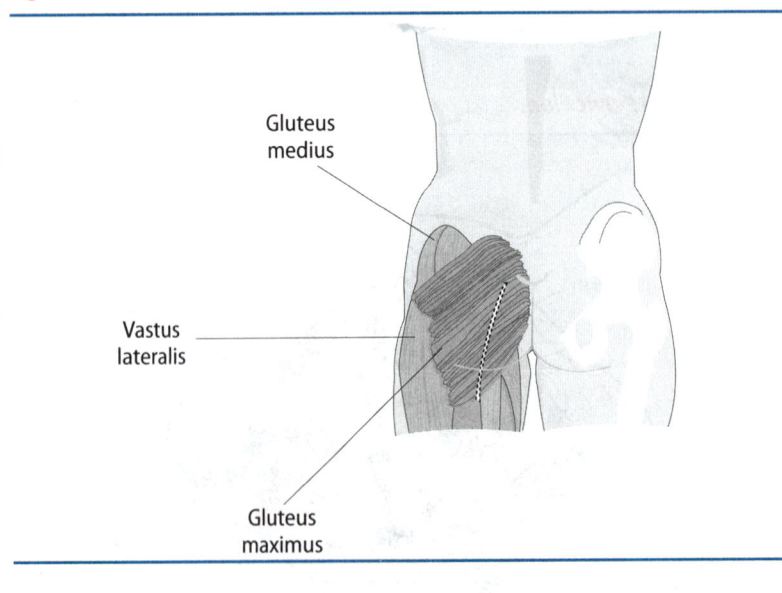

Moving from the medial part of the anterior thigh outward, the first muscle encountered is the gracilis, running from the lower edge of the ischium section of the coxal bones to the tibia, serving to adduct the thigh and flex the knee. The adductor magus and adductor longus are the next two muscles moving medially across the thigh. These muscles adduct the thigh and assist in lateral rotation of the leg. The longus is also a flexor, whereas the magus is an extensor. Cutting across the anterior thigh, connecting the outer hipbone to the medial portion of the knee, is the sartorius muscle. It flexes, abducts, and laterally rotates the thigh.

The group of muscles lateral to the sartorius muscle is sometimes referred to as the quadriceps femoris group. This group of muscles makes up the meaty part of the front and side of the thighs. It consists of four extensor muscles: the rectus femoris, vastus lateralis, vastus medialis, and vastus intermedius. They function together to extend the leg at the knee. The vastus lateralis is covered in a layer of fascia on the outside of the thigh.

Figure 4.20: Anterior View of Thigh

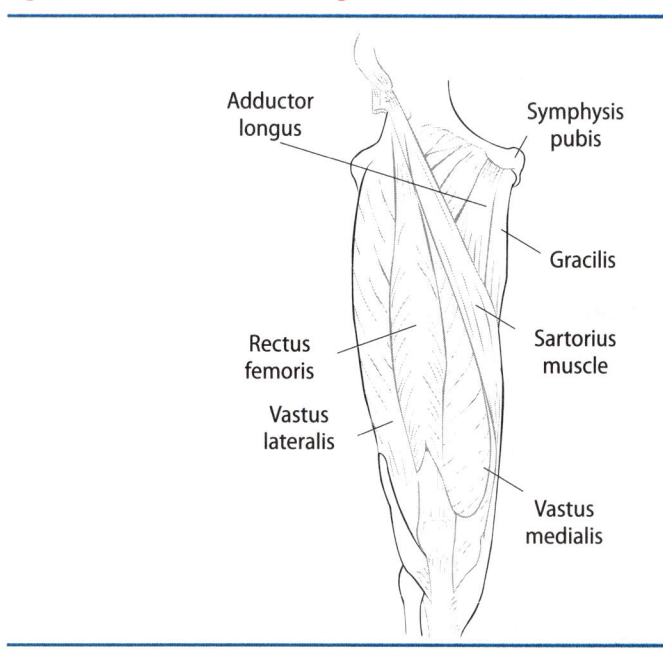

The posterior part of the thigh is commonly referred to as the hamstrings. The hamstrings are a group of three muscles that extend from the ischium to the tibia. The three muscles that compose the hamstrings are the biceps femoris, semitendinosus, and semimembranosus.

Figure 4.21: Gluteus Maximus

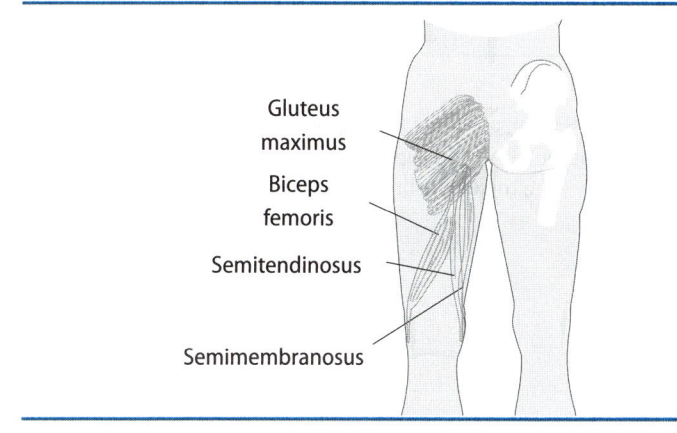

The muscles in the lower part of the leg can be divided by the foot actions for which they are responsible, *dorsiflexion* or *plantar flexion*. Those responsible for dorsiflexion are:

- **Tibialis anterior:** Stretches from the lateral part of the knee to the medial part of the foot; it also assists in *inversion*.
- **Peroneus tertius:** Located on the anterior part of the fibula; it also assists in *eversion*.
- **Extensor digitorum longus:** Between the tibia and fibula; it also assists in eversion and extension of the toes.

The plantar flexors include:

- **Gastrocnemius:** Located in the calf area, it is the most predominant muscle of the posterior lower leg; it also assists in the flexing of the knee.
- **Soleus:** Located underneath the calcaneal tendon, which runs from the gastrocnemius to the calcaneus.
- **Flexor digitorum longus:** Located on the posterior side of the tibia, ending at the distal phalanges of the toes; it also assists in inversion and flexion of the four lateral toes.
- **Tibialis posterior:** Located on the back of the leg and is the deepest muscle; it also assists in inversion.
- **Peroneus longus:** Located on the anterior lateral side of the calf; it also assists in eversion and supports the arch of the foot.

Figure 4.22: Lower Leg

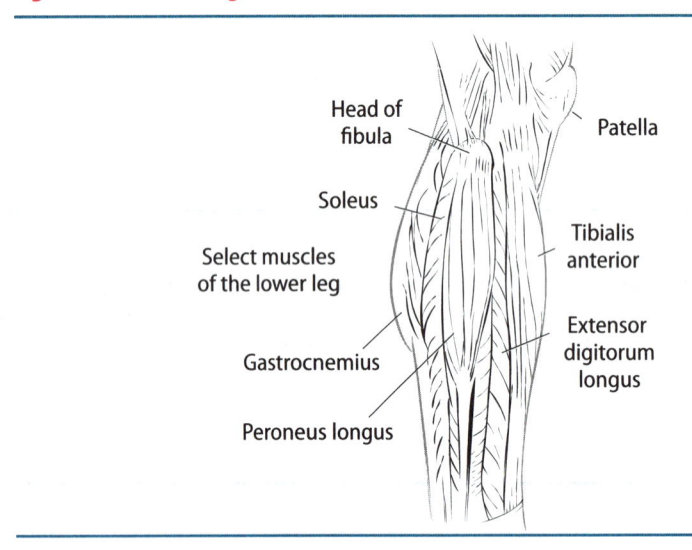

Similar to the hand, the foot has muscles that are responsible for the more specific actions of the foot, such as ambulation and support of the entire body. There is only one muscle on the top of the foot, the extensor digitorum brevis. It extends the toes.

DEFINITIONS

dorsiflexion. Bending of the foot upward.

eversion. Movement in which the sole of the foot faces laterally.

inversion. Movement in which the sole of the foot faces medially.

plantar flexion. Bending of the foot downward.

Figure 4.23: Foot

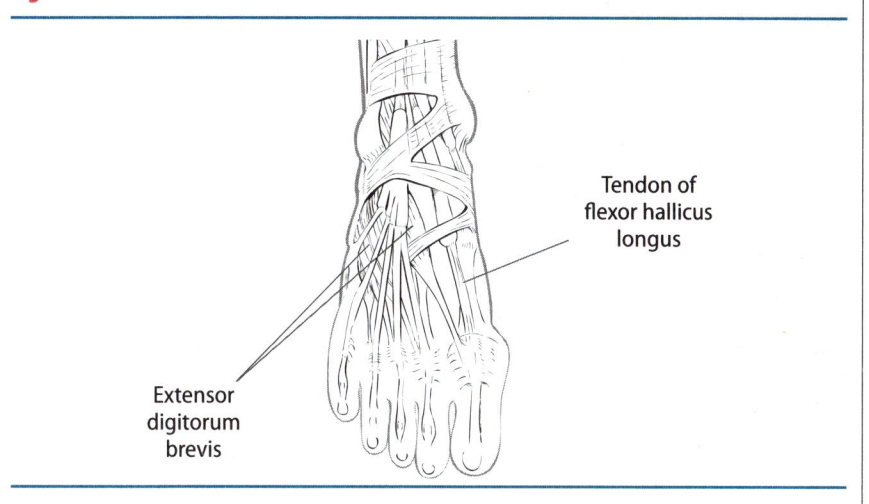

There are four layers of muscles on the plantar side of the foot. The first and most superficial layer includes the abductor hallucis, the flexor digitorum brevis, and the abductor digiti minimi. The next layer includes the quadratus plantae and the lumbricals. There are three muscles in the third layer, the flexor hallucis brevis, adductor hallucis, and flexor digiti minimi brevis. The deepest layer includes the dorsal and plantar interossei, the arrangement of which resembles that of the interossei muscles in the hands.

Figure 4.24: Foot

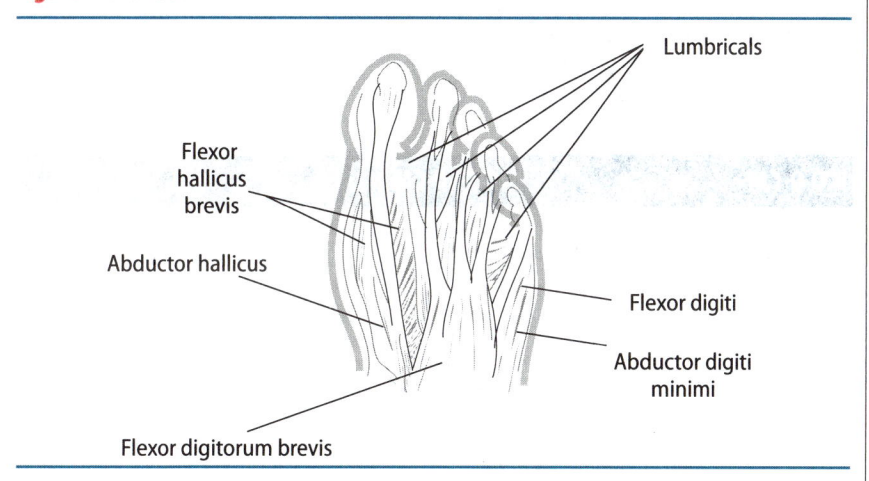

Anatomy and Pathophysiology and the ICD-10-CM Code Set

Knowing the basic anatomy of the muscles is imperative for assigning codes in both ICD-9-CM and ICD-10-CM. To select the appropriate codes in ICD-10-CM, additional, advanced information regarding not only the anatomy but also the action of the skeletal muscles is necessary.

Injuries

Because muscles are soft organs just beneath the subcutaneous tissue and because they absorb and generate force and movement, not only are injuries to them common, but the types of injuries are varied. This chapter highlights the types of injuries for which in-depth knowledge is needed to assign an appropriate code in ICD-10-CM.

It is important to note that ICD-10-CM requires seven characters to completely describe most traumatic injuries. The most common seventh characters used in conjunction with the muscles are "A"—Initial encounter, "D"—Subsequent encounter, and "S"—Sequela.

A "pulled" muscle, or muscle or tendon strain, is a fairly generic type of injury, and ICD-9-CM treats it as such. In the older classification system, sprains and strains are synonymous; however, physiologically they are very different injuries to a synovial joint. A sprain occurs when there is a stretch or tear of a ligament, the tissue that connects bone to bone. A strain is an injury to a muscle or tendon, usually due to overexertion, twisting, or pulling. ICD-10-CM not only provides separate categories for the two injuries, but also identifies the site and type of action for which the muscle and tendon are responsible.

The differences in the classification systems are best seen when looking at the ICD-9-CM codes for sprains and strains of other specified sites of shoulder and upper arm, 840.8, and sprains and strains of other specified sites of hip and thigh, 843.8.

Coding for Strains

ICD-9-CM		ICD-10-CM	
840.8	Sprain and strain of other specified sites of shoulder and upper arm	S43.49[1,2,9]A	Other sprain of shoulder joint, initial encounter
		S43.60XA	Sprain of sternoclavicular joint, unspecified side, initial encounter
		S43.61XA	Sprain of right sternoclavicular joint, initial encounter
		S43.62XA	Sprain of left sternoclavicular joint, initial encounter
		S46.01[1,2,9]A	Strain of muscle(s) and tendon(s) of the rotator cuff of shoulder, initial encounter
		S46.11[1,2,9]A	Strain of muscle, fascia and tendon of long head of biceps, initial encounter
		S46.21[1,2,9]A	Strain of muscle, fascia and tendon of other parts of biceps, initial encounter
		S46.31[1,2,9]A	Strain of muscle, fascia and tendon of triceps, initial encounter
		S46.81[1,2,9]A	Strain of other muscle, fascia and tendons at shoulder and upper arm level, initial encounter

6th Character meanings for codes as indicated
1 right   2 left   9 unspecified

ICD-9-CM		ICD-10-CM	
843.8	Sprains and strains of other specified sites of hip and thigh	S73.19[1,2,9]A	Other sprain of hip, initial encounter
		S76.01[1,2,9]A	Strain of muscle, fascia and tendon of hip, initial encounter
		S76.21[1,2,9]A	Strain of adductor muscle, fascia and tendon of thigh, initial encounter
		S76.31[1,2,9]A	Strain of muscle, fascia and tendon of the posterior muscle group at thigh level, initial encounter
		S76.81[1,2,9]A	Strain of other specified muscles, fascia and tendons at thigh level, initial encounter
		6th Character meanings for codes as indicated 1 right 2 left 9 unspecified	

A rotator cuff tear in the shoulder region is a very common injury and is sometimes classified as a sprain. This injury usually involves the supraspinatus muscle but can occur in the other muscles or tendons in the shoulder. In the younger population (younger than 40), the tear is usually due to an earlier trauma to the area, such as a fracture or dislocation, or excessive overhead, repetitive movements required in certain occupations and sports. In the older population, this injury occurs as a result of normal wear and tear on the aging body. The majority of these injuries occur in the older population.

In ICD-9-CM, if rotator cuff tear is the only documentation by the physician, it is assumed to be traumatic, coding to an acute, traumatic injury by default of the Volume 2 index. This is the first and most obvious difference between the two classification systems. ICD-10-CM assumes with no further documentation that the injury is nontraumatic, following the clinical findings that the majority of rotator cuff tears are nontraumatic.

Both classification systems give the option to differentiate between the traumatic and nontraumatic if the documentation supports it; however, when the tear is specified as nontraumatic, ICD-10-CM further differentiates the injury by identifying the muscle or type of tendon (flexor or extensor) injured, using the terminology rotator cuff syndrome for a complete or incomplete tear of the supraspinous muscle but giving various codes for tears of the shoulder that do not include this muscle.

ICD-9-CM also describes a degenerative rotator cuff tear with a nonspecific code, whereas ICD-10-CM assumes that degenerative and nontraumatic are the same.

Coding for Rotator Cuff Tears

ICD-9-CM		ICD-10-CM	
840.4	Sprains and strains of rotator cuff (capsule)	S43.421A	Sprain of right rotator cuff capsule, initial encounter
		S43.422A	Sprain of left rotator cuff capsule, initial encounter
		S43.429A	Sprain of unspecified rotator cuff capsule, initial encounter
727.61	Complete rupture of rotator cuff, nontraumatic	M75.120	Complete rotator cuff tear or rupture of unspecified shoulder, not specified as traumatic
		M75.121	Complete rotator cuff tear or rupture of right shoulder, not specified as traumatic
		M75.122	Complete rotator cuff tear or rupture of left shoulder, not specified as traumatic

Comprehensive Anatomy and Physiology for ICD-10-CM and ICD-10-PCS Coding

ICD-9-CM		ICD-10-CM	
726.10	Disorders of **bursae** and tendons in shoulder region, unspecified (degenerative rotator cuff tear)	M75.100	Unspecified rotator cuff tear or rupture of unspecified shoulder, not specified as traumatic
		M75.101	Unspecified rotator cuff tear or rupture of right shoulder, not specified as traumatic
		M75.102	Unspecified rotator cuff tear or rupture of left shoulder, not specified as traumatic

> **DEFINITIONS**
>
> **bursa.** Cavity or sac containing fluid that occurs between articulating surfaces and reduces friction from moving parts. An anatomical structure frequently referenced in orthopedic notes, as it may become diseased or need removal.

Another common injury to the muscular system occurs during a laceration, which is usually considered a skin injury. Occasionally, a cut goes below the subcutaneous tissue and severs or injures the fascia, muscle, and tendons. This happens most frequently on injuries of the hand, as the surrounding tissues are thin and don't protect the tendons well.

When assigning a code for tendon injuries in ICD-9-CM, the only necessary information is the site of the injury and tendon involvement. ICD-10-CM goes much farther into the details of the location, not only the anatomical location of the laceration but also the digit the muscle controls. It also differentiates between intrinsic versus extrinsic muscles and tendons, and the movement type (flexor or extensor) of the muscle or tendon that is injured. Separate codes are required to report both the site of the open traumatic laceration and the tendon laceration. A detailed crosswalk between ICD-9-CM and ICD-10-CM outlines how to report tendon laceration injuries of the hand.

Coding for Tendon Laceration of the Hand

ICD-9-CM		ICD-10-CM	
882.2	Open wound of hand except finger(s) alone with tendon involvement	S66.021A	Laceration of long flexor muscle, fascia and tendon of right thumb at wrist and hand level, initial encounter
		S66.022A	Laceration of long flexor muscle, fascia and tendon of left thumb at wrist and hand level, initial encounter
		S66.029A	Laceration of long flexor muscle, fascia and tendon of unspecified thumb at wrist and hand level, initial encounter
		S66.12[0-9]A	Laceration of flexor muscle, fascia and tendon of finger at wrist and hand level, initial encounter
		S66.221A	Laceration of extensor muscle, fascia and tendon of right thumb at the wrist and hand level, initial encounter
		S66.222A	Laceration of extensor muscle, fascia and tendon of left thumb at the wrist and hand level, initial encounter
		S66.229A	Laceration of extensor muscle, fascia and tendon of unspecified thumb at the wrist and hand level, initial encounter
		S66.32[0-9]A	Laceration of extensor muscle, fascia and tendon of finger at the wrist and hand level, initial encounter
		S66.421A	Laceration of intrinsic muscle, fascia and tendon of right thumb at wrist and hand level, initial encounter
(Continued on next page)			

ICD-9-CM		ICD-10-CM	
882.2	Open wound of hand except finger(s) alone with tendon involvement *(Continued)*	S66.422A	Laceration of intrinsic muscle, fascia and tendon of left thumb at wrist and hand level, initial encounter
		\multicolumn{2}{l	}{**6th Character meanings for codes as indicated** 0 right index 1 left index 2 right middle 3 left middle 4 right ring 5 left ring 6 right little 7 left little 8 other 9 unspecified}
		S66.429A	Laceration of intrinsic muscle, fascia and tendon of unspecified thumb at wrist and hand level, initial encounter
		S66.52[0-9]A	Laceration of intrinsic muscle, fascia and tendon of other and unspecified finger at wrist and hand level, initial encounter
		S66.821A	Laceration of other specified muscles, fascia and tendons at right wrist and hand level, initial encounter
		S66.822A	Laceration of other specified muscles, fascia and tendons at left wrist and hand level, initial encounter
		S66.829A	Laceration of other specified muscles, fascia and tendons at unspecified wrist and hand level, initial encounter
		S66.921A	Laceration of unspecified muscles, fascia and tendons at right wrist and hand level, initial encounter
		S66.922A	Laceration of unspecified muscle, fascia and tendon at left wrist and hand level, initial encounter
		S66.929A	Laceration of unspecified muscle, fascia and tendon at wrist and hand level of unspecified side, initial encounter
		\multicolumn{2}{l	}{**6th Character meanings for codes as indicated** 0 right index 1 left index 2 right middle 3 left middle 4 right ring 5 left ring 6 right little 7 left little 8 other 9 unspecified}

Infections and Inflammations

In addition to injuries, tendons and tendon sheaths can suffer from inflammation due to other disease processes such as infection. Inflammation of the tendon and tendon sheath is called tenosynovitis. This occurs most often in the tendons of the wrist, ankle, and feet. A flare-up due to overuse of the tendons of the abductor pollicis longus and extensor pollicis brevis of the wrist at the base of the thumb is called de Quervain tenosynovitis. Because these muscles and tendons cross over the **radial styloid process**, the condition can also be called radial stylus tenosynovitis. Transient tenosynovitis is inflammation of the hip joint in children from 3 to 10 years of age that dissipates within a week.

ICD-9-CM recognizes the most common anatomical locations of tenosynovitis by providing specific codes for the hand and wrist and the foot and ankle, but does not distinguish the cause of the inflammation. In ICD-10-CM, the most common causes of tenosynovitis are given specific categories, each of which includes the major joints of the body, rather than just the most likely joints to be affected.

> **DEFINITIONS**
>
> **radial styloid process.** Projection of the distal lateral radial bone.

Coding for Tenosynovitis

ICD-9-CM		ICD-10-CM	
727.04	Radial styloid tenosynovitis	M65.4	Radial styloid tenosynovitis [de Quervain]
727.05	Other tenosynovitis of hand and wrist	M65.831	Other synovitis and tenosynovitis, right forearm
		M65.832	Other synovitis and tenosynovitis, left forearm
		M65.839	Other synovitis and tenosynovitis, unspecified forearm
		M65.841	Other synovitis and tenosynovitis, right hand
		M65.842	Other synovitis and tenosynovitis, left hand
		M65.849	Other synovitis and tenosynovitis, unspecified hand
727.06	Tenosynovitis of foot and ankle	M65.871	Other synovitis and tenosynovitis, right ankle and foot
		M65.872	Other synovitis and tenosynovitis, left ankle and foot
		M65.879	Other synovitis and tenosynovitis, unspecified ankle and foot
727.09	Other synovitis and tenosynovitis	M65.10	Other infective (teno)synovitis, unspecified site
		M65.11[1,2,9]	Other infective (teno)synovitis, shoulder
		M65.12[1,2,9]	Other infective (teno)synovitis, elbow
		M65.13[1,2,9]	Other infective (teno)synovitis, wrist
		M65.14[1,2,9]	Other infective (teno)synovitis, hand
		M65.15[1,2,9]	Other infective (teno)synovitis, hip
		M65.16[1,2,9]	Other infective (teno)synovitis, knee
		M65.17[1,2,9]	Other infective (teno)synovitis, ankle and foot
		M65.18	Other infective (teno)synovitis, other site
		M65.19	Other infective (teno)synovitis, multiple sites
		M65.80	Other synovitis and tenosynovitis, unspecified site
		M65.81[1,2,9]	Other synovitis and tenosynovitis, shoulder
		M65.82[1,2,9]	Other synovitis and tenosynovitis, upper arm
		M65.85[1,2,9]	Other synovitis and tenosynovitis, thigh
		M65.86[1,2,9]	Other synovitis and tenosynovitis, lower leg
		M65.88	Other synovitis and tenosynovitis, other site
		M65.89	Other synovitis and tenosynovitis, multiple sites
		M67.30	Transient synovitis, unspecified site
		M67.31[1,2,9]	Transient synovitis, shoulder
		M67.32[1,2,9]	Transient synovitis, elbow
		M67.33[1,2,9]	Transient synovitis, wrist
		M67.34[1,2,9]	Transient synovitis, hand
		M67.35[1,2,9]	Transient synovitis, hip
		M67.36[1,2,9]	Transient synovitis, knee

6th Character meanings for codes as indicated
1 right   2 left   9 unspecified

(Continued on next page)

ICD-9-CM	ICD-10-CM	
727.09 Other synovitis and tenosynovitis *(Continued)*	M67.37[1,2,9]	Transient synovitis, ankle and foot
	M67.38	Transient synovitis, other site
	M67.39	Transient synovitis, multiple sites
	6th Character meanings for codes as indicated 1 right 2 left 9 unspecified	

Slightly different from tenosynovitis, in that it affects only the tendon without swelling of the tendon sheath, is tendinitis. This condition is usually reported with a vague set of **enthesopathy** ICD-9-CM codes. These code sets include inflammation of the bursa, also called bursitis and various other joint afflictions, such as **osteophytes** and bone spurs, for which ICD-10-CM has assigned specific codes. The table below outlines the more specific conditions that were once reported in a general manner.

Coding for Enthesopathy

ICD-9-CM		ICD-10-CM	
726.30	Unspecified enthesopathy of elbow	M25.721	Osteophyte, right elbow
		M25.722	Osteophyte, left elbow
		M25.729	Osteophyte, unspecified elbow
726.39	Other enthesopathy of elbow region	M70.30	Other bursitis of elbow, unspecified elbow
		M70.31	Other bursitis of elbow, right elbow
		M70.32	Other bursitis of elbow, left elbow
726.4	Enthesopathy of wrist and carpus	M25.731	Osteophyte, right wrist
		M25.732	Osteophyte, left wrist
		M25.739	Osteophyte, unspecified wrist
		M25.741	Osteophyte, right hand
		M25.742	Osteophyte, left hand
		M25.749	Osteophyte, unspecified hand
		M70.10	Bursitis, unspecified hand
		M70.11	Bursitis, right hand
		M70.12	Bursitis, left hand
		M77.20	**Periarthritis,** unspecified wrist
		M77.21	Periarthritis, right wrist
		M77.22	Periarthritis, left wrist
726.5	Enthesopathy of hip region	M25.751	Osteophyte, right hip
		M25.752	Osteophyte, left hip
		M25.759	Osteophyte, unspecified hip
		M70.6[0,1,2]	Trochanteric bursitis, hip
		M70.7[0,1,2]	Other bursitis of hip
		M76.0[0,1,2]	Gluteal tendinitis, hip
		M76.1[0,1,2]	Psoas tendinitis, hip
		M76.2[0,1,2]	Iliac crest spur, hip
		M76.3[0,1,2]	Iliotibial band syndrome, leg
		5th Character meanings for codes as indicated 0 unspecified 1 right 2 left	
726.60	Unspecified enthesopathy of knee	M25.761	Osteophyte, right knee
		M25.762	Osteophyte, left knee
		M25.769	Osteophyte, unspecified knee
		M70.50	Other bursitis of knee, unspecified knee
		M70.51	Other bursitis of knee, right knee
		M70.52	Other bursitis of knee, left knee
726.69	Other enthesopathy of knee	M76.899	Other specified enthesopathies of unspecified lower limb, excluding foot

> **DEFINITIONS**
>
> **enthesopathy.** Disorders that occur at points where muscle, tendons, and ligaments attach to bones or joint capsules.
>
> **osteophytes.** Bony outgrowth.
>
> **periarthritis.** Inflammation of tissues around a joint.

Comprehensive Anatomy and Physiology for ICD-10-CM and ICD-10-PCS Coding

📖 **DEFINITIONS**

metatarsalgia. Foot condition in the metatarsal region of the foot.

ICD-9-CM	ICD-10-CM	
726.70 Unspecified enthesopathy of ankle and tarsus	M25.771	Osteophyte, right ankle
	M25.772	Osteophyte, left ankle
	M25.773	Osteophyte, unspecified ankle
	M25.774	Osteophyte, right foot
	M25.775	Osteophyte, left foot
	M25.776	Osteophyte, unspecified foot
	M76.899	Other specified enthesopathies of unspecified lower limb, excluding foot
	M77.40	*Metatarsalgia,* unspecified foot
	M77.41	Metatarsalgia, right foot
	M77.42	Metatarsalgia, left foot
726.79 Other enthesopathy of ankle and tarsus	M76.70	Peroneal tendinitis, unspecified leg
	M76.71	Peroneal tendinitis, right leg
	M76.72	Peroneal tendinitis, left leg
	M77.50	Other enthesopathy of unspecified foot
	M77.51	Other enthesopathy of right foot
	M77.52	Other enthesopathy of left foot

Another cause of tendinitis and bursitis is a buildup of calcium deposits within the tissues. ICD-9-CM has a vague code assignment for these conditions, not distinguishing what tissue is affected or the site. ICD-10-CM codes, however, reflect whether the deposits are in the tendon or bursa and the anatomical location.

Coding for Calcium Deposits in the Tendons and Bursa

ICD-9-CM	ICD-10-CM	
727.82 Calcium deposits in tendon and bursa	M65.20	Calcific tendinitis, unspecified site
	M65.22[1,2,9]	Calcific tendinitis, upper arm
	M65.23[1,2,9]	Calcific tendinitis, forearm
	M65.24[1,2,9]	Calcific tendinitis, hand
	M65.25[1,2,9]	Calcific tendinitis, thigh
	M65.26[1,2,9]	Calcific tendinitis, lower leg
	M65.27[1,2,9]	Calcific tendinitis, ankle and foot
	M65.28	Calcific tendinitis, other site
	M65.29	Calcific tendinitis, multiple sites
	M71.40	Calcium deposit in bursa, unspecified site
	M71.42[1,2,9]	Calcium deposit in bursa, elbow
	M71.43[1,2,9]	Calcium deposit in bursa, wrist
	M71.44[1,2,9]	Calcium deposit in bursa, hand
	M71.45[1,2,9]	Calcium deposit in bursa, hip
	M71.46[1,2,9]	Calcium deposit in bursa, knee
	M71.47[1,2,9]	Calcium deposit in bursa, ankle and foot
	M71.48	Calcium deposit in bursa, other site
	M71.49	Calcium deposit in bursa, multiple sites
	6th Character meanings for codes as indicated	
	1 right 2 left 9 unspecified	

Most of the other inflammations and infections that affect the muscular system are reported similarly between the two classification systems. The main variance is that in ICD-10-CM, the laterality of the disorder is specified.

Other Abnormalities

Sometimes, muscle tissue becomes more like bone or cartilage and hardens, or ossifies. There are multiple types of this disease, called generally myositis ossificans. The most common type, known as myositis ossificans traumatica, is a localized ossification usually occurring after trauma to the muscle. This disease is most commonly seen in the arms or muscles of the quadriceps. Hardening that occurs locally without mention of trauma is called myositis ossificans circumscripta. Occasionally, second- and third-degree burns cause the muscles in the area of the burns to calcify.

A more serious and often fatal type of muscle hardening is myositis ossificans progressiva. In this rare genetic disease, each muscle progressively becomes ossified until the patient is completely stiff. Most patients with this condition suffer from fatal respiratory infections and pneumonias due to the hardening of the muscles involved in lung function.

It is more important in ICD-10-CM than in ICD-9-CM to know the type or cause of the ossification to assign the code. ICD-9-CM automatically assumes unspecified myositis ossificans is traumatic, as this is the most common type of the condition. ICD-10-CM, however, defaults to a vague code of "other," making understanding the underlying cause important to code selection. Both classification systems distinguish between the three main types of the disease, circumscripta, traumatica, and progressiva, using similar terminology. ICD-10-CM also provides the detail of the body site and laterality for each category, making this a key detail, especially in myositis progressiva, in reporting and tracking the progression of the disease over time. The addition of "in (due to)" in the ICD-10-CM index provides further division of myositis ossificans, clarifying if the condition is due to burn or paralysis.

It is noteworthy that ICD-9-CM treats calcification and ossification as one and the same disease. However, as is clinically correct, ICD-10-CM gives each general term its own category. Ossification is the forming of new bone tissue within the muscles or tendons, whereas calcification is the formation of crystals, usually calcium based, in the soft tissue. The process of calcification occurs during the ossification process, but they are not synonymous. Calcification can occur without ossification.

Coding for Myositis Ossificans

ICD-9-CM		ICD-10-CM	
728.10	Unspecified calcification and ossification	M61.20	Paralytic calcification and ossification of muscle, unspecified site
		M61.21[1,2,9]	Paralytic calcification and ossification of muscle, shoulder
		M61.22[1,2,9]	Paralytic calcification and ossification of muscle, upper arm
		M61.23[1,2,9]	Paralytic calcification and ossification of muscle, forearm
		M61.24[1,2,9]	Paralytic calcification and ossification of muscle, hand
		M61.25[1,2,9]	Paralytic calcification and ossification of muscle, thigh
		M61.26[1,2,9]	Paralytic calcification and ossification of muscle, lower leg
		M61.27[1,2,9]	Paralytic calcification and ossification of muscle, ankle and foot
		M61.28	Paralytic calcification and ossification of muscle, other site
		M61.29	Paralytic calcification and ossification of muscle, multiple sites
		M61.9	Calcification and ossification of muscle, unspecified
		6th Character meanings for codes as indicated 1 right 2 left 9 unspecified	

ICD-9-CM		ICD-10-CM	
728.19	Other muscular calcification and ossification	M61.30	Calcification and ossification of muscles associated with burns, unspecified site
		M61.31[1,2,9]	Calcification and ossification of muscle associated with burns, shoulder
		M61.32[1,2,9]	Calcification and ossification of muscle associated with burns, upper arm
		M61.33[1,2,9]	Calcification and ossification of muscle associated with burns, forearm
		M61.34[1,2,9]	Calcification and ossification of muscle associated with burns, hand
		M61.35[1,2,9]	Calcification and ossification of muscle associated with burns, thigh
		M61.36[1,2,9]	Calcification and ossification of muscle associated with burns, lower leg
		M61.37[1,2,9]	Calcification and ossification of muscle associated with burns, ankle and foot
		M61.38	Calcification and ossification of muscle associated with burns, other site
		M61.39	Calcification and ossification of muscle associated with burns, multiple sites
		M61.40	Other calcification of muscle, unspecified site
		M61.41[1,2,9]	Other calcification of muscle, shoulder
		M61.42[1,2,9]	Other calcification of muscle, upper arm
		M61.43[1,2,9]	Other calcification of muscle, forearm
		M61.44[1,2,9]	Other calcification of muscle, hand
		M61.45[1,2,9]	Other calcification of muscle, thigh
		M61.46[1,2,9]	Other calcification of muscle, lower leg
		M61.47[1,2,9]	Other calcification of muscle, ankle and foot
		M61.48	Other calcification of muscle, other site
		M61.49	Other calcification of muscle, multiple sites
		M61.50	Other ossification of muscle, unspecified site
		M61.51[1,2,9]	Other ossification of muscle, shoulder
		M61.52[1,2,9]	Other ossification of muscle, upper arm
		M61.53[1,2,9]	Other ossification of muscle, forearm
		M61.54[1,2,9]	Other ossification of muscle, hand
		M61.55[1,2,9]	Other ossification of muscle, thigh
		M61.56[1,2,9]	Other ossification of muscle, lower leg
		M61.57[1,2,9]	Other ossification of muscle, ankle and foot
		M61.58	Other ossification of muscle, other site
		M61.59	Other ossification of muscle, multiple sites

6th Character meanings for codes as indicated
1 right   2 left   9 unspecified

Some abnormalities in muscle function are considered manifestations of an underlying condition. Many of these are reported with general codes in ICD-9-CM. For example, there are many types of abnormal, involuntary movements. ICD-9-CM lumps all of them into a single code, although these different movements can indicate a disease. ICD-9-CM codes therefore do not convey all of the information about the type of abnormal movement. In contrast, ICD-10-CM has unbundled these symptoms into four unique types of movement:

- **Abnormal head movements:** Include flopping, nodding, tic, chorea, and myoclonic jerks of the head and neck.

Chapter 5. ICD-10-CM: Nervous System

Anatomic Overview

The nervous system is a complex network of specialized organs, tissues, and cells that coordinate the body's actions and functions. It consists of two main subdivisions: the central nervous system and the peripheral nervous system. The central nervous system includes the brain and the spinal cord, and the peripheral nervous system includes the sense organs and the nerves that link the organs, muscles, and glands to the central nervous system. Nerves designated as cranial nerves originate in the brain and branch through the structures of the head, including the face and cranial sense organs (e.g., eyes, ears). Four groups of peripheral nerves branch from the spinal cord at cervical, thoracic, lumbar, and sacral levels and innervate the corresponding regions of the body.

The central nervous system (CNS) is composed of the brain, the spinal cord, and their associated connective tissues. The brain and spinal cord function as central processing units to receive, integrate, and interpret information, as well as to formulate a response to stimuli.

Figure 5.1: Brain

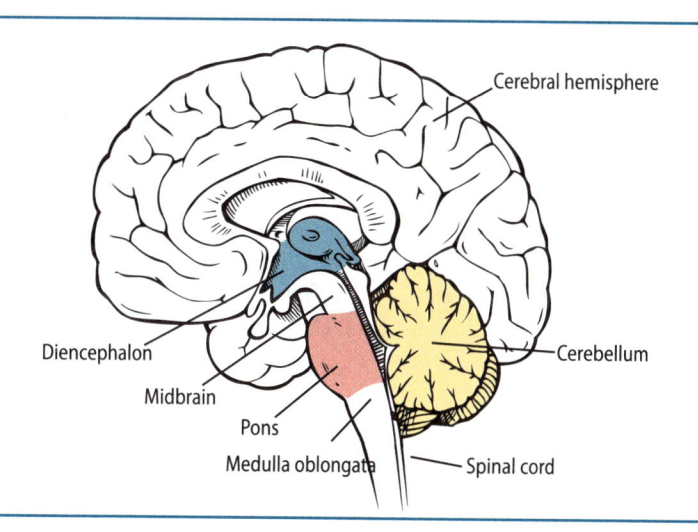

The brain can be divided into several regions:

- **Cerebral hemispheres:** These form the largest part of the brain, occupying the anterior and middle cranial fossae in the skull.
- **Diencephalon:** This includes the thalamus, hypothalamus, epithalamus, and subthalamus, and forms the central core of the brain.
- **Midbrain:** The midbrain is located at the junction of the middle and posterior cranial fossae.
- **Pons:** This part of the brain is in the anterior part of the posterior cranial fossa; fibers within the pons connect the cerebral hemisphere with its opposite cerebellar hemisphere.

- **Medulla oblongata:** This region is continuous with the spinal cord and controls the respiratory and cardiovascular systems.
- **Cerebellum:** The cerebellum overlies the pons and medulla and controls motor functions that regulate muscle tone, coordination, and posture.

The spinal column, which encloses the spinal cord, consists of vertebrae linked by cartilaginous intervertebral discs held together by ligaments. The spinal cord extends from the first lumbar vertebrae to the medulla at the base of the brain. The outer layer of the spinal cord consists of myelin-sheathed nerve fibers that are bundled and that conduct impulses triggered by pressure, pain, heat, and other sensory stimuli or conduct motor impulses activating muscles and glands. The inner layer (i.e., gray matter) is primarily composed of nerve cell bodies. The central canal, within the gray matter, circulates the cerebrospinal fluid.

Three connective layers of meninges wrap around the spinal cord and cover the brain. The pia mater is the innermost layer, the arachnoid lies in the middle, and the dura mater is the outside layer, to which the spinal nerves are attached. The 31 pairs of spinal nerves deliver impulses to the spinal cord, which in turn relays them to the brain. Conversely, motor impulses generated in the brain are relayed by the spinal cord to spinal nerves, which pass the impulses to muscles and glands. Nerve fibers in the spinal cord usually do not regenerate if injured by trauma or disease.

Figure 5.2: Spinal Column

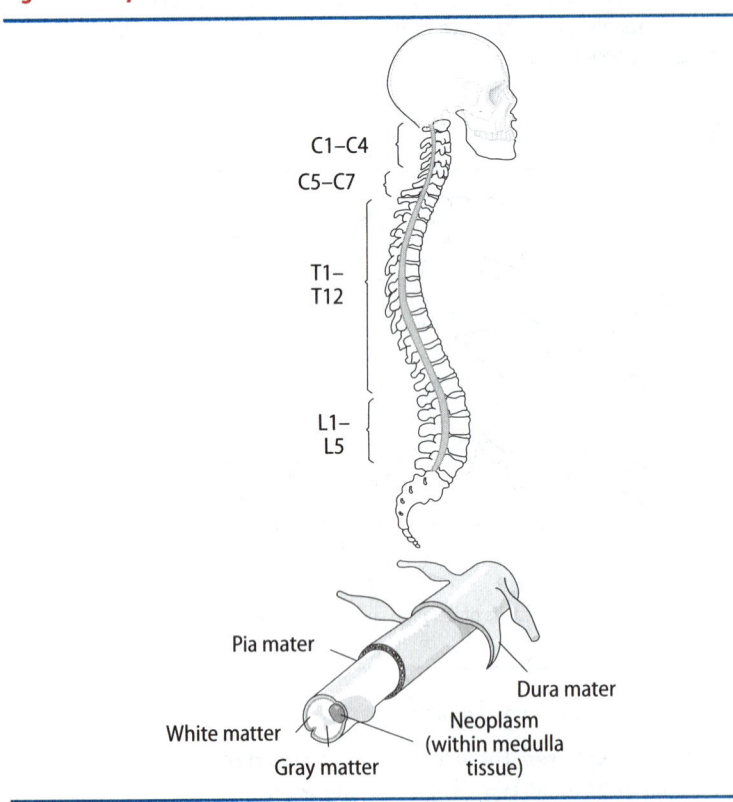

The structures of the peripheral nervous system (PNS) consist of cranial and spinal nerves, which serve as communication lines between the CNS and the rest of the body. The PNS may be subdivided into the autonomic and somatic nervous systems.

The autonomic nervous system facilitates automatic bodily processes—parasympathetic and sympathetic. These processes convey sensory impulses from the blood vessels, heart, and all of the organs in the chest, abdomen, and pelvis through nerves to the central nervous system (specifically the medulla, pons, and hypothalamus within the brain). These impulses are automatic by nature—reflex responses that occur largely without conscious thought. The efferent autonomic nerves affect reactions in the cardiovascular system and organs of the body in response to stimuli, such as environmental temperature, posture, food intake, stressful experiences, and other changes to which all individuals are exposed. The parasympathetic division of the autonomic nervous system controls anabolism (energy storage); an anabolic activity occurs in normal, nonstressful situations, such as initiating digestion after eating. In general, sympathetic processes reverse parasympathetic responses in defense or in response to stress. In defense situations, for example, catabolism (energy use) produces an increased heart rate, an expansion of the lungs to hold more energy, dilated pupils, and blood flow to the muscles and tissues.

Figure 5.3: Peripheral Nervous System

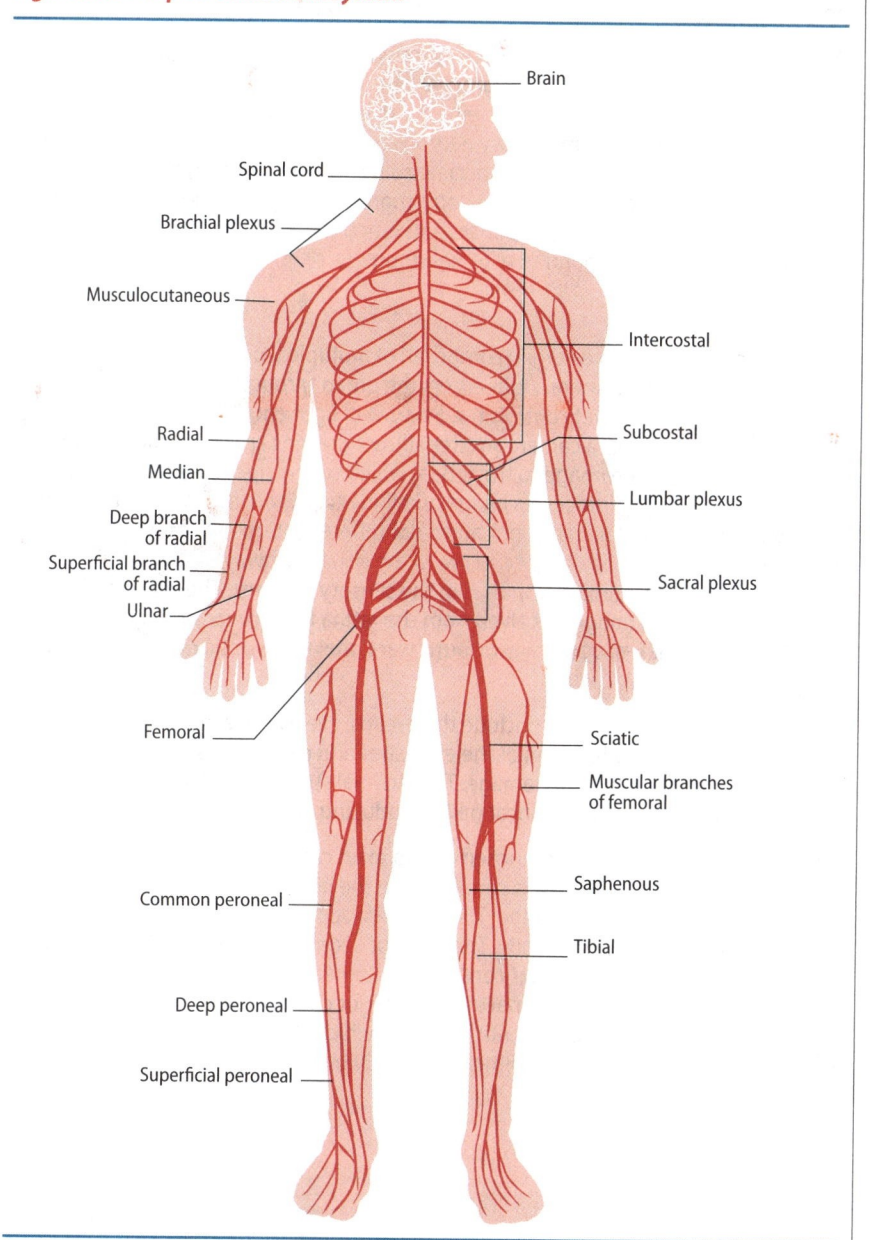

> **INTERESTING A & P FACT**
>
> The left side of the human brain controls the right side of the body and vice-versa.

As the PNS is composed of nerves that project to the limbs, heart, skin, and other organs outside the brain, it controls the somatic (or bodily) nervous system. This system regulates voluntary control over skeletal muscles in response to stimuli. The SNS processes sensory stimuli and controls voluntary muscle systems within the body by neurotransmission of signals within the efferent, or motor, nerves. This process contrasts with the autonomic nervous system, which generally functions involuntarily, independent of conscious control.

The sympathetic and parasympathetic divisions work together to process and facilitate response to stimuli. These structures control voluntary actions and transmit sensation from the skin (somatic nervous system) and sense organs. Two chemicals, acetylcholine and norepinephrine, act as neurotransmitters that facilitate communication with the autonomic nervous system. Specifically, cholinergic nerve fibers secrete acetylcholine, and adrenergic nerve fibers secrete norepinephrine. In general, whereas acetylcholine causes parasympathetic (inhibiting) effects, norepinephrine causes sympathetic (stimulating) effects.

> **INTERESTING A & P FACT**
>
> It is estimated that there are more nerve cells in the human brain than there are stars in the Milky Way.

At the cellular level, efferent neurons relay messages away from the brain or spinal cord to the muscles and organs. In contrast, sensory (afferent) neurons relay stimuli from nerve receptors to the brain or spinal cord. Interneurons are specialized nerve cells that relay impulses from sensory neurons to motor neurons. These specialized cells all make up a complex, highly-specialized network in the body that may be considered the "control" center of the body, monitoring conditions within the body to regulate and control bodily responses and functions, while transmitting signals to receive, interpret, and respond to external stimuli.

Eye and Adnexa

The human eye is a complex organ composed of multiple working parts that function together similarly to a camera. Light enters the organ through the cornea. The iris (colored portion of the eye) controls the amount of light entering by constricting or dilating the pupil, just as a camera shutter adjusts the lens aperture. The lens adjusts the focus and sends the image to the retina, which covers the posterior two-thirds of the interior eyeball and processes images similarly to camera film. Within the retina, the rod and cone cells facilitate light and color differentiation and depth perception. The image is then sent via the optic nerve to the visual pathways of the brain with the assistance of electrochemical impulses in the sensory neurons. The visual pathways that facilitate optical images received from the retina to be processed by the brain include the optic nerve, optic chiasm, optic tract, thalamus, optic radiations, and primary visual cerebral cortex.

Accessory structures of the eye include the eyelids, eyelashes, eyebrows, and lacrimal apparatus. The primary function of the eyelashes and eyebrows is to protect the eye from foreign matter and light damage. The lacrimal structures (glands, ducts, and puncta) facilitate protective lubrication by producing and draining tears.

The eye is a spherical organ composed of two main compartments: a smaller, curved section (anterior segment) that is connected to the larger spherical region (posterior segment) by the scleral membrane. The posterior segment contains a gelatinous substance called the vitreous body. The anterior segment is the fluid-filled (aqueous humor) front third of the eye that contains the cornea, iris, ciliary body, and lens. The anterior segment contains two spaces: the anterior chamber, which lies between the cornea and the iris, and the posterior chamber, which lies between the iris and vitreous. The lens is connected to the ciliary body by fine, transparent fibers and a suspensory ligament.

Figure 5.4: Adnexa

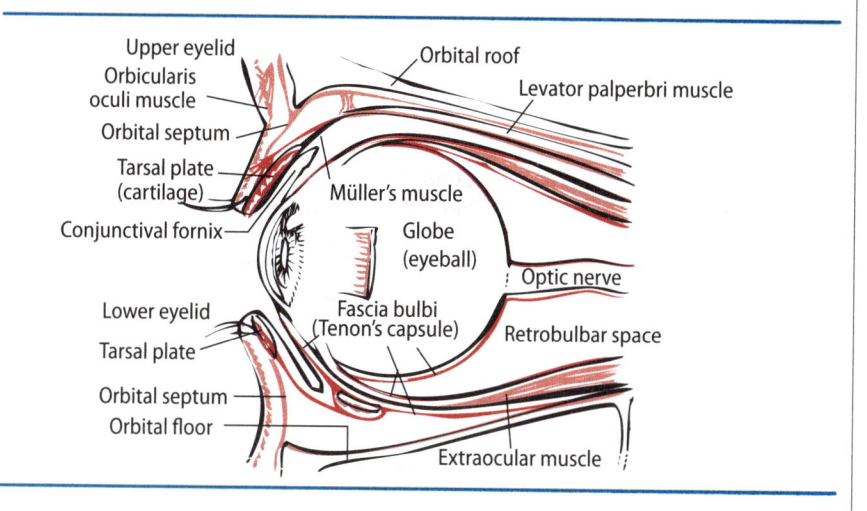

Although the sclera connects the two chambers of the eye, the organ is surrounded by multiple membranes. The outermost layer contains the cornea (anterior segment) and the sclera (posterior segment); the middle layer contains the choroid (vascular layer), ciliary body, and the iris. The innermost layer is the retina, a highly vascularized photosensitive membrane. These inner layers of the eye can be visualized with an ophthalmoscope during dilated eye examination.

The eyes adjust to the motions of the head by a set of extraocular muscles connected to the outer surface of each eye. These muscles allow the eye to focus and receive images, while adjusting to motion on a small area of the retina called the fovea, which facilitates visual acuity. Extraocular muscles include the lateral, medial, and superior recti, and the inferior and superior obliques. These muscles allow the eyes to rotate and are responsible for coordinating and rotating both eyes synchronously. Images are stabilized during movement of the head by the vestibulo-ocular reflex, which allows the image to remain situated at the center of the visual field.

Figure 5.5: Eye Musculature

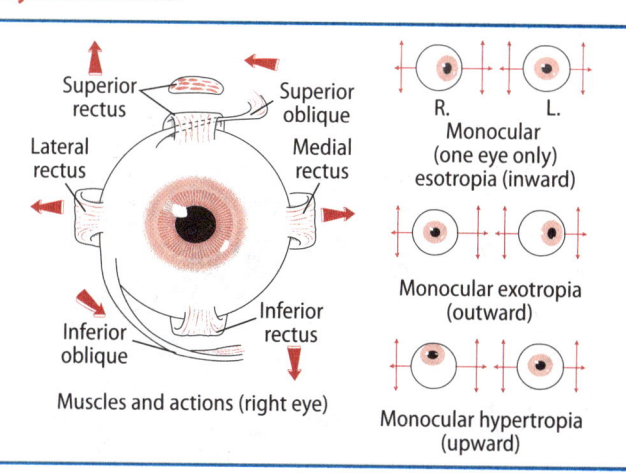

Close-range visual adjustment involves three processes to facilitate image focus on the retina. For two eyes to converge at the same point to visualize an object, the eyes rotate to allow projection of the image on the center of the retina in both eyes. Convergence describes the ability to focus a nearby object by means of rotating the eyes together, whereas divergence is the rotation of the eyes apart to focus on an object in the distance. Disorders of accommodation occur when vergence

Comprehensive Anatomy and Physiology for ICD-10-CM and ICD-10-PCS Coding

> **DEFINITIONS**
>
> **refract (vision).** Alteration of light waves as they pass from one medium into another of unequal optical density.

movements are impaired and the normal process of focus and accommodation are disrupted. Accommodation is the process by which the eye changes the convergence or divergence of light to maintain focus upon an image as the proximity or distance changes. This process is controlled by the ciliary muscles that surround the lens and contract and relax to *refract* light as needed to maintain an object in focus.

There are many diseases, disorders, injuries, congenital anomalies, and age-related changes that affect the eyes and surrounding structures. These conditions vary widely in cause, severity, and onset. While some conditions are of sudden, acute onset (e.g., infection, trauma) others entail anatomic and physiologic processes that follow a progressive or gradual decline. The presence of genetic predisposition, congenital anomalies, or systemic disease contributes to eye disorders and vision problems. For example, diabetes mellitus is a disease increasing in incidence in the United States that can lead to potentially serious retinal damage and precipitate cataract formation and early-onset glaucoma. The natural aging process also contributes to certain degenerations within the ocular structures that facilitate vision, the most common of which include eyelid laxity, liquefaction of the vitreous with opacification, retinal degeneration, cataract formation, and normal age-related pupillary changes. Although the cause of myopia may be multifactorial if not uncertain, it has been estimated that the prevalence of near-sightedness in the United States affects one out of 10 children and two out of 10 adults.

Ear

In human anatomy, the ear detects sound and facilitates equilibrium of balance and body position. The ear can be anatomically divided into external, middle, and inner sections. The outer ear (also called the pinna or auricle) is made up of cartilaginous and cutaneous tissue. It acts as a funnel for sound waves, which travel through the pinna into the external auditory canal, a short tube that terminates at the tympanic membrane, or eardrum. The external auditory canal contains tiny hairs and specialized sebaceous (oil) glands that secrete a protective, waxy substance called cerumen.

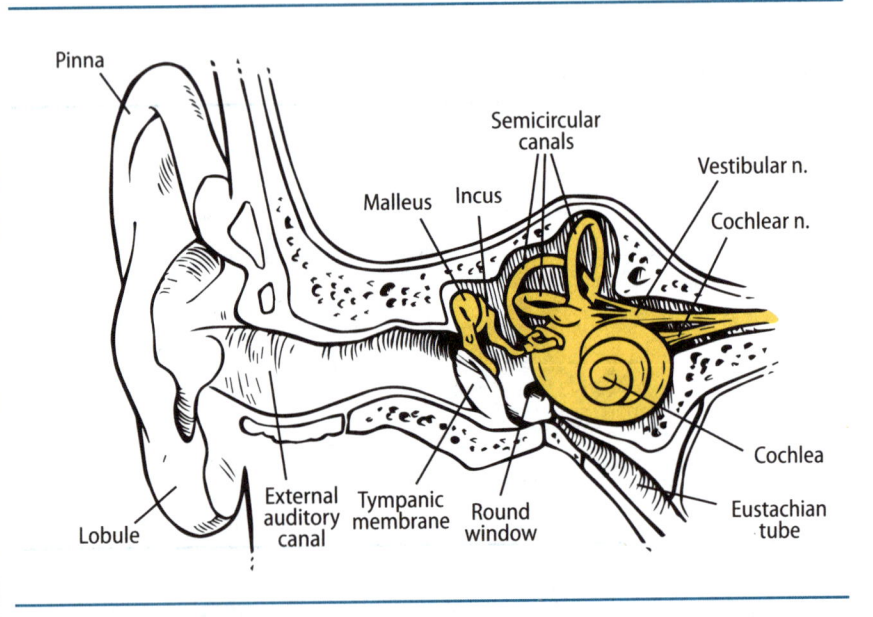

Figure 5.6: Ear Anatomy

The middle ear is an air-filled cavity behind the tympanic membrane. Three tiny ear bones (ossicles) vibrate in response to sound waves. These bones include the malleus (hammer), incus (anvil), and stapes (stirrup), which vibrate and strike against the tympanic membrane to amplify the sound waves. The malleus resembles a hammer, in that it contains a long process that is attached to the mobile portion of the tympanic membrane (eardrum). The incus connects the malleus and stapes. The three bones are arranged so that movement of the tympanic membrane causes movement of the malleus, which causes movement of the incus, which causes movement of the stapes. Two tiny ligaments (tensor tympani, tensor stapedius) adjust the tension of the tympanic membrane to protect the inner ear from loud noises. The stapes strikes against the oval window, which is in front of another membranous opening, the round window. The movement of the stapes against these membranes moves the fluid within the cochlea (a portion of the inner ear). The vibrations of the ossicles stimulate the fluid-filled cochlea of the inner ear to transform sound into nerve impulses that are passed on to the brain via the eighth cranial (auditory) nerve.

Also within the middle ear is the eustachian (auditory) tube, the primary functions of which are to drain fluid from the middle ear into the pharynx and to equalize pressure between the outer and middle ears. It is a hollow, tubular structure that normally remains collapsed but expands in response to changes in air pressure.

The inner ear contains a series of canals: the cochlea, the vestibule, and the semicircular canals. These structures are encased within the temporal bone of the skull. The cochlea is a spiral-shaped (snail-like) structure filled with fluid. The semicircular canals (labyrinths) contain receptor cells to facilitate balance together with the vestibular apparatus (semicircular ducts, utricle, and saccule). Specialized epithelial and ciliary cells (microscopic hairs) within the cochlea release chemical neurotransmitters to a portion of the temporal lobe within the cerebral cortex that processes sound sensory input. The eighth cranial (auditory) nerve originates from the brainstem, with its point of insertion in the inner ear. Sound waves are received by the structures of the external ear, pass through the vibrating structures within the middle ear, and are transferred to the oval window of the cochlea in the inner ear, as described above. The fluid inside the ducts flows against specialized sensory cells in the organ of Corti, which is situated on the basilar membrane in the cochlea and stimulates the auditory nerve to transmit the information to the brain. The stimulation of thousands of tiny, specialized hair cells in the semicircular canals not only plays a part in auditory processing, but is also key in the sensation of equilibrium. The hair cells, microvilli, release neurotransmitters to the sensory neurons, which are passed to the vestibulocochlear nerve. These impulses are then passed on to the brainstem, cerebellum, thalamus, and cerebral cortex for processing, translation, and stimulation of responsive mechanisms.

> **INTERESTING A & P FACT**
>
> The stapes is the smallest bone that has a name in the human body.

Anatomy and Pathophysiology and the ICD-10-CM Code Set

The nervous system can be affected by many types of disease. The tissues that make up or protect portions of the nervous system are susceptible to degeneration, neoplasm, infection, and other pathology.

The nervous system works closely with other organ systems within the body to maintain homeostatic function. For example, the nervous system sends and receives information from the endocrine system to produce and inhibit secretion of hormones to perform a variety of bodily functions, including regulating metabolism. For this reason, endocrine manifestations may be commonly associated with certain nervous system diseases, and vice versa. Additionally, the nervous system is vulnerable to infectious agents such as bacteria, parasites, and viruses, resulting in conditions such as encephalomyelitis, meningitis, and certain infectious neuropathies.

See the *ICD-10-CM Official Guidelines for Coding and Reporting* for specific guidance regarding coding certain nervous system disorders, including pain, and reporting conditions that affect the **dominant** versus the **nondominant** side.

> **DEFINITIONS**
>
> **dominant (side).** Exercising the most influence or control (left-handed versus right-handed).
>
> **nondominant (side).** Pertaining to that with the least influence or control.

Inflammatory Diseases of the Central Nervous System

As in ICD-9-CM, certain conditions are described by multiple codes or the codes describing them must be sequenced in a particular way. However, because ICD-10-CM has greater data granularity, there are fewer manifestation code edits. For example, code section G00–G09 Inflammatory diseases of the central nervous system, contains only five codes in ICD-10-CM, down from 18 such codes in ICD-9-CM. A manifestation code is not allowed to be reported as a principal or first-listed diagnosis because it describes a manifestation of some other underlying disease, not the disease itself. This is important to understand when reporting CNS infections, since additional codes often are assigned for the causal infection or organism. Certain CNS infections represent a primary infection, one originating within the central nervous system. Other CNS infections present as secondary sites from an infection that originated elsewhere within the body. Therefore, it is important to understand the clinical terminology as it applies to many of the disease classifications included in this chapter.

Generally, the ICD-10-CM code set describes conditions in a more clinically or anatomically specific manner than the ICD-9-CM system. However, it is interesting to note that at the time of this publication, there are some instances in which ICD-10-CM is less specific than ICD-9-CM:

ICD-9-CM:

320.81 **Anaerobic meningitis**
Bacteroides (fragilis)
Gram-negative anaerobes

ICD-10-CM:

G00.8 **Other bacterial meningitis**
Meningitis due to Escherichia coli
Meningitis due to Friedländer's bacillus
Meningitis due to Klebsiella
Use additional code to further identify organism (B96.-)

In this example, ICD-9-CM provides a single, specific classification code for anaerobic meningitis, whereas ICD-10-CM reclassifies the condition to a general "other" category, requiring an additional code to identify the organism. In this example, ICD-10-CM requires multiple codes, and ICD-9-CM classifies the condition to a single, specific classification code. Certain conditions represented with unique classification codes in ICD-9-CM require more than one code in ICD-10-CM. In these instances, manifestation-etiology edits indicate that the manifestation code must be sequenced secondary to the underlying disease or condition:

Coding for Meningitis

ICD-9-CM		ICD-10-CM	
321.1	Meningitis in other fungal diseases	G02	Meningitis in other infectious and parasitic diseases classified elsewhere
321.2	Meningitis due to viruses not elsewhere classified	G02	Meningitis in other infectious and parasitic diseases classified elsewhere
321.3	Meningitis due to trypanosomiasis	G02	Meningitis in other infectious and parasitic diseases classified elsewhere

ICD-10-CM:

G02   **Meningitis in other infectious and parasitic diseases classified elsewhere**
        Code first underlying disease, such as:
            African trypanosomiasis (B56.-)
            poliovirus infection (A80.-)

The examples above illustrate reclassification of infectious meningitis to the causal infectious disease code in chapter 1 of ICD-10-CM, thereby conserving space within the classification for future expansion and minimizing redundancies. The less specific code description in ICD-10-CM does not mean that coders do not need to be knowledgeable about these other infectious and parasitic diseases. In fact, it means that coders must watch for additional information in the medical record to make sure the underlying disease is coded first. Now instead of one combination code, two or more codes must be used.

Certain ICD-10-CM classifications differentiate specific conditions that were previously classified together. For example, 323.9 Unspecified causes of encephalitis, myelitis, and encephalomyelitis, is equivalent to two possible codes in ICD-10-CM:

ICD-9-CM:

323.9   **Unspecified causes of encephalitis, myelitis, and encephalomyelitis**

ICD-10-CM:

G04.90   **Encephalitis and encephalomyelitis, unspecified**

G04.91   **Myelitis, unspecified**

When coding and reporting conditions classified to section G00–G09 Inflammatory diseases of the central nervous system, it is important to distinguish between the site and type of infection as specified in the diagnosis. For this reason, a clear understanding of the terminology associated with central nervous system inflammatory conditions is essential.

Infections and inflammatory conditions of the CNS are serious and potentially fatal. The associated cerebral edema can cause irreversible brain damage or intracerebral hemorrhage. Infections included in this code section include meningitis, encephalitis, encephalomyelitis, and myelitis.

- **Meningitis:** Meningitis is inflammation of the CNS meninges, the protective membranes surrounding the brain and spinal cord. Causal factors include toxic effects viruses, bacteria, or other microorganisms, and infection with viruses, bacteria, or other microorganisms. Presenting symptoms include headache, cervicalgia, fever, confusion, photophobia, nausea, and vomiting.
- **Encephalitis:** This is an inflammatory condition of the brain and is most commonly caused by a viral infection. Primary encephalitis is a direct viral infection of the brain, whereas secondary encephalitis occurs as a result of an infection originating elsewhere in the body.
- **Myelitis:** This condition is inflammation of the spinal cord most commonly caused by viral infection. Symptoms vary by region of the spinal cord affected and most commonly include fever, headaches, neuralgia, paresthesia, or impaired bladder or bowel control.
- **Encephalomyelitis:** This is a general term describing an inflammatory condition of the brain and spinal cord. Presenting symptoms overlap those of other CNS infections. Treatment focuses on eradicating the causal infection or stabilizing the causal condition.
- **Encephalopathy:** Encephalopathy is a nervous system dysfunction due to toxicity, trauma, disease, or other pathology affecting the brain. It may be permanent or reversible and varies widely in severity, depending on the etiology. The most common symptom is altered mental state, which may be accompanied by a host of additional neurological signs and symptoms.

Comprehensive Anatomy and Physiology for ICD-10-CM and ICD-10-PCS Coding

ICD-10-CM requires coders to understand anatomy, physiology, and pathology to code accurately. Code section G00–G09 contains certain codes that require multiple coding, as do many of their ICD-9-CM counterparts. In general, code structure within this rubric is similar between systems, with a few exceptions.

Coding for Cerebral Cryptococcus

ICD-9-CM		ICD-10-CM	
117.5	Cryptococcosis	B45.0	Pulmonary cryptococcosis
		B45.1	Cerebral cryptococcosis
		B45.2	Cutaneous cryptococcosis
		B45.3	Osseous cryptococcosis
		B45.7	Disseminated cryptococcosis
		B45.8	Other forms of cryptococcosis
321.0	Cryptococcal meningitis	B45.1	Cerebral cryptococcosis

> **CLINICAL NOTE**
>
> Cryptococcal infection occurs due to contact with a rare pathogen, most commonly caused by inhaling the spores into the lungs, resulting in pneumonia. It can also affect the CNS, manifesting as meningitis or focal brain lesions (cryptococcomas), which may cause hydrocephalus, seizures, and focal neurological deficits.

Understanding the terminology and pathological disease processes inherent in the nervous system is vital to understanding the process of ICD-10-CM coding, especially in making the switch from ICD-9-CM.

Lipoidosis is a general term describing several inherited disorders of fat metabolism. These disorders are characterized by the abnormal accumulation of specific lipids (fat cells) in the body that result in progressive debility due to the associated destruction of the brain and nervous system tissue. Leukodystrophy is a condition in which inherited deficiencies in protein synthesis disrupt the growth or maintenance of the myelin sheath. The myelin (e.g., myelin sheath) is a fatty-appearing insulating membrane that covers and protects nerve axons while serving as a conducting mechanism for transmitting electrical signals between nerve cells. In effect, disorders of the myelin sheath can be loosely equated to problems with electrical wire insulation. These disruptions cause multiple deleterious nervous system effects.

Depending on the causal metabolic abnormality, deficiency of certain fat metabolizing enzymes cause various multisystemic disease processes. Codes have been created based on causal genetic defects and associated systemic manifestations.

Coding for Cerebral Lipoidoses and Leukodystrophies

ICD-9-CM		ICD-10-CM	
330.0	Leukodystrophy	E75.23	Krabbe disease
		E75.25	Metachromatic leukodystrophy
		E75.29	Other sphingolipidosis
330.1	Cerebral lipoidoses	E75.00	GM2 **gangliosidosis**, unspecified
		E75.01	Sandhoff disease
		E75.02	Tay-Sachs disease
		E75.09	Other GM2 gangliosidosis
		E75.10	Unspecified gangliosidosis
		E75.11	**Mucolipidosis** IV
		E75.19	Other gangliosidosis
		E75.4	Neuronal ceroid **lipofuscinosis**

> **DEFINITIONS**
>
> **gangliosidosis.** Abnormal harmful accumulation of certain lipids (gangliosides) due to enzyme deficiency, causing progressive destruction of nervous system tissues.
>
> **lipofuscinosis (ceroid).** Abnormal accumulation of lipopigments in the nervous system tissues causing neurodegeneration.
>
> **mucolipidosis.** Abnormal harmful accumulation of lipids in cells manifested by damage to the motor nerve and ocular tissues.

Specific codes have been created in ICD-10-CM for certain cerebral degenerative diseases of childhood onset to reflect medical advances in identifying genetic links to disease.

Coding for Degenerative Diseases

ICD-9-CM		ICD-10-CM	
330.8	Other specified cerebral degenerations in childhood	F84.2	Rett's syndrome
		G31.81	Alpers disease
		G31.82	Leigh's disease

Rett's syndrome is an inherited disorder caused by mutations in the X chromosome linked MECP2 gene and therefore occurs almost exclusively in females. Onset of symptoms occurs most commonly between 6 and 18 months of age and includes progressive problems with movement, coordination, and communication. Additional symptoms include breathing problems, arrhythmias, seizures, and constipation. Genetic testing establishes the diagnosis, which is often evasive and may be confused with autism, cerebral palsy, or other developmental delay.

Leigh's disease is an inherited neurometabolic disorder of the central nervous system that occurs due to mutations of the mitochondrial DNA (mtDNA). These mutations impair the growth and development of essential brainstem cells, which inhibits motor skills. The disease is characterized by the patient's inability to control movement. In infants, early symptoms include poor sucking ability, inability to control head movements, and seizure. As the disease progresses, organ function and development are delayed or regress, resulting in failure to thrive. Prognosis varies widely in accordance with age of onset and severity.

Alpers disease is an inherited autosomal recessive disorder caused by mutations in the mtDNA, specifically identified as the POLG gene. Initial symptoms in infancy include developmental delay, hypotonia, and spasticity. Disease progression is marked by progressive paralysis, dementia, and mental retardation. Myoclonic seizures are characteristic of Alpers disease. Diagnostic imaging of the central nervous system often displays status spongiosis degeneration of the cerebrum. Prognosis is poor. Patients often expire within the first decade of life.

Alzheimer's and Parkinson's Disease and Related Syndromes

ICD-9-CM contains a specific code for Alzheimer's disease; ICD-10-CM has been expanded to provide information regarding onset within the code set itself.

Coding for Alzheimer's Disease

ICD-9-CM		ICD-10-CM	
331.0	Alzheimer's disease	G30.0	Alzheimer's disease with early onset
		G30.1	Alzheimer's disease with late onset
		G30.8	Other Alzheimer's disease
		G30.9	Alzheimer's disease, unspecified

Alzheimer's disease is a chronic, progressive form of dementia caused by the destruction of subcortical white matter in the brain with plaque formations. Diagnostic imaging typically reveals shrinkage of white matter and an increase in the size of the ventricles.

In a normally functioning process, the ends of nerve cells (synapses) release neurotransmitter molecules that bind to neurotransmitter receptors, thus converting a nerve impulse into a chemical signal. The neurotransmitter receptor receives the transmitter signal and, in turn, generates a responsive nerve impulse. In Alzheimer's disease, there is a deficit in the levels of acetylcholine and degeneration of cholinergic neurons, neurotransmitter proteins, and cells within the brain. The debilitating and ultimately fatal disease is manifested by cognitive and memory decline and other neuropsychiatric symptoms and behavioral dysfunctions. Patients exhibit progressive behavioral changes, including loss of interest and memory problems. The associated frustration and aggressiveness can be treated with sedative or neuroleptic therapies.

Figure 5.7: Neuromuscular Junction

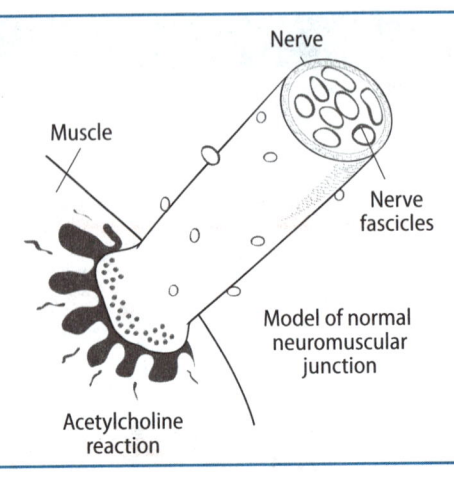

Parkinson's disease (paralysis agitans) is an idiopathic neurological condition marked by degeneration and dysfunction within the basal ganglia, clusters of nerve cells (neurons) at the base of the cerebrum, on both sides of the thalamus, above the brainstem. The basal ganglia may also be referred to as separate structures that include the caudate nucleus, putamen, and globus pallidus. This disease involves the degeneration of the nigral neurons, a group of specialized cells in the midbrain that contain neuromelanin and manufacture the neurotransmitter dopamine. When 75 to 80 percent of the dopamine innervation is destroyed, signs and symptoms of parkinsonism begin to manifest. These symptoms include tremor, rigidity, shuffling gait, drooling, "pill rolling" hand movement, and impaired control of facial muscles.

Figure 5.8: Parkinson's Disease

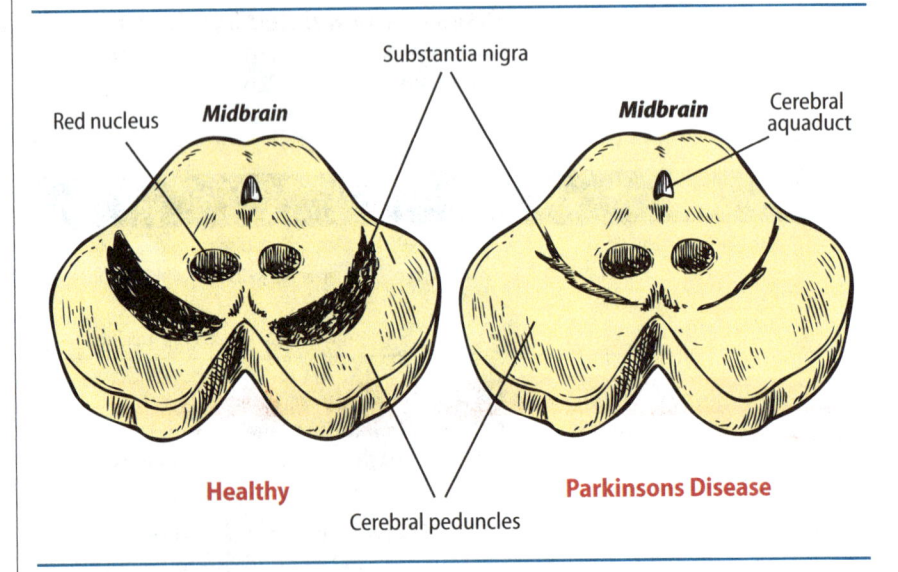

Secondary parkinsonism occurs due to the adverse effects of certain disease processes, drugs, or chemicals. These may include exposure to toxic chemicals, adverse effects of anesthesia, and overdose or prolonged use of certain medications or drugs, including narcotics. Additional causal factors include secondary effects of infectious or inflammatory disease (e.g., encephalitis, meningitis), cerebrovascular disease (stroke), or diseases that damage dopamine neurons. ICD-10-CM expands to a number of codes for diseases of the basal ganglia. Certain related conditions may be classified elsewhere (e.g., G31.83 Lewy body disease). Whereas ICD-9-CM provided a single code for secondary parkinsonism, ICD-10-CM differentiates between certain causal factors.

Coding for Parkinsonism

ICD-9-CM		ICD-10-CM	
332.1	Secondary Parkinsonism	G21.11	**Neuroleptic** induced parkinsonism
		G21.19	Other drug induced secondary parkinsonism
		G21.2	Secondary parkinsonism due to other external agents
		G21.3	Postencephalitic parkinsonism
		G21.8	Other secondary parkinsonism
		G21.9	Secondary parkinsonism, unspecified

ICD-10-CM can be much more specific than ICD-9-CM when it comes to clinical differentiation of conditions. For example:

Coding for Degenerative Diseases of the Basal Ganglia

ICD-9-CM		ICD-10-CM	
333.0	Other degenerative diseases of the basal ganglia	G23.0	**Hallervorden-Spatz disease**
		G23.1	Progressive supranuclear ophthalmoplegia
		G23.2	**Striatonigral degeneration**
		G23.8	Other specified degenerative diseases of the basal ganglia
		G23.9	Degenerative disease of basal ganglia, unspecified
		G90.3	Multi-system degeneration of the autonomic nervous system

Chorea and Movement Disorders

Chorea describes a group of abnormal involuntary movement disorders characterized by overactivity of the neurotransmitter dopamine, causing irregular muscle contractions known as dyskinesias. Pathophysiology is thought to originate from a malfunction in the regulation of basal ganglia neurotransmission that causes an excess of thalamo-cortical output. The movements are nonrepetitive and nonrhythmic. Rather, they occur as irregular, abrupt, and seemingly random involuntary movements that vary in severity and affected anatomic site.

Mild cases may manifest as restlessness or fidgeting, whereas more severe movements may include wild, violent flinging of the extremities (ballism). Multiple types of chorea have been identified, including certain inherited forms (e.g., **Huntington's chorea**), those due to adverse effects of drugs (e.g., hormonal therapies, neuroleptics), and underlying endocrine disease (e.g., thyroid).

Associated contributing factors include pregnancy (e.g., chorea gravidarum), infection (e.g., rheumatic fever), or autoimmune disease (e.g., systemic lupus erythematosus). Certain choreas can interfere with speech, swallowing, gait, or posture and may become exacerbated during periods of anxiety or stress, abating during rest or sleep. Prognosis and treatment options vary, depending on the type of chorea, causal factors, and associated disease processes. Symptomatic treatment may include neuroleptic medications, dopamine inhibitors, and benzodiazepines.

Disorders specified as "**extrapyramidal**" affect the areas of the brain that coordinate muscle movement. They are so named for the complex pathways and feedback loops that lie outside the tracts of the **motor cortex**, which extend through the pyramid-shaped regions of the medulla. Certain pyramidal pathways innervate

> **DEFINITIONS**
>
> **extrapyramidal.** Neural pathways situated outside of or independent from corticospinal pyramidal tracts.
>
> **Hallervorden-Spatz disease.** Demyelination of the nerves between the stratum and pallidum.
>
> **Huntington's chorea.** Fatal hereditary disease in which degeneration of the cerebral cortex and basal ganglia result in chronic, progressive mental deterioration; dementia and death occur within 15 years of onset.
>
> **motor cortex.** Regions of the cerebral cortex of the brain that coordinate and control motor functions.
>
> **neuroleptic (drug).** Antipsychotic, tranquilizing medication.
>
> **striatonigral degeneration.** Neurodegeneration caused by localized abnormalities in the striatum and substantia nigra (mesencephalon) causing difficulty with balance and movement.

motor neurons of the brainstem or spinal cord, whereas the extrapyramidal tracts conduct and modulate motor activity indirectly, transmitting nerve impulses from the pons and medulla of the brain using motor neurons of the basal ganglia, cerebellum, and thalamus to the spinal cord. These pathways help regulate automatic movements that affect muscle tone, balance, and posture. The complexity of the neural circuitry that indirectly achieves motor control through routes other than the direct innervation of the pyramidal system has made it difficult to establish a cohesive, collaborative definition of the extrapyramidal pathways.

Figure 5.9: Pyramidal Pathways

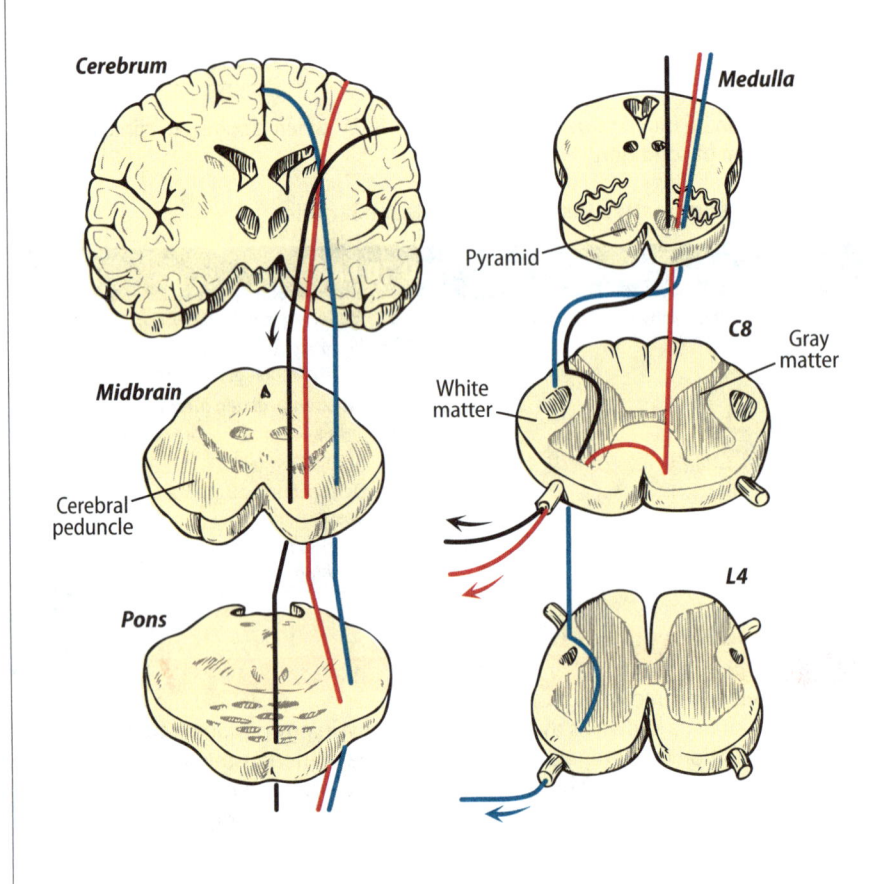

Many of these conditions are identified in association with the anatomic location of the disease or disease characteristics. In general, extrapyramidal symptoms may be described as *akathisia*, *akinesia*, and muscle spasms. Causal factors may include adverse effects of antipsychotic or other medications (e.g., neuroleptics), or as sequelae of brain injury. Unique codes have been established throughout this chapter to differentiate drug-induced nervous system disorders from those otherwise specified, including extrapyramidal and abnormal movement disorders.

DEFINITIONS

akathisia. Motor restlessness.
akinesia. Inability to initiate movement.

ICD-10-CM:

G25.1	Drug-induced tremor
G25.61	Drug-induced tics
G25.4	Drug-induced chorea
G24.02	Drug-induced acute dystonia
G24.09	Other drug-induced dystonia
G25.70	Drug-induced movement disorder
G25.71	Drug-induced akathisia
G25.79	Other drug-induced movement disorders

Demyelinating Diseases

Demyelinating diseases of the central nervous system previously coded to categories 340–341 in ICD-9-CM have been expanded in the ICD-10-CM coding system, and will have their own distinct section (rubric), G35–G37. Included within these categories are multiple sclerosis (G35), other acute **disseminated** demyelination (G36), and other demyelinating diseases of the central nervous system (G37).

Demyelinating diseases affect both the central and peripheral nervous systems. Pathogenesis of demyelination may be summarized as the abnormal loss of myelin, the protective white matter substance that insulates nerve endings and facilitates neuroreception and neurotransmission. When this substance is damaged, nerve function is short-circuited, resulting in impaired or loss of function. As a result, patches of scar tissue (sclerosis) develop where the protective myelin has been damaged at the nerve endings. Although healing remyelination can occur in certain disease processes, there could be permanent damage in the form of sequelae and long-term effects. The anatomic location of demyelination may be associated with certain types or manifestations of disease. For example, patients with transverse myelitis usually exhibit demyelination at the thoracic spine level, with associated lower extremity, bowel, and bladder impairments. Causal factors include genetic predisposition, certain infections, autoimmune disease, and exposures to certain drugs or chemicals.

Multiple sclerosis is a chronic demyelinating disease affecting the white matter of the spinal cord and brain. It is characterized by the breaking down of the myelin fibers of the nervous system; patches of scarred nervous fibers develop at these sites. The etiology is unknown, but recent studies suggest the condition may be a cell-mediated autoimmune disease due to an inherited disorder of immune regulation. The disease affects adults between ages 20 and 40 and occurs more often in women. Signs and symptoms of multiple sclerosis include vision disturbances (e.g., acute optic neuritis, **diplopia**), poor muscle control and coordination (e.g., clumsiness, stumbling, or falling), incontinence, paresthesias, and mental changes. Therapies include corticosteroids to lessen the intensity and duration of acute exacerbations, physical and occupational therapy to preserve muscle strength and maintain motor function, and muscle relaxant and transcutaneous electrical nerve stimulation (TENS) units to treat spasm and pain.

DEFINITIONS

diplopia. Double vision.

disseminated. Widely spread or distributed; dispersed throughout a large area or region.

CODING AXIOM

Guillain-Barre syndrome is coded to G61.0 Acute inflammatory demyelinating polyneuropathy.

Coding Clinic, 2Q, 14, 4

Figure 5.10: Myelin and Nerve Structure

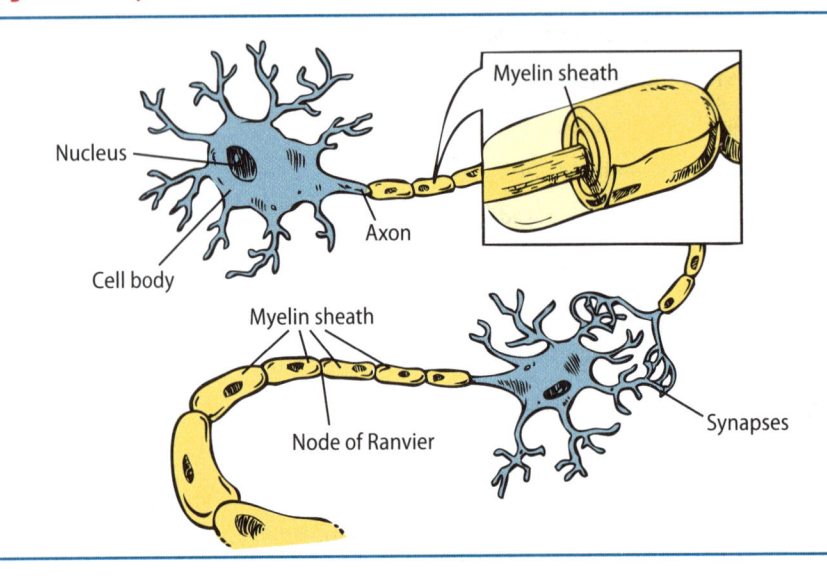

Definitions

epilepsy. Brain disorder characterized by electrical-like disturbances; may include occasional impairment or loss of consciousness, abnormal motor phenomena, and psychic or sensory disturbances.

intractable. Difficult to manage, change, or resolve; strong-willed or resistant.

migraine. Benign vascular headache of extreme pain; commonly associated with irritability, nausea, vomiting, and often photophobia; premonitory visual hallucination of a crescent in the visual field (scotoma).

Headache, Migraine, and Epilepsy

Classifications for *epilepsy*, *migraine*, and headache are generally similar between systems. However, ICD-10-CM includes expanded subclassifications that differentiate headache as "*intractable*" or "not intractable," by type similar to existing classifications for epilepsy and migraine. A note at category G40 Epilepsy and recurrent seizures, and G43 Migraine, provides synonymous terms for the classification of "intractable," including:

- Pharmacoresistant (pharmacologically resistant)
- Treatment resistant
- Refractory (medically)
- Poorly controlled

Coding for Cluster Headache

ICD-9-CM		ICD-10-CM	
339.00	Cluster headache syndrome, unspecified	G44.001	Cluster headache syndrome, unspecified, intractable
		G44.009	Cluster headache syndrome, unspecified, not intractable
339.01	Episodic cluster headache	G44.011	Episodic cluster headache, intractable
		G44.019	Episodic cluster headache, not intractable
339.02	Chronic cluster headache	G44.021	Chronic cluster headache, intractable
		G44.029	Chronic cluster headache, not intractable

Differentiating between the various types of headache, such as cluster headache and migraine, can be difficult. To further complicate matters, patients may experience overlapping types of headache, such as a migraine and cluster headache combination. However, cluster headaches can be differentiated from migraine in that:

- There are no discernible phases in cluster headaches (i.e., prodrome, aura, headache, and postdrome).
- Cluster headaches typically occur spontaneously, while migraine headaches are often precipitated by sentinel symptoms such as aura or other warning.

- Gastrointestinal symptoms are rarely reported with cluster headaches, while 40 percent of migraine patients report nausea or vomiting symptoms.
- Cluster headaches are comparatively short in duration.
- Cluster headaches may go into remission for an extended period of time where the patient is pain-free.
- Cluster headaches are commonly nocturnal and may wake the patient from sleep.
- Patients generally prefer to remain upright during a cluster headache. During migraine attacks, movement is often reported to worsen the pain.
- Cluster headaches are more common in men than in women. Migraines are more common in women than in men.

ICD-10-CM classifications for headache syndromes map directly to their ICD-9-CM counterparts, with the exception of a sixth-character severity indicator that differentiates between intractable versus not intractable presentations. However, there are many clinical variations of headache pain with distinct characteristics and treatments. Treatment relies on accurate diagnosis; therefore, differentiation between headache syndromes is essential. Classification distinctions include the following:

- **Cluster headaches:** Incorporating a "clock" mechanism, cluster headaches occur most frequently at night and are associated with rapid eye movement (REM). Approximately half of cluster headache patients are awakened from sleep by paroxysmal pain, usually within two hours of falling asleep.
- **Drug-induced headache:** Headaches caused by the frequent use of certain over-the-counter (OTC) or prescription drugs. When the effect of one dose wears off, a withdrawal effect occurs, triggering the next headache and another round of medication, perpetuating the cycle.
- **Hemicrania continua:** Previously defined as a persistent primary unilateral headache of unknown causation, this type of headache is characteristically responsive to indomethacin, differentiating hemicrania continua from migraine or cluster headache. Other medications, including Triptans, are not effective.
- **New daily persistent headache (NDPH):** Developing rapidly (over less than three days), this new, unrelenting headache occurs daily at the same time. NDPH is not a continuum of a migraine or tension headache but may present with similar features. The cause is unknown, but it may be associated with viral infection. NDPH is typically unresponsive to traditional medical therapies.
- **Post-traumatic headache:** This type of headache occurs commonly following head trauma. Although the headache has the potential to persist for months or even years, frequency and severity of post-traumatic headache usually resolve within six to 12 months of injury. Associated symptoms may include dizziness, insomnia, difficulties in concentration, and mood and personality changes. Chronic headache after trauma is commonly caused by sustained muscle contractions of the neck and scalp or by vascular changes caused by previous injury. Emotional stress and reactions to the headache occurrences and initial injury can complicate treatment by creating a situational anxiety cycle.
- **Tension type (or stress) headaches:** The most common type of headache among adults, tension headaches are idiopathic but may be triggered by or associated with various factors, including stress, sleep habits, and emotional state.
- **Trigeminal autonomic cephalgia (TAC):** This group of primary headache disorders is characterized by unilateral distribution of pain along the fifth cranial nerve occurring in association with characteristic autonomic ipsilateral cranial features.

Comprehensive Anatomy and Physiology for ICD-10-CM and ICD-10-PCS Coding

==Epilepsy is a disorder characterized by recurrent transient disturbances of the cerebral function.== An abnormal paroxysmal neuronal discharge in the brain usually causes convulsive seizures but may result in loss of consciousness, abnormal behavior, and sensory disturbances in any combination. Epilepsy may be secondary to prior trauma, hemorrhage, intoxication (toxins), chemical imbalances, anoxia, infections, neoplasms, or congenital defects. Signs and symptoms of epilepsy include momentary interruption of activity, staring, and mental blankness. More severe symptoms include complete loss of consciousness, sudden momentary loss or contracture of muscle tone, rolling of the eyes, stiffness, violent jerking movements, and incontinence.

Clinical classification of seizures is based on whether the origin or source of the seizure is localized (partial or focal, involving one part of the brain) or generalized (distributed throughout multiple areas of the brain). These classifications can progress or overlap, in which case certain seizures may manifest as partial and progress to generalized. Localized or partial seizures are further differentiated by the extent to which consciousness is affected. For example, consciousness is impaired in a complex partial seizure, whereas in simple localized seizures, consciousness is unaffected. Although all generalized seizures lead to impairment or loss of consciousness, ICD-10-CM differentiates among them by specifying whether they are idiopathic in origin, associated with an underlying cause (e.g., drugs, hormones), or distinguished as inherent to certain identifiable syndromes (e.g., **Lennox-Gastaut**, **West's**).

Although coding for migraine is generally similar between systems, ICD-10-CM includes expanded subclassifications that differentiate certain identifiable migraine variants.

Coding for Migraine

ICD-9-CM		ICD-10-CM	
346.21	Variants of migraine, NEC without status migrainosus	G43.819	Other migraine, intractable, without status migrainosus
		G43.A1	Cyclical vomiting, intractable
		G43.B1	Ophthalmoplegic migraine, intractable
		G43.C1	Periodic headache syndromes in child or adult, intractable
		G43.D1	Abdominal migraine, intractable

Migraine is a common type of vascular headache. Migraine headaches appear to be caused by blood vessels that overreact to various triggers, such as stress, or an allergic reaction that creates vasoconstrictive spasm. The spasm reduces blood flow and therefore oxygen supply to the brain. In response, vasodilation occurs, triggering the release of pain-producing substances called prostaglandins. The result is a throbbing pain in the head. Diagnosis of migraine may be made based on clinical presentation.

Status migrainosus describes a severe migraine attack that lasts for more than 72 hours and is often associated with nausea and vomiting. Certain symptoms, collectively known as "*aura*," may include flashing lights, bright spots, loss of part of one's field of vision, *scotoma*, geometric visual patterns, or numbness or tingling in the hand, tongue, or side of the face. Aura may precede various types of migraine, including classical or common migraine. Other symptoms may include:

- Moderate to severe throbbing pain for up to 72 hours; pain may be localized to a specific part or region of the head
- Nausea, with or without vomiting
- Sensitivity to light (*photophobia*) and sound
- Visual or auditory hallucinations

📖 DEFINITIONS

aura. Warning symptoms that precede migraine headache or seizure.

Lennox-Gastaut syndrome. Severe epilepsy with onset in early childhood; seizures occur frequently and vary in type.

photophobia. Sensitivity to light.

scotoma. Blind spot within the visual field or an area of lost or diminished vision.

West's syndrome. Serious severe infantile epilepsy often due to anoxic brain injury, birth trauma, or other disease process; characterized by a triad of infantile spasms, specific EEG pattern changes, and developmental regression.

👉 INTERESTING A & P FACT

The term "aura" derives from the Greek word for wind. An aura may precede a migraine or seizure as a strong wind may precede a storm.

Common migraine pain can last three to four days. In addition to classic and common, migraine headache can take several other forms:

- **Basilar artery migraine:** Disturbance of the basilar artery; occurs primarily in adolescent and young adult women.
- **Hemiplegic migraine:** Characterized by temporary paralysis on one side of the body. Familial hemiplegic migraine (FHM) has been linked to mutations of specific genes on chromosomes 1 and 19. Sporadic hemiplegic migraine (SHM) is FHM without the familial connection and that particular genetic mutation.
- **Menstrual migraine:** Associated with hormonal changes inherent to the menstrual cycle.
- **Ophthalmoplegic migraine:** Presents with pain around the eye; often is associated with a droopy eyelid, double vision, and other visual problems.

Migraine complications may include associated cerebral infarction in which the migraine adversely disrupts circulation, resulting in significant ischemia with subsequent infarction (stroke).

Neurological Effects of Vascular Conditions

Many vascular conditions with neurologic effects previously coded as circulatory conditions in ICD-9-CM will now be coded as nervous system conditions. Conversely, paralytic sequelae of cerebral infarct/stroke are classified in ICD-10-CM to chapter 9, "Diseases of the Circulatory System." Code categories G45 and G46 contain expanded subclassifications that include specific types of vascular conditions with updated terminology. In some cases, conditions previously separately classified have been combined and in other cases conditions previously classified to other specified (.8) codes or "ill-defined" codes in ICD-9-CM have been assigned unique codes in ICD-10-CM. These reclassifications provide greater specificity by which to differentiate certain TIA syndromes by type or affected anatomic site.

Coding for Neurovascular Effects of Vascular Conditions

ICD-9-CM		ICD-10-CM	
435.8	Other specified transient cerebral ischemias	G45.1	Carotid artery syndrome (hemispheric)
		G45.2	Multiple and bilateral **precerebral artery** syndromes
435.2	Subclavian steal syndrome	G45.8	Other transient cerebral ischemic attacks and related syndromes
435.8	Other specified transient cerebral ischemias	G45.8	Other transient cerebral ischemic attacks and related syndromes
		G46.0	Middle cerebral artery syndrome
		G46.1	Anterior cerebral artery syndrome
		G46.2	Posterior cerebral artery syndrome
437.8	Other ill-defined cerebrovascular disease	G46.3	Brain stem stroke syndrome
		G46.4	Cerebellar stroke syndrome
		G46.5	Pure **motor lacunar** syndrome
		G46.6	Pure **sensory** lacunar syndrome
		G46.7	Other lacunar syndromes
		G46.8	Other vascular syndromes of brain in cerebrovascular diseases

Transient cerebral ischemia or attack (TIA) describes episodes of focal neurological symptoms. A typical transient ischemic event may last between two and 15 minutes, yet resolve within 24 hours. The most common cause of a TIA-type event is **embolization** due to cardiovascular causes, including rheumatic heart disease, arrhythmia, valve disease, endocarditis, and myocardial infarction. Transient cerebral ischemia may be identified by affected vessel, such as the **basilar** or **vertebral**

🖝 INTERESTING A & P FACT

The term hemicrania derives from the Greek word hemicranios, meaning half of the head.

📖 DEFINITIONS

basilar artery. Major cerebral artery (origin) inferior to the pons that (insertion) divides into the posterior cerebral arteries and the superior cerebellar artery.

embolization. Forming of a circulatory obstruction out of circulating matter or particle (e.g., blood clot or plaque) and associated physiologic disruptions.

lacunar. Pertaining to discontinuity of space within an anatomical structure; pits, depressions, or hollows.

motor. Of or relating to a motor nerve; one that causes or imparts motion.

precerebral artery. Artery that flows to the cerebrum but is not located within the cerebrum.

sensory. Of or relating to the senses; including vision, hearing, tactile sense, or taste.

vertebral artery. Major cervical artery (origin) branching from the subclavian arteries to (insertion) the basilar artery.

Comprehensive Anatomy and Physiology for ICD-10-CM and ICD-10-PCS Coding

> **DEFINITIONS**
>
> **circle of Willis.** Circular network of arteries that supply blood to the brain.

arteries. The primary function of the vertebral and basilar arteries is to supply the brain with oxygen-rich blood. The paired vertebral arteries (right and left) together with the basilar artery are often referred to as the vertebrobasilar system. These vessels connect with the **circle of Willis**, a vascular network of five bilateral arteries.

Figure 5.11: Circle of Willis

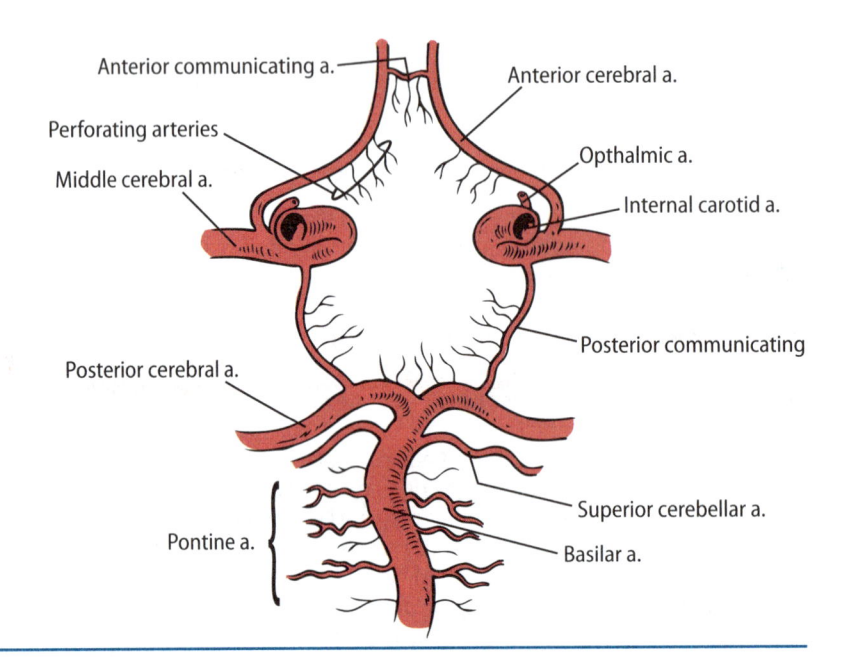

- Anterior communicating a.
- Anterior cerebral a.
- Perforating arteries
- Opthalmic a.
- Middle cerebral a.
- Internal carotid a.
- Posterior communicating
- Posterior cerebral a.
- Superior cerebellar a.
- Pontine a.
- Basilar a.

> **CODING AXIOM**
>
> ICD-10-CM Official Coding Guideline I. C. 6. a. states "Dominant/Nondominant Side—Should the affected side be documented, but not specified as dominant or nondominant, and the classification system does not indicate a default, code selection is as follows:
>
> - For ambidextrous patients, the default should be dominant.
> - If the left side is affected, the default is non-dominant.
> - If the right side is affected, the default is dominant."

Vascular syndromes specified as middle, anterior, or posterior artery in nature indicate conditions in which the blood supply from the affected artery is restricted, leading to a reduction of the function of the portions of the brain supplied by that vessel. Presenting symptoms are often represented by impairment in the brain functions performed by the affected area of the brain. For example, cerebellar stroke syndrome is so named for the characteristic manifestations associated with cerebellum-mediated functions. When disease compromises the vasculature of the cerebellum, the associated physiological functions of the cerebellum that control hearing and balance are disrupted, resulting in hearing loss, dizziness, and ataxia.

Lacunar strokes, ischemic attacks, and other vascular syndromes originate due to disease processes in intracerebral vessels, most commonly occlusions of the branches of a larger artery (e.g., middle cerebral, posterior cerebral, basilar). Lacunar cerebrovascular events tend to occur in the deeper, smaller vessel branches within the brain.

Figure 5.12: Cerebrovascular Arteries

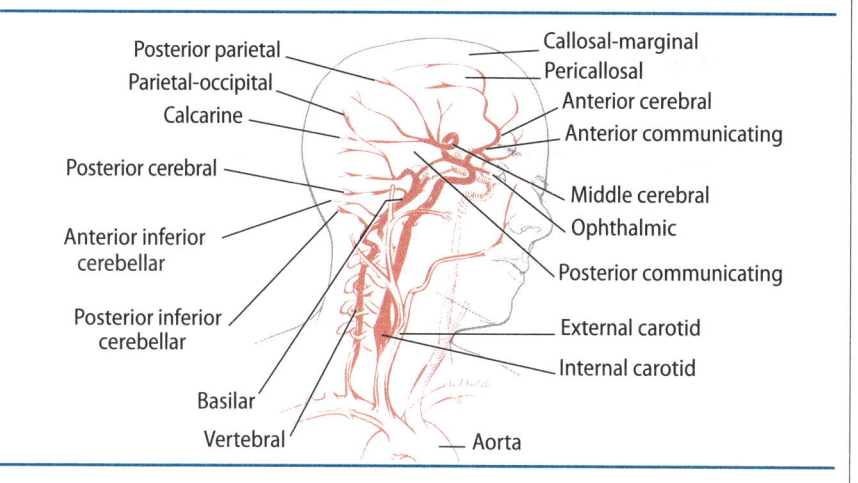

Labels: Posterior parietal, Parietal-occipital, Calcarine, Posterior cerebral, Anterior inferior cerebellar, Posterior inferior cerebellar, Basilar, Vertebral, Callosal-marginal, Pericallosal, Anterior cerebral, Anterior communicating, Middle cerebral, Ophthalmic, Posterior communicating, External carotid, Internal carotid, Aorta

Lacunar syndromes described as "pure motor" are a common type of transient cerebrovascular disease characterized by hemiparesis, weakness on one side of the body that may include the face and/or the extremities. Speech, vision, and other sensory symptoms may also be present, though often relatively minor and transient. By contrast, those cerebrovascular syndromes described as "pure sensory" are characterized by sensory abnormalities that may include visual or auditory disturbances, numbness, and variations in the perceptions of pain, temperature, and pressure. Anatomic sites affected in lacunar cerebrovascular disease with motor manifestations may include the vasculature of the internal capsule or the basis pontis, the anterior portion of the pons, whereas sensory syndromes typically arise from pathology affecting the thalamus. Overlapping "motor" and "sensory" symptoms occur when cerebrovascular disease affects vessels that supply the thalamus and the adjacent interior capsule. In such cases, sensory and motor symptoms may manifest on the same side of the body.

Multiple clinical variations of brainstem stroke syndrome have been identified that may be differentiated by the pattern of deficits caused by the interruption of specific affected cranial nerves. A brainstem stroke may be potentially life-threatening if the cranial nerves that control respiration and cardiac function are disrupted. Similarly, certain brainstem strokes may cause double vision, ataxia, impaired speech, and gastrointestinal symptoms.

Certain syndromes identified elsewhere in ICD-9-CM will be coded as cerebrovascular syndromes in ICD-10-CM. For example, ICD-10-CM code G46.3 Brain stem stroke syndrome, includes:

- Benedikt's, Foville's, Weber, and Millard-Gubler syndromes (344.89), and Claude syndrome (352.6), characterized by oculomotor nerve palsy, contralateral hemiparesis, ataxia, and hemiplegia of the face and upper extremities
- Paraplegia and anesthesia over part of the body caused by lesions in the brain or spinal cord
- Wallenberg syndrome (436), characterized by dysphagia, hoarseness, loss of taste, and paralysis of the ipsilateral vocal cord and tongue due to lesions of the glossopharyngeal (IX) & vagus (X) nerves.

> **INTERESTING A & P FACT**
>
> The term "cerebellum" may be translated to mean "little brain." Situated posterior to the cerebrum, above the medulla oblongata, its main function is to coordinate fine motor skills and learning, equilibrium, and balance.

Figure 5.13: Trigeminal and Facial Nerve Branches

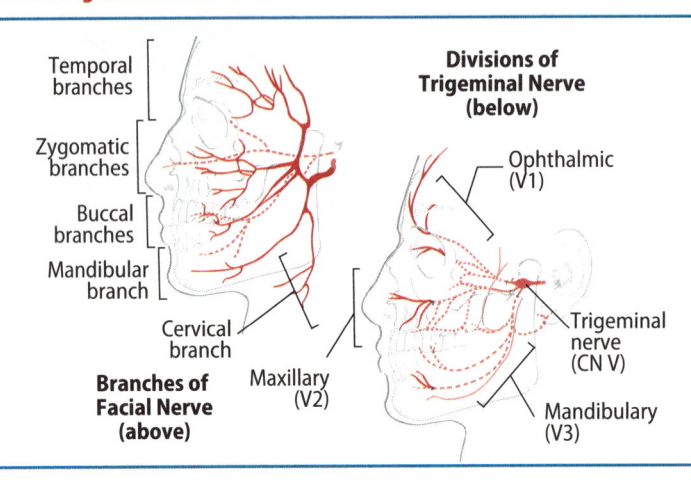

Facial Nerve Disorders

Although many codes are mapped directly between the systems (e.g., trigeminal neuralgia is coded as 350.1 in ICD-9-CM and G50.0 in ICD-10-CM), ICD-10-CM provides unique codes to identify certain facial nerve disorders that were previously included in "other specified" (.8) ICD-9-CM classifications.

Coding for Facial Nerve Disorders

ICD-9-CM		ICD-10-CM	
351.8	Other facial nerve disorders	G51.2	Melkersson's syndrome
		G51.3	Clonic hemifacial spasm
		G51.4	Facial myokymia
		G51.8	Other disorders of facial nerve

Melkersson (-Rosenthal) syndrome is a genetic condition with onset in childhood or adolescence. It is characterized by chronic facial swelling, localized particularly to the lips, and recurrent facial palsy. Recurrent attacks may become permanent, with a hardening, discoloration, and cracking of labial tissue. Associated conditions include fissured tongue and ophthalmic symptoms, including lagophthalmos, blepharochalasis, corneal opacities, retrobulbar neuritis, and exophthalmos.

Facial *myokymia* may be described as a form of involuntary movement, or "quivering," in which the affected muscle appears to spasm in continuous, rippling motions. Causal conditions include neoplasm (typically a brainstem glioma), demyelinating diseases (e.g., multiple sclerosis), or certain polyneuropathies (e.g., Guillain Barré syndrome).

Clonic facial spasm is an idiopathic disorder with onset in the fifth or sixth decade of life. Presentation is most commonly unilateral, although bilateral presentations have been observed in severe cases. Characteristic clonic facial muscle spasm occurs on one side of the face, with abnormally rapid periods of alternating muscular contractions and relaxations. Facial muscles typically affected include the corrugator, frontalis, orbicularis oris, platysma, and zygomaticus.

INTERESTING A & P FACT

Clonic derives from the Greek word klonos, which means "turmoil."

DEFINITIONS

clonic. Neuromuscular abnormality characterized by rapidly alternating muscular contraction and relaxation.

myokymia. Involuntary, spontaneous muscle contractions characterized by undulating or rippling-appearing muscle spasms.

Figure 5.14: Facial Nerves

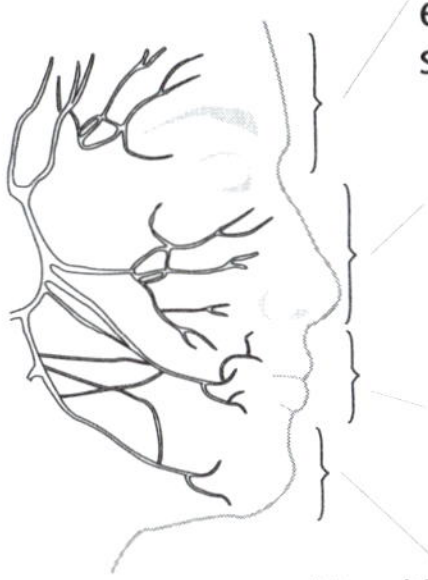

Schematic of select branches of the facial nerve and facial muscle groups

Temporal branches: Muscles of forehead, eyelids, and surrounding tissue

Zygomatic branches: Muscles of nose, cheeks, and surrounding tissue

Buccal branches: Muscles of lips and surrounding tissue

Mandibular branch: Muscles of chin and surrounding tissue

Sustained tonic contractions can result in chronic irritation of the facial nerve, hyperexcitability, and disruptions in neurotransmission. Causal conditions include compressive lesions (e.g., tumor), stroke, multiple sclerosis, and infection.

Coma

ICD-9-CM treats coma as a symptom or condition secondary to various other conditions, such as diabetes or epilepsy. ICD-10-CM still has codes representing coma secondary to various conditions, but also requires coders to delve into the record a bit further with regards to coma and traumatic brain injury codes, acute cerebrovascular disease codes, or sequelae of cerebrovascular disease codes. The Glasgow coma scale (GCS) is now represented though a series of codes found in category R4Ø of ICD-10-CM. These codes are assigned in conjunction with code categories such SØ2.- fracture of skull or SØ6.- intracranial injury.

The Glasgow coma scale measures response to stimuli in three different areas, including eye opening response, verbal response, and motor response. The patient is assigned a score in each of these three areas, and these scores are added up to create a total Glasgow coma scale score.

Eye Opening Response

Response	Points
Spontaneous and open with blinking at baseline	4
Responds to verbal stimuli, command, speech	3
Responds to pain only (stimuli not applied to face)	2
No response to stimuli	1

Verbal Response

Response	Points
Oriented	5
Has confused conversation, but patient was able to answer questions	4
Patient uses inappropriate words	3
Patient uses incomprehensible speech	2
No response	1

> **CODING AXIOM**
>
> The EMT and other nonphysician documentation on the prehospital report may be used in determining the Glasgow coma score.
>
> *Coding Clinic,* 1Q, 14, 19

Motor Response

Response	Points
Obeys commands for movement	6
Purposeful movement to painful stimulus	5
Withdraws from painful stimulus	4
Abnormal (spastic) flexion, decorticate posture	3
Extensor (rigid) response, decerebrate posture	2
No response to painful stimuli	1

Source: Adapted from Glasgow Coma Scale, Womack Army Medical Center, Fort Bragg, NC.

The points across the three areas are added up to determine an overall GCS score, which will be represented by a code in subcategory R40.24-. If individual scores are documented, they can be represented via codes found in subcategories R40.21--R40.23-. As coders were not likely seeking this information in the record previously, it is important to become familiar with the GCS and its components. If a patient is in a comatose state without a GCS score and it appears one should be assigned, query the provider for additional information. Coders in many specialties will be using these codes, such as neurology, trauma registry, and inpatient rehabilitation, just to name a few.

> **CODING AXIOM**
>
> Codes from subcategories R40.21-, R40.22-, and R40.23- for individual Glasgow coma scores (GCS) may be assigned based on documented individual score(s) or numeric values rather than the actual description of the codes if the provider's documentation clearly shows that the specific scores or numeric values are for the Glasgow scale. The 7th character indicates when the scale was recorded and should match for all three codes.
>
> R40.24- Glasgow coma scale, total score is assigned when only the total score is documented in the medical record and not the individual score(s).
>
> *Coding Clinic,* 2Q, 15, 16

Eye and Adnexa

ICD-10-CM separates the nervous system disease classifications from those of the sense organs (eye and ear), creating three separate chapters. Perhaps one of the most significant changes in the ICD-10-CM system is the incorporation of laterality; that is, the codes reflect paired organs and anatomic sites. Some code classifications indicate right, left, bilateral, and unspecified laterality. This is particularly evident in chapter 7, "Diseases of the Eye and Adnexa (H00–H59)."

ICD-10-CM associates certain ophthalmic diseases with closely related manifestations separately. For example, parasitic endophthalmitis has been expanded to include separate classifications for parasitic cyst, by affected anatomic site. Previously, ICD-9-CM provided a single code for parasitic endophthalmitis and parasitic cyst, regardless of affected site.

Coding for Endophthalmitis

ICD-9-CM		ICD-10-CM	
360.13	Parasitic endophthalmitis, NOS	H21.331	Parasitic cyst of iris, ciliary body or anterior chamber, right eye
		H21.332	Parasitic cyst of iris, ciliary body or anterior chamber, left eye
		H21.333	Parasitic cyst of iris, ciliary body or anterior chamber, bilateral
		H21.339	Parasitic cyst of iris, ciliary body or anterior chamber, unspecified eye
		H33.121	Parasitic cyst of retina, right eye
		H33.122	Parasitic cyst of retina, left eye
		H33.123	Parasitic cyst of retina, bilateral
		H33.129	Parasitic cyst of retina, unspecified eye
		H44.121	Parasitic endophthalmitis, unspecified, right eye
		H44.122	Parasitic endophthalmitis, unspecified, left eye
		H44.123	Parasitic endophthalmitis, unspecified, bilateral
		H44.129	Parasitic endophthalmitis, unspecified, unspecified eye

Figure 5.15: Anterior Chamber

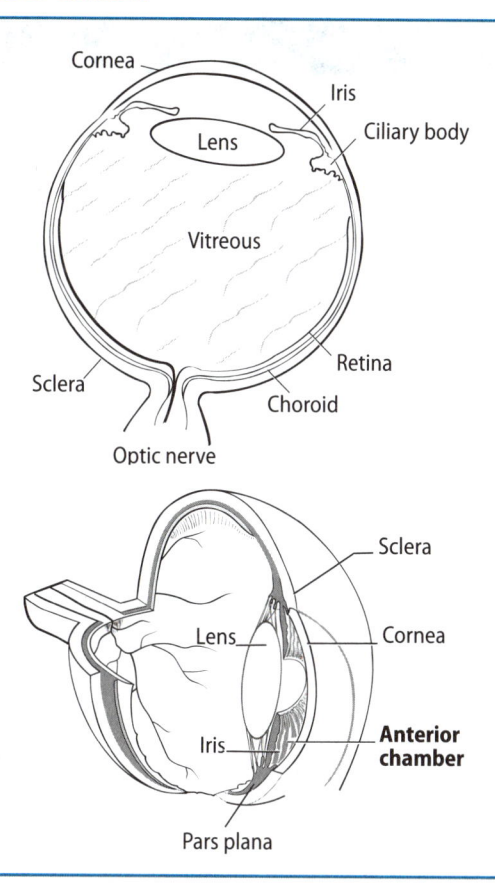

Endophthalmitis is an infection or inflammation of the tissues and internal structures of the eye. The anterior or posterior chamber, or both, may be affected. Parasitic endophthalmitis describes an infection of the eye due to invasion by a parasitic microorganism through direct exposure to the parasite or through blood-borne transportation to the eye or adjacent structures. There are multiple parasites that can invade the eye that for coding purposes may be classifiable elsewhere, depending on the nature of the organism and anatomic site of infection. Signs of infection include white nodules on the lens capsule, iris, retina, or choroid, or inflammation of all of the ocular tissues, which leads to a globe of full, purulent exudates. General symptoms may include impairment of visual acuity and the visual field, pain, excessive tearing, ocular discharge, and photophobia. If the infection is inadequately treated, inflammation may spread to the orbital soft tissue.

Some ICD-10-CM code descriptions have been updated to reflect current clinical terminology and in response to a better understanding of conditions through advancing medical technologies. For example, the diagnoses blind hypotensive eye and blind hypertensive eye have been revised to atrophy of the globe and absolute glaucoma, respectively.

Coding for Hypotensive and Hypertensive Eyes

ICD-9-CM		ICD-10-CM	
360.41	Blind hypotensive eye	H44.521	Atrophy of globe, right eye
		H44.522	Atrophy of globe, left eye
		H44.523	Atrophy of globe, bilateral
		H44.529	Atrophy of globe, unspecified eye
360.42	Blind hypertensive eye	H44.511	Absolute glaucoma, right eye
		H44.512	Absolute glaucoma, left eye
		H44.513	Absolute glaucoma, bilateral
		H44.519	Absolute glaucoma, unspecified eye

Definitions

atrophy. Wasting away or decrease in the size of a body organ or part due to malnutrition or other damage.

enucleation. Surgical removal of the eye.

phthisis. Wasting disease; a disease or condition characterized by wasting.

Atrophy of the globe (*phthisis* bulbi) describes vision loss due to extremely low intraocular pressure (IOP). Phthisical eye occurs when disease or damage causes the ciliary body to stop producing aqueous fluid, resulting in a loss of IOP (hypotony). Prolonged low pressure can distort and cause degeneration of the chorioretinal vascular, cornea, and optic disc. Phthisis bulbi is an end-stage severity presentation of ocular hypotony characterized by a soft, atrophic, and nonfunctional eye.

Normal IOP is between 10 and 20 mm Hg (millimeters of mercury). Hypotony of the eye is an IOP of less than 10 mm Hg, although it may not be considered problematic until the pressure drops below 6 mm Hg. Causal factors for hypotony include postsurgical wound leak, inflammatory eye diseases (e.g., uveitis), and chorioretinal detachments. In the past, hypotony was a common complication of trabeculectomy procedures used to treat glaucoma. However, advances in surgical technique have rendered incidence to minimal, although leakage around the scleral flap incision occasionally occurs. Certain eye conditions, such as chronic inflammations and retinal defects, alter the osmotic state of the eye, resulting in hypotony. Other associated conditions include glaucoma, neoplasm, ocular injury, postoperative complications, and certain inflammatory eye diseases.

Characteristics of the phthisical eye include a small, shrunken globe with marked thickening of the sclera, metaplasia of the retinal pigment epithelium, displacement or atrophy of the intraocular contents, and ossification. At the advanced stages inherent to phthisis bulbi, prognosis is poor, resulting in a small shrunken globe of tissue with no function. Treatment options include *enucleation* with replacement of the globe or fitting a scleral shell prosthesis.

The ciliary body produces aqueous humor, which is integral to maintaining intraocular pressure. The lens and anterior eye structures separate the aqueous humor from the posterior segment of the eye. The anterior segment is divided into the anterior and posterior chambers. The aqueous humor flows into the posterior chamber through the pupil of the iris and the anterior chamber. It proceeds through the trabecular meshwork to enter the normal body circulation. Ocular hypertension, or increased IOP, may be caused by increased production or decreased outflow of aqueous humor.

Ocular hypertension is a significant finding of multifactorial etiology. Patients with a history of myopia or diabetes have an increased incidence of elevated IOP. Although ocular hypertension is not typically synonymous with glaucoma, increased IOP is a characteristic sign of glaucoma. Ocular hypertension is typically defined as an IOP greater than 21 mm Hg, with absolute glaucoma representing vision loss due to the severity and progression of ocular hypertension.

In its initial stages, ocular hypertension is quiescent; it often has no discernible signs or symptoms. It is often noted upon routine eye exam by tonometry. Not all patients with increased IOP develop glaucoma—ocular hypertension is a physical finding and glaucoma represents a myriad of intraocular diseases characterized by increased IOP. General symptoms may include vision loss, eye pain, increased eye pressure sensation and an abnormally hardened texture to the globe. The diagnosis of "blind

Interesting A & P Fact

Increased IOP is a characteristic sign of glaucoma but does not necessarily indicate the disease.

hypertensive eye" represents the end stage of intraocular hypertensive disease, whereby the ocular structures have sustained irreparable damage.

ICD-10-CM includes unique codes for conditions not previously identified by ICD-9-CM. In the classification of retinoschisis and retinal cysts, new subcategory codes have been created to specifically identify cyst ora serrata, the junction between the retina and the ciliary body.

Coding for Cyst Ora Serrata

ICD-9-CM		ICD-10-CM	
361.19	Other retinoschisis and retinal cysts	H33.111	Cyst of ora serrata, right eye
		H33.112	Cyst of ora serrata, left eye
		H33.113	Cyst of ora serrata, bilateral
		H33.119	Cyst of ora serrata, unspecified eye
		H33.191	Other retinoschisis and retinal cysts, right eye
		H33.192	Other retinoschisis and retinal cysts, left eye
		H33.193	Other retinoschisis and retinal cysts, bilateral
		H33.199	Other retinoschisis and retinal cysts, unspecified eye

Subcategory H33.1 classifies acquired retinoschisis and other retinal cysts. These include primary and secondary retinal cysts and pseudocysts, similar to ICD-9-CM. However, ICD-10-CM includes a unique code subcategory to identify ora serrata cysts. In normal anatomy, the ora serrata is the serrated junction between the retina and the ciliary body. The ciliary body is part of the uvea and connects anteriorly to the root of the iris and posteriorly to the choroid at the ora serrata retinae. It is divided into the pars plana and the pars plicata. Cysts in this area of the eye may form as part of a degenerative retinoschisis, which typically originates at the periphery of the retina and extends into the ora serrata as the condition progresses. However, primary and secondary retinal cysts increase the patient's risk for retinal detachment. Secondary cysts form as a result of other (primary) ophthalmic disease. Pseudocyst describes an area of fluid accumulation without an encasing membranous lining. Retinoschisis, which can be hereditary or acquired, is an abnormal splitting of the retinal layers. It most commonly occurs in the outer plexiform layer of nervous tissue, causing vision loss in the affected area. Degenerative retinoschisis (e.g., flat, bullous) is the most common presentation. It is easily confused with retinal detachment but must be differentiated, since the management and treatment options are different.

Coding for Diabetic Ophthalmic Disease

ICD-9-CM		ICD-10-CM	
362.01	Background diabetic retinopathy	E08.311	Diabetes mellitus due to underlying condition with unspecified diabetic retinopathy with macular edema
		E08.319	Diabetes mellitus due to underlying condition with unspecified diabetic retinopathy without macular edema
		E09.311	Drug or chemical induced diabetes mellitus with unspecified diabetic retinopathy with macular edema
		E09.319	Drug or chemical induced diabetes mellitus with unspecified diabetic retinopathy without macular edema
		E09.331	Drug or chemical induced diabetes mellitus with moderate nonproliferative diabetic retinopathy with macular edema
		E10.311	Type 1 diabetes mellitus with unspecified diabetic retinopathy with macular edema
		E11.311	Type 2 diabetes mellitus with unspecified diabetic retinopathy with macular edema
366.41	Diabetic cataract	E08.36	Diabetes mellitus due to underlying condition with diabetic cataract
		E09.36	Drug or chemical induced diabetes mellitus with diabetic cataract
		E10.36	Type 1 diabetes mellitus with diabetic cataract
		E11.36	Type 2 diabetes mellitus with diabetic cataract
		E13.36	Other specified diabetes mellitus with diabetic cataract
362.07	Diabetic macular edema	E08.311	Diabetes mellitus due to underlying condition with unspecified diabetic retinopathy with macular edema
		E09.311	Drug or chemical induced diabetes mellitus with unspecified diabetic retinopathy with macular edema
		E10.311	Type 1 diabetes mellitus with unspecified diabetic retinopathy with macular edema
		E11.311	Type 2 diabetes mellitus with unspecified diabetic retinopathy with macular edema
		E13.311	Other specified diabetes mellitus with unspecified diabetic retinopathy with macular edema

In the previous example, the ICD-10-CM chapter 4 code (E00–E88) includes the causal disease (diabetes mellitus), type of disease, specific ophthalmic manifestation, and associated conditions or complications. ICD-10-CM codes for diabetes mellitus no longer indicate whether the disease is controlled. See the *ICD-10-CM Official Guidelines for Coding and Reporting* for specific guidance regarding coding and reporting diabetes as multiple codes are required to report conditions in several cases. The previous table is a sample of the possible code mapping combinations for diabetic eye conditions. For more detailed information on ICD-9-CM to ICD-10-CM mapping, see Optum360's *ICD-10-CM Mappings*.

Diabetes mellitus is a complex metabolic disorder with multisystemic manifestations, many of which affect various portions of the nervous system. It can be a primary disease or occur secondary to infection, drug or chemical exposures, or other disease processes. Diabetes is clinically categorized as Type 1 or Type 2. Type 1 indicates inadequate secretion of insulin by the pancreas, whereas Type 2 is the body's inability to respond to insulin, called insulin resistance. Both have similar symptoms, including excessive thirst, hunger, and urination. Laboratory tests that detect glucose in the urine and elevated levels of glucose in the blood usually confirm the diagnosis.

Diabetes may manifest in a wide range of problems that affect the eyes, in particular the retina, lens, and trabecular meshwork. Visual changes can be minimal to severe and temporary or permanent depending on the type, location, and extent of damage.

Diabetic retinopathy (DR) is a frequent and common complication of the retinal vasculature that eventually affects most diabetic patients. Leakage and scar tissue caused by damaged retinal vessels distort and blur vision. The retina is sensitive nervous tissue that sends messages via the optic nerve to the brain and one of three layers of the eyeball. The outer, white layer is the sclera, which is the true wall of the eyeball. Lining the sclera is the choroid, a thin membrane that supplies nutrients to part of the retina. The retina, the innermost layer, begins posterior to the iris, just behind the area called the pars plana, and lines the inner wall of the eye. The central portion of the retina is the macula, which is roughly the area inside of the arcade vessels that extend from the optic nerve and around the macula. The *macula* is the area of the retina where central vision is the clearest for color and reading vision. The true focal point of the eye is the foveal avascular zone (FAZ), which is only 400 microns wide (0.4 mm). The single-layer retinal pigment epithelium (RPE) outside the retina provides nutrients to the photoreceptors; it is also dark with melanin, which decreases light scatter within the eye. The rods and cones are photoreceptors; the cone system dominates vision in daytime, whereas the rod system dominates night vision. Below the RPE is a multilayered membrane called Bruch's membrane, which separates the RPE and retina from the choroid, a vascular layer that provides most of the oxygen to the photoreceptors and RPE. The vitreous is a clear, gel-like substance that fills up most of the inner space of the eyeball. It lies behind the lens and is in contact with the retina.

Diabetic retinopathy represents a continuum of disease, a progression of pathologic changes in the retina due to microvascular complications inherent in diabetes mellitus. Nonproliferative diabetic retinopathy indicates early stage of the disease. Microaneurysms form, retinal hemorrhages occur, and blind spots are characteristic. Increased vessel leakage occurs as the disease progresses, resulting in further vision impairment. The disease progresses from mild to moderate to severe nonproliferative retinopathy and becomes proliferative in its more advanced stage, characterized by new blood vessel formation in the retina due to significant ischemia from the damaged vessels. Diabetic macular edema (DME) occurs when leakage from the blood vessels causes swelling of the central portion of the retina, which impairs vision. Exudates or plaques may develop in the posterior pole of the retina due to the breakdown of retinal vasculature, which can precipitate vision loss.

Retinal vascular occlusion is a potentially blinding blockage that occurs in any of the blood vessels in the retina, the light-sensitive membrane in the back of the eye. Central retinal artery occlusion is blockage of the central retinal artery. The blockage is often caused by a tiny embolus in the bloodstream that obstructs circulation and oxygen supply to the retina, causing sudden, complete vision loss. In some cases, antecedent amaurosis fugax has been reported before complete occlusion and loss of vision. In the past, the term amaurosis fugax referred to symptomatic temporary blindness. However, clinical studies suggest that the underlying anatomic origin of retinal *ischemia* should be distinguished from the pathophysiologic origin to ensure optimal treatment. Recently, amaurosis fugax has been attributed in the majority of cases to internal carotid artery stenosis. This condition is considered a risk factor for permanent occlusion of the central retinal artery and stroke.

> **DEFINITIONS**
>
> **ischemia.** Decrease in blood supply to the organs or tissues.
>
> **macula.** Central part of the retina that provides sharp vision, the ability to discern fine detail, and color.

> **INTERESTING A & P FACT**
>
> Diabetic retinopathy is the third leading cause of legal blindness in adults in the United States.

Figure 5.16: Posterior Segment of Eye

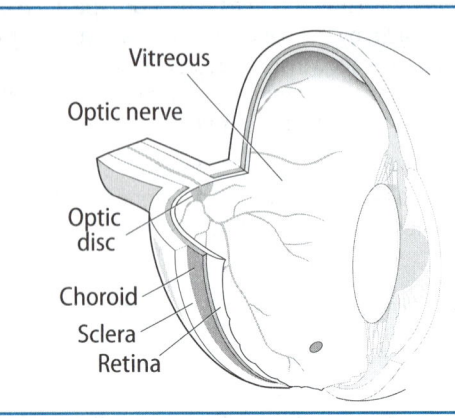

(Diagram labels: Vitreous, Optic nerve, Optic disc, Choroid, Sclera, Retina)

> **DEFINITIONS**
>
> **endothelial.** Related to flat cells that make up the inner linings of cavities and organ structures.
>
> **foveal.** Related to the center of the retinal macula, where light falls directly on the cones.

The central retinal artery enters the eye through the optic disc and divides into multiple branches to perfuse the inner layers of the retina. If circulation remains in the cilioretinal arteries to supply the macula, central vision may be preserved. However, there is a small window of opportunity to treat central retinal artery occlusion, as irreversible retinal damage occurs rapidly after onset. Occlusion of a branch of the retinal artery is often caused by a tiny embolus in the bloodstream that blocks circulation and oxygen supply to the retina, resulting in visual field loss. Loss of visual acuity indicates *foveal* involvement.

Disease progression for retinal artery occlusion is determined by the anatomical location, area of supply, drainage, arterial or venous supply, and the extent of occlusion. For central retinal artery occlusion, outcomes improve dramatically if treatment is sought within 24 hours of onset. If vision does not improve after 72 hours, the retina may have infarcted (tissue died because of partial occlusion of a vessel), in which case blindness may be permanent. Studies suggest that early detection and pathogenic differentiation between transient and permanent eye and brain ischemic syndromes can lead to more effective mechanisms for stroke prevention.

Coding for Retinal Degeneration

ICD-9-CM		ICD-10-CM	
362.64	Senile reticular degeneration of the peripheral retina	H35.441	Age-related reticular degeneration of retina, right eye
		H35.442	Age-related reticular degeneration of retina, left eye
		H35.443	Age-related reticular degeneration of retina, bilateral
		H35.449	Age-related reticular degeneration of retina, unspecified eye

ICD-10-CM classifications for retinal dystrophies primarily involving the Bruch's membrane have been reclassified as choroidal degenerations and atrophies. The alphabetic index directs the coder to "see choroid" for conditions affecting the Bruch's membrane.

The Bruch's membrane is the stratified inner layer of the choroid that separates the choroid from the pigmented layer of the retina (RPE) and the **endothelial** cells of the choriocapillaris. It has inner and outer collagenous layers rich in elastin and elastin-associated proteins.

In normal anatomy, the retinal pigment epithelium transports metabolic waste from the photoreceptors across Bruch's membrane to the choroid. Similar to the age-related forms of disease, the Bruch's membrane thickens abnormally and the transportation of metabolites becomes less efficient, which may lead to *drusen* or age-related macular degeneration. As a result, certain inflammatory and neovascular processes may occur as the membrane fragments, leading to destruction of the retinal architecture with progressive vision loss. Conditions such as pseudoxanthoma elasticum, myopia, and trauma can also cause defects in Bruch's membrane, with associated choroidal neovascularization. As the Bruch's membrane thickens, accumulation of debris and calcification (hardening) commonly occurs. Complications may include the formation of drusen and basal *laminar* deposits.

In ICD-10-CM, conditions previously classified separately as preglaucoma or borderline glaucoma are now classified to a single ICD-10-CM code.

Coding for Glaucoma

ICD-9-CM		ICD-10-CM	
365.00	Unspecified preglaucoma	H40.001	Preglaucoma, unspecified, right eye
		H40.002	Preglaucoma, unspecified, left eye
		H40.003	Preglaucoma, unspecified, bilateral
		H40.009	Preglaucoma, unspecified, unspecified eye
365.01	Borderline glaucoma, open angle with borderline findings	H40.011	Open angle with borderline findings, low risk, right eye
		H40.012	Open angle with borderline findings, low risk, left eye
		H40.013	Open angle with borderline findings, low risk, bilateral
		H40.019	Open angle with borderline findings, low risk, unspecified eye
365.02	Borderline glaucoma, anatomical narrow angle	H40.031	Anatomical narrow angle, right eye
		H40.032	Anatomical narrow angle, left eye
		H40.033	Anatomical narrow angle, bilateral
		H40.039	Anatomical narrow angle, unspecified eye
365.03	Borderline glaucoma, steroid responders	H40.041	Steroid responder, right eye
		H40.042	Steroid responder, left eye
		H40.043	Steroid responder, bilateral
		H40.049	Steroid responder, unspecified eye
365.04	Borderline glaucoma, ocular hypertension	H40.051	Ocular hypertension, right eye
		H40.052	Ocular hypertension, left eye
		H40.053	Ocular hypertension, bilateral
		H40.059	Ocular hypertension, unspecified eye

The diagnosis of "glaucoma suspect" describes a patient with borderline signs and symptoms of glaucoma, such as a suspicious-looking optic nerve, a borderline high IOP (intraocular pressure), and associated visual field deficits. Ocular hypertension is an increase in the pressure inside the eye (IOP) and is higher than normal. Normal eye pressure ranges from 10 to 21 mm Hg. Eye pressure is measured in millimeters of mercury (mm Hg). The eye pressure for ocular hypertension is greater than 21 mm Hg. Codes in subcategory H40.0 describe high intraocular pressures, including those with no apparent cause, that may create a minor block in aqueous outflow from the eye when a definitive diagnosis of glaucoma is suspected but has not yet been established.

Conditions once coded separately in ICD-9-CM as pseudoexfoliation glaucoma (365.52) are now coded as open angle, primary *capsular glaucoma* with pseudoexfoliation of the lens. The alphabetic index directs the coder accordingly.

> **DEFINITIONS**
>
> **capsular glaucoma.** Glaucoma occurring in association with widespread deposit of cellular organelles on the lens capsule, ocular blood vessels, iris, and ciliary body.
>
> **drusen.** Accumulation of extracellular material on the Bruch's membrane of the choroid.
>
> **laminar.** Having to do with a thin, flat membrane or layer of a larger structure.

> **CODING AXIOM**
>
> ICD-10-CM Official Coding Guidelines I.C.7.a.1-5. address the use of codes from category H40 Glaucoma. One of these guidelines state to "assign as many codes from category H40 Glaucoma, as needed to identify the type of glaucoma, the affected eye, and the glaucoma stage." It is important for the user to follow these guidelines to ensure that all elements of the documented glaucoma are captured.

Figure 5.17: Glaucoma

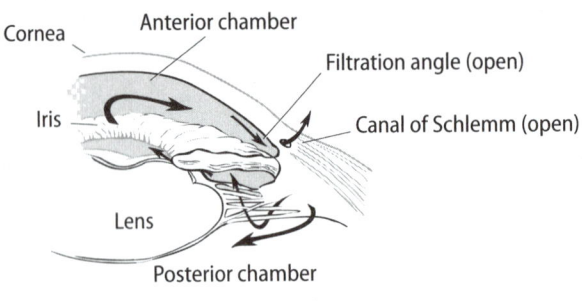

Cornea — Anterior chamber
Iris — Filtration angle (open)
— Canal of Schlemm (open)
Lens
Posterior chamber

Normal aqueous flow and pressure

Tonometry indirectly measures the intraocular pressure by determining the amount of pressure within the eye

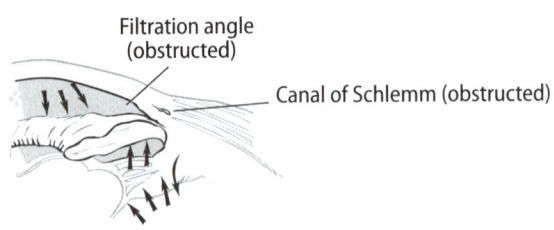

Filtration angle (obstructed)
Canal of Schlemm (obstructed)

Obstructed aqueous flow and abnormal pressure in the chambers

In glaucoma, pseudoexfoliation of the lens capsule is characterized by small, grayish particles deposited on the pupillary margin of the iris, anterior chamber, and lens. This occurs when cells within the eye release dandruff-like flakes as the outer layers of the lens slough off and block normal flow of the aqueous humor. Material deposited on the front surface of the lens in the eye may be partially rubbed off as the pupil moves over the lens. This exfoliation may occlude the outflow track (trabecular meshwork) and cause intraocular pressure to rise. Left untreated, this condition could lead to subsequent damage to the optic nerve, causing visual field loss and progressive blindness. Pseudoexfoliation syndrome-associated glaucoma commonly affects elderly patients with coexisting cataracts. It typically presents unilaterally but can progress to a bilateral presentation within several years.

Primary angle-closure glaucoma occurs when aqueous outflow is obstructed by occlusion of the trabecular meshwork, resulting in optic nerve damage and visual field loss. The pressure from secretion of aqueous into the posterior chamber by the ciliary body pushes the peripheral iris anteriorly, closing the angle. Clinical presentation varies from gradual and progressive to rapid and emergent. Symptoms of open-angle glaucoma include progressive loss of peripheral vision over a span of years, blurred or foggy vision, seeing halos around lights, reduced night vision, and aching in the eyes.

ICD-10-CM code descriptions for cataract classifications have been updated (as with other ocular disorders) by replacing the term "senile" with "age-related," where appropriate, since the term "senile" has been confused with an age-related dementia, cognitive decline, or other degenerative mental health conditions beyond that associated with the normal aging process. ICD-10-CM has also revised terminology within the cataract classification categories, changing "*after-cataract*" to "secondary cataract" and denoting hypermature senile cataract (366.18) as an age-related cataract, *morgagnian type* (H25.2-).

DEFINITIONS

after-cataract. Cataract characterized by opacifications of the posterior capsule occurring subsequent to extracapsular cataract extraction.

morgagnian-type cataract. Mature, age-related cataract with lens opacification and a soft, liquefied or flattened fragile lens, causing nuclear shifts to the bottom of the lens capsule.

Coding for Cataracts

ICD-9-CM		ICD-10-CM	
366.18	Hypermature senile cataract	H25.20	Age-related cataract, morgagnian type, unspecified eye
		H25.21	Age-related cataract morgagnian type, right eye
		H25.22	Age-related cataract, morgagnian type, left eye
		H25.23	Age-related cataract, morgagnian type, bilateral

By definition, a morgagnian-type cataract is a hypermature, age-related cataract with lens opacification characterized by a soft, liquefied, or flattened lens that is prone to leakage of cortical matter through the capsule. The nucleus shifts to the bottom of the lens capsule, which may cause swelling and irritation of other structures in the eye.

Figure 5.18: Cataract

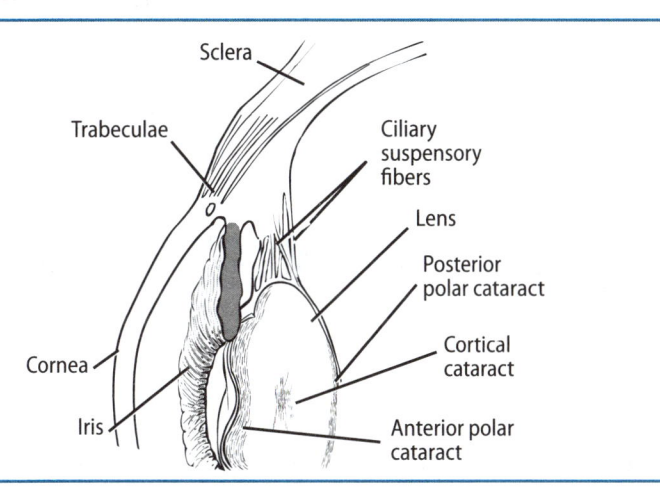

A senile (age-related) cataract involves partial or total opacity of the lens due to degenerative changes associated with the aging process. Age-related cataracts form gradually and often bilaterally in patients 55 to 70 years of age. Signs and symptoms of a senile cataract include a slow, progressive, and painless loss of vision, leukocoria (white reflection from the pupil), difficulty in night driving, altered color perception, and strabismus. Cataracts can be clinically classified by the zones of the lens involved in the opacity: anterior and posterior cortical, equatorial cortical, and supranuclear and nuclear. Age-related cataracts may include specific types of cataract, including cuneiform, nuclear, or posterior subcapsular cataract, or those with overlapping characteristics. Most age-related cataracts are identified by increased opacity of the lens followed by its softening and shrinkage associated with degeneration.

ICD-9-CM required two codes in specific sequence to report ophthalmic infection with *Acanthamoeba,* whereas ICD-10-CM has a single code:

Coding for *Acanthamoeba* Infection

ICD-9-CM		ICD-10-CM	
136.21	Specific infection due to Acanthamoeba	B60.13	Keratoconjunctivitis due to Acanthamoeba
370.8	Other forms of keratitis		
136.21	Specific infection due to Acanthamoeba	B60.12	Conjunctivitis due to Acanthamoeba
372.15	Parasitic conjunctivitis		

Diseases caused by the free-living (not parasitic) ameboid protozoan *Acanthamoeba* include amoebic keratoconjunctivitis and meningoencephalitis. *Acanthamoeba* infection is a rare but potentially blinding affliction of the cornea. It primarily affects otherwise healthy persons who improperly store, handle, or disinfect their contact lenses (e.g., by using tap water or homemade solutions for cleaning). Symptoms are similar to those of other eye infections, but targeted treatment is necessary to be effective. Complications include corneal scarring and vision loss. Long-term therapy and management are often required.

Certain ICD-10-CM code descriptions have been updated and code classifications further specified by creating unique codes for conditions once listed as inclusion terms under less-specific ICD-9-CM codes. For example, ICD-9-CM listed **arcus senilis** as an inclusion term under code 371.41 Senile corneal changes. ICD-10-CM has created a separate subcategory classification for arcus senilis (H18.41-), distinct from other specified corneal degenerative disorders (H18.4-).

Coding for Arcus Senilis

ICD-9-CM		ICD-10-CM	
371.41	Senile corneal changes	H18.411	Arcus senilis, right eye
		H18.412	Arcus senilis, left eye
		H18.413	Arcus senilis, bilateral
		H18.419	Arcus senilis, unspecified eye

Arcus senilis is the appearance of a white or gray opaque ring in the corneal margin due to cholesterol deposits on the corneal stroma. It may be described as a peripheral corneal opacity, one in which an abnormal white ring appears around the iris. Although other forms of corneal arcus may be present at birth or in childhood (i.e., arcus juvenilis), they often fade. If the condition persists earlier in life, it may herald an underlying lipid disorder. In the aged population, arcus senilis is commonly due to hypercholesterolemia but may also occur as a sign of corneal ischemia secondary to other ocular disease. Normally, arcus senilis does not adversely affect vision or require treatment other than to precipitate treatment of the underlying disease (e.g., ischemia, lipid disorder).

DEFINITIONS

arcus senilis. Abnormal white or gray opaque ring appearing at the periphery of the corneal margin; occurring in older adults and often associated with hypercholesterolemia.

Figure 5.19: Arcus Senilis

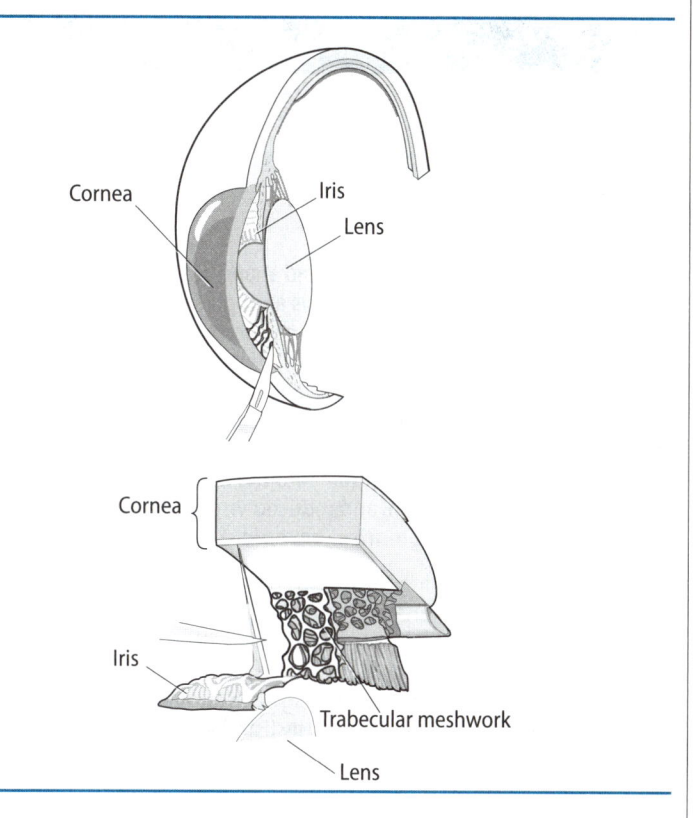

The cornea is the transparent tissue that covers the front of the eye and is composed of three layers:

1. The epithelium blocks the passage of foreign material and provides a smooth surface that absorbs oxygen and other needed cell nutrients that are contained in tears.

2. The stroma gives the cornea its strength and elasticity, and the protein fibers of the stroma produce the cornea's light-conducting transparency.

3. The endothelium pumps excess water out of the stroma.

Unlike most tissues in the body, the cornea contains no blood vessels to protect it against infection. The cornea is a physical barrier that shields the inside of the eye from germs, dust, and other foreign objects. It also acts as the eye's outermost lens; when light strikes the cornea, it refracts the incoming light onto the crystalline lens. The lens focuses the light onto the retina. Although much thinner than the lens, the cornea provides about 65 percent of the eye's power to bend light. Most of this power resides in the center of the cornea, which is rounder and thinner than the outer part of the tissue and is better suited to bending light waves.

Although certain ICD-10-CM codes that separate conditions according to severity of presentation are similar to those of ICD-9-CM, terminology has been updated to reflect current clinical language. For example, keratoconus was previously classified as unspecified (371.60), stable (371.61), or with acute hydrops (371.62). In ICD-10-CM, the term "unstable" replaces the less frequently documented "acute hydrops."

Coding for Keratoconus

ICD-9-CM		ICD-10-CM	
371.62	Keratoconus, acute hydrops	H18.621	Keratoconus, unstable, right eye
		H18.622	Keratoconus, unstable, left eye
		H18.623	Keratoconus, unstable, bilateral
		H18.629	Keratoconus, unstable, unspecified eye

> ### DEFINITIONS
>
> **astigmatism.** Condition causing blurred vision due to the irregular shape of the cornea or curvature of the lens.
>
> **chloasma.** Patchy tan to brown skin discolorations, often secondary to melanocyte stimulation; may be associated with hormonal fluctuation or imbalance.
>
> **Descemet's membrane.** Collagenous inner layer of the corneal endothelium.
>
> **madarosis.** Loss of eyelashes, congenital or acquired; most commonly occurs secondary to other medical conditions.
>
> **myopia.** Impairment of distant vision; nearsightedness.
>
> **vitiligo.** Tan to white patches of skin discoloration from the loss or impairment of cutaneous melanocytes.

Keratoconus causes the normally round shape of the cornea to thin and take on a bulging, cone-shaped appearance. It is a progressive, noninflammatory, usually bilateral disease of the cornea. Onset may occur in the teens and early 20s, progressing for five to 15 years, and sometimes longer. When progression stops, the disease is considered stable and typically remains so for the remainder of the patient's life. During rapid progression, sudden visual disturbances can spontaneously occur. In acute or unstable presentations, a break in *Descemet's membrane* allows aqueous to drain into the cornea, resulting in an immediate edema, corneal opacification, and reduced visual acuity. Vision loss is attributed primarily to resultant *astigmatism*, *myopia*, and secondary corneal scarring.

Certain conditions affecting the eyelids have been differentiated in ICD-10-CM not only by laterality, but by anatomic site: upper eyelid or lower eyelid. For example, the following ophthalmic conditions have been further specified in ICD-10-CM by creating unique codes for conditions once listed as inclusion terms under less-specific ICD-9-CM codes, specifying both laterality and anatomic site. *Chloasma*, *vitiligo* and *madarosis* were previously listed as inclusion terms under comparatively general ICD-9-CM code descriptions.

Coding for Eyelid Disorders

ICD-9-CM		ICD-10-CM	
374.52	Hyperpigmentation of eyelid	H02.711	Chloasma of right upper eyelid and periocular area
		H02.712	Chloasma of right lower eyelid and periocular area
		H02.713	Chloasma of right eye, unspecified eyelid and periocular area
		H02.714	Chloasma of left upper eyelid and periocular area
		H02.715	Chloasma of left lower eyelid and periocular area
		H02.716	Chloasma of left eye, unspecified eyelid and periocular area
		H02.719	Chloasma of unspecified eye, unspecified eyelid and periocular area
374.53	Hypopigmentation of eyelid	H02.731	Vitiligo of right upper eyelid and periocular area
		H02.732	Vitiligo of right lower eyelid and periocular area
		H02.733	Vitiligo of right eye, unspecified eyelid and periocular area
		H02.734	Vitiligo of left upper eyelid and periocular area
		H02.735	Vitiligo of left lower eyelid and periocular area
		H02.736	Vitiligo of left eye, unspecified eyelid and periocular area
		H02.739	Vitiligo of unspecified eye, unspecified eyelid and periocular area

ICD-9-CM		ICD-10-CM	
374.55	Hypotrichosis of eyelid	H02.721	Madarosis of right upper eyelid and periocular area
		H02.722	Madarosis of right lower eyelid and periocular area
		H02.723	Madarosis of right eye, unspecified eyelid and periocular area
		H02.724	Madarosis of left upper eyelid and periocular area
		H02.725	Madarosis of left lower eyelid and periocular area
		H02.726	Madarosis of left eye, unspecified eyelid and periocular area
		H02.729	Madarosis of unspecified eye, unspecified eyelid and periocular area

Ear and Mastoid Process

ICD-10-CM classifies disorders of the ear and mastoid process by anatomic site, according to those conditions that affect the external (H60–H62), middle (H65–H75), or inner (H80–H83) ear. Additional classification sections group together other disorders of ear (H90–H94) and intraoperative or postprocedural disorders (H95). In addition, code titles were revised to uniquely classify certain types of disease previously included within a code category.

Coding for Otitis Media

ICD-9-CM		ICD-10-CM	
381	Nonsuppurative otitis media and eustachian tube disorders	H65	Nonsuppurative otitis media
382	Suppurative and unspecified otitis media	H66	Suppurative and unspecified otitis media
		H67	Otitis media in diseases classified elsewhere

These unique codes enable condition details to be more specific, making the granularity of data greater than in the ICD-9-CM system. This is particularly evident in ICD-10-CM classification of ear infections, in which code categories have been differentiated and expanded, not only to further specify site, laterality, and severity of presentation (i.e., acute, chronic, unspecified), but also to distinguish between specific types and characteristics of infection.

Coding for Ear Infections

ICD-9-CM		ICD-10-CM	
380.10	Unspecified infective otitis externa	H60.01	**Abscess** of right external ear
		H60.11	**Cellulitis** of right external ear
		H60.311	**Diffuse** otitis externa, right ear
		H60.321	**Hemorrhagic** otitis externa, right ear
380.22	Other acute otitis externa	H60.511	Acute actinic otitis externa, right ear
		H60.521	Acute chemical otitis externa, right ear
		H60.531	Acute contact otitis externa, right ear
		H60.541	Acute eczematoid otitis externa, right ear
		H60.551	Acute reactive otitis externa, right ear

> **DEFINITIONS**
>
> **abscess.** Enclosed, localized collection of pus.
>
> **cellulitis.** Inflammation of the cells caused by infection of the tissue just below the skin surface.
>
> **diffuse.** Scattered or spread throughout an area.
>
> **hemorrhagic.** Characterized by bleeding (hemorrhage).

Furthermore, ICD-10-CM separately classifies recurrent acute otitis media. ICD-9-CM does not identify recurrent acute conditions specifically. ICD-10-CM, however, describes certain recurrent forms of allergic otitis media in code category H65.11 Acute and subacute allergic otitis media. Separately classified as mucoid, sanguinous, or serous in ICD-9-CM, acute otitis media is identified instead by laterality and presentation (recurrent or nonrecurrent) in ICD-10-CM.

Coding for Otitis Media

ICD-9-CM		ICD-10-CM	
381.01	Acute serous otitis media	H65.01	Acute serous otitis media, right ear
		H65.04	Acute serous otitis media, recurrent, right ear
381.02	Acute mucoid otitis media	H65.111	Acute and subacute allergic otitis media (mucoid) (sanguinous) (serous), right ear
		H65.114	Acute and subacute allergic otitis media (mucoid) (sanguinous) (serous), recurrent, right ear
381.03	Acute sanguinous otitis media	H65.111	Acute and subacute allergic otitis media (mucoid) (sanguinous) (serous), right ear
		H65.114	Acute and subacute allergic otitis media (mucoid) (sanguinous) (serous), recurrent, right ear
381.04	Acute allergic serous otitis media	H65.111	Acute and subacute allergic otitis media (mucoid) (sanguinous) (serous), right ear
		H65.114	Acute and subacute allergic otitis media (mucoid) (sanguinous) (serous), recurrent, right ear
381.05	Acute allergic mucoid otitis media	H65.111	Acute and subacute allergic otitis media (mucoid) (sanguinous) (serous), right ear
		H65.114	Acute and subacute allergic otitis media (mucoid) (sanguinous) (serous), recurrent, right ear
381.06	Acute allergic sanguinous otitis media	H65.111	Acute and subacute allergic otitis media (mucoid) (sanguinous) (serous), right ear
		H65.114	Acute and subacute allergic otitis media (mucoid) (sanguinous) (serous), recurrent, right ear

Disorders of the external ear include those of the auricle (pinna) and external auditory meatus. The auricle consists of the helix, anthelix, scapha, concha, tragus, antitragus, intertragic notch, and lobule. The auricle is a single, elastic cartilage covered in skin and normal adnexal features (hair follicles, sweat glands, and sebaceous glands). The ridges in the auricle channel sounds into the acoustic meatus. The semicircular depression leading to the ear is named the concha, Latin for shell. The external auditory meatus consists of cartilaginous and osseous portions with the canal lined with epidermis, hair, and ceruminous glands that extend to the tympanic membrane.

Figure 5.20: External Ear

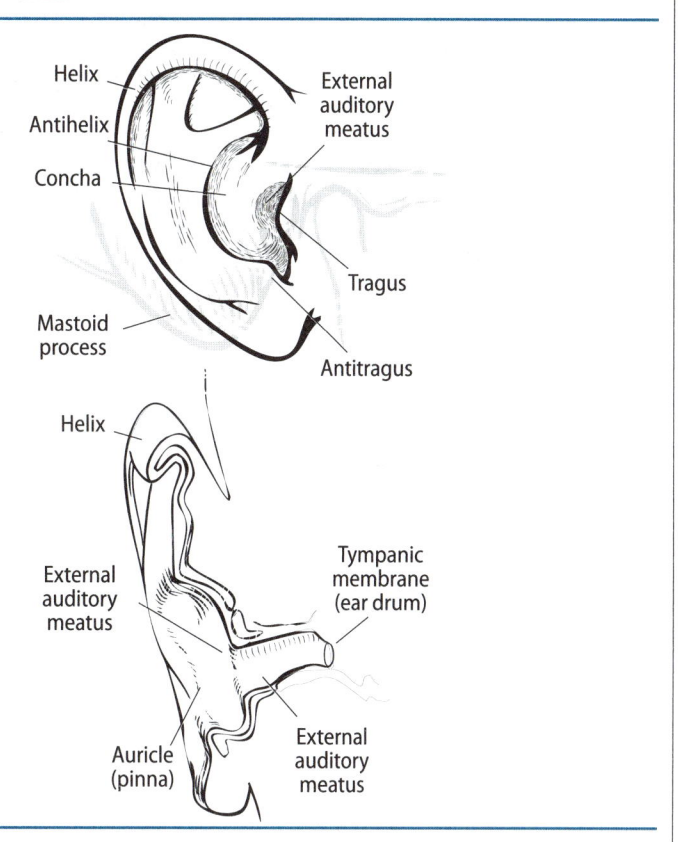

Otitis externa is an inflammation or infection of the auricle and external **meatus**. Although otitis externa is most commonly caused by infection, it may also be associated with noninfectious local or systemic conditions. Infective otitis externa indicates the presence of bacteria as the etiology of the inflammation. Causal organisms may include *Pseudomonas, Proteus vulgaris, Streptococci,* and *Staphylococcus aureus,* or fungal infections such as *Candida albicans.* Bacterial overgrowth can often be attributed to excessive exposure to moisture or trauma, both of which compromise the natural homeostasis within the ear. Cerumen provides a natural defense against the overgrowth of bacteria and creates a barrier for excess moisture; however, an imbalance in the amount of cerumen can impair these defensive processes and create an environment vulnerable to pathogenesis. Signs and symptoms of infective otitis externa include pain, redness, and swelling that can obstruct the meatus, serous or purulent drainage, external ear tenderness, and enlarged regional lymph nodes. Diagnostic tests include culture and sensitivity to identify the infective organism. An otoscopy reveals inflammation and ceruminous impaction. Therapies include antimicrobials (topically, systemically, or both), heat therapy to relieve pain, and gentle ear cleansing.

Noninfectious otitis externa can precipitate infectious otitis externa or occur independently of infection. Both systemic and local dermatologic conditions can result in an inflammation of the ear. Causal conditions may include certain types of dermatitis (e.g., eczematous, atopic, contact, *seborrheic*), lupus erythematosus, **psoriasis**, and acne. Similarly, localized inflammation can occur secondary to exposures to allergens or other irritants. Allergic dermatitis is commonly acute in presentation, with characteristic redness, pruritus, and edema. Contact dermatitis is often similar in presentation but with epidermal thickening and hardening. Tissue irritation due to noninfectious causes can precipitate secondary bacterial infection. Treatment depends on identifying and removing the irritant. Topical steroids are often beneficial in reducing inflammation and facilitating healing.

DEFINITIONS

meatus. Body opening or passage (e.g., the external opening of a canal).

otitis externa. Inflammation or infection of the auricle and external auditory meatus.

psoriasis. Chronic, painful skin disease characterized by inflamed, reddened patches on the skin and thickened, silvery scales.

seborrheic. Characterized by the overproduction of sebum, the oily secretion of sebaceous glands.

Disorders of the middle ear affect the structures inside the tympanic membrane, extending to the oval window of the cochlea. The middle ear (tympanic cavity) lies within the temporal bone and contains the ossicles, the trio of auditory bones connected by synovial joints and suspended by specialized ligaments and muscles. The eustachian tube connects the tympanic and nasal cavities to help equalize pressure within the cavities with the atmospheric pressure. Equalized pressure allows the tympanic membrane to vibrate freely. Disproportionate pressure can result in severe pain, hearing impairment, "ringing" in the ears, and vertigo. Middle ear infections often occur as a result of pathogens migrating from the nasopharynx through the eustachian tube to the auditory canal.

Figure 5.21: Middle and Inner Ear

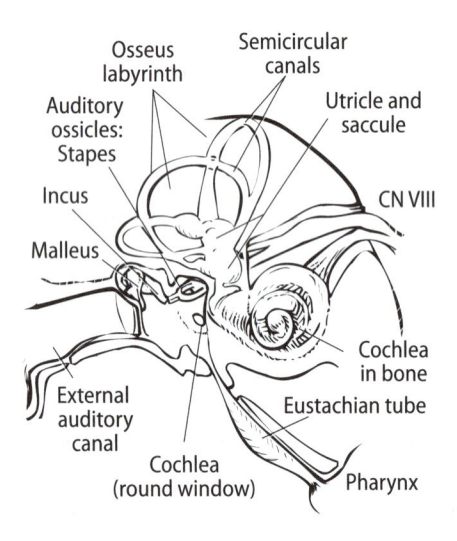

Exposed view of middle and inner ear

> **DEFINITIONS**
>
> **ankylosis (ossicles).** Abnormal stiffness, adhesion, rigidity, or hardening of the auditory ossicles, decreasing mobility and conduction.
>
> **necrotic.** Pertaining to the deterioration or death of tissue in response to disease or injury.
>
> **suppurative.** Characterized by the formation and discharge of pus.
>
> **tympanosclerosis.** Characterized by the accumulation of hardened, dense tissue or plaque in the middle ear, adversely affecting the mobility of the tympanic membrane and ossicles.

Otitis media is a painful inflammation of the tympanic membrane characterized by a build-up of fluids in the middle ear. Signs and symptoms may be similar to an upper respiratory infection and include chills and fever, malaise, deep throbbing ear pain, nausea and vomiting, dulled or impaired hearing, ear drainage, bulging of tympanic membrane, and a tender, swollen mastoid process. Untreated otitis media can progress to a suppurative presentation in which the tympanic membrane becomes thinned and **necrotic**, which leads to perforation.

Suppurative otitis media is most commonly caused by a bacterial infection (e.g., *Streptococcus pneumoniae, Haemophilus influenza, Moraxella catarrhalis*). Complications of otitis media are often associated with chronic or subacute disease. Acute and chronic otitis media infection may spread beyond the temporal bone and cause intratemporal (e.g., mastoiditis, petrositis, labyrinthitis, and facial nerve paralysis) and intracranial (e.g., extradural abscess, brain abscess, subdural abscess, otic hydrocephalus, and meningitis) complications. Associated conditions include adenoiditis or tonsillitis, colds or sinusitis, cholesteatoma, adhesions or scarring of middle ear structures, conductive hearing loss, abscesses, and jugular vein thrombosis. **Tympanosclerosis** is a common sequela after acute and chronic otitis media; the pathological calcified plaques are found in the tympanic membrane and the middle ear ossicles. These accumulation of plaques decreases the mobility of the tympanic membrane (tympanic sclerosis) and of the ossicles (**ankylosis**), impairing hearing.

Diagnosis includes use of a pneumatoscopy to ascertain whether there is fluid behind the eardrum or an otomicroscopy using the operating microscope to visualize depth and three-dimensional structure. Antibiotics are usually prescribed for infection. Once osteitis is diagnosed, mastoidectomy is generally warranted to remove the infected, often necrotic bone. If there is an abscess, surgery is performed to drain pus and remove the infected bone.

Therapies include systemic antibiotics, nasal decongestants, and analgesics such as aspirin to control pain and fever, and myringotomy with aspiration of the middle ear fluid if the tympanic membrane is in danger of rupture. Surgery may be performed (tympanoplasty, myringoplasty, mastoidectomy, excision of cholesteatomas) for chronic otitis media.

Although ICD-10-CM generally is far more specific than ICD-9-CM, certain classifications have been made less specific. For example, certain forms of vertigo, labyrinthitis, labyrinthine fistula, and dysfunction once separately classified according to type have been grouped together within revised subcategories and are instead identified by general diagnosis and laterality.

Coding for Vertigo, Labyrinthitis, and Fistula

ICD-9-CM		ICD-10-CM	
386.19	Other and unspecified peripheral vertigo	H81.311	Aural vertigo, right ear
386.31	Serous labyrinthitis	H83.01	Labyrinthitis, right ear
386.32	Circumscribed labyrinthitis		
386.33	Suppurative labyrinthitis		
386.41	Round window fistula	H83.11	Labyrinthine fistula, right ear
386.42	Oval window fistula		
386.43	Semicircular canal fistula		
386.51	Hyperactive labyrinth, unilateral	H83.2X1	Labyrinthine dysfunction, right ear
386.55	Loss of labyrinthine reactivity, unilateral	H83.2X1	Labyrinthine dysfunction, right ear

The inner ear consists of a system of fluid-filled tubes and sacs called the labyrinth, as well as the nerves that connect the labyrinth to the brain. Impulses for equilibrium are transmitted along the vestibular cochlear nerve to the brain. The vestibular system lies within the temporal bone of the skull and contains the labyrinth and the cochlea. The cochlea contains fluid-filled channels and membranes that transmit sound vibrations via thousands of tiny, specialized hairs to the vestibulocochlear nerve. The vestibular apparatus of the inner ear contains the semicircular ducts, utricle, and saccule, which work together to maintain dynamic equilibrium. The nerve impulses transmitted to the brain are relayed to the medulla, pons, and cerebellum. The cerebellum receives the sensory information from the vestibular apparatus and makes the corrective adjustments to maintain static and dynamic equilibrium.

Figure 5.22: Schematic of Labyrinth and Semicircular Ducts

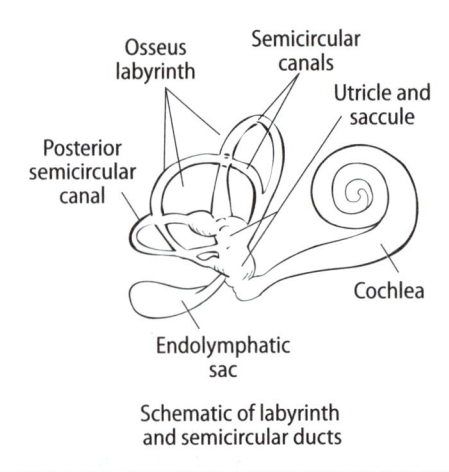

Schematic of labyrinth and semicircular ducts

Classification systems differentiate between aural vertigo and Ménière's disease, although clinical definitions for both conditions overlap. For classification purposes, vertigo specified as "aural" or "otogenic" describes peripheral vertigo of inner ear origin, not specified as Ménière's disease. Peripheral vertigo refers to a group of conditions in which the vertigo symptoms are of inner-ear origin, whereas "central" vertigo refers to a group of conditions in which the symptoms originate in the central nervous system.

Ménière's disease is a disorder of the inner ear that causes episodes of vertigo, tinnitus, a feeling of fullness or pressure in the ear, and fluctuating hearing loss that can last two to four hours. Episodes may occur in clusters, or weeks, months, or years may pass between episodes. Between the acute attacks, most people are free of symptoms or note only mild imbalance and tinnitus. Between attacks, medication may be prescribed to help regulate the fluid pressure in the inner ear, reducing the severity and frequency of episodes. Treatment includes medical or surgical measures to relieve the pressure on the inner ear or to block the transmission of information from the affected ear to the brain.

Labyrinthitis and neuronitis are inflammatory conditions of the inner ear commonly caused by viral or bacterial infection. Inflammation of the cochlea can cause disturbances in hearing, such as tinnitus. Dizziness, unsteadiness, or imbalance when walking and nausea are the most common symptoms of vestibular disorders. Because the vestibular system interacts with other parts of the nervous system, concurrent visual disturbances, cognitive difficulties, amnesia, and motor function impairment may occur with such disorders. Patients with vestibular disorders often report fatigue, loss of stamina, and an inability to concentrate. Trauma and ear infections (e.g., otitis media, labyrinthitis) may reduce blood flow to the inner ear, which can damage the vestibular apparatus. High doses or long-term use of certain antibiotics can also cause permanent damage to the inner ear. Other drugs, such as aspirin, caffeine, alcohol, nicotine, sedatives, and tranquilizers can cause temporary dizziness but do not permanently damage the vestibular system.

Benign paroxysmal positional vertigo is commonly induced upon repositioning the head or body (e.g., getting out of bed, standing up from a sitting or lying position) and is often attributed to calcium-impacted inner ear canals. Treatment includes removing the impaction.

Labyrinthine fistula is an abnormal opening between the inner and middle ear through which the inner ear fluid drains into the middle ear cavity. Symptoms include dizziness and hearing loss. Causal conditions include dislocation of the inner ear structures (e.g., trauma or infection), congenital malformation, or **cholesteatoma** (abnormal overgrowth of granulation tissue).

DEFINITIONS

cholesteatoma. Abnormal overgrowth of granulation tissue in the middle ear and/or mastoid process.

Labyrinthine dysfunction is a general term describing a malfunction of the labyrinth that disrupts neurotransmission to the brain regarding body position. As a result, the labyrinth does not respond properly to movement. Trauma and infection are common causal factors. The dysfunction is often characterized by the sensation of *oscillopsia*, the illusion that the environment is moving. Symptoms may include vertigo, disequilibrium, motion sickness, nausea and vomiting, visual disturbances, and difficulty with memory and concentration.

ICD-10-CM codes for abnormal auditory perception disorders separately identify certain conditions (e.g., temporary auditory threshold shift), whereas other conditions (e.g., impairment of auditory discrimination) are grouped into general code subcategories such as H93.29 Other abnormal auditory perceptions.

> **DEFINITIONS**
>
> **oscillopsia.** Illusion that the environment is moving caused by disrupted neurotransmission from the labyrinth to the brain.

Coding for Auditory Misperception

ICD-9-CM		ICD-10-CM	
315.32	Mixed receptive-expressive language disorder	H93.25	Central auditory processing disorder
388.40	Unspecified abnormal auditory perception	H93.241	Temporary auditory threshold shift, right ear
		H93.242	Temporary auditory threshold shift, left ear
		H93.243	Temporary auditory threshold shift, bilateral
		H93.249	Temporary auditory threshold shift, unspecified ear
		H93.291	Other abnormal auditory perceptions, right ear
		H93.292	Other abnormal auditory perceptions, left ear
		H93.293	Other abnormal auditory perceptions, bilateral
388.43	Impairment of auditory discrimination	H93.299	Other abnormal auditory perceptions, unspecified ear
388.45	Acquired auditory processing disorder		

The ear has a number of defense mechanisms that protect its complex sensory structures from damage. For example, vasoconstriction of the auditory blood vessels in response to loud sound reduces the blood supply to the organ of Corti, thereby reducing the sensitivity and response of the sensory hair cells and protecting these structures from damage. Under normal conditions, the ear's sensitivity adjusts according to sound exposure. Sound vibrations are detected by the sensory apparatus of the inner ear and transmitted to the brain where they can be interpreted to yield meaningful information. Advances in diagnostic medicine continue to identify certain disorders pertaining to physiological interpretation and processing of sound, which were previously overlooked or misdiagnosed. These conditions may overlap or coexist with those classified elsewhere, such as ototoxic disorders secondary to adverse effects of medication, trauma, infection, or other systemic disease.

In auditory medicine, the term "auditory perception" may be defined as the ability to identify, interpret, and attach meaning to sound. Disorders of auditory perception can be difficult to diagnose because they can occur independently or secondary to infection, stroke, trauma, or other health problems. In children, these auditory perception and processing disorders may be associated with learning difficulties and therefore may be misdiagnosed as attention deficit disorder or certain forms of autism.

Auditory processing and perception disorders are not synonymous with deficits in general attention, language, or cognitive function, although such conditions may coexist or overlap. For example, individuals with auditory discrimination difficulties are unable to denote the differences between sounds, which is integral to language development. Auditory discrimination also is necessary in distinguishing between foreground and background noise. If this process is not functioning properly, the individual may become confused or overwhelmed when they are unable to ignore irrelevant noise. This state can impair learning and be misinterpreted as an inability to focus or concentrate.

Auditory synthesis facilitates language comprehension by combining sounds into understandable units. The term "auditory sequencing" may also refer to the process by which one understands and remembers the order in which sounds occur. Auditory synthesis and sequencing are integral to auditory perception and memory.

Disorders of auditory perception may be congenital or acquired. The onset of either form in early childhood can pose learning challenges. Individuals with impaired auditory perception may seem not to respond well to auditory or verbal cues or understand what they hear, or require that auditory cues be repeated before giving the desired response. These conditions are generally attributed to a disorder or dysfunction of the auditory nerve, which most appropriately identifies the underlying physiological causal factors.

Auditory processing disorder is a general term describing various disorders that often arise from impaired neural function. Manifestations may include problems differentiating between related speech sounds, and speech and environmental sounds; or relating spoken word with intent. Coping mechanisms may include depending on visual cues such as body language, eye contact, or lip reading.

Diplacusis describes a cochlear dysfunction in which the patient hears a single auditory stimulus as two sounds. This condition may be colloquially described as being "tone deaf." Acquired diplacusis may be attributed to allergies, head trauma, infection, exposure to toxins, or neoplasms (e.g., leukemia, acoustic neuromas).

Hyperacusis is a condition of acute hearing sensitivity that may or may not be accompanied by pain. Causal conditions include migraine, Asperger syndrome, Bell's palsy, and many other conditions.

Auditory recruitment describes the abnormal perception of volume of speech or sound. It is often associated with certain degrees of sensorineural hearing loss or labyrinthitis, in which hearing is not sensitive to quiet sounds, yet is overly sensitive to loud sounds.

Auditory threshold shift is the process by which the ear protects itself by adjusting its sensitivity when exposed to noise. When this occurs, only sounds louder than a certain level are heard. Also known as "aural fatigue," the duration of shift can be temporary or permanent. Temporary auditory threshold shift often implies a temporary hearing loss to low-level sounds and may be associated with tinnitus. If the sensory hair cells of the inner ear are not allowed to recover through reduced exposure to loud sounds, they can become permanently damaged.

Coding for Conductive Hearing Loss

ICD-9-CM		ICD-10-CM	
389.03	Conductive hearing loss, middle ear	H90.0	Conductive hearing loss, bilateral
		H90.11	Conductive hearing loss, unilateral, right ear, with unrestricted hearing on the contralateral side
		H90.12	Conductive hearing loss, unilateral, left ear, with unrestricted hearing on the contralateral side

Chapter 6. ICD-10-CM: Endocrine System

Anatomic Overview

The endocrine system is comprised of **glands** that produce and secrete **hormones** with a varied array of vital functions. These hormones are chemical substances released by organs or individual cells within an organ. The hormones are then carried through the bloodstream to other organs or tissues. A hormone's purpose is varied and includes the regulation of growth, metabolism, and sexual development and function. Hormones are often referred to as the "chemical messengers" because they transfer information from one set of cells to another to synchronize the body's functions.

The major glands of the endocrine system are the hypothalamus, pituitary, thymus, thyroid, parathyroid, adrenal, pineal body, ovaries, testes, and pancreas. Many organs and tissues within the body work with the endocrine system even though they are not fully functioning parts of the system. These organs and tissues contain cells that also secrete hormones, including but not limited to adipose tissue, heart, liver, kidneys, placenta, skin, small intestine, and stomach.

The endocrine system is made up of two different types of glandular tissue: exocrine and endocrine. Exocrine glands release secretions into ducts, which distribute the secretions to other areas of the body. Exocrine glands include digestive, mucus, oil, and sweat glands. Endocrine glands secrete hormones into the fluid surrounding the secretory cells. The blood then carries the hormones throughout the body.

Approximately 50 hormones are produced within the endocrine system. Hormones move throughout the body but can react only with certain cells, referred to as "**target cells**." These cells contain specific protein receptors that allow the hormone to chemically bind to the cells. Receptors are continuously being created and broken down within the body. When certain hormone imbalances occur, the body may produce excessive amounts of a hormone. The receptors automatically respond by reducing the number of receptors reacting to the target cells and by making the target cells less sensitive to the hormone. When there is a decrease in hormone production, the target tissue becomes more sensitive and more receptors appear in the cells.

Hormones are released when the body is stimulated by the nervous system (e.g., anxiety, fear, or stress) or from chemical changes in the blood, such as sugar level. For example, after ingesting a meal, glucose levels rise and the pancreas responds by releasing the hormone insulin into the bloodstream. The insulin circulates throughout the body until glucose levels return to normal.

Hormones are divided into different classifications based on chemical structure. Some are soluble in water, and others are soluble in fats or lipids. Water-soluble hormones typically include **amines** and **peptide** hormones. Lipid-soluble hormones include steroids, thyroid hormones, and nitric oxide.

Examples of water-soluble hormones grouped to amines include:

- Epinephrine (Epi) (adrenaline)
- Histamine
- Melatonin
- Norepinephrine (NE) (noradrenaline, NA)
- Serotonin (5-HT)

INTERESTING A & P FACT

The endocrine glands are sometimes referred to as ductless glands.

DEFINITIONS

amines. Chemical compound that is derived from ammonia and contains nitrogen.

endocrine glands. Group of glands that secrete hormones directly into the blood and not through a duct.

hormone. Chemical substance produced by the body that has a regulatory effect on the function of its specific target organ(s).

peptide. Molecule consisting of two or more amino acids.

target cell. Specific collection of cells that responds to a given hormone treatment or tissue against which any type of immunity is directed.

> **DEFINITIONS**
>
> **amino acid.** One of the building blocks of protein that contains a basic amino (NH2), an acidic carboxyl (COOH), and a variable side chain (R) attached to an alpha carbon atom.

Peptide hormones are the largest class of hormones and include all of the hormones secreted by the hypothalamus, pituitary, heart, kidneys, thymus, digestive tract, and pancreas. Peptide and protein hormones are grouped together depending upon the number of *amino acids* the hormone contains.

A few examples of these types of hormones include:

- Alpha-fetoprotein
- Antidiuretic hormone (vasopressin)
- Erythropoietin (EPO)
- Follicle stimulating hormone (FSH)
- Gastrin
- Glucagon
- Growth hormone (GH)
- Human chorionic gonadotropin
- Insulin
- Luteinizing hormone (LH)
- Oxytocin
- Prolactin
- Secretin
- Somatostatin
- Thyrotropin (TSH)

Examples of lipid-soluble hormones include:

- Steroids:
    - aldosterone
    - androgen
    - calcitriol
    - cortisol
    - estrogen
    - progesterone
    - testosterone
- Thyroid hormones:
    - triiodothyronine (T^3)
    - thyroxine (T^4)
- Gas:
    - nitric oxide (NO)

Figure 6.1: Endocrine System

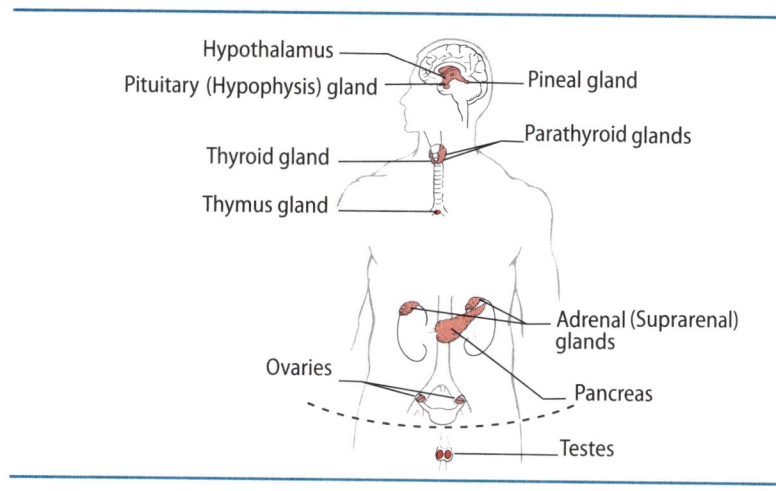

Pancreas Gland

The pancreas is a fish-shaped gland that extends horizontally behind the stomach from the curve of the duodenum to the spleen. The pancreas has two types of glandular tissue: the exocrine, which secretes digestive enzymes, and the endocrine, which produces hormones. However, it is primarily an exocrine organ.

The major part of the pancreas, called the exocrine pancreas, secretes digestive enzymes into the gastrointestinal tract. Distributed through the pancreas are clusters of endocrine cells that secrete insulin, glucagon, and somatostatin. These specialized cells are needed to maintain stable blood sugar levels in the body. Insulin helps body cells use glucose for energy, therefore reducing the amount of sugar in the bloodstream. At the same time, the hormone glucagon stimulates the liver to release its stored sugar into the blood, which raises the blood sugar levels.

Figure 6.2: Pancreas

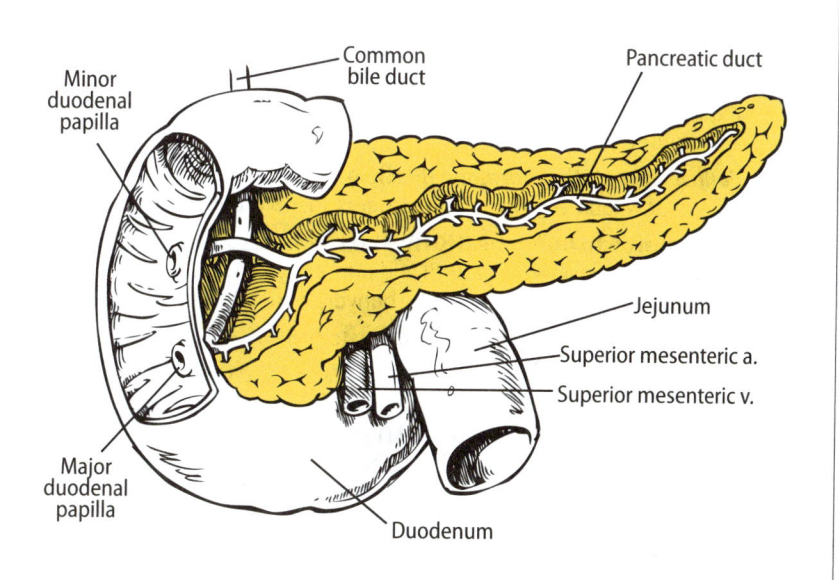

> **DEFINITIONS**
>
> **pancreatitis.** Inflammation of the pancreas that may be acute or chronic, symptomatic or asymptomatic, due to the autodigestion of pancreatic tissue by its own enzymes that have escaped into the pancreas, most often as a result of alcoholism or biliary tract disease such as calculi in the pancreatic duct.

Figure 6.3: Pituitary Gland

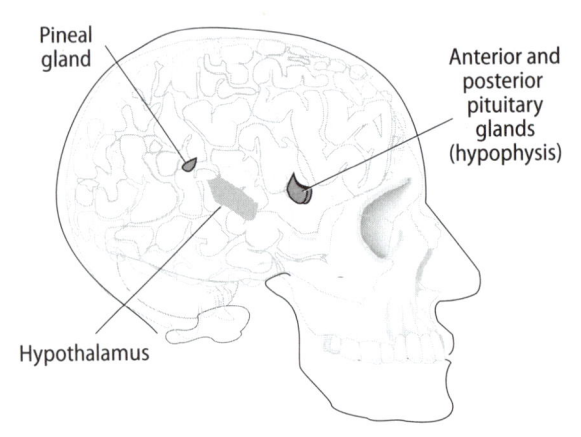

The pituitary gland and its controller, the hypothalamus, control body growth and stimulate and regulate other glands

Pituitary Gland

The pituitary gland, also referred to as hypophysis, is a pea-shaped structure located in the sella turcica of the sphenoid bone in the skull. The gland is attached to the undersurface of the hypothalamus by a short, slender stalk called the infundibulum. The pituitary gland contains endocrine cells surrounded by an extensive capillary network. It is also part of the hypophyseal portal system and provides entry into the circulatory system. It secretes several hormones that control the function of the other endocrine glands and regulates growth and fluid balance.

The pituitary gland is divided into two parts: the anterior and posterior lobes, each having separate functions. It is further subdivided into the distal part pars distalis and the intermediate part pars intermedia. The majority of the endocrine cells are found in the pars distalis. The anterior lobe regulates the activity of the thyroid, adrenal, and reproductive glands. It also regulates the body's growth and stimulates milk production in women who are breast-feeding.

Hormones secreted by the anterior lobe include:

- *Adrenocorticotropic hormone* (**ACTH**): Triggers the adrenal glands, which regulate stress response, to release hormones such as cortisol and aldosterone.
- *Follicle-stimulating hormone* (**FSH**): In females, this hormone controls oocyte development; in males, it triggers sperm production.
- **Human growth hormone (HGH):** Also known as somatotropin, HGH is primarily responsible for growth and maturation. In addition, this hormone helps control protein, lipid, and carbohydrate metabolism.
- **Lipotropins (LPH):** Reduces sensitivity to pain.
- *Luteinizing hormone* (**LH**): Controls ovulation and the menstrual cycle. After ovulation occurs, this hormone helps form the **corpus luteum** and the secretion of progesterone. Jointly LH and FSH trigger the ovarian follicle to secrete estrogen, which is needed along with progesterone for implantation of the fertilized ovum into the uterus.
- **Melanocyte-stimulating hormone (MSH):** This hormone stimulates melanocytes of the skin.
- **Prolactin:** Stimulates milk production.
- **Thyrotropic hormone (TSH):** Stimulates the thyroid gland to release thyroid hormones. These hormones control the basal metabolic rate and play an important role in growth and maturation.

DEFINITIONS

adrenocorticotropic hormone. Hormone secreted by the anterior pituitary that acts on the adrenal cortex and its secretion of corticosteroids. ACTH is used in hormone replacement therapy and as a diagnostic aid.

corpus luteum. Yellowish mass of endocrine tissue in the ovary that secretes progesterone, formed by a mature follicle that has released its ovum. The corpus luteum dissolves after about 10 days if there is no fertilization but persists for several months if the ovum is impregnated.

follicle-stimulating hormone. Gonadotropic hormone secreted by the anterior lobe of the pituitary gland. In women, it stimulates growth and maturation of the ovum and its enclosing cells, the production of estrogen, and the endometrial changes that occur in the first phase of the menstrual cycle. In men, the hormone stimulates the production of sperm.

luteinizing hormone. Gonadotropic hormone secreted by the pituitary gland. In women, it promotes ovulation, the release of the egg from the ovary, and sustains the luteal (second) phase of the menstrual cycle. It also promotes the secretion of progesterone. In men, the hormone stimulates the development of testicular Leydig's cells.

The posterior lobe of the pituitary gland contains the nerve endings (axons) from the hypothalamus, which stimulate or suppress hormone production. This lobe secretes antidiuretic hormones (ADH), which control water balance in the body. ADH secretion is stimulated by a rise of electrolytes or a decrease in blood volume or blood pressure. Also secreted is oxytocin, which controls muscle contractions in the uterus. In males, oxytocin stimulates muscle contraction of the prostate gland, which is essential in the release of semen before ejaculation.

Hypothalamus Gland

The hypothalamus controls the pituitary gland from deep within the brain. Although it is part of the brain, the hypothalamus is considered part of the endocrine system because it secretes several hormones. It is the primary link between the brain and the pituitary gland, and the primary link between the endocrine and nervous systems. The hypothalamus contains nerve cells that control the pituitary gland by producing chemicals that stimulate or suppress hormone secretions from the pituitary. Many factors, such as emotions and seasonal changes, can influence the production and secretion of pituitary hormones. This information (such as environmental temperature, light exposure patterns, and feelings) is sensed by the brain and relayed by the hypothalamus to the pituitary.

The hypothalamus also regulates blood sugar levels, body temperature, metabolism, and body rhythms (e.g., activity and rest, appetite and digestion, sexual behavior, and menstrual and reproductive cycles).

Pineal Gland

The pineal gland is a small, cone-shaped gland located in the middle of the brain. It secretes only one hormone, melatonin, which regulates the body's *circadian* rhythm. The gland's production of melatonin varies according to the time of day and with age, with production dramatically increased during the nighttime hours and decreased during the day. Melatonin contributes to the release of female reproductive hormones. It helps determine when a woman starts to menstruate, the frequency and duration of the menstrual cycle, and when a woman enters *menopause*. It has been found that melatonin levels drop significantly just before puberty and are lower still in adults. Melatonin seems to suppress a child's body from undergoing sexual maturation, since sex hormones such as luteotropin that play a role in the development of sexual organs emerge only after melatonin levels have declined.

DEFINITIONS

circadian. Relating to a cyclic, 24-hour period.

menopause. Cessation of menstruation involving four physical stages: premenopause, in which periods may be irregular but without classic menopausal symptoms; perimenopause, the onset of symptoms that indicate a drop in estrogen, such as erratic periods, hot flashes, and vaginal dryness—this stage lasts approximately four years, counting the first two years before and after the last period; menopause, referring to the final menstrual period, marked once the female has had no periods for one year; and postmenopause, the phase in which a woman has been free of periods for at least one year.

Figure 6.4: Thyroid

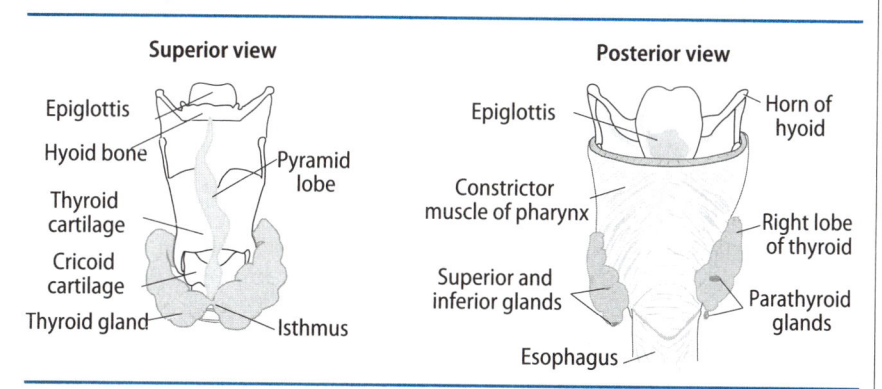

Superior view
- Epiglottis
- Hyoid bone
- Thyroid cartilage
- Cricoid cartilage
- Thyroid gland
- Pyramid lobe
- Isthmus

Posterior view
- Epiglottis
- Constrictor muscle of pharynx
- Superior and inferior glands
- Esophagus
- Horn of hyoid
- Right lobe of thyroid
- Parathyroid glands

Thyroid Gland

The thyroid gland is located in the front part of the lower neck. Its right and left lobes lie on each side of the trachea, connected in the middle by a mass of tissue called the isthmus. The thyroid is filled with microscopic circular sacs called thyroid follicles that store the thyroid hormones. It derives its blood supply from the superior and interior thyroid arteries. Although a separate gland, the thyroid is controlled by the pituitary gland. When thyroid hormone levels decrease, the pituitary gland sends a signal to the thyroid by producing thyroid-stimulating hormone (TSH), which in turn stimulates the thyroid gland to produce more hormones. Under the influence of TSH, the thyroid manufactures and secretes thyroxine (T4) and triiodothyronine (T3). These hormones regulate growth and metabolism and play a role in brain development during childhood.

Nestled between the thyroid follicles are parafollicular cells. These cells produce calcitonin, which lowers the concentration of calcium in the blood when it rises above the normal value.

Figure 6.5: Dorsal View of Parathyroid Glands

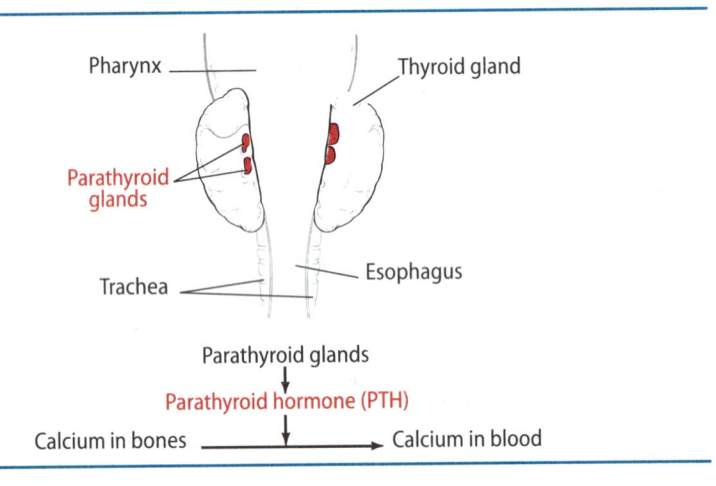

☞ INTERESTING A & P FACT

As many as 14 percent of the population have five parathyroid glands; and a few are known to have six.

📖 DEFINITIONS

osteopenia. Decreased calcification that is less severe than that resulting from osteoporosis, caused by the resorption of bone at a rate that exceeds bone synthesis.

osteoporosis. Bone degeneration caused by the breakdown of the bony matrix without equivalent regeneration, resulting in a weak, porous, fragile bone structure.

Parathyroid Gland

The parathyroid is located behind the thyroid gland at the front of the neck. There are four glands: a superior pair and an inferior pair.

There are two types of cells in the parathyroid glands: oxyphil cells and chief cells. Oxyphil cells appear at the onset of puberty, although their function is unknown. The chief cells are responsible for producing the parathyroid hormone (PTH), which regulates the level of calcium in the bones and the rest of the body. Calcium is the primary element that causes muscle contraction and is also very important to the normal conduction of electrical currents along nerves. The PTH hormone is responsible for the bones releasing calcium into the bloodstream, which keeps the calcium in the blood at a normal level. If there is too much PTH, the bones release excessive amounts of calcium and leave the bones with too little calcium, leading to conditions such as *osteopenia* and *osteoporosis*.

Another way PTH acts to increase calcium in the blood is through the intestines. The PTH makes the lining of the intestine more efficient at absorbing calcium found in foods. In addition to regulating the amount of calcium in the blood from bone and intestine, PTH also controls the excretion of calcium in urine, thus conserving calcium in blood.

Adrenal Glands

The adrenal glands, also called suprarenal glands, are located on the top of each kidney and have two distinct parts. The outer part, called the adrenal cortex, produces a variety of hormones called corticosteroids. Chief among the corticosteroids is cortisol, which regulates salt and water balance in the body, prepares the body for stress, regulates metabolism, interacts with the immune system, and influences sexual function. The inner part, the adrenal medulla, is considered an extension of the sympathetic nervous system (SNS); therefore, the hormones it secretes are called sympathomimetic hormones. The medulla produces catecholamines, epinephrine (adrenaline), and norepinephrine (noradrenaline). During times of stress these hormones increase blood pressure and heart rate, they facilitate blood flow to the muscles and brain, cause relaxation of **smooth muscles**, and help with conversion of glycogen to glucose in the liver.

Figure 6.6: Uterus and Ovaries

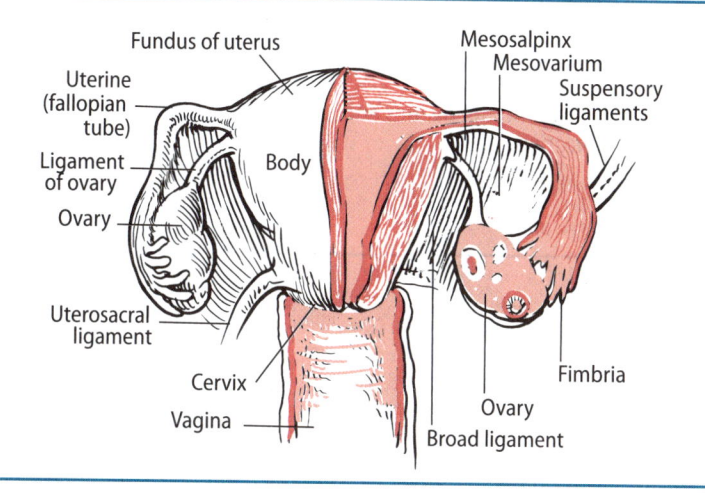

Gonad Gland

The gonads are the main source of sex hormones. Female gonads (ovaries) secrete sex hormones in response to stimulation from the pituitary gland. Located in the pelvis, the ovaries produce eggs. They also secrete female sex hormones, **estrogen** and **progesterone,** which regulate development of the reproductive organs, female secondary sex characteristics, and menstruation and pregnancy.

Male gonads (**testes**) are located in the scrotum. They produce sperm and secrete **androgens**. The androgens, the most important of which is testosterone, regulate the sexual and reproductive functions in males. Among other things, testosterone also regulates body changes associated with puberty, including enlargement of the penis, the growth spurt that occurs during puberty, and characteristics such as deepening of the voice, growth of facial and pubic hair, and the increase in bone and muscle mass.

DEFINITIONS

androgen. Male sex hormone. Testosterone is the primary androgen. In the fetus, androgens cause the formation of external male genitalia.

estrogen. Group of estrus-stimulating hormones produced by the ovaries, possibly the adrenal cortex and testes, that have different functions in both sexes. They are the main female sex hormones (estradiol, estrone, and estriol) responsible for the maturation and development of female secondary sex characteristics and that act on the reproductive organs to prepare for fertilization, implantation, and nourishment of the embryo. Estrogens also have nonreproductive actions such as minimizing calcium loss from bones by antagonizing the effects of parathyroid hormone and promoting blood clotting.

progesterone. Steroid hormone, secreted by the corpus luteum of the ovary and by the placenta, that acts to prepare the uterus for implantation of the fertilized ovum, to maintain pregnancy, and to promote development of the mammary glands.

smooth muscle. Thin layers of muscle tissue that move involuntarily as part of the body's natural processes. Smooth muscle lines the walls of hollow organs, such as the uterus and gastrointestinal tract.

testes. Male gonadal paired glands located in the scrotum that secrete testosterone and contain the seminiferous tubules where sperm is produced.

Figure 6.7: Male Pelvic Organs

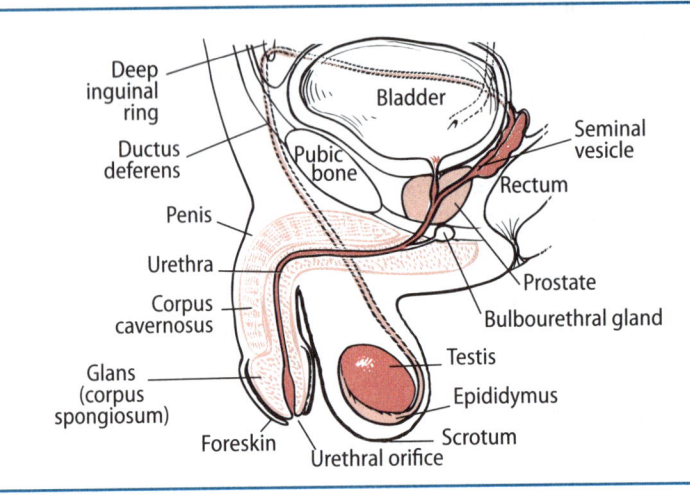

More information regarding the ovaries and testes can be found in the reproductive chapter of this publication.

Figure 6.8: Thymus Gland

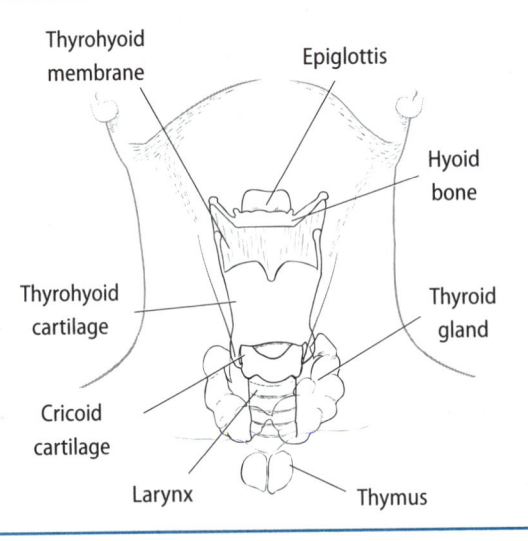

Thymus Gland

The thymus gland is located just under the breast bone in the anterior, superior mediastinum, and is composed of lymphatic and epithelial tissue (Hassall's corpuscles). It has two lobes, each divided into lobules by a **septum**. Hormones produced within the gland are collectively known as thymosins. These hormones play a key role in the development and maintenance of immune defenses by controlling white blood cell maturation. White blood cells (WBC), known as **lymphocytes**, pass through the thymus and are transformed into T cells. The T cells' primary role is to fight infection. The role of the thymus is not entirely understood, though it seems to be most important from infancy through puberty, after which the lymphatic tissue diminishes and is replaced by fat. In adults, the thymus can be removed without a significant health impact.

DEFINITIONS

lymphocytes. White blood cells formed in the body's lymph system.

septum. Anatomical partition or dividing wall.

Anatomy and Pathophysiology and the ICD-10-CM Code Set

The endocrine system regulates many body functions and, as such, it can be affected by many different disease states. It is imperative to understand the terminology describing the disease states as the ICD-10-CM code set describes them in a much more detailed way than does ICD-9-CM.

Disorders of the Endocrine Gland

A number of endocrine gland disorders result from conditions that affect thyroid gland function, including goiter, malignancy, Grave's disease, and inflammation.

Figure 6.9: Goiter

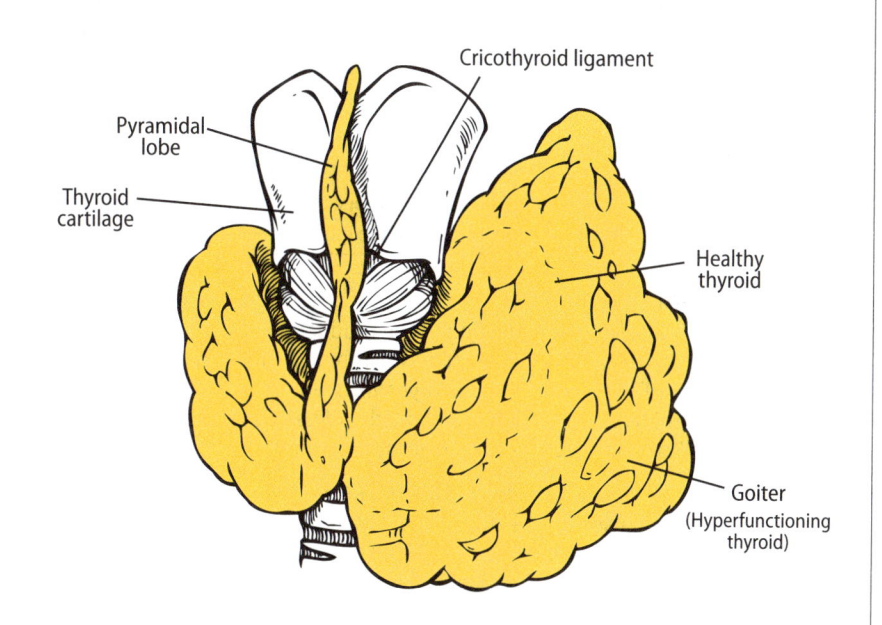

Goiter

A goiter is an abnormal enlargement of the thyroid gland commonly caused by a deficiency of dietary iodine. Goiters can be simple or nontoxic nodular. If a goiter has enough mass, it may cause compression that may lead to airway restriction, swallowing difficulty, or problems with venous flow.

In simple goiter, the thyroid gland is enlarged, but the thyroid hormone secretions are still within normal limits and not associated with malignancy. A simple goiter can have several causes, such as iodine deficiency. The thyroid of a person whose diet has insufficient iodine, which is essential to thyroid hormone secretion, becomes enlarged so that it can produce more of the hormone. Iodine deficiency is the most common cause of simple goiter, but as there is no deficiency in the United States, this cause is rarely seen here. Simple goiter can also occur during puberty, pregnancy, or during menses as a result of hormonal imbalances.

An endemic goiter is the swelling of the thyroid gland due to inadequate amounts of dietary iodine. This deprivation leads to diminished production and secretion of thyroid hormone by the gland. Endemic goiter occurs from time to time in adolescents at puberty and widely in population groups in geographic areas in which limited amounts of iodine are present in soil, water, and food. This type of goiter is without apparent signs of hyperthyroidism or hypothyroidism of the gland.

Coding for Goiters

ICD-9-CM		ICD-10-CM	
240.0	Goiter, specified as simple	E04.0	Nontoxic diffuse goiter
240.9	Goiter, unspecified	E01.0	Iodine-deficiency related diffuse (endemic) goiter
		E01.2	Iodine-deficiency related (endemic) goiter unspecified
		E04.9	Nontoxic goiter, unspecified

In a nontoxic nodular goiter, the thyroid gland exhibits palpable nodules that do not affect thyroid hormone secretion. Goiters are classified as having a singular nodule or multiple nodules. This type of goiter may be malignant.

Coding for Goiter

ICD-9-CM		ICD-10-CM	
241.0	Nontoxic uninodular goiter	E04.1	Nontoxic single thyroid nodule
241.1	Nontoxic multinodular goiter	E01.1	Iodine-deficiency related multinodular (endemic) goiter
		E04.2	Nontoxic multinodular goiter
241.9	Unspecified nontoxic nodular goiter	E04.8	Other specified nontoxic goiter
		E04.9	Nontoxic goiter, unspecified

Hyperthyroidism

Hyperthyroidism is a broad term referring to the production of too much of the thyroid hormone thyroxine (T4) and/or triiodothyronine (T3). Hyperthyroidism has several causes, including thyroid nodules, **thyroiditis**, and Graves' disease. Another cause of hyperthyroidism is ingestion of too much iodine or overmedicating with synthetic thyroid hormone used to treat hypothyroidism.

Graves' disease, also referred to as **toxic diffuse goiter**, is an autoimmune disease. It is the most common cause of hyperthyroidism. In this disease, the immune system produces an antibody called thyroid stimulating immunoglobulin (TSI), which acts much like TSH and causes the thyroid to produce too much thyroid hormone.

A nodule, or fluid-filled cyst, is a growth within the thyroid that can be benign or malignant. Nodules have many causes, including **Hashimoto's disease**, genetic defects, a lack of iodine, and radiation treatments.

Thyrotoxicosis is a toxic condition caused by an excess of thyroid hormones in the blood. It is often related to hyperthyroidism, where the thyroid gland is overproducing hormones. There are many factors that can contribute to thyrotoxicosis, including goiters, benign tumors, and thyroid adenomas, which can become toxic and cause excess hormones to be produced. Medications and radiation may also lead to this condition.

A thyrotoxic crisis or storm is a sudden, life-threatening crisis in which symptoms of hyperthyroidism are exacerbated and new symptoms develop. It is most likely to occur at the time of infection, surgical procedure, or trauma in a patient with undertreated or untreated hyperthyroidism. The patient may develop a fever, emotional instability or psychosis, heart complications, and an enlarged liver.

DEFINITIONS

diffuse toxic goiter. Diffuse thyroid enlargement seen mostly in women that stems from the autoimmune process. It is accompanied by the secretion of excessive thyroid hormone, goiter, and bulging eyes.

Hashimoto's disease. Autoimmune disorder marked by goiter, chronic inflammation of the thyroid, and often hypothyroidism.

thyroiditis. Inflammation of the thyroid gland.

Coding for Thyrotoxicosis

ICD-9-CM		ICD-10-CM	
242.00	Toxic diffuse goiter without mention of thyrotoxic crisis or storm	E05.00	Thyrotoxicosis with diffuse goiter without thyrotoxic crisis or storm
242.01	Toxic diffuse goiter with mention of thyrotoxic crisis or storm	E05.01	Thyrotoxicosis with diffuse goiter with thyrotoxic crisis or storm
242.10	Toxic uninodular goiter without mention of thyrotoxic crisis or storm	E05.10	Thyrotoxicosis with toxic single thyroid nodule without thyrotoxic crisis or storm
242.11	Toxic uninodular goiter with mention of thyrotoxic crisis or storm	E05.11	Thyrotoxicosis with toxic single thyroid nodule with thyrotoxic crisis or storm
242.20	Toxic multinodular goiter without mention of thyrotoxic crisis or storm	E05.20	Thyrotoxicosis with toxic multinodular goiter without thyrotoxic crisis or storm
242.21	Toxic multinodular goiter with mention of thyrotoxic crisis or storm	E05.21	Thyrotoxicosis with toxic multinodular goiter with thyrotoxic crisis or storm
242.30	Toxic nodular goiter, unspecified type, without mention of thyrotoxic crisis or storm	E05.20	Thyrotoxicosis with toxic multinodular goiter without thyrotoxic crisis or storm
242.31	Toxic nodular goiter, unspecified type, with mention of thyrotoxic crisis or storm	E05.21	Thyrotoxicosis with toxic multinodular goiter with thyrotoxic crisis or storm
242.40	Thyrotoxicosis from *ectopic* thyroid nodule without mention of thyrotoxic crisis or storm	E05.30	Thyrotoxicosis from ectopic thyroid tissue without thyrotoxic crisis or storm
242.41	Thyrotoxicosis from ectopic thyroid nodule with mention of thyrotoxic crisis or storm	E05.31	Thyrotoxicosis from ectopic thyroid tissue with thyrotoxic crisis or storm

> **DEFINITIONS**
>
> **ectopic.** Relating to an organ or other structure that is aberrant or out of place.

Hypothyroidism

The most common cause of congenital hypothyroidism is absence of a thyroid gland at birth. This requires lifelong hormone therapy since thyroxine regulates metabolism and growth. Untreated, congenital hypothyroidism causes serious problems in the central nervous system, developmental delay, and problems with somatic growth. By providing replacement thyroid hormones, almost all of the complications of congenital hypothyroidism are avoidable.

Neurological-type hypothyroidism includes endemic cretinism, which is defined as having impaired physical and mental development with dystrophy of bones and soft tissues. This is due to congenital lack of thyroid secretion. Additionally, patients may have deaf-mutism, spasticity, and motor dysfunction.

A diffuse goiter, which is nontoxic, is a diffuse or nodular enlargement of the thyroid that is not associated with abnormal thyroid function and does not result from an inflammatory or neoplastic process.

An endemic goiter, also called a colloid goiter, is a thyroid enlargement that occurs in groups of people who live in areas with iodine-poor soil.

A myxedematous type-goiter is marked by dry skin and swellings around the lips and nose, in addition to abnormal deposits of mucin in the skin and other tissues.

In the ICD-10-CM code set, an additional code (F70–F79) should be used if applicable, to identify associated mental retardation.

Coding for Congenital Hypothyroidism

ICD-9-CM		ICD-10-CM	
243	Congenital hypothyroidism	E00.0	Congenital iodine-deficiency syndrome, neurological type
		E00.1	Congenital iodine-deficiency syndrome, myxedematous type
		E00.2	Congenital iodine-deficiency syndrome, mixed type
		E00.9	Congenital iodine-deficiency syndrome, unspecified
		E03.0	Congenital hypothyroidism with diffuse goiter
		E03.1	Congenital hypothyroidism without goiter

Acquired Hypothyroidism

Hypothyroidism is a deficiency of thyroid hormone. Primary (acquired) hypothyroidism usually develops in older adults, usually after age 40. There are many causes of this type of hypothyroidism, the most common due to any condition that causes inflammation of the gland. For example, the most frequent cause of hypothyroidism is inflammation of the thyroid gland, which damages the gland's cells. Autoimmune and Hashimoto's *thyroiditis* are good examples of diseases in which the immune system attacks the thyroid gland. *Postpartum* thyroiditis may also develop in some women.

Other causes of hypothyroidism include:

- Certain drugs (such as amiodarone, lithium, methimazole, and propylthiouracil [PTU])
- Iodine, resulting from administration or ingestion of iodine
- Postsurgical/postprocedural, due to removal of partial or total thyroid gland
- Radioactive iodine used to treat an overactive thyroid (hyperthyroidism)
- Viral thyroiditis, which may cause hyperthyroidism and is often followed by temporary or permanent hypothyroidism

Coding for Acquired Hypothyroidism

ICD-9-CM		ICD-10-CM	
244.0	Postsurgical hypothyroidism	E89.0	Postprocedural hypothyroidism
244.1	Other postablative hypothyroidism		
244.2	Iodine hypothyroidism	E03.2	Hypothyroidism due to medicaments and other exogenous substances
244.3	Other *iatrogenic* hypothyroidism		
244.8	Other specified acquired hypothyroidism	E01.8	Other iodine- deficiency related thyroid disorders and allied conditions
		E02	Subclinical iodine-deficiency hypothyroidism
		E03.3	Postinfectious hypothyroidism
		E03.8	Other specified hypothyroidism
244.9	Unspecified hypothyroidism	E03.9	Hypothyroidism, unspecified

---

DEFINITIONS

iatrogenic. Adversely induced in the patient; caused by medical treatment.

postpartum. Period of time following childbirth.

thyroiditis. Inflammation of the thyroid gland.

Hypoparathyroid Conditions

Hypoparathyroidism is a condition in which one or more of the parathyroid glands secrete an abnormally low amount of the parathyroid hormone (PTH). This condition causes decreased levels of calcium and increased levels of phosphorus in the blood, muscle cramping, increased frequency of urination, and cataracts. The most common cause of hypoparathyroidism is injury to the glands during head and neck surgery. Occasionally, hypoparathyroidism is a side-effect of radioactive iodine treatment.

Coding for Hypoparathyroidism

ICD-9-CM		ICD-10-CM	
252.1	Hypoparathyroidism	E20.0	*Idiopathic* hypoparathyroidism
		E20.8	Other hypoparathyroidism
		E20.9	Hypoparathyroidism, unspecified
		E89.2	Postprocedural hypoparathyroidism

Secondary Diabetes Mellitus

Secondary diabetes mellitus (SDM) presents with the same symptoms as diabetes mellitus (discussed in the subsequent section), manifesting with elevated blood sugar levels and resulting in the inability to successfully metabolize carbohydrates, fats, and proteins. Secondary diabetes develops when defects in insulin production and secretion, or defects in the action of insulin occur, but as a result of another, underlying primary cause. This may be caused, for instance, when the islets of Langerhans, responsible for the production of insulin, are absent or destroyed by events such as chronic disease, trauma, or surgical removal of the pancreas. Secondary diabetes can also result from hormonal disturbances, such as **Cushing's syndrome** (described in more detail later in this chapter in the pituitary section) or excessive growth hormone production that results in **acromegaly**.

Nonketotic hyperglycemic-hyperosmolar coma (NKHHC), also referred to as diabetic hyperglycemic hyperosmolar syndrome (HHS), is a complication of secondary diabetes mellitus that is associated with high mortality. This type of coma generally follows an infection, myocardial infarction, stroke, or acute illness. Sometimes it may occur in patients who have not been diagnosed with diabetes or in patients with uncontrolled diabetes. The patient usually presents with a glucose of 600 mg/dL or greater without the presence of ketones.

Hyperglycemia is abnormally high blood sugar, usually greater than 140 mg/dl in a nonfasting, nondiabetic patient. Hyperglycemia in a diabetic patient is not easily quantified; levels vary from patient to patient.

Hyperosmolarity is the increase in osmolarity or the concentration of ions and chemicals in blood or a solution.

Ketoacidosis is an abnormal increase in the acidity of body fluids and tissues (acidosis) caused by the increased accumulation of ketone bodies, most often seen in Type 1 diabetes or excessive alcohol consumption.

Secondary diabetes mellitus is divided into two separate categories in ICD-10-CM. Codes under category E08 Diabetes mellitus due to underlying condition, and E09 Drug or chemical induced diabetes mellitus, identify complications and/or manifestations associated with secondary diabetes mellitus. Codes should be assigned according to the instructions found in the ICD-10-CM tabular section. For example, in category E08 Diabetes mellitus due to underlying condition, code first the underlying condition. In category E09 Drug or chemical induced diabetes mellitus, code first poisoning due to a drug or toxin, if applicable (T36–T65 with fifth or sixth character 1–4 or 6). Use an additional code for adverse effect, if applicable, to identify the drug itself (T36–T50 with fifth or sixth character 5).

> **DEFINITIONS**
>
> **acromegaly.** Chronic condition caused by overproduction of the pituitary growth hormone that results in enlarged skeletal parts and facial features.
>
> **Cushing's syndrome.** Abdominal striae, acne, hypertension, decreased carbohydrate tolerance, moon face, obesity, protein catabolism, and psychiatric disturbances resulting from increased adrenocortical secretion of cortisol caused by ACTH-dependent adrenocortical hyperplasia or tumor, or by effects of steroids.
>
> **idiopathic.** Having no known cause.

> **CODING AXIOM**
>
> ICD-10-CM Official Coding Guideline I.C.4.a.6.(b).(i). states, "for post pancreatectomy diabetes mellitus (lack of insulin due to the surgical removal of all or part of the pancreas), assign code E89.1 Postprocedural hypoinsulinemia. Assign a code from category E13 and a code from subcategory Z90.41- Acquired absence of pancreas, as additional codes."

Coding for Secondary Diabetes Mellitus

ICD-9-CM		ICD-10-CM	
249.20	Secondary diabetes mellitus with hyperosmolarity not stated as uncontrolled, or unspecified	E08.00	Diabetes mellitus due to underlying condition with hyperosmolarity without nonketotic hyperglycemic-hyperosmolar coma (NKHHC)
		E08.01	Diabetes mellitus due to underlying condition with hyperosmolarity with coma
		E09.00	Drug or chemical induced diabetes mellitus with hyperosmolarity without nonketotic hyperglycemic- hyperosmolar coma (NKHHC)
		E09.01	Drug or chemical induced diabetes mellitus with hyperosmolarity with coma
249.21	Secondary diabetes mellitus with hyperosmolarity uncontrolled	E08.01	Diabetes mellitus due to underlying condition with hyperosmolarity with coma
		E08.65	Diabetes mellitus due to underlying condition with hyperglycemia
		E09.01	Drug or chemical induced diabetes mellitus with hyperosmolarity with coma
249.30	Secondary diabetes mellitus with other coma not stated as uncontrolled, or unspecified	E08.11	Diabetes mellitus due to underlying condition with ketoacidosis with coma
		E08.641	Diabetes mellitus due to underlying condition with hypoglycemia with coma
249.31	Secondary diabetes mellitus with other coma uncontrolled	E09.11	Drug or chemical induced diabetes mellitus with ketoacidosis with coma
		E09.641	Drug or chemical induced diabetes mellitus with hypoglycemia with coma

Secondary diabetes mellitus may be complicated by the presence of nephropathy or chronic kidney disease. Chronic kidney disease is decreased renal efficiencies resulting in the kidney's reduced ability to filter waste. The National Kidney Foundation's classification includes five clinical stages, based on the glomerular filtration rate (GFR). The stages of CKD are as follows: stage 1, some kidney damage with a normal or slightly increased GFR value (> 90); stage 2, mild kidney damage with a GFR value of 60 to 89; stage 3, moderate kidney damage with a GFR value of 30 to 59; stage 4, severe kidney damage and a GFR value of 15 to 29; and stage 5, severe kidney damage that has progressed to a GFR value of less than 15. Dialysis or transplantation is required at stage 5.

Nephropathy is defined as a disease or abnormality of the kidney. The following table is an example of some of the mapping crosswalks between ICD-9-CM and ICD-10-CM for secondary diabetes with renal manifestations. For the complete mapping, please see Optum360's *ICD-10-CM Mappings*.

Coding for Secondary Diabetes Mellitus with Renal Manifestations

ICD-9-CM		ICD-10-CM	
249.40	Secondary diabetes mellitus with renal manifestations not stated as uncontrolled, unspecified	E08.21	Diabetes mellitus due to underlying condition with diabetic nephropathy
		E08.22	Diabetes mellitus due to underlying condition with diabetic chronic kidney disease
		E08.29	Diabetes mellitus due to underlying condition with other diabetic kidney complication
		E09.21	Drug or chemical induced diabetes mellitus with diabetic nephropathy
		E09.22	Drug or chemical induced diabetes mellitus with diabetic chronic kidney disease
		E09.29	Drug or chemical induced diabetes mellitus with other diabetic kidney complication

Secondary diabetes mellitus may also have **ophthalmic** complications, including cataracts, retinopathy, and macular edema.

Figure 6.10: Cataract

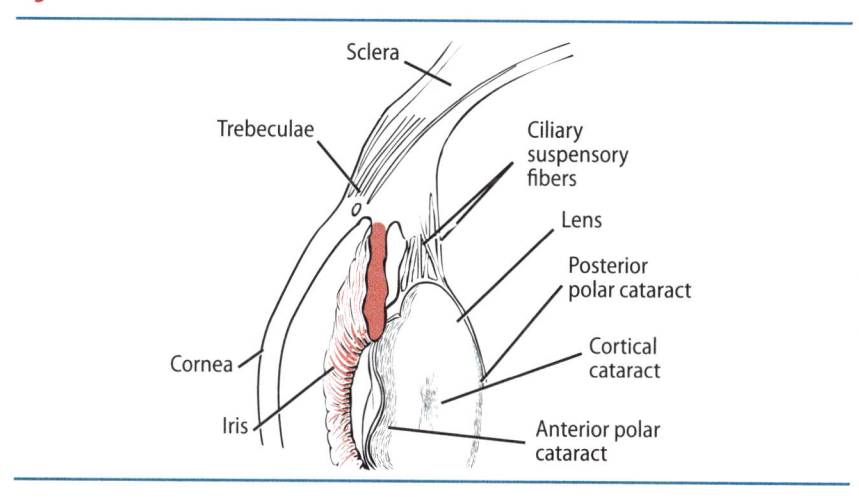

A cataract is a clouding or opacity of the lens that prevents clear images from forming on the **retina**, causing vision impairment or blindness. The classification and coding of cataracts are dependent upon size, shape, location, and etiology.

Diabetic macular edema (DME) occurs when leakage from the blood vessels causes the retina to swell. In DME, the central portion of the retina, the macula, swells and impairs vision. Exudates or plaques may develop in the posterior pole of the retina due to the breakdown of retinal vasculature, which can precipitate vision loss.

Retinopathy usually occurs in diabetes of long duration. It represents a continuum of disease; a progression of pathologic changes in the retina due to microvascular complications inherent in diabetes mellitus. Nonproliferative diabetic retinopathy is indicative of early stage disease. Microaneurysms form, retinal **hemorrhages** occur, and blind spots are characteristic. Increased vessel leakage occurs as the disease progresses, resulting in further vision impairment. The disease progresses from mild to moderate to severe nonproliferative retinopathy and becomes proliferative in its more advanced stage, characterized by new blood vessel formation in the retina due to significant ischemia from the damaged vessels.

ICD-9-CM codes 249.50 and 249.51 crosswalk to the same group of ICD-10-CM codes. In ICD-9-CM, two or more codes are needed to accurately describe secondary diabetes mellitus with ophthalmic manifestations. However, combination codes have been created in ICD-10-CM. For example, ICD-9-CM codes 249.50, 362.10, and 362.07 are needed to identify secondary diabetes mellitus with retinopathy and macular edema. ICD-10-CM requires only code E08.311 or E09.311.

Amyotrophy is muscular wasting and weakening that generally occurs in patients with diabetes. It usually affects the thighs and pelvic region.

Autonomic neuropathy describes a disease complication that has affected one or more nerves in the **autonomic nervous system**.

Mononeuropathy is a disease process of severe inflammation of one nerve; inflammation of multiple nerves is called **poly**neuropathy.

ICD-9-CM codes 249.60 and 249.61 crosswalk to the same group of ICD-10-CM codes. These codes describe diabetes complications involving the neurological system.

DEFINITIONS

autonomic nervous system. Portion of the nervous system that controls involuntary body functions. The fibers of the autonomic nervous system regulate the iris of the eye and the smooth-muscle action of the heart, blood vessels, lungs, glands, stomach, colon, bladder, and other visceral organs that are not under conscious control by the individual. The autonomic nerve fibers exit from the central nervous system and branch out into the sympathetic and parasympathetic nervous systems.

hemorrhage. Internal or external bleeding with loss of significant amounts of blood.

mono-. One or single.

ophthalmic. Relating to the eye.

poly-. Much or many.

retina. Layer of tissue located at the back of the eye that is sensitive to light similar to film in a camera.

Coding for Secondary Diabetes Mellitus with Neurological Manifestations

ICD-9-CM		ICD-10-CM	
249.60	Secondary diabetes mellitus with neurological manifestations, not stated as uncontrolled, or unspecified	E08.40	Diabetes mellitus due to underlying condition with diabetic neuropathy, unspecified
		E08.41	Diabetes mellitus due to underlying condition with diabetic mononeuropathy
		E08.42	Diabetes mellitus due to underlying condition with diabetic polyneuropathy
		E08.43	Diabetes mellitus due to underlying condition with diabetic autonomic (poly)neuropathy
		E08.44	Diabetes mellitus due to underlying condition with diabetic amyotrophy
		E08.49	Diabetes mellitus due to underlying condition with other diabetic neurological complication
		E08.610	Diabetes mellitus due to underlying condition with diabetic neuropathic arthropathy
		E09.40	Drug or chemical induced diabetes mellitus with neurological complications with diabetic neuropathy, unspecified
		E09.41	Drug or chemical induced diabetes mellitus with neurological complications with diabetic mononeuropathy
		E09.42	Drug or chemical induced diabetes mellitus with neurological complications with diabetic polyneuropathy
		E09.43	Drug or chemical induced diabetes mellitus with neurological complications with diabetic autonomic (poly)neuropathy
		E09.44	Drug or chemical induced diabetes mellitus with neurological complications with diabetic amyotrophy
		E09.49	Drug or chemical induced diabetes mellitus with neurological complications with other diabetic neurological complication
249.61	Secondary diabetes mellitus with neurological manifestations, uncontrolled	E08.40	Diabetes mellitus due to underlying condition with diabetic neuropathy, unspecified
		E08.65	Diabetes mellitus due to underlying condition with hyperglycemia
		E09.40	Drug or chemical induced diabetes mellitus with neurological complications with diabetic neuropathy, unspecified

The following section describes complications of secondary diabetes mellitus involving the circulatory system.

Gangrene frequently occurs when a large area of tissue dies, usually resulting from a loss of vascular supply, followed by a bacterial attack or onset of disease.

An angiopathy is any disease of the blood or lymph vessels.

Coding for Secondary Diabetes Mellitus with Circulatory Manifestations

ICD-9-CM		ICD-10-CM	
249.70	Secondary diabetes mellitus with **peripheral** circulatory disorders, not stated as uncontrolled, or unspecified	E08.51	Diabetes mellitus due to underlying condition with diabetic peripheral angiopathy without gangrene
249.71	Secondary diabetes mellitus with peripheral circulatory disorders, uncontrolled	E08.52	Diabetes mellitus due to underlying condition with diabetic peripheral angiopathy with gangrene
		E09.51	Drug or chemical induced diabetes mellitus with diabetic peripheral angiopathy without gangrene
		E09.52	Drug or chemical induced diabetes mellitus with diabetic peripheral angiopathy with gangrene

The following section describes complications of secondary diabetes mellitus of other specified manifestations, including:

- **Arthropathy:** Joint disease.
- **Dermatitis:** Inflammation of the skin.
- **Ulcer:** Open sore or excavating lesion of skin or the tissue on the surface of an organ from the sloughing of chronically inflamed and necrosing tissue.

Hypoglycemia is abnormally low blood glucose levels. Excessive insulin produced by the pancreas, sometimes associated with tumors, or an overdose of insulin to treat diabetes may be a cause.

Hyperglycemia is just the opposite—abnormally high blood sugar, usually greater than 140 mg/dl in a nonfasting, nondiabetic patient. Hyperglycemia in a diabetic patient is not easily quantified; levels vary from patient to patient.

Note that ICD-9-CM codes 249.80 and 249.81 crosswalk to the same group of ICD-10-CM codes: E08.618–E08.638, E08.649–E08.69, and E09.618–E09.69.

Diabetes Mellitus

Diabetes mellitus (DM) is a complex metabolic disease with multisystem manifestations. It is characterized by high glucose (blood sugar) levels. Normally the hormone insulin controls glucose levels. In patients with diabetes mellitus, insulin is not produced normally or the body has a resistance to it, resulting in elevated blood sugar levels.

Diabetes mellitus has two forms. Diabetes mellitus Type 1 is caused by inadequate secretion of insulin by the pancreas. Type 1, also referred to as Type 1 insulin-dependent diabetes mellitus (IDDM), is classified as an autoimmune disease wherein the patient's immune system incorrectly produces antibodies, resulting in damage to the body's tissues. This type is most often seen at a young age, usually at 6 to 7 years of age, and sometimes in early adulthood as well. The patient requires regular insulin injections due to the autoimmune destruction of pancreatic beta cells, which cease to produce insulin. It is unknown what triggers the autoimmune response.

Diabetes mellitus Type 2 is caused by the body's inability to respond to insulin, called **insulin resistance**. DM Type 2 is also referred to as non-insulin-dependent diabetes mellitus (NIDDM) or adult-onset diabetes mellitus (AODM). Type 2 accounts for 90 to 95 percent of all cases and is usually diagnosed in adulthood as the pancreas gradually loses the ability to produce insulin or the body becomes more resistant to that which is being produced. An increasing number of children are being diagnosed with Type 2 diabetes due to the increase of childhood obesity. Children are developing Type 2 DM at an older age than is common with Type 1 DM, usually around 12 years of age, and they usually have a family history of DM.

> **DEFINITIONS**
>
> **insulin resistance syndrome.** Group of health risks that increase the likelihood of developing heart disease, stroke, and diabetes. Diagnosis of insulin resistance syndrome is made if one has three or more of the following: waist measurement of 40 or more inches for men and 35 or more inches for women; blood pressure of 130/85 mm or higher; triglyceride level greater than 150 mg/dl; fasting blood sugar of more than 100 mg/dl; HDL level less than 40 mg/dl in men or less than 50 mg/dl in women.
>
> **peripheral.** Outside of a structure or organ.

Comprehensive Anatomy and Physiology for ICD-10-CM and ICD-10-PCS Coding

> **CODING AXIOM**
>
> ICD-10-CM Official Coding Guideline I.C.4.a.2. states, "if the type of diabetes mellitus is not documented in the medical record the default is E11.- Type 2 diabetes mellitus."

The primary factor that distinguishes Type 1 from Type 2 is the absence of naturally occurring insulin within the body. Type 1 diabetics require insulin injections to survive. Type 2 diabetics may improve their health with insulin injections and may even come to require insulin, but the administration of insulin has no bearing on code selection for diabetes, nor does the age of onset. A patient with Type 2 diabetes is always coded as having Type 2, even when the medical record states the patient requires insulin.

Diabetes can cause a variety of complications, including kidney problems, pain due to nerve damage, blindness, and coronary heart disease.

Many of the terms used in this category to describe complications are the same as those used in secondary diabetes. Please see the definitions in the previous section.

In ICD-10-CM, this category of codes is classified according to Type 1 or Type 2, the body system affected, and the type of complication. The status and the presence of diabetic control are not indicated. Multiple codes within a particular category may be necessary to describe all of the complications of the disease. They should be sequenced based on the reason for a particular encounter.

Coding for Diabetes Mellitus

ICD-9-CM		ICD-10-CM	
250.20	Diabetes with hyperosmolarity, Type II or unspecified type, not stated as uncontrolled	E11.00	Type 2 diabetes mellitus with hyperosmolarity without nonketotic hyperglycemic-hyperosmolar coma (NKHHC)
		E11.01	Type 2 diabetes mellitus with hyperosmolarity with coma
		E13.00	Other specified diabetes mellitus with hyperosmolarity without nonketotic hyperglycemic-hyperosmolar coma (NKHHC)
		E13.01	Other specified diabetes mellitus with hyperosmolarity with coma

Diabetes mellitus may be complicated by the presence of nephropathy or chronic kidney disease. These conditions are described in more detail above in the secondary diabetes section.

Combination codes have been created in ICD-10-CM. For example, in ICD-9-CM, codes 250.41 and 583.81 are needed to accurately identify diabetes mellitus, Type 1 with nephropathy. ICD-10-CM requires only code, E10.21.

Coding for Diabetes Mellitus with Renal Manifestations

ICD-9-CM		ICD-10-CM	
250.40	Diabetes with renal manifestations, Type II or unspecified type, not stated as uncontrolled	E11.21	Type 2 diabetes mellitus with diabetic nephropathy
		E11.22	Type 2 diabetes mellitus with diabetic chronic kidney disease
		E11.29	Type 2 diabetes mellitus with other diabetic kidney complication
		E13.21	Other specified diabetes mellitus with diabetic nephropathy
		E13.22	Other specified diabetes mellitus with diabetic chronic kidney disease
		E13.29	Other specified diabetes mellitus with other diabetic kidney complication

ICD-9-CM		ICD-10-CM	
250.41	Diabetes with renal manifestations, Type I [juvenile type], not stated as uncontrolled	E10.21	Type 1 diabetes mellitus with diabetic nephropathy
		E10.22	Type 1 diabetes mellitus with diabetic chronic kidney disease
		E10.29	Type 1 diabetes mellitus with other diabetic kidney complication

Like secondary diabetes, diabetes mellitus may also have ophthalmic complications, including cataract, retinopathy, and macular edema. The following table is not a complete mapping of all of the types of ophthalmic manifestations that may occur in diabetes, but gives the coder an idea of what may be seen in ICD-10-CM. For detailed information on ICD-9-CM to ICD-10-CM mapping, see Optum360's *ICD-10-CM Mappings*.

Coding for Diabetes Mellitus with Ophthalmic Manifestations

ICD-9-CM		ICD-10-CM	
250.50	Diabetes with ophthalmic manifestations, Type II or unspecified type, not stated as uncontrolled	E11.321	Type 2 diabetes mellitus with mild nonproliferative diabetic retinopathy with macular edema
		E11.329	Type 2 diabetes mellitus with mild nonproliferative diabetic retinopathy without macular edema
		E11.331	Type 2 diabetes mellitus with moderate nonproliferative diabetic retinopathy with macular edema
		E11.339	Type 2 diabetes mellitus with moderate nonproliferative diabetic retinopathy without macular edema
		E11.341	Type 2 diabetes mellitus with severe nonproliferative diabetic retinopathy with macular edema
		E11.349	Type 2 diabetes mellitus with severe nonproliferative diabetic retinopathy without macular edema
		E11.351	Type 2 diabetes mellitus with proliferative diabetic retinopathy with macular edema
		E11.359	Type 2 diabetes mellitus with proliferative diabetic retinopathy without macular edema
		E11.36	Type 2 diabetes mellitus with diabetic cataract
250.51	Diabetes with ophthalmic manifestations, Type I [juvenile type], not stated as uncontrolled	E10.321	Type 1 diabetes mellitus with mild nonproliferative diabetic retinopathy with macular edema
		E10.329	Type 1 diabetes mellitus with mild nonproliferative diabetic retinopathy without macular edema
		E10.331	Type 1 diabetes mellitus with moderate nonproliferative diabetic retinopathy with macular edema
		E10.339	Type 1 diabetes mellitus with moderate nonproliferative diabetic retinopathy without macular edema
		E10.341	Type 1 diabetes mellitus with severe nonproliferative diabetic retinopathy with macular edema
		E10.349	Type 1 diabetes mellitus with severe nonproliferative diabetic retinopathy without macular edema
(Continued on next page)		E10.351	Type 1 diabetes mellitus with proliferative diabetic retinopathy with macular edema

ICD-9-CM		ICD-10-CM	
250.51	Diabetes with ophthalmic manifestations, Type I [juvenile type], not stated as uncontrolled *(Continued)*	E10.359	Type 1 diabetes mellitus with proliferative diabetic retinopathy without macular edema
		E10.36	Type 1 diabetes mellitus with diabetic cataract
		E10.39	Type 1 diabetes mellitus with other diabetic ophthalmic complication

In ICD-9-CM, two or more codes are needed to accurately describe Type 1 diabetes mellitus with neurological manifestations. However, combination codes have been created in ICD-10-CM. For example, ICD-9-CM codes 250.51, 362.01, and 362.07 are needed to identify diabetes mellitus Type 1 with retinopathy and macular edema. ICD-10-CM requires only code, E10.311.

The following codes describe complications involving the neurological system. These conditions are described in more detail in the secondary diabetes section above.

Coding for Diabetes Mellitus with Neurological Manifestations

ICD-9-CM		ICD-10-CM	
250.60	Diabetes with neurological manifestations, Type II or unspecified type, not stated as uncontrolled	E11.40	Type 2 diabetes mellitus with diabetic neuropathy, unspecified
		E11.41	Type 2 diabetes mellitus with diabetic mononeuropathy
		E11.42	Type 2 diabetes mellitus with diabetic polyneuropathy
		E11.43	Type 2 diabetes mellitus with diabetic autonomic (poly)neuropathy
		E11.44	Type 2 diabetes mellitus with diabetic amyotrophy
		E11.49	Type 2 diabetes mellitus with other diabetic neurological complication
		E13.40	Other specified diabetes mellitus with diabetic neuropathy, unspecified
		E13.41	Other specified diabetes mellitus with diabetic mononeuropathy
		E13.42	Other specified diabetes mellitus with diabetic polyneuropathy
		E13.43	Other specified diabetes mellitus with diabetic autonomic (poly)neuropathy
		E13.44	Other specified diabetes mellitus with diabetic amyotrophy
		E13.49	Other specified diabetes mellitus with other diabetic neurological complication
250.61	Diabetes with neurological manifestations, Type I [juvenile type], not stated as uncontrolled	E10.40	Type 1 diabetes mellitus with diabetic neuropathy, unspecified
		E10.41	Type 1 diabetes mellitus with diabetic mononeuropathy
		E10.42	Type 1 diabetes mellitus with diabetic polyneuropathy
		E10.43	Type 1 diabetes mellitus with diabetic autonomic (poly)neuropathy
		E10.44	Type 1 diabetes mellitus with diabetic amyotrophy
		E10.49	Type 1 diabetes mellitus with other diabetic neurological complication

The following codes describe complications involving the circulatory system. Many of the terms used in this category to describe complications are the same as those used in secondary diabetes. Please see the definitions in the previous section.

Chapter 6. ICD-10-CM: Endocrine System

Coding for Diabetes Mellitus with Circulatory Manifestations

ICD-9-CM		ICD-10-CM	
250.70	Diabetes with peripheral circulatory disorders, Type II or unspecified type, not stated as uncontrolled	E11.51	Type 2 diabetes mellitus with diabetic peripheral angiopathy without gangrene
		E11.52	Type 2 diabetes mellitus with diabetic peripheral angiopathy with gangrene
		E11.59	Type 2 diabetes mellitus with other circulatory complications
		E13.51	Other specified diabetes mellitus with diabetic peripheral angiopathy without gangrene
		E13.52	Other specified diabetes mellitus with diabetic peripheral angiopathy with gangrene
		E13.59	Other specified diabetes mellitus with other circulatory complications
250.71	Diabetes with peripheral circulatory disorders, Type I [juvenile type], not stated as uncontrolled	E10.51	Type 1 diabetes mellitus with diabetic peripheral angiopathy without gangrene
		E10.52	Type 1 diabetes mellitus with diabetic peripheral angiopathy with gangrene
		E10.59	Type 1 diabetes mellitus with other circulatory complications

> **CODING AXIOM**
>
> When uncontrolled Type 1 diabetes mellitus with ketoacidosis is diagnosed, an additional code for Type 1 diabetes mellitus with hyperglycemia is not needed as ketoacidosis denotes uncontrolled.
>
> *Coding Clinic,* 3Q, 13, 20

The following section of diabetes mellitus codes encompasses complications that did not have a category assigned in the other sections previously discussed. Many of the terms used in this category to describe complications are the same as those used in secondary diabetes. Please see the definitions in the previous section.

Coding for Diabetes Mellitus with Other Specified Manifestations

ICD-9-CM		ICD-10-CM	
250.80	Diabetes with other specified manifestations, Type II or unspecified type, not stated as uncontrolled	E11.618	Type 2 diabetes mellitus with other diabetic arthropathy
		E11.620	Type 2 diabetes mellitus with diabetic dermatitis
		E11.621	Type 2 diabetes mellitus with foot ulcer
		E11.622	Type 2 diabetes mellitus with other skin ulcer
		E11.628	Type 2 diabetes mellitus with other skin complications
		E11.630	Type 2 diabetes mellitus with periodontal disease
		E11.638	Type 2 diabetes mellitus with other oral complications
		E11.649	Type 2 diabetes mellitus with hypoglycemia without coma
		E11.65	Type 2 diabetes mellitus with hyperglycemia
		E13.618	Other specified diabetes mellitus with other diabetic arthropathy
		E13.620	Other specified diabetes mellitus with diabetic dermatitis
		E13.621	Other specified diabetes mellitus with foot ulcer
		E13.622	Other specified diabetes mellitus with other skin ulcer
		E13.628	Other specified diabetes mellitus with other skin complications
		E13.630	Other specified diabetes mellitus with *periodontal* disease
(Continued on next page)		E13.638	Other specified diabetes mellitus with other oral complications

> **DEFINITIONS**
>
> **periodontal.** Relating to the tissues that support and surround the teeth.

© 2015 Optum360, LLC

ICD-9-CM		ICD-10-CM	
250.80	Diabetes with other specified manifestations, Type II or unspecified type, not stated as uncontrolled *(Continued)*	E13.641	Other specified diabetes mellitus with hypoglycemia with coma
		E13.649	Other specified diabetes mellitus with hypoglycemia without coma
		E13.65	Other specified diabetes mellitus with hyperglycemia
250.81	Diabetes with other specified manifestations, Type I [juvenile type], not stated as uncontrolled	E10.618	Type 1 diabetes mellitus with other diabetic arthropathy
		E10.620	Type 1 diabetes mellitus with diabetic dermatitis
		E10.621	Type 1 diabetes mellitus with foot ulcer
		E10.622	Type 1 diabetes mellitus with other skin ulcer
		E10.628	Type 1 diabetes mellitus with other skin complications
		E10.630	Type 1 diabetes mellitus with periodontal disease
		E10.638	Type 1 diabetes mellitus with other oral complications
		E10.649	Type 1 diabetes mellitus with hypoglycemia without coma
		E10.65	Type 1 diabetes mellitus with hyperglycemia
		E10.69	Type 1 diabetes mellitus with other specified complication

Pituitary Gland Disorders

Acromegaly and gigantism are caused by a **benign** tumor of the pituitary that stimulates production of excessive growth hormone, causing abnormal growth in particular parts of the body. Acromegaly is a rare, chronic, metabolic disorder and usually develops over many years in adults. Gigantism occurs when excess growth hormone begins to be secreted in childhood.

In ICD-10-CM, code E34.4 Constitutional tall stature is also appropriate for constitutional gigantism.

Coding for Acromegaly and Gigantism

ICD-9-CM		ICD-10-CM	
253.0	Acromegaly and gigantism	E22.0	Acromegaly and pituitary gigantism
		E34.4	Constitutional tall stature

Cushing's syndrome, sometimes called hypercortisolism, is caused when the body is exposed to high levels of the hormone cortisol for a long period of time. This can be the result of glucocorticoid medications or over-secretion of adrenal cortisol. Cushing's syndrome is relatively rare and most commonly affects adults aged 20 to 50. The most common cause of Cushing's syndrome is glucocorticoids. These steroid hormones are chemically similar to naturally produced cortisol and are present in prednisone used for **asthma**, **rheumatoid arthritis**, **lupus**, and other inflammatory diseases.

Cushing's syndrome may also be referred to as Cushing's disease. However, the terms are not synonymous. Cushing's disease is specific to one cause of Cushing's syndrome, a benign **tumor** or **hyperplasia** in the pituitary gland that produces large amounts of adrenocorticotropic hormone (ACTH), which subsequently elevates cortisol.

Ectopic **ACTH** syndrome is a condition in which a tumor forms outside the pituitary or adrenal glands and produces ACTH. Such tumors are usually found in the lung, pancreas, thyroid, or thymus gland and can be benign or malignant. The most common forms of these tumors are small-cell lung cancer and **carcinoid tumors**.

DEFINITIONS

ACTH. Adrenocorticotropic hormone. Hormone secreted by the anterior pituitary that acts on the adrenal cortex and its secretion of corticosteroids. ACTH is used in hormone replacement therapy and as a diagnostic aid.

asthma. Narrowing or inflammation of the airway causing obstructed, labored breathing.

benign. Mild or nonmalignant in nature.

carcinoid tumor. Benign or malignant tumor that arises from neuroendocrine cells located throughout the body. The most common sites are the appendix, bronchi, rectum, small intestine, and stomach.

hyperplasia. Abnormal proliferation in the number of normal cells in regular tissue arrangement.

rheumatoid arthritis. Autoimmune disease causing pain, stiffness, inflammation, and possibly joint destruction.

systemic lupus. Inflammatory connective tissue disease.

tumor. Pathological swelling or enlargement; a neoplastic growth of uncontrolled, abnormal multiplication of cells.

Other less common types of tumors that can produce ACTH are medullary carcinomas of the thyroid, pancreatic islet cell tumors, and thymomas.

The ICD-10-CM classification code for pituitary-dependent Cushing's disease is appropriate to use for Cushing's disease caused by an overproduction of ATCH by tumors of the pituitary (pituitary-dependent).

Note: Codes have also been introduced in ICD-10-CM to indicate Cushing's syndrome as a result of alcohol or drugs.

Coding for Cushing's Syndrome

ICD-9-CM		ICD-10-CM	
255.0	Cushing's syndrome	E24.0	Pituitary-dependent Cushing's disease
		E24.2	Drug-induced Cushing's syndrome
		E24.3	Ectopic ACTH syndrome
		E24.4	Alcohol-induced *pseudo*-Cushing's syndrome
		E24.8	Other Cushing's syndrome
		E24.9	Cushing's syndrome, unspecified

> **DEFINITIONS**
>
> **dehydration.** Condition resulting from an excessive loss of water from the body.
>
> **pseudo.** Indicates false or imagined.
>
> **subcutaneous.** Below the skin.

Addison's disease is caused by decreased function of the adrenal cortex as a result of some sort of damage. In this disease, the adrenal glands produce too little cortisol and often insufficient levels of aldosterone. Adrenal cortex damage can result from such things as autoimmune disease, fungal infections, HIV, tuberculosis, tumors, and the use of anticoagulants.

Addisonian crisis occurs when a person with Addison's disease is under extreme physical stress, such as illness, physical shock (e.g., a car accident), or previously undiagnosed Addison's disease.

Coding for Addison's Disease

ICD-9-CM		ICD-10-CM	
255.41	Glucocorticoid deficiency	E27.1	Primary adrenocortical insufficiency
		E27.2	Addisonian crisis
		E27.3	Drug-induced adrenocortical insufficiency
		E89.6	Postprocedural adrenocortical (-medullary) hypofunction

Nutritional Deficiencies

Ingestion of imbalanced amounts of nutrients can disrupt the balance of nutrients required for proper health and endocrine function. One example of this is a goiter, commonly caused by a deficiency of dietary iodine. In the United States, nutritional and vitamin deficiencies are usually the result of poverty, prolonged parenteral feeding, chronic substance abuse, food fads, or extreme diets.

ICD-10-CM has expanded the available categories used to describe nutritional deficiencies. A few will be discussed in the following section.

Kwashiorkor

Kwashiorkor is an African word meaning "first-child, second-child." It refers to the protein-deficit illness that affects the first child when it is weaned to make room for the second child. Instead of protein-rich breast milk, the first child is fed a thin gruel made from sweet potato, banana, or cassava. The gruel is starchy, so there is no energy deficit, but the lack of protein causes edema, lethargy, and impaired growth. Kwashiorkor is considered a third-degree malnutrition disorder.

Marasmic kwashiorkor is a condition in which there is a deficiency of both calories and protein; it is the most severe form of protein-energy malnutrition. It is accompanied by severe tissue wasting, loss of **subcutaneous** fat, and usually **dehydration.**

DEFINITIONS

ataxia. Defect in muscular coordination, seen especially when voluntary muscular movements are attempted.

edema. Swelling due to fluid accumulation in the intercellular spaces.

malabsorption. Body's inability to absorb a substance or nutrient, usually occurring in the small intestine.

neuritis. Inflammation of a nerve or group of nerves, often manifested by loss of function and reflexes, pain, and numbness or tingling.

Coding for Kwashiorkor

ICD-9-CM		ICD-10-CM	
260	Kwashiorkor	E40	Kwashiorkor
		E42	Marasmic kwashiorkor

Thiamine and Niacin Deficiencies

Alcoholism is the main cause of thiamine (vitamin B1) deficiency in the United States. It is also common in people with *malabsorption* problems, which sometimes occur after bariatric surgery. In other countries, it can result from eating a diet of highly polished rice. Infants can develop a thiamine deficiency when breast-fed by thiamine-deficient mothers. Thiamine deficiency causes beriberi, with manifestations of *neuritis*, *edema*, and heart disease.

Wet beriberi describes a thiamine deficiency that involves the cardiovascular system.

Dry beriberi is a thiamine deficiency that also affects the nervous system.

Wernicke's encephalopathy is brain damage in lower parts of the brain called the thalamus and hypothalamus, caused by a lack of thiamine. Symptoms include confusion, *ataxia*, and vision changes.

Niacin deficiency is called pellagra and is characterized by a light-sensitive rash, diarrhea, glossitis, and psychosis. Pellagra is most common in countries in which corn is the main food source and is rare in the United States.

Coding for Beriberi

ICD-9-CM		ICD-10-CM	
265.0	Beriberi	E51.11	Dry beriberi
		E51.12	Wet beriberi
265.1	Other and unspecified manifestations of thiamine deficiency	E51.2	Wernicke's encephalopathy
		E51.8	Other manifestations of thiamine deficiency
		E51.9	Thiamine deficiency, unspecified
265.2	Pellagra	E52	Niacin deficiency [pellagra]

B-group Deficiencies

Ariboflavinosis is riboflavin, or vitamin B2, deficiency that causes inflammation of the lips, tongue fissures, corneal vascularization, and anemia. Ariboflavinosis is associated with milk deficiency, though the disease can also occur secondarily in patients with chronic diseases affecting nutritional absorption.

Pyridoxine, or vitamin B6, is important in blood, the central nervous system, and skin metabolism. It is uncommon to find a primary deficiency of vitamin B6, but secondary deficiency can result in chronic diseases affecting nutritional absorption in patients using oral contraceptives or in alcoholism. Vitamin B6 deficiency causes skin, lip, and tongue disturbances, peripheral neuropathy, and, in infants, convulsions.

Coding for Deficiency of B-complex Components

ICD-9-CM		ICD-10-CM	
266.0	Ariboflavinosis	E53.0	Riboflavin deficiency
266.1	Vitamin B6 deficiency	E53.1	Pyridoxine deficiency
266.2	Other B-complex deficiencies	D81.818	Other biotin-dependent carboxylase deficiency
		D81.819	Biotin-dependent carboxylase deficiency, unspecified
		E53.8	Deficiency of other specified B group vitamins

Ascorbic Acid Deficiency

Vitamin C, or ascorbic acid, is essential for wound healing and connective tissue health, and it facilitates absorption of iron. A deficiency in this vitamin is commonly called scurvy or Cheadle-Moller-Barlow syndrome. Vitamin C is common to many fruits and vegetables. Symptoms of scurvy include bleeding gums, weight loss, myalgias, and slowing of the healing process. The symptoms are reversed with ascorbic acid therapy.

ICD-10-CM has further classified vitamin C deficiency with the addition of code E64.2 Sequelae of vitamin C deficiency. When using this code, the condition resulting from the malnutrition or deficiency should be reported first.

Coding for Ascorbic Acid Deficiency

ICD-9-CM		ICD-10-CM	
267	Ascorbic acid deficiency	E54	Ascorbic acid deficiency
		E64.2	Sequelae of vitamin C deficiency

ICD-10-CM has expanded the ICD-9-CM categories used to identify other nutritional deficiencies. Many deficiencies reported as not elsewhere classified or other in ICD-9-CM now have their own code description in ICD-10-CM.

Coding for Other Deficiencies

ICD-9-CM		ICD-10-CM	
269.0	Deficiency of vitamin K	E56.1	Deficiency of vitamin K
269.1	Deficiency of other vitamins	E56.0	Deficiency of vitamin E
		E56.8	Deficiency of other vitamins
269.2	Unspecified vitamin deficiency	E56.9	Vitamin deficiency, unspecified
269.3	Mineral deficiency, not elsewhere classified	E58	Dietary calcium deficiency
		E59	Dietary selenium deficiency
		E60	Dietary zinc deficiency
		E61.0	Copper deficiency
		E61.1	Iron deficiency
		E61.2	Magnesium deficiency
		E61.3	Manganese deficiency
		E61.4	Chromium deficiency
		E61.5	Molybdenum deficiency
		E61.6	Vanadium deficiency
269.8	Other nutritional deficiency	E61.7	Deficiency of multiple nutrient elements
		E61.8	Deficiency of other specified nutrient elements
		E63.0	Essential fatty acid [EFA] deficiency
		E63.1	Imbalance of constituents of food intake
		E63.8	Other specified nutritional deficiencies
		E64.8	Sequelae of other nutritional deficiencies
269.9	Unspecified nutritional deficiency	E61.9	Deficiency of nutrient element, unspecified
		E63.9	Nutritional deficiency, unspecified
		E64.9	Sequelae of unspecified nutritional deficiency

ICD-10-CM has expanded the ICD-9-CM categories used to identify metabolic and immunity disorders. Many disorders reported under one broad category in ICD-9-CM now have their own classification in ICD-10-CM. A few examples follow.

Cystinosis is a genetic metabolic disease that causes the amino acid cystine to accumulate in various organs of the body. The cystine crystallizes and commonly accumulates within the brain, eyes, kidneys, liver, muscles, pancreas, and white blood cells.

Comprehensive Anatomy and Physiology for ICD-10-CM and ICD-10-PCS Coding

> **DEFINITIONS**
>
> **albinism.** Genetic condition with absence of pigment in skin, hair, and eyes that is often accompanied by astigmatism, photophobia, and nystagmus.
>
> **calculus.** Abnormal, stone-like concretion of calcium, cholesterol, mineral salts, or other substances that forms in any part of the body.
>
> **cataract.** Clouding or opacities of the lens that stop clear images from forming on the retina, causing vision impairment or blindness. The classification and coding of cataracts are dependent upon size, shape, location, and etiology.
>
> **Fanconi (-de Toni) (-Debré) syndrome.** Renal tubular malfunction, including cystinosis and osteomalacia caused by inherited disorders, the result of multiple myeloma, or proximal epithelial growth.
>
> **glaucoma.** Rise in intraocular pressure, restricting blood flow and decreasing vision.
>
> **hypotonia.** Diminished muscle tone and stretching resistance.

Cystinosis is an autosomal recessive genetic disease. In simple terms, both parents are carriers of the abnormal gene. The parents do not show any of the symptoms of cystinosis, but the odds are that one in four of their children will have cystinosis. Cystinosis is a rare disease primarily affecting children, although it can develop in adults. If this condition is left untreated, eventually complete kidney failure will result and other complications, such as **Fanconi syndrome**, may develop.

Cystinuria is a hereditary metabolic disorder characterized by the abnormal transfer of amino acids, such as cystine, lysine, arginine, and ornithine, in the intestines and kidneys. Excessive amounts of cystine in the urine cause the formation of **calculus** in the kidney, bladder, and/or ureter.

Hartnup's disease is an inherited inborn error of metabolism of amino acids in addition to a niacin deficiency. People with this disease are not able to absorb some of the amino acids in their intestines. One of the main amino acids that is not absorbed is tryptophan, which the body uses to make its own form of niacin. Generally individuals with this disease do not have symptoms, but exposure to sunlight, fever, stress, or poor nutrition can cause skin problems, coordination impairment, vision problems, mild mental retardation, gastrointestinal problems, and central nervous system abnormalities. Frequency of attacks usually diminishes with age.

Lowe's syndrome, also referred to as OCRL (oculo-cerebro-renal) syndrome, is a rare genetic condition characterized by anomalies affecting the eye, the nervous system, and the kidney. This disorder occurs almost exclusively in males. Infants with this syndrome are born with congenital **cataracts**, infantile **glaucoma**, neonatal or infantile **hypotonia**, intellectual impairment, and renal tubular dysfunction (Fanconi syndrome).

Phenylketonuria (PKU) is a genetic disorder characterized by an inability to process a part of protein called phenylalanine (Phe). Phe is found in almost all foods. Because of a genetic abnormality, affected individuals lack or have very low levels of an enzyme (phenylalanine hydroxylase or PAH) that converts Phe to other substances the body needs. Extremely elevated Phe levels can cause brain damage and severe mental retardation.

Coding for Disorders of Amino-acid Transport and Metabolism

ICD-9-CM		ICD-10-CM	
270.0	Disturbances of amino-acid transport	E72.00	Disorders of amino-acid transport, unspecified
		E72.01	Cystinuria
		E72.02	Hartnup's disease
		E72.04	Cystinosis
		E72.09	Other disorders of amino-acid transport
270.1	Phenylketonuria (PKU)	E70.0	Classical phenylketonuria
		E70.1	Other hyperphenylalaninemias

Tyrosinemia is a genetic disorder in which the body cannot effectively break down the amino acid tyrosine. Increased levels of tyrosine and its byproducts build up in tissues and organs, leading to serious medical problems such as liver and kidney disturbances and mental retardation. Untreated, tyrosinemia can be fatal.

X-linked ocular albinism (XLOA), which occurs almost exclusively in males, is caused by a gene mutation of the X chromosome. People with XLOA have the developmental and functional vision problems of **albinism.** However, eye, hair, and skin color are usually the same as others in the family or slightly lighter.

Autosomes are the chromosomes that contain genes for general body characteristics. Generally each individual inherits two of these chromosomes: one from the mother and one from the father. In autosomal recessive ocular albinism, albinism is an inherited recessive trait, obvious only when two copies of the gene for that trait are present. In other words, if one parent carries a mutated chromosome and the other does not, the child will not have albinism but instead be a carrier. However, if both parents (that are only carriers) have mutated chromosomes that are passed on, the child will have albinism. In this situation, there is a one in four chance that the child will have albinism.

Tyrosinase negative oculocutaneous albinism type IA (OCA1A) results from a genetic defect in an enzyme called tyrosinase. This enzyme helps the body transform the amino acid tyrosine into pigment. The enzyme is inactive and no melanin is produced; therefore, there is a complete absence of pigment in the skin, hair, and eyes. These individuals also present with **photophobia**, moderate-to-severe reduced **visual acuity**, and **nystagmus**.

In tyrosinase positive oculocutaneous albinism type II (OCA2), the enzyme tyrosinase is present. Generally OCA2 manifests with a minimal-to-moderate amount of pigment remaining in the skin, hair, and eyes. Many patients can develop pigmented freckles, lentigines, and/or **nevi** with age. Individuals with OCA2 have the usual visual anomalies associated with albinism, including decreased acuity and nystagmus. OCA2 is the most prevalent form of oculocutaneous albinism. The occurrence of this disorder is greatly increased in patients with **Willi-Prader** or **Angelman syndrome**.

Chediak-Higashi syndrome is an autosomal recessive immunodeficiency disorder. Individuals with this disorder inherit a defective gene from each parent. This gene affects multiple body areas but has the biggest impact on the immune system. It prevents white blood cells from functioning properly, leaving them unable to fight viruses and bacteria. This disease also manifests symptoms of oculocutaneous albinism (light pigmentation of eyes, hair, and skin, and vision problems), prolonged bleeding times, easy bruisability, and peripheral **neuropathy**.

Hermansky-Pudlak syndrome is an autosomal recessive type of albinism that includes a **coagulation** defect and lung disease. This disease also manifests symptoms of oculocutaneous albinism (light pigmentation of eyes, hair, and skin, and vision problems), in addition to **colitis** and kidney failure.

Coding for Disorders of Aromatic Amino-acid Metabolism

ICD-9-CM		ICD-10-CM	
270.2	Other disturbances of aromatic amino-acid metabolism	E70.20	Disorder of tyrosine metabolism, unspecified
		E70.21	Tyrosinemia
		E70.29	Other disorders of tyrosine metabolism
		E70.30	Albinism, unspecified
		E70.310	X-linked ocular albinism
		E70.311	Autosomal recessive ocular albinism
		E70.318	Other ocular albinism
		E70.319	Ocular albinism, unspecified
		E70.320	Tyrosinase negative oculocutaneous albinism
		E70.321	Tyrosinase positive oculocutaneous albinism
		E70.328	Other oculocutaneous albinism
		E70.329	Oculocutaneous albinism, unspecified
		E70.330	Chediak-Higashi syndrome
(Continued on next page)		E70.331	Hermansky-Pudlak syndrome

Definitions

Angelman syndrome. Emergence in early childhood of a pattern of interrupted development, stiff jerky gait, absence or impairment of speech, excessive laughter, and seizures.

coagulation. Clot formation.

colitis. Inflammation of the colon, caused by any number of infections, external influences such as laxatives or radiation, and antibiotics.

neuropathy. Abnormality, disease, or malfunction of the nerves.

nevus. plural of nevi. Benign, pigmented skin lesion that includes congenital lesions of the skin such as birthmarks, telangiectasias (permanent dilations of small blood vessels), vascular spider veins, hemangiomas, and moles.

nystagmus. Rapid, rhythmic, involuntary movements of the eyeball in vertical, horizontal, rotational, or mixed directions that can be congenital, acquired, physiological, neurological, or due to ocular disease.

photophobia. Sensitivity to light.

visual acuity. Clarity of vision.

Willi-Prader syndrome. Typified by rounded face, almond-shaped eyes, strabismus, low forehead, hypogonadism, hypotonia, mental retardation, and an insatiable appetite.

ICD-9-CM		ICD-10-CM	
270.2	Other disturbances of aromatic amino-acid metabolism *(Continued)*	E70.338	Other albinism with hematologic abnormality
		E70.339	Albinism with hematologic abnormality, unspecified
		E70.39	Other specified albinism
		E70.5	Disorders of tryptophan metabolism
		E70.8	Other disorders of aromatic amino-acid metabolism
		E70.9	Disorder of aromatic amino-acid metabolism, unspecified

Summary

The endocrine system, which is vital to many daily functions, can be affected by numerous conditions. This chapter reviews many of these conditions, and outlines the increased specificity included in the ICD-10-CM code set. In order to be well prepared to transition to ICD-10-CM, it is important to be aware of the basic anatomy and physiology of the endocrine system, as well as the specific disease pathologies that are described in both code sets.

Chapter 7. ICD-10-CM: Cardiovascular System

Anatomic Overview

The cardiovascular system houses some of the most important components needed for day-to-day survival. The heart and the approximately 60,000 miles of blood vessels in the circulatory system provide oxygen-rich blood, nutrients such as amino acids and electrolytes, and important hormones to all of the body's cells and carry off carbon dioxide and other waste products of metabolism. In addition, the cardiovascular system stabilizes body temperature and pH. Other body systems work closely with the cardiovascular system to ensure proper functioning and homeostasis, which is the ability of an organism to obtain and maintain internal stability by adjusting its physiological processes. For instance, the digestive system provides needed nutrients to the body by way of the cardiovascular system.

Anatomy of the Heart

The heart, itself, is a small organ, approximately the size of a fist. It is located in the mediastinum, with the majority of it to the left of the body's midline. It is enclosed in a protective, two-layer membrane that positions it in the chest but also allows for expansion as needed for contractions. The outer layer, the fibrous pericardium, is made up of dense connective tissue. The serous pericardium is double layered, with the outermost parietal layer adherent to the fibrous pericardium and the inner visceral layer (epicardium) adherent to the heart's surface. Between these two layers, the pericardial cavity contains lubricating pericardial fluid that decreases friction caused by the beating of the heart.

Figure 7.1: Sections of Heart Muscle

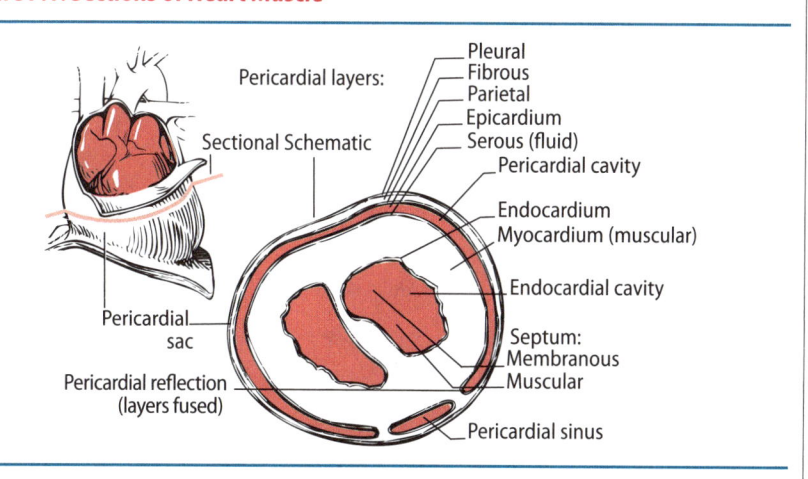

The heart wall comprises three layers: the external epicardium (also called the visceral serous pericardial layer), the middle myocardium, and the endocardium, which is the innermost layer covering the four chambers of the heart, the valves, and the lining of large blood vessels connected to the heart.

The four chambers of the heart include the right and left atria on the upper side and the left and right ventricles on the lower side. The outermost surface of the heart contains channels known as sulci. These sulci, which contain some fat and the coronary blood vessels, delineate the outside margins of the heart chambers.

Each of the four valves of the heart, although located in different areas, function in the same way. The valves open and close in response to pressure differences caused by contraction and relaxation of the heart chambers. This allows blood to flow from areas with higher pressure to those with lower pressure. Valves allow blood to flow in one direction only, preventing backflow when closed.

Between the right atrium and the right ventricle lies the tricuspid valve, through which blood flows. From the right ventricle, blood passes through the pulmonary valve into the pulmonary trunk where it is carried to the lungs for oxygenation. After oxygenation occurs, the blood returns to the left atrium through the four pulmonary veins. It passes from the left atrium through the bicuspid (mitral) valve to the left ventricle. The blood is then passed through the aortic valve into the ascending aorta where some flows into the coronary arteries and the rest passes into the aortic arch and descending aorta where other arteries carry the blood throughout the body.

Collectively, the bicuspid and the tricuspid valves are referred to as the atrioventricular (AV) valves, while the pulmonary and aortic valves are referred to as the semi-lunar (SL) valves.

Figure 7.2: Anatomy

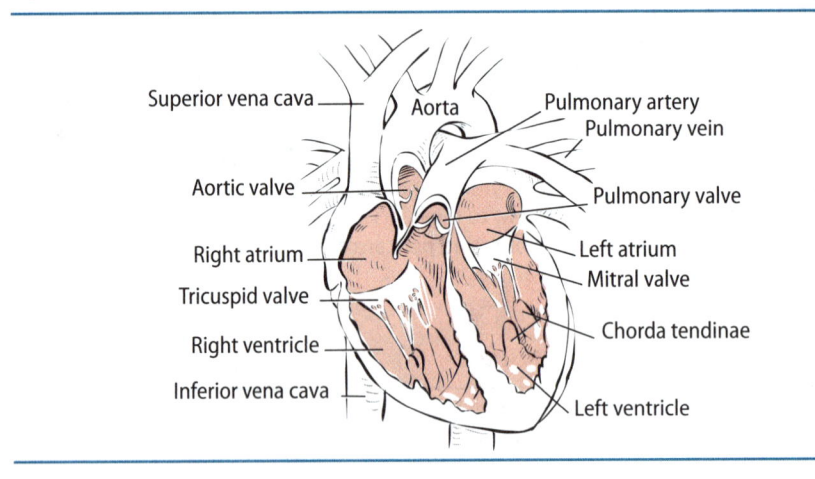

Figure 7.3: Blood Flow

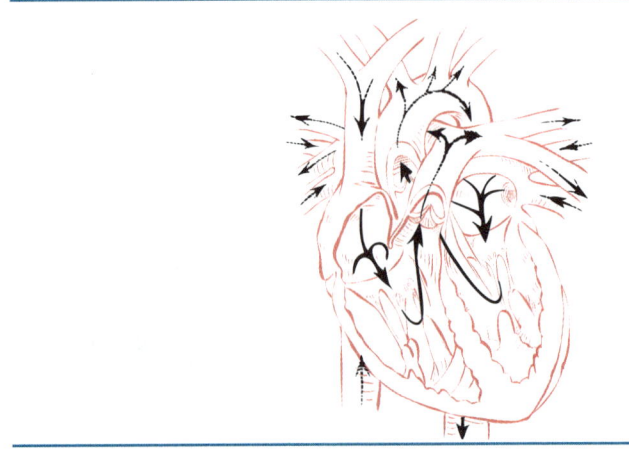

Conduction System of the Heart

Specialized autorhythmic cells in the cardiac muscle not only produce the electrical stimulation that initiates the heartbeat, but also form the conduction system that stimulates the contraction of the heart to make it pump effectively. Inherent in the heart's muscle tissue are the physiological properties of:

- **Automaticity:** Property of a cell to reach a threshold potential and generate an impulse on its own without stimulation from another source.
- **Conductivity:** Ability to transfer an impulse from cell to cell.
- **Contractility:** Property that allows shortening of the muscle when stimulated.
- **Excitability:** Capacity of a cell to respond to a stimulus.

Figure 7.4: Conduction System of the Heart

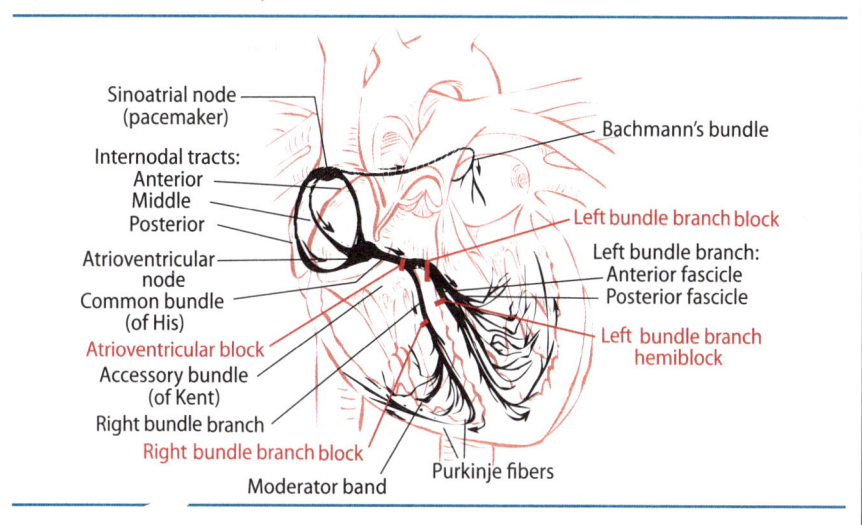

In a normal heart, the muscle is stimulated by impulses that originate in the sinoatrial (SA) node, also referred to as the sinus node and the heart's pacemaker. The impulse goes from the sinus node, through the atria, to the atrioventricular (AV) node, which is positioned between the atria and the ventricles, through the bundle branches, and ends in the Purkinje fibers of the ventricles' walls to initiate systole.

The SA node, under control of the autonomic nervous system, is innervated by parasympathetic nervous system fibers, as well as sympathetic nervous system fibers. Stimulation of the sympathetic nervous system increases the heart rate, raises blood pressure, and increases the force of myocardial contraction. On the other hand, parasympathetic stimulation slows the heart rate, lowers blood pressure, and decreases the force of contraction. The manipulation of the autonomic nervous system by drugs such as beta adrenergic blocking drugs (beta blockers) takes advantage of these effects. Blocking the sympathetic nervous system relieves stress on the heart, causing it to slow down, decreases the force of the heart's contraction, and reduces blood vessel contraction as well. These drugs are useful following myocardial infarction and for treating cardiac dysrhythmias and hypertension.

Cardiac Cycle

A cardiac cycle is the sequence of events that occur during each heartbeat. An impulse from the SA node causes the atria to contract first (atrial systole), while the ventricles relax (ventricular diastole). Atria contraction forces blood through the open AV valves to the ventricles. Since the SL valves are closed, the ventricle is able to fill with approximately 130 cc of blood, a volume referred to as the end-diastolic volume (EDV). When the ventricles contract (ventricular systole), the atria relax (atria diastole). The increased ventricular pressure forces the SL valves open, ejecting blood from the heart. Ventricular ejection is the period of time when the SL valves are open. Each ventricle ejects about 70 cc of blood, leaving approximately 60 cc in the ventricle, referred to as the end systolic volume (ESV). The four chambers of the heart then relax, and the cycle begins again.

Coronary Circulation

The heart has its own system of blood vessels, referred to as coronary or cardiac circulation. The left main and right main coronary arteries supply oxygenated blood to the myocardium. They originate at the base of the aorta from openings called the coronary ostia, which are behind the leaflets of the aortic valve. The left coronary artery divides into the left anterior descending (LAD) artery, also called the anterior interventricular branch and circumflex branches. The LAD artery carries blood to both ventricular walls, and the circumflex branch provides oxygenated blood to the left atrial walls and the left ventricle. The right coronary artery divides into branches that carry blood to the right atrium and further divide into the posterior interventricular and marginal branches. These vessels provide blood to both ventricular walls and to the right ventricular myocardium, respectively. The myocardium has many connections where blood may be received from more than one artery, which enables the heart's tissue to receive adequate oxygen even when a coronary artery is blocked.

Figure 7.5: Arteries of the Heart

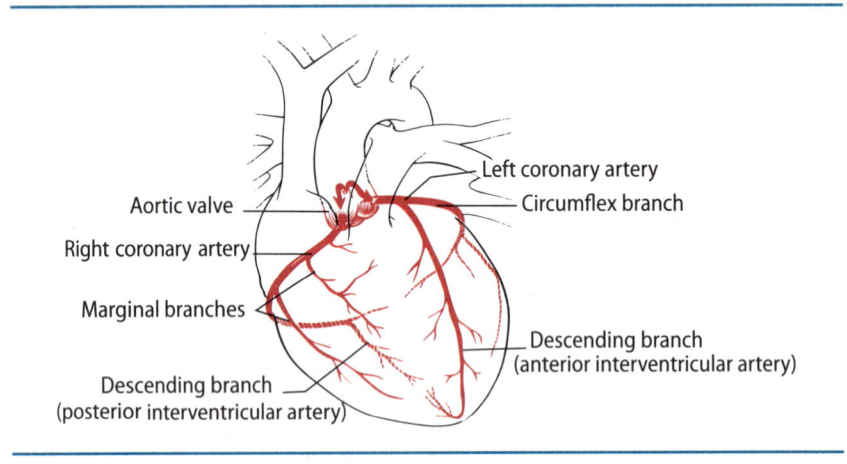

Labels: Left coronary artery, Circumflex branch, Aortic valve, Right coronary artery, Marginal branches, Descending branch (anterior interventricular artery), Descending branch (posterior interventricular artery)

> **INTERESTING A & P FACT**
>
> A healthy heart is seemingly tireless, beating approximately 100,000 times a day and pumping 30 times its own weight in blood every minute.

Once the blood has completed its circuit through the arteries, it continues to the capillaries, delivering oxygen and nutrients and collecting CO_2 and any waste product before it drains into the coronary sinus. On the venous side of the coronary circulation are veins that empty deoxygenated blood into the coronary sinus and ultimately into the right atrium, including:

- **Anterior cardiac veins:** Drain the right ventricle.
- **Great cardiac vein:** Drains the left atrium and both ventricles.
- **Middle cardiac vein:** Drains both ventricles.
- **Small cardiac vein:** Drains the right atrium and ventricle.

Circulatory Pathways

The heart and the blood vessels form two distinct, but parallel, circulatory pathways that nourish all of the organs and cells of the body. The systemic circulation includes all of the arteries and arterioles that branch off the aorta as it emerges from the left ventricle to deliver oxygen-rich blood to the body, as well as the veins and venules that eventually drain into the superior and inferior vena cava and the coronary sinus that empties oxygen-poor blood into the right atrium. The blood then goes to the right ventricle, where it is picked up by the pulmonary circulation to be reoxygenated. Blood leaves the right ventricle via the pulmonary trunk, which splits into the right and left pulmonary arteries. These branches further divide, becoming successively smaller until they become pulmonary capillaries surrounding the alveoli in the lungs. The layers of cells that line the alveoli and the surrounding capillaries are very thin and in close proximity to each other. It is here that carbon dioxide is passed from the blood to the alveoli to be exhaled and oxygen from the air is passed from the lungs into the blood, a process known as alveolar capillary exchange. As this cycle continues, the tiny capillaries join together to form venules and ultimately the four (two left, two right) pulmonary veins bring oxygen-rich blood to the left atrium, then the left ventricle, where the oxygenated blood is pumped into the systemic circulation.

Blood Vessel Anatomy: Artery, Veins, Arterioles, Venules, and Capillaries

Although there are variations in the function of each particular blood vessel, the walls of most have the following three layers:

- **Tunica interna:** Innermost layer of the vessel that contains a single layer of endothelium on the inner surface that helps influence blood flow, secretes chemicals that affect capillary permeability, and aids in vessel contraction.
- **Tunica media:** Thick middle layer of mostly smooth muscle cells and extensive elastic fibers. The primary function of this layer is to regulate blood pressure and flow by contraction and dilation.
- **Tunica externa:** Outermost layer of the vessel, its function is to attach the vessel to the surrounding tissue. It is made up of collagen, elastic fibers, and many nerves. In the case of larger vessels, the tunica externa also contains very small vessels that supply blood to the vessel wall.

Arteries transport blood away from the heart to all organs and cells of the body and are divided into two types: elastic and muscular. Elastic, or conducting, arteries have the largest diameter of all arteries in the body and include the aorta, pulmonary trunk, brachiocephalic, common carotid, common iliac, and subclavian arteries. They drive blood forward while the ventricles are relaxed, pushing blood toward smaller arteries. Muscular (distributing) arteries are mid-size arteries that are branches of the elastic arteries. Varying in size from the pencil-sized axillary and femoral arteries to the small, string-size arteries that carry blood to organs, the thick walls of these arteries are able to regulate blood flow with vasoconstriction and vasodilatation. Some examples of muscular arteries include the brachial and radial arteries of the arm. Branching into increasingly smaller arteries, the muscular arteries eventually branch out into the microscopic arterioles that control blood flow into the capillary networks. Changes at this level can impact blood pressure, with arteriole vasodilatation decreasing blood pressure and arteriole vasoconstriction increasing blood pressure.

Upon entering the tissue, arterioles branch off further into capillaries, which are the body's smallest blood vessels. They exchange substances in the blood and interstitial fluid of the body's cells. They are not present in cartilage or in the cornea or lens of the eye, but they are found in abundance in connection with tissues that have high metabolic requirements, such as the nervous system, liver, and muscles.

Figure 7.6: Capillary Bed

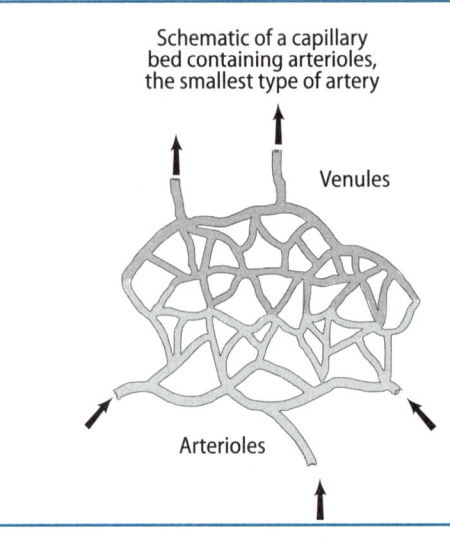

Capillaries function as part of a capillary bed, comprising 10 to 100 capillaries through which blood flows and capillary exchange takes place. Diffusion is the primary mechanism of this process, allowing oxygen, hormones, nutrients, and byproducts of metabolism to cross the capillary walls. Transcytosis may also take place, particularly with larger or lipid-insoluble materials, such as antibodies and proteins. Transcellular transport takes place when the substance becomes enclosed in the wall of the cell and is moved across the cell and expelled through the cell wall on the opposite side.

After capillary exchange takes place, the tiny postcapillary venules continue the exchange of nutrients and waste products, especially for larger molecules. The venules then begin to reunite and become successively larger veins, eventually returning the blood to the right atrium via the inferior and superior vena cava.

Brain Circulation

The carotid and vertebral arteries supply oxygenated blood to the brain. The carotid arteries are easily palpated under the jaw: one on the left and one on the right. At the top of the neck, the carotids **bifurcate** into the external and internal carotid arteries. The external carotid arteries provide blood and nutrients to the face and scalp, while the internal carotid arteries supply the anterior three-fifths of the cerebrum, with the exception of parts of the temporal and occipital lobes.

The vertebral arteries course along the spinal column, joining together to create the single basilar artery (vertebrobasilar arteries) near the brain stem at the skull base. These arteries nourish the posterior two-fifths of the cerebrum, part of the cerebellum, and the brain stem.

DEFINITIONS

bifurcation. Point of division into two separate branches or structures, such as the site where the trachea divides into the right and left main bronchi or the common carotid artery becomes the external and internal carotid arteries.

Figure 7.7: Cerebrovascular Arteries

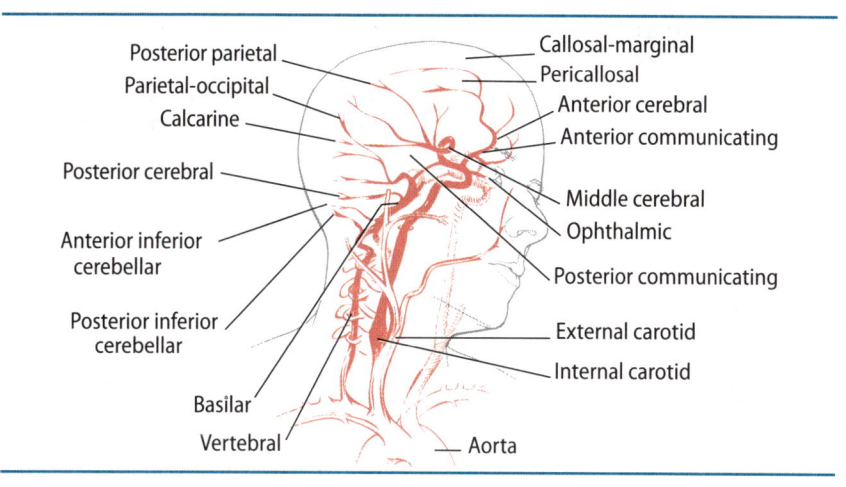

The internal-carotid and vertebral arteries converge at the Circle of Willis. It is from the circle of Willis that other arteries—the anterior cerebral artery (ACA), the middle cerebral artery (MCA), and the posterior cerebral artery (PCA)—arise and travel to all parts of the brain. One of the shortcomings of the circle of Willis is that cerebral aneurysms are inclined to develop at the arterial junctions. Deoxygenated blood is removed from the brain via the jugular vein.

Figure 7.8: Head Veins

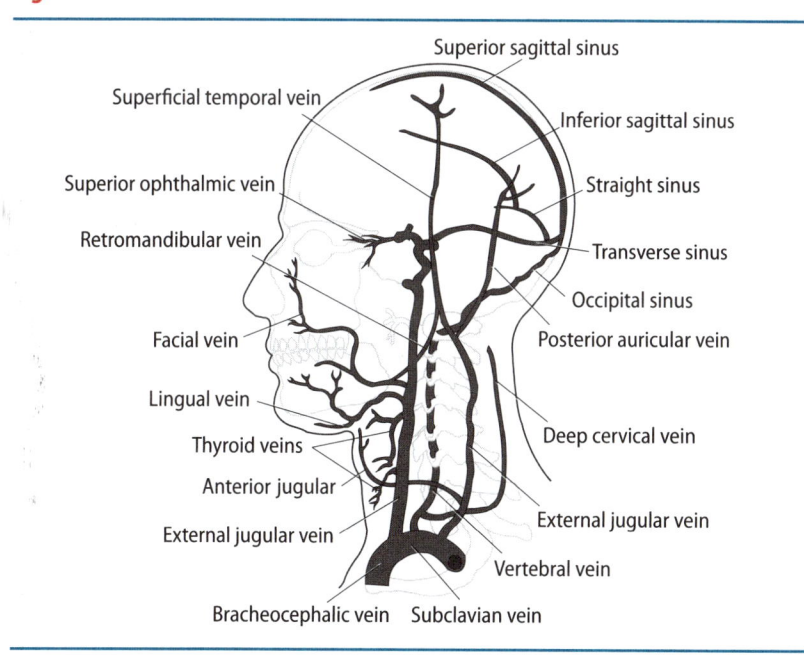

Systemic Circulation

The aorta, which is approximately one inch in diameter, is the largest artery in the body. From every part of the aorta, other arteries branch off into a network of successively smaller arteries until they eventually divide into arterioles and finally capillaries, where the exchange of oxygen, nutrients, and waste products takes place within the individual organs.

Comprehensive Anatomy and Physiology for ICD-10-CM and ICD-10-PCS Coding

The aorta is divided into four segments:

- **Ascending aorta:** Arises from the left ventricle and is the site of the coronary arteries.
- **Aortic arch:** First arching to the left, the aorta descends through the diaphragm. This segment includes arteries that travel to the head, neck, and upper extremities.
- **Thoracic aorta:** Part of the aorta between the arch and the diaphragm that contains arterial branches that supply the bronchi, esophagus, pericardium, mediastinum, intercostal muscles, muscles of the chest, and a portion of the diaphragm.
- **Abdominal aorta:** Portion of the aorta between the diaphragm and the branches of the common iliac arteries that supplies part of the diaphragm, intestines, all of the visceral organs, lower limbs, reproductive organs, bladder, and buttock muscles.

Figure 7.9: Arterial System

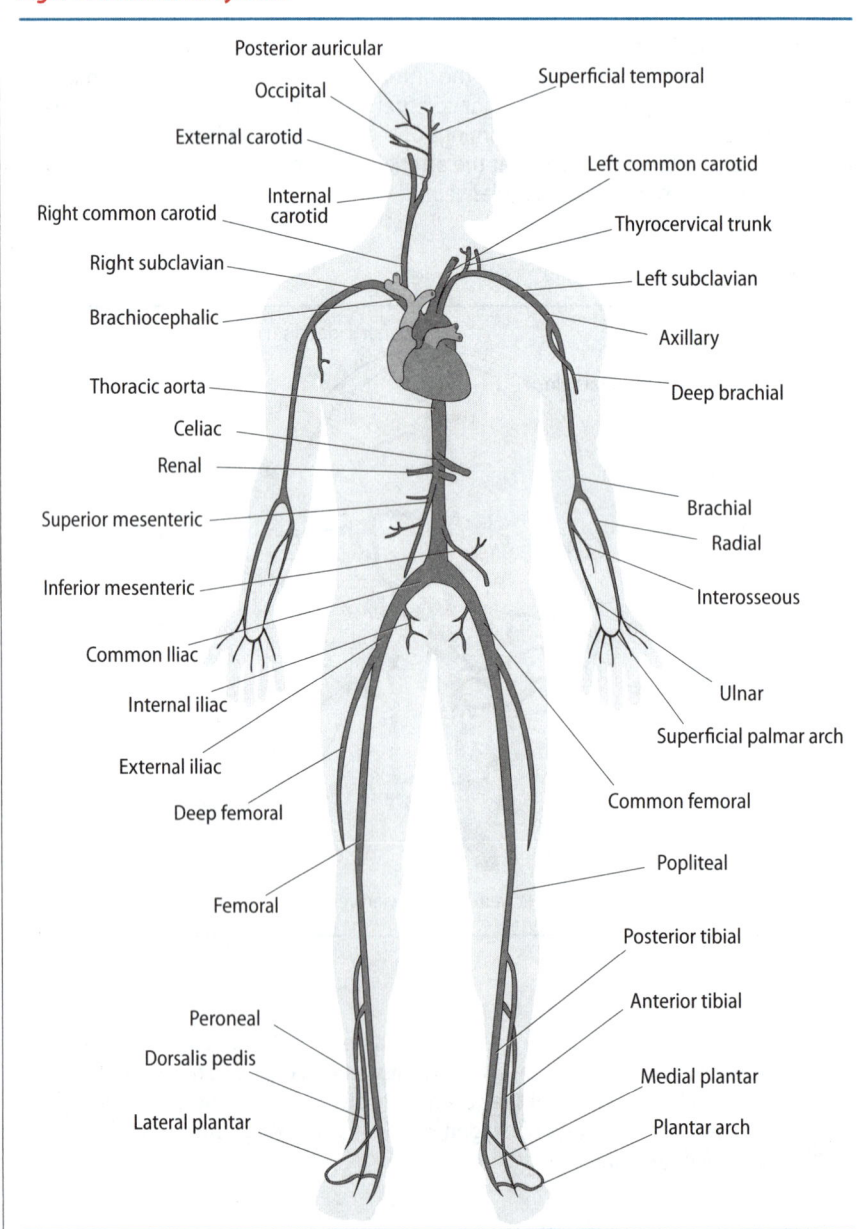

Hepatic Portal System

Simply put, a portal system consists of a network of blood vessels through which blood is transported after passing through one capillary bed to another network of capillaries prior to being returned to systemic circulation. The portal venous system channels blood from parts of the digestive tract, spleen, and pancreas to the liver for processing prior to returning to the heart.

Blood flow to the liver differs from that in the general circulation since the liver receives oxygenated blood, as well as partially deoxygenated blood. Oxygenated blood from the hepatic artery mixes with the nutrient rich blood from the portal vein in the liver sinusoids.

The large veins that make up the portal venous system are:

- Hepatic portal vein
- Inferior mesenteric vein
- Splenic vein
- Superior mesenteric vein

Figure 7.10: Portal System

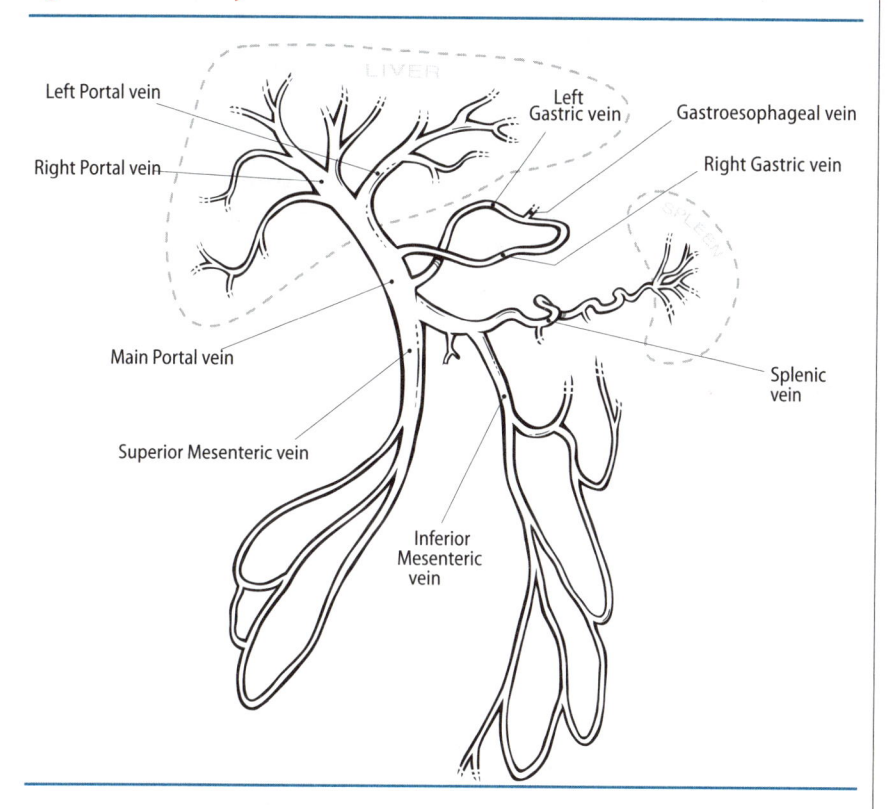

Anatomy and Pathophysiology and the ICD-10-CM Code Set

In ICD-10-CM, diagnosis coding of conditions affecting the cardiovascular system is much more detailed than it is in ICD-9-CM. In many cases, there is one ICD-9-CM code describing a diagnosis, whereas there are several ICD-10-CM codes. Details such as specific anatomical site or the severity of a condition have been incorporated into ICD-10-CM that didn't exist in ICD-9-CM.

For example, ICD-9-CM has one specific code to classify cardiac arrest:

> 427.5   Cardiac arrest

In ICD-10-CM, however, more specific codes are available to classify the cardiac arrest, including:

> I46.2   Cardiac arrest due to underlying cardiac condition
>
> I46.8   Cardiac arrest due to other underlying condition
>
> I46.9   Cardiac arrest, cause unspecified

The increased specificity of ICD-10-CM makes it imperative that physicians document more detailed information and that coders are able to determine from documentation the code or codes appropriate for the patient's condition.

Valvular Disorders

Acute rheumatic fever, a complication of strep pharyngitis in children, results in various cardiac conditions in more than a third of patients affected. Depending on the extent of heart inflammation involved, patients with the acute form of the disease may develop heart failure, **pericarditis**, myocarditis, and endocarditis, which is manifested as insufficiency of the mitral (65 to 70 percent of cases) and aortic valves (25 percent of cases).

DEFINITIONS

pericarditis. Inflammation affecting the pericardium.

Figure 7.11: Valvular Function

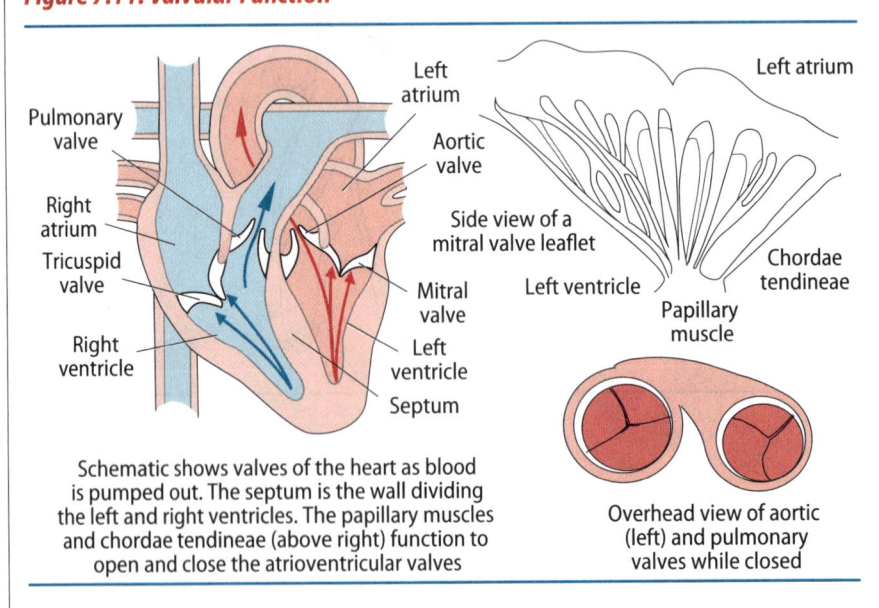

Schematic shows valves of the heart as blood is pumped out. The septum is the wall dividing the left and right ventricles. The papillary muscles and chordae tendineae (above right) function to open and close the atrioventricular valves

Overhead view of aortic (left) and pulmonary valves while closed

Chronic disease may result in arrhythmias, ventricular dysfunction, and dilation of the atria. In adults, acute rheumatic fever is the most common cause of mitral valve stenosis and the leading cause for valvular replacement surgery. Although the mitral valve is most commonly affected, the aortic and tricuspid valves may also be involved.

Chronic manifestations due to protracted disease and continued valve deformity occur in an estimated 9 to 39 percent of adults with previous rheumatic heart disease. Two to 10 years after an acute episode of rheumatic fever, the valve apparatus may fuse, with resulting stenosis or stenosis with insufficiency. Each recurrent episode can extend the valvular damage.

For acute rheumatic heart conditions, there is a one-to-one mapping of the appropriate ICD-9-CM code to the appropriate ICD-10-CM code. For instance, ICD-9-CM code 391.0 for acute rheumatic pericarditis directly correlates to code I01.0 in ICD-10-CM. This is also true for some valvular diseases resulting from rheumatic fever. Although ICD-9-CM does classify some conditions as rheumatic in nature, ICD-10-CM has distinguished, in large part, specific valvular diseases caused by rheumatic fever versus those not related to the disease, as well as the specific valve involved as shown in the following table. This differentiation does not always result in additional ICD-10-CM codes, as demonstrated by ICD-9-CM codes 396.0 through 396.8, which map to ICD-10-CM code I08.0.

Coding for Diseases of the Heart Valves

ICD-9-CM		ICD-10-CM	
Rheumatic			
394.0	Mitral stenosis	I05.0	Rheumatic mitral stenosis
394.2	Mitral stenosis with insufficiency	I05.2	Rheumatic mitral stenosis with insufficiency
394.9	Other and unspecified mitral valve diseases	I05.8	Other rheumatic mitral valve diseases
		I05.9	Rheumatic mitral valve disease, unspecified
396.0	Mitral valve stenosis and aortic valve stenosis	I08.0	Rheumatic disorders of both mitral and aortic valves
396.1	Mitral valve stenosis and aortic valve insufficiency	I08.0	Rheumatic disorders of both mitral and aortic valves
396.2	Mitral valve insufficiency and aortic valve stenosis		
396.3	Mitral valve insufficiency and aortic valve insufficiency		
397.0	Diseases of tricuspid valve	I07.0	Rheumatic tricuspid stenosis
		I07.1	Rheumatic tricuspid insufficiency
		I07.2	Rheumatic tricuspid stenosis and insufficiency
		I07.8	Other rheumatic tricuspid valve diseases
		I07.9	Rheumatic tricuspid valve disease, unspecified
397.1	Rheumatic diseases of pulmonary valve	I09.89	Other specified rheumatic heart diseases
397.9	Rheumatic diseases endocardium, valve unspecified	I08.1	Rheumatic disorders of both mitral and tricuspid valves
		I08.2	Rheumatic disorders of both aortic and tricuspid valves
		I08.3	Combined rheumatic disorders of mitral, aortic and tricuspid valves
		I08.8	Other rheumatic multiple valve diseases
		I08.9	Rheumatic multiple valve disease, unspecified
		I09.1	Rheumatic diseases of endocardium, valve unspecified

There are many differences between the ICD-9-CM and ICD-10-CM terminology used for valvular disorders. Key differences can be as simple as a "disorder" code in ICD-9-CM becoming more specific in ICD-10-CM; however, there are some important terms to be aware of.

Insufficiency is, in general, the inability to perform a function adequately or to the level necessary for the human body. When using the term with regard to valve

> **DEFINITIONS**
>
> **insufficiency.** Inadequate closure of the valve, allowing abnormal backward blood flow.

function, it typically means the valve isn't functioning as well as it should be, allowing blood to flow back into the chamber inappropriately.

Prolapse, specifically mitral valve prolapse, occurs when the cusps of the mitral valve protrude into the left atrium during ventricular systole. It is sometimes referred to as mitral valve prolapse syndrome.

Stenosis means narrowing or contracted. Regarding the valves, it describes a condition in which there has been a narrowing or a stricture caused by a multitude of factors, such as calcification or a congenital malformation.

Understanding these three terms helps when reporting valve disorders in ICD-10-CM. It is not known how payers will handle unspecified codes under the ICD-10-CM code set, so it is important to always code to the highest level of specificity. This may mean querying the provider for additional information.

> **DEFINITIONS**
>
> **stenosis.** Narrowing or constriction of a passage.

Coding for Diseases of the Heart Valves

ICD-9-CM		ICD-10-CM	
Nonrheumatic			
424.0	Mitral valve disorders	I34.0	Nonrheumatic mitral (valve) insufficiency
		I34.1	Nonrheumatic mitral (valve) prolapse
		I34.2	Nonrheumatic mitral (valve) stenosis
		I34.8	Other nonrheumatic mitral valve disorders
		I34.9	Nonrheumatic mitral valve disorder unspecified
424.1	Aortic valve disorders	I35.0	Nonrheumatic aortic (valve) stenosis
		I35.1	Nonrheumatic aortic (valve) insufficiency
		I35.2	Nonrheumatic aortic (valve) stenosis with insufficiency
		I35.8	Other nonrheumatic aortic valve disorders
		I35.9	Nonrheumatic aortic valve disorder, unspecified
424.2	Tricuspid valve disorders specified as nonrheumatic	I36.0	Nonrheumatic tricuspid (valve) stenosis
		I36.1	Nonrheumatic tricuspid (valve) insufficiency
		I36.2	Nonrheumatic tricuspid (valve) stenosis with insufficiency
		I36.8	Other nonrheumatic tricuspid valve disorders
		I36.9	Nonrheumatic tricuspid valve disorder, unspecified
424.3	Pulmonary valve disorders	I37.0	Nonrheumatic pulmonary valve stenosis
		I37.1	Nonrheumatic pulmonary valve insufficiency
		I37.2	Nonrheumatic pulmonary valve stenosis with insufficiency
		I37.8	Other nonrheumatic pulmonary valve disorders
		I37.9	Nonrheumatic pulmonary valve disorder, unspecified

Acute Coronary Syndromes

Obstruction of a coronary artery can result in a number of conditions that make up acute coronary syndrome. Depending on the percentage of the artery obstructed, as well as the specific location of the obstruction, the diagnosis may range from unstable angina to non-ST-segment elevation MI (NSTEMI), ST-segment elevation MI (STEMI), or sudden cardiac death. Symptoms for angina and myocardial infarctions (MI) are comparable and include chest discomfort with or without dyspnea, nausea, and diaphoresis. A diagnosis is made by ECG, as well as by the use of specific serologic markers. Treatment may include antiplatelet drugs, anticoagulants, nitrates, and beta-blockers. For STEMI, treatment may also include emergency reperfusion using fibrinolytic drugs, percutaneous intervention, or coronary artery bypass graft surgery.

Myocardial Infarction

Figure 7.12: Acute Myocardial Infarction

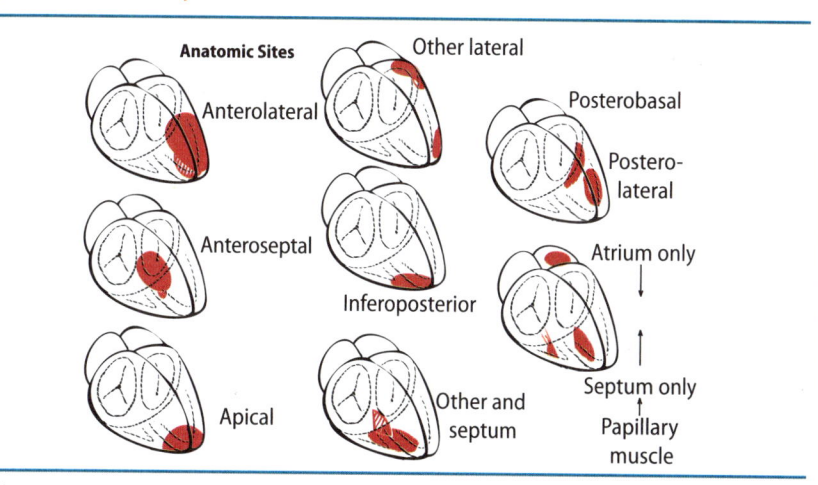

Myocardial infarction, also referred to as a heart attack, may be caused by several conditions but is most frequently attributed to narrowing of the coronary blood vessels due to atheromatous plaques. With rupture of the plaques, thrombi may form in the coronary vessel and vasospasm of the arteries occurs, causing complete or partial vessel occlusion. With the flow of oxygen and nutrients required by the heart blocked, myocardial ischemia begins in the endocardium and extends to the epicardium. Permanent heart damage, most of which occurs in the first two to three hours after infarction, must be quickly reversed to save the heart muscle.

The size and site of the infarction are primary factors in determining death and debility. For instance, anterior infarcts are likely to be larger and have a poorer prognosis than do inferoposterior infarcts. They are most often due to obstruction of the left coronary artery, particularly the anterior descending artery. Inferoposterior infarcts, on the other hand, are indicative of right coronary or dominant left circumflex artery obstruction.

While an MI most often affects the left ventricle, damage may also extend into the right ventricle or the atria. Right ventricular infarction commonly results from obstruction of the right coronary or a dominant left circumflex artery. A right ventricular infarction that complicates a left ventricular infarction represents a grave clinical situation with considerable increase in mortality risk.

Transmural infarcts involve the entire thickness of the myocardium from epicardium to endocardium and are most often distinguished by abnormal Q waves on the patient's ECG. Nontransmural or subendocardial infarcts do not extend through the ventricular wall and result in ST-segment and T-wave (ST-T) abnormalities. The quicker the oxygen supply is restored, the better the chance of saving the heart and minimizing damage. After a period of four to six hours, however, the ischemia caused by an occlusion can cause necrosis to the heart that cannot be reversed.

Other causes of myocardial infarction include:

- Acute anemia due to hemorrhage
- Anomalies such as aneurysms of the coronary arteries
- Aortic dissection, with retrograde involvement of the coronary arteries
- Arteritis

> **INTERESTING A & P FACT**
>
> In the United States, myocardial infarction is the foremost cause of morbidity and mortality, with more than 500,000 cases each year. There is also an estimated 1.3 million cases of nonfatal MI every year. On a global scale, MIs result in 12 million deaths each year.

- Chest trauma
- Drugs such as amphetamines, cocaine, and ephedrine
- Emboli of the coronary arteries, due to air, cholesterol, sepsis, and heart valve infection
- Hypoxia secondary to acute pulmonary conditions or carbon monoxide poisoning
- Pediatric coronary artery disease, such as seen with Marfan syndrome and progeria
- Vasospasm of the coronary arteries
- Ventricular hypertrophy (e.g., left ventricular hypertrophy [LVH], idiopathic hypertrophic subaortic stenosis [IHSS], or underlying valve disease)

> **CODING AXIOM**
>
> Left atrial thrombus is a thrombosis in the heart, not the coronary vessels, and is coded as I51.3 Intracardiac thrombosis, not elsewhere classified.
>
> *Coding Clinic, 1Q, 13, 24*

The risk factors for the formation of atherosclerotic plaque are well documented and include:

- Age
- Diabetes mellitus
- Family history
- Hypercholesterolemia and hypertriglyceridemia (includes inherited lipoprotein disorders)
- Hypertension
- Male gender
- Smoking
- Sedentary lifestyle
- Type A personality

The increased specificity of ICD-10-CM coding is evident in the classification of MIs. For this reason, it is important to understand the details of the condition.

Symptoms indicative of an MI require rapid emergency intervention to restore blood flow to the heart as quickly as possible. An electrocardiogram (ECG) is performed to evaluate the electrical activity of the heart to determine if blood flow through heart tissue has been compromised. One component of an ECG is the ST segment, which is found on the ECG following the QRS complex and continuing into the T wave. Depression or elevation of the ST segment is characteristic of ischemia or injury to the myocardium. The ST segment differentiates between two types of myocardial infarction: ST segment elevation myocardial infarction (STEMI) and non-ST-segment elevation myocardial infarction (NSTEMI). Although both types indicate damage to the heart's blood flow, patients with STEMI are more likely to be candidates for thrombolytic drug (clot buster) therapy, while those with NSTEMI are not. An elevated ST segment signifies a comparatively large amount of damage to the heart muscle is taking place due to total occlusion of a coronary artery. The milder NSTEMI results in a partly occluded artery, which affects only part of the heart muscle. STEMIs account for 30 to 45 percent of all heart attacks.

> **CODING AXIOM**
>
> Acute MIs specified by site (with the exception of subendocardial and non-transmural), but not specified as STEMI or NSTEMI, should be coded to acute STEMI by specific site.
>
> Assign code I21.3, ST elevation (STEMI) myocardial infarction, unspecified site, when neither the site of the MI nor whether the MI is STEMI or NSTEMI, is specified.
>
> *Coding Clinic, 1Q, 13, 25-26*

The ICD-9-CM code book distinguishes between STEMIs and NSTEMIs using inclusion notes under the MI code descriptors. In ICD-10-CM, the code descriptor itself includes the designation of STEMI or NSTEMI. Although ICD-9-CM and ICD-10-CM have specific codes that identify the area of the heart the MI affected, guidelines for MIs vary quite a bit in how they define an episode of care and in the reporting of subsequent MIs.

For instance, ICD-9-CM defines an acute episode of care as a period of eight weeks or less. In ICD-10-CM, this has been redefined as a period of four weeks. In ICD-9-CM, a fifth-digit subclassification of 1 indicates the first episode of care and is used to report the MI whether or not the patient is transferred to another facility. A fifth digit of 2 indicates a patient was admitted for additional treatment of the cardiac condition at any time during the eight-week period following the initial MI. However, if a patient sustains a second MI during the admission for treatment of the initial MI, a fifth digit of 1 is still reported.

ICD-10-CM guidelines indicate that a code from category I21 should be reported when a patient has an initial MI. However, if the patient has another MI within the four-week period of the initial MI, a code from category I22 is reported as well. In this type of scenario, the sequencing of codes indicates the reason for the encounter or admission. For instance, a patient has an MI and is admitted to the hospital, where he suffers a second MI on day five of the hospitalization. In this case, a code from category I21 is sequenced first, and code I22 is sequenced as the secondary diagnosis.

However, if a patient has an MI, is treated, and is discharged home, a code from category I21 is reported. If the same patient has a second MI, a code from category I22 is sequenced first, with a code from category I21 listed as a secondary code to demonstrate the patient is within the four-week time period from the original MI.

In the following table, ICD-10-CM designates each MI as STEMI or NSTEMI, as well as initial or subsequent.

> **CODING AXIOM**
>
> ICD-10-CM Official Coding Guideline I.C.9.e.4. provides the following instruction on how to code a subsequent acute myocardial infarction. "A code from category I22 Subsequent ST elevation (STEMI) and non ST elevation (NSTEMI) myocardial infarction, is to be used when a patient who has suffered an AMI has a new AMI within the 4 week time frame of the initial AMI. A code from category I22 must be used in conjunction with a code from category I21. The sequencing of the I22 and I21 codes depends on the circumstances of the encounter."

Coding for Myocardial Infarctions

ICD-9-CM		ICD-10-CM	
410.01	AMI of anterolateral wall, initial episode of care	I21.09	ST elevation (STEMI) MI involving other coronary artery of anterior wall
		I22.0	Subsequent ST elevation (STEMI) MI of anterior wall
410.11	AMI of other anterior wall, initial episode of care	I21.01	ST elevation (STEMI) MI involving left main coronary artery
		I21.02	ST elevation (STEMI) MI involving left anterior descending coronary artery
		I21.09	ST elevation (STEMI) MI involving other coronary artery of anterior wall
		I22.0	Subsequent ST elevation (STEMI) MI of anterior wall
410.21	AMI of inferolateral wall, initial episode of care	I21.19	ST elevation (STEMI) MI involving other coronary artery of inferior wall
		I22.1	Subsequent ST elevation (STEMI) MI of inferior wall
410.31	AMI of inferoposterior wall, initial episode of care	I21.11	ST elevation (STEMI) MI involving right coronary artery
		I22.1	Subsequent ST elevation (STEMI) MI of inferior wall
410.41	AMI of other inferior wall, initial episode of care	I21.19	ST elevation (STEMI) MI involving other coronary artery of inferior wall
		I22.1	Subsequent ST elevation (STEMI) MI of inferior wall
410.51	AMI of other lateral wall, initial episode of care	I21.29	ST elevation (STEMI) MI involving other sites
		I22.8	Subsequent ST elevation (STEMI) MI of other sites
410.61	AMI, true posterior wall infarction, initial episode of care	I21.29	ST elevation (STEMI) MI involving other sites
		I22.8	Subsequent ST elevation (STEMI) MI of other sites
410.71	AMI, subendocardial infarction, initial episode of care	I21.4	Non-ST elevation (NSTEMI) MI
		I22.2	Subsequent non-ST elevation (NSTEMI) MI
410.81	AMI of other specified sites, initial episode of care	I21.21	ST elevation (STEMI) MI involving left circumflex coronary artery
		I21.29	ST elevation (STEMI) MI involving other sites
		I22.8	Subsequent ST elevation (STEMI) MI of other sites

ICD-9-CM		ICD-10-CM	
410.91	AMI, unspecified site, initial episode of care	I21.3	ST elevation (STEMI) MI of unspecified site
		I22.9	Subsequent ST elevation (STEMI) MI of unspecified site

Atherosclerosis

Arteriosclerosis, also referred to as "hardening of the arteries," occurs when the arteries become narrowed due to **atherosclerosis** and then become hardened by fibrous tissue and calcification. As this process continues, it results in a decrease in blood and oxygen supply to the affected organ. Eventually, the plaque may cause severe or complete obstruction of the artery, causing tissue necrosis. Although this process is often associated with the heart, it may occur in any of the organs, including the brain, kidneys, intestines, eyes, and limbs. Chronic hypertension may also cause arteriosclerosis, with the elevated blood pressure contributing to the thickening of the muscular arterial walls.

In the heart, atherosclerosis may lead to coronary artery disease, while in the brain, it may lead to a stroke. In the lower extremities, arterial constriction results in pain, numbness, and the sensation of cold legs or feet. Peripheral artery disease (PAD) limits physical movement due to pain, and severe complications such as nonhealing ulcers and gangrene may occur resulting in limb amputation.

Angina

As a general definition, angina is chest pain that occurs due to inadequate blood flow to the heart. In stable angina, rest and mild activity fail to elicit symptoms. However, an increase in activity that puts stress on the heart and increases oxygen demand does cause pain. This occurs because partial blockage of a coronary artery restricts blood flow to the myocardium. The term "stable" is attributed to this type of angina since the pattern or pain is predictable in the sense that it occurs only when the heart is under stress. While plaque is present and causing diminished blood flow, plaque growth is slow and collateral circulation may occur.

"Unstable" angina shares many of the characteristics of myocardial infarction and is included in the range of acute coronary syndromes. It is most commonly caused by atherosclerotic coronary artery disease. In this condition, there is rupture or disruption of the plaque, thrombosis, and vasoconstriction. It often precedes an MI, cardiac arrhythmias, or, in some cases, sudden death. Other names for this condition include acute coronary insufficiency, preinfarction angina, and intermediate syndrome.

Prinzmetal's (variant) angina is a rare form caused by vasospasm. Pain, which occurs most often at rest, may be intense but is treatable with medications.

Microvascular angina causes chest pain in patients seemingly without occlusions of a coronary artery. Pain results when the tiny blood vessels nourishing the heart, as well as the limbs, do not function property. This type of angina is also treated with medications.

In ICD-9-CM, unstable angina is classified to code 411.1 but only when the underlying cause is not identified and when surgery is not performed. If a patient is admitted for bypass surgery or angioplasty to avoid the progression of unstable angina to an infarction, an appropriate code reporting the underlying coronary atherosclerosis is reported first, with unstable angina reported as a secondary code. ICD-10-CM, however, has two subcategories that specifically classify atherosclerosis with angina using combination codes, making the assumption about a causal relationship between the two conditions. These codes are further classified according to whether the condition involves native coronary artery disease, a bypass graft, or a transplanted heart. In addition, ICD-10-CM specifies whether a spasm is documented, a factor not addressed in ICD-9-CM. The following table compares the coding of unstable angina with and without atherosclerotic heart disease in ICD-9-CM and ICD-10-CM.

Definitions

arteriosclerosis. Condition causing thickening of the artery walls.

atherosclerosis. Buildup of yellowish plaques composed of cholesterol and lipoid material within the arteries.

Interesting A & P Fact

Arteriosclerosis has been found to start as early as childhood, with streaks of fat developing in the aorta not long after birth. These streaks of fat increase and then start to diminish as the individual reaches age 30. Around age 40, these fat streaks are progressively replaced by atheromas and fibrous plaques that cause complications such as thrombosis, which can eventually lead to MIs and strokes.

The following table is not a complete mapping of all of the types of unstable angina and coronary atherosclerosis, but gives the coder an idea of what may be seen in ICD-10-CM. For detailed information on ICD-9-CM to ICD-10-CM mapping, see Optum360's *ICD-10-CM Mappings*.

Coding for Unstable Angina and Coronary Atherosclerosis

ICD-9-CM		ICD-10-CM	
411.1	Intermediate coronary syndrome	I20.0	Unstable angina
		I25.110	Atherosclerotic heart disease of native coronary artery with unstable angina pectoris
		I25.710	Atherosclerosis of autologous vein coronary artery bypass graft(s) with unstable angina pectoris
		I25.720	Atherosclerosis of autologous artery coronary artery bypass graft(s) with unstable angina pectoris
		I25.730	Atherosclerosis of nonautologous biological coronary artery bypass graft(s) with unstable angina pectoris
		I25.750	Atherosclerosis of native coronary artery of transplanted heart with unstable angina
413.9	Other and unspecified angina pectoris	I20.8	Other forms of angina pectoris
		I20.9	Angina pectoris, unspecified
		I25.111	Atherosclerotic heart disease of native coronary artery with angina pectoris with documented spasm
		I25.118	Atherosclerotic heart disease of native coronary artery with other forms of angina pectoris
		I25.119	Atherosclerotic heart disease of native coronary artery with unspecified angina pectoris
		I25.701	Atherosclerosis of coronary artery bypass graft(s), unspecified, with angina pectoris with documented spasm
		I25.708	Atherosclerosis of coronary artery bypass graft(s), unspecified, with other forms of angina pectoris
414.01	Coronary atherosclerosis native coronary artery	I25.10	Atherosclerotic heart disease of native coronary artery without angina pectoris
		I25.110	Atherosclerotic heart disease of native coronary artery with unstable angina pectoris
		I25.111	Atherosclerotic heart disease of native coronary artery with angina pectoris with documented spasm
		I25.118	Atherosclerotic heart disease of native coronary artery with other forms of angina pectoris
		I25.119	Atherosclerotic heart disease of native coronary artery with unspecified angina pectoris

ICD-9-CM		ICD-10-CM	
414.02	Coronary atherosclerosis autologous vein bypass graft	I25.710	Atherosclerosis of autologous vein coronary artery bypass graft(s) with unstable angina pectoris
		I25.711	Atherosclerosis of autologous vein coronary artery bypass graft(s) with angina pectoris with documented spasm
		I25.718	Atherosclerosis of autologous vein coronary artery bypass graft(s) with other forms of angina pectoris
		I25.719	Atherosclerosis of autologous vein coronary artery bypass graft(s) with unspecified angina pectoris

Atherosclerosis of Extremity Arteries

The primary cause of arterial disease of the lower extremities is atherosclerosis. Once the plaque begins to build up in the artery, not only is blood flow reduced, but the arterial walls become stiffer and unable to dilate. This means the leg muscles don't receive adequate blood and oxygen when demand is increased, such as by walking and exercising. Symptoms include pain, fatigue, aching, burning, and discomfort of the calves, feet, or thighs, which subside with rest. If the condition progresses, symptoms begin to appear sooner and during less strenuous activity. Pain and ulceration often limit physical activity. If the condition continues to progress, there is an inadequate supply of blood and oxygen at rest and symptoms do not resolve. Complications most often include unhealed ulcer, gangrene, and amputation of the affected limb.

As the disease progresses, patients may experience:

- Arterial bruits
- Atrophy of calf muscles
- Diminished blood pressure in the affected limb
- Hair loss on feet or legs
- Impotence
- Limb pulses that are weak or absent altogether
- Non-healing ulcers
- Pain and cramps in the legs at night
- Pain or tingling in the feet/toes so severe that the weight of clothes or bed sheets is painful
- Increased pain with leg elevation that improves when the leg is dangled
- Cyanotic or pale, shiny, or tight skin of the feet or toes
- Thickened toenails

Peripheral artery disease (PAD) is a common disorder that primarily affects men older than age 50. A history of any of the following conditions puts the individual at higher risk:

- Abnormal cholesterol level
- Cerebrovascular disease (stroke)
- Coronary artery disease
- Diabetes
- Heart disease (coronary artery disease)
- Hypertension
- Kidney disease with hemodialysis
- Smoking

Growth of an atherosclerotic lesion occurs in three stages. In the first stage, a fatty streak develops with no impediment to blood flow in the vessel. In the second stage, fibrous plaques form. Often located at arterial bifurcations, the lesion can, at this stage, impede blood flow. In the third stage, a complicated lesion develops where the plaque is distorted by calcification, hemorrhage, and mural thrombus. This can lead to embolism and is the underlying cause of vessel obstruction.

Coding atherosclerosis of the extremities is similar in ICD-9-CM and ICD-10-CM. Both systems specify the symptoms of:

- Intermittent *claudication*
- Pain at rest
- Ulceration
- Gangrene

Both classification systems also differentiate between atherosclerosis of a native artery, an autologous bypass graft, or a nonautologous biological bypass graft. However, ICD-10-CM requires the coder to indicate the affected leg (right or left), as well as the specific site of an ulcer (e.g., heel and midfoot or calf). ICD-10-CM also has specific codes to indicate bilateral disease. The following table compares ICD-9-CM and ICD-10-CM coding of atherosclerosis of a native artery of the extremities with an ulcer.

> **DEFINITIONS**
>
> **claudication.** Lameness, pain, and weakness occurring in the arms or legs during exercise due to muscles not receiving the needed oxygen and nutrients.

Coding for Atherosclerosis of Native Arteries of the Extremities

ICD-9-CM		ICD-10-CM	
440.23	Atherosclerosis of the extremities with ulceration	I70.231	Atherosclerosis of native arteries of right leg with ulceration of thigh
		I70.232	Atherosclerosis of native arteries of right leg with ulceration of calf
		I70.233	Atherosclerosis of native arteries of right leg with ulceration of ankle
		I70.234	Atherosclerosis of native arteries of right leg with ulceration of heel and midfoot
		I70.235	Atherosclerosis of native arteries of right leg with ulceration of other part of foot
		I70.238	Atherosclerosis of native arteries of right leg with ulceration of other part of lower right leg
		I70.239	Atherosclerosis of native arteries of right leg with ulceration of unspecified site
		I70.241	Atherosclerosis of native arteries of left leg with ulceration of thigh
		I70.242	Atherosclerosis of native arteries of left leg with ulceration of calf
		I70.243	Atherosclerosis of native arteries of left leg with ulceration of ankle
		I70.244	Atherosclerosis of native arteries of left leg with ulceration of heel and midfoot
		I70.245	Atherosclerosis of native arteries of left leg with ulceration of other part of foot
		I70.248	Atherosclerosis of native arteries of left leg with ulceration of other part of lower left leg
		I70.249	Atherosclerosis of native arteries of left leg with ulceration of unspecified site
		I70.25	Atherosclerosis of native arteries of other extremities with ulceration

> **INTERESTING A & P FACT**
>
> Peripheral emboli are atheroemboli that result from small abdominal aortic aneurysms (AAA), which produce livedo reticularis of the feet, or blue toe syndrome.

Diseases of the Aorta

Like other arteries, the aorta and its major branches may also be affected by arteriosclerosis. In fact, the most common cause of thoracic aortic aneurysms, particularly in the descending part, is arteriosclerosis. Although this condition can be an expected part of the aging process, the condition is highly variable. In some patients, the loss of elasticity in the tissue results in dilation, which causes the aorta to become tortuous. On the other hand, advanced dilation may result in a ruptured aneurysm that leads to certain death.

Figure 7.13: Thoracic and Abdominal Aortic Aneurysm

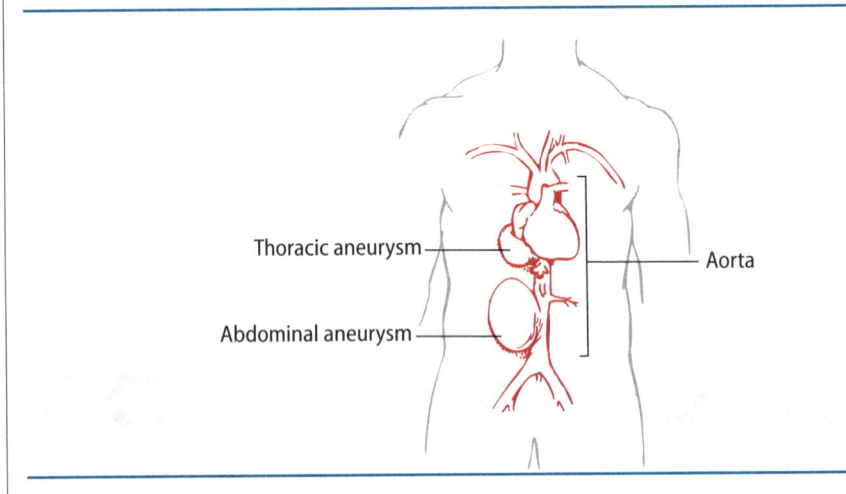

Arteriosclerosis may diminish blood flow to the aortic branches as well and result in a range of conditions due to insufficient blood flow to a given area. For instance, if the renal vessels are involved, the kidneys may become ischemic and possibly lead to renal failure.

Calcium deposits in the aorta also occur due to arteriosclerosis or other conditions. Treatment and outcome of arteriosclerosis vary.

Aortic Dissection

A dissecting aneurysm occurs when the middle arterial layer (media) deteriorates (medial necrosis). Hypertension and arteriosclerosis play a role in this process, causing further damage until a rupture occurs in the innermost arterial layer, which allows blood to fill the wall of the aorta, causing separation of the layers. When the rupture extends through the outermost wall, fatal hemorrhage occurs.

Aortic dissections are seen in individuals with hypertension or arteriosclerosis, or with a family history of aortic (or thoracic) dissection. Less often, it is seen in patients with congenital diseases such as Marfan's syndrome, Ehlers-Danlos syndrome, and congenital valvular disorders. Other conditions that may cause aortic dissection include Takayasu disease, giant cell arteritis, tertiary syphilis, relapsing polychondritis, fungal infections from heart valve surgeries, immunodeficiency, and intravenous drug abuse.

ICD-9-CM and ICD-10-CM classify aortic aneurysms and aortic dissection in much the same way: according to the specific site and whether a rupture or a dissection has occurred.

> **CLINICAL NOTE**
>
> Two types of aortic dissections are recognized:
> - **Type A:** Dissection to the ascending aorta; may be treated medically for a period of time with interventional catheterization or using open surgical techniques.
> - **Type B:** Dissection of the descending aorta; may be treated medically with regular monitoring and medications that include antihypertensive and cholesterol lowering agents.

Venous Phlebitis and Thrombophlebitis

Venous thrombosis may occur in surface veins (superficial thrombophlebitis) or in the deeper veins (deep venous thrombosis, or DVT). When there is an injury to the most inner layer of the vein, hypercoagulability occurs, and a clot may form. The combination of these three conditions is referred to as the Virchow triad. Thrombophlebitis refers to a thrombus that causes vein inflammation (phlebitis) at the site of the injury, reducing venous flow (venous stasis). This condition may be chronic or acute in nature.

Figure 7.14: Venous System

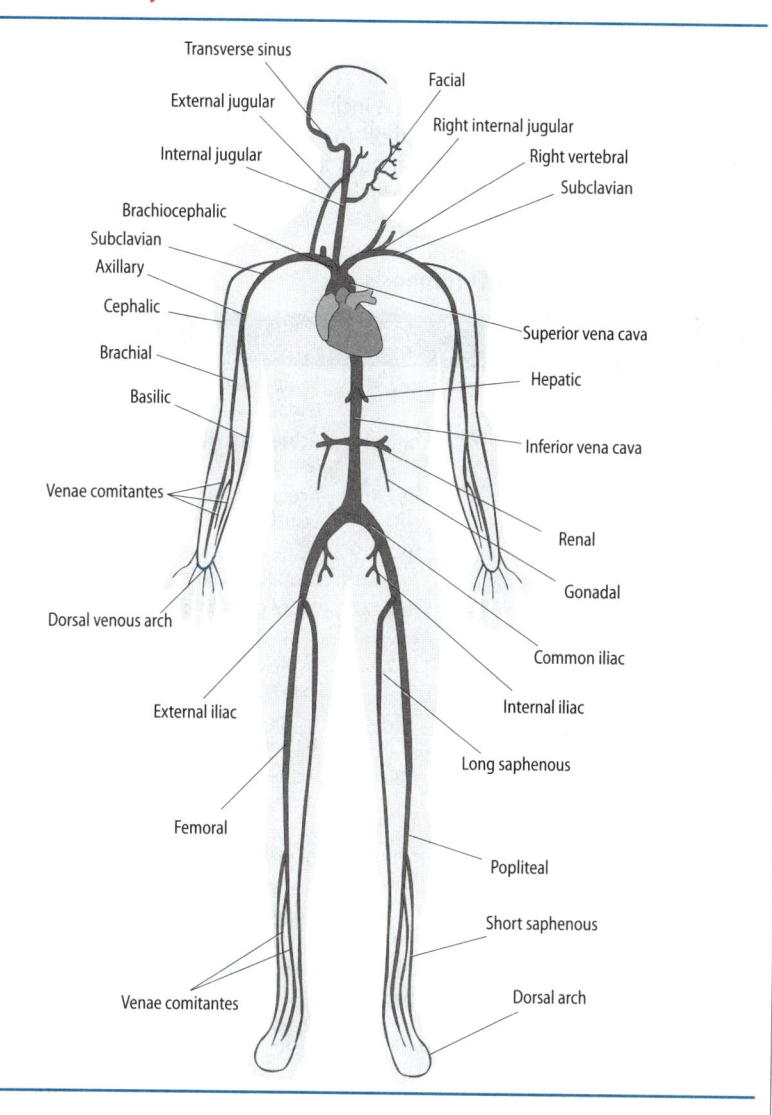

> **CLINICAL NOTE**
>
> The terms thrombosis and thrombitis are often used interchangeably.

Embolism refers to a condition whereby a ***thrombus*** or a piece of one breaks off from where it has formed in the vein and migrates through the bloodstream. Emboli seldom develop with superficial thrombophlebitis. However, emboli that occur with DVT, most often found in the veins of the legs, is of utmost concern since they may travel to the lungs (pulmonary embolus), which demands emergent medical treatment to prevent death.

Although the greatest single risk factor for superficial venous thrombosis and DVT is a past medical history of these conditions, other risk factors include:

- Aging

> **DEFINITIONS**
>
> **thrombus.** Stationary blood clot inside a blood vessel.

- Abdominal cancer
- Blood coagulation disorders
- Extended bed rest or sitting (e.g., such as on an airplane)
- Heart failure
- Intravenous (IV) catheter usage/use of irritating medications in the IV
- Oral contraceptives
- Pregnancy
- Stroke
- Trauma
- Varicose veins

As is the common theme when comparing the classification systems, greater specificity regarding these conditions is included in ICD-10-CM. Laterality is key in ICD-10-CM, as well as the specific embolism or thrombosis vein site. Similar to ICD-9-CM, the ICD-10-CM system continues to differentiate between acute and chronic, distal and proximal, and superficial versus deep vessels. A few examples have been included in the following tables.

Coding for Embolism and Thrombosis

ICD-9-CM		ICD-10-CM	
453.41	Acute venous embolism and thrombosis of deep vessels proximal lower extremity	I82.411	Acute embolism and thrombosis of right femoral vein
		I82.412	Acute embolism and thrombosis of left femoral vein
		I82.413	Acute embolism and thrombosis of femoral vein, bilateral
		I82.419	Acute embolism and thrombosis of unspecified femoral vein
		I82.421	Acute embolism and thrombosis of right iliac vein
		I82.422	Acute embolism and thrombosis of left iliac vein
		I82.423	Acute embolism and thrombosis of iliac vein, bilateral
		I82.429	Acute embolism and thrombosis of unspecified iliac vein
		I82.431	Acute embolism and thrombosis of right popliteal vein
		I82.432	Acute embolism and thrombosis of left popliteal vein
		I82.433	Acute embolism and thrombosis of popliteal vein, bilateral
		I82.439	Acute embolism and thrombosis of unspecified popliteal vein

Coding for Acute Venous Embolism and Thrombosis of Axillary Veins

ICD-9-CM		ICD-10-CM	
453.84	Acute venous embolism and thrombosis of axillary veins	I82.A11	Acute embolism and thrombosis of right axillary vein
		I82.A12	Acute embolism and thrombosis of left axillary vein
		I82.A13	Acute embolism and thrombosis of axillary vein, bilateral
		I82.A19	Acute embolism and thrombosis of unspecified axillary vein

Varicose Veins

Varicose veins are abnormal, permanently distended, or stretched veins. Once the vein becomes thickened and tortuous, the affected parts of the veins are referred to as varicosities. Most often found in the legs, they may occur in any area of the body, such as hemorrhoids and esophageal varices.

Figure 7.15: Map of Major Veins

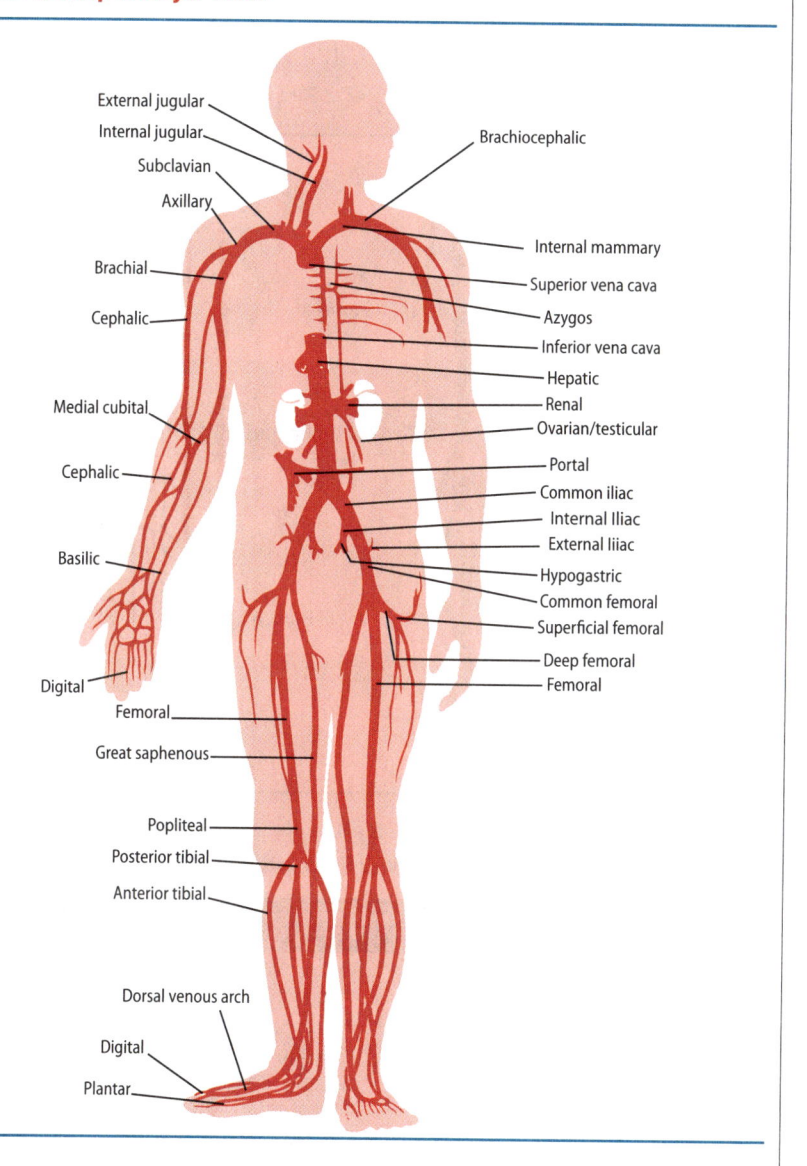

The superficial veins closest to the surface of the skin are the ones that most often develop varicosities. The largest superficial vein is the greater saphenous vein running from the ankle to the thigh on the medial aspect of the leg. Varicosities can also originate from the communicating veins that join the superficial veins to the deep veins.

Although there is much speculation as to why varicosities occur, it is thought to be due to damaged or defective valves in the veins. There are many factors associated with this condition, including:

- Age
- Obesity

- Pregnancy
- Previous leg surgery or trauma
- Spending too much time on one's feet

Although varicose veins of the lower extremities may be asymptomatic, they are often seen in conjunction with inflammation, skin ulcers, or both. Correct code assignment depends on the existence (or not) of one of these complications. ICD-10-CM adds detail by including laterality and the location of the leg ulcer, as is evident in the following table.

Figure 7.16: Veins of Lower Extremities

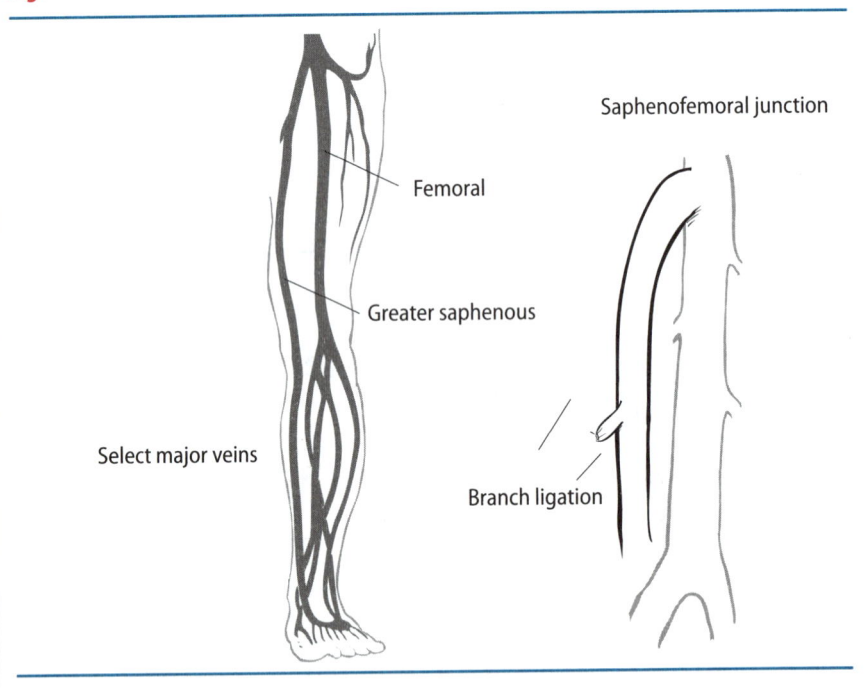

Coding for Varicose Veins of the Lower Extremities

ICD-9-CM		ICD-10-CM	
454.0	Varicose veins of lower extremities with ulcer	I83.001	Varicose veins of unspecified lower extremity with ulcer of thigh
		I83.002	Varicose veins of unspecified lower extremity with ulcer of calf
		I83.003	Varicose veins of unspecified lower extremity with ulcer of ankle
		I83.004	Varicose veins of unspecified lower extremity with ulcer of heel and midfoot
		I83.005	Varicose veins of unspecified lower extremity with ulcer other part of foot
		I83.008	Varicose veins of unspecified lower extremity with ulcer other part of lower leg
		I83.009	Varicose veins of unspecified lower extremity with ulcer of unspecified site
		I83.011	Varicose veins of right lower extremity with ulcer of thigh
		I83.012	Varicose veins of right lower extremity with ulcer of calf
(Continued on next page)		I83.013	Varicose veins of right lower extremity with ulcer of ankle

ICD-9-CM		ICD-10-CM	
454.0	Varicose veins of lower extremities with ulcer *(Continued)*	I83.014	Varicose veins of right lower extremity with ulcer of heel and midfoot
		I83.015	Varicose veins of right lower extremity with ulcer other part of foot
		I83.018	Varicose veins of right lower extremity with ulcer other part of lower leg
		I83.019	Varicose veins of right lower extremity with ulcer of unspecified site
		I83.021	Varicose veins of left lower extremity with ulcer of thigh
		I83.022	Varicose veins of left lower extremity with ulcer of calf
		I83.023	Varicose veins of left lower extremity with ulcer of ankle
		I83.024	Varicose veins of left lower extremity with ulcer of heel and midfoot
		I83.025	Varicose veins of left lower extremity with ulcer other part of foot
		I83.028	Varicose veins of left lower extremity with ulcer other part of lower leg
		I83.029	Varicose veins of left lower extremity with ulcer of unspecified site

Hypertension

Blood pressure is the measurement of the force exerted against the arterial walls produced by the left ventricle during contraction (systole), and pressure that remains in the arteries when the ventricle relaxes (diastole). Blood pressure readings are measured in millimeters of mercury (mmHg) and expressed as two numbers (e.g., 120/80). Either one or both of these numbers may be too high (hypertension). The difference between the two pressures, the systolic and the diastolic, is referred to as the pulse pressure. Normal pulse pressure is 40 mmHg, and if this is increased it provides valuable information about the health of the cardiovascular system. Atherosclerosis is one of the conditions that causes increased pulse pressure. Hypertension is often associated with arterial disease, as well as an increased risk of stroke, heart attack, and heart failure.

Systolic pressure is considered:

- High if over 140 mmHg for the majority of the time
- Normal if below 120 mmHg for the majority of the time

Diastolic pressure is considered:

- High if over 90 mmHg for the majority of the time
- Normal if below 80 mmHg for the majority of the time

Prehypertension may be a concern when:

- Systolic pressure is between 120 and 139 for the majority of the time
- Diastolic blood pressure is between 80 and 89 for the majority of the time

The most common type of hypertension is primary hypertension, previously referred to as "essential" hypertension. Primary hypertension is identified in 85 to 95 percent of all cases, and has no known cause. Although genetics may predispose an individual to this condition, the exact process is not known. Environmental factors such as obesity, dietary sodium, and stress appear to affect only those individuals with genetic predisposition.

Benign hypertension is defined as a mild to moderate elevation of blood pressure for a protracted period but with no damage to target organs (kidneys, retina, heart).

Risk factors include:

- African American heritage
- Diabetes
- Family history
- High levels of stress or anxiety
- Obesity
- High dietary sodium intake
- Smoking

Hypertension with an identified cause (secondary hypertension) is usually due to a renal disorder. Usually no symptoms develop unless hypertension is severe or long-standing. Diagnosis is by sphygmomanometry. Tests may be done to determine cause, assess damage, and identify other cardiovascular risk factors. Treatment involves lifestyle changes and medication.

High blood pressure resulting from another medical condition or due to a medication is secondary hypertension. This condition may be attributed to conditions such as:

- Atherosclerosis
- Autoimmune diseases
- Chronic kidney disease
- Coarctation of the aorta
- Cocaine use
- Connective tissue disease
- Diabetes with kidney damage
- Endocrine disorders (e.g., adrenal tumors [pheochromocytoma, aldosteronism], Cushing syndrome, thyroid disease)
- Excessive alcohol use
- Medications:
  - appetite suppressants
  - cold medications
  - corticosteroids
  - migraine medications
  - oral contraceptives
- Polycystic kidney disease
- Polynephritis
- Renovascular disease
- Stenosis of renal artery

Examining the dilated retina is integral to assessing damage from hypertension. Examination of the retinal microvascular allows a view of the inner arterial and venous systems and can detect the onset of systemic diseases before symptoms appear. Manifestations of arteriosclerosis include narrowing of the arterioles and sclerosis of the vessels. Cotton wool spots and flame-shaped hemorrhages are often found in hypertensive retinopathy. Edema of the disc indicates malignant hypertension. In many instances, the retinal examination provides the first clue the patient has hypertension.

A hypertensive emergency exists when blood pressure is high enough to damage target organs, such as the cardiovascular system, kidneys, and the central nervous system. A diagnosis of malignant hypertension includes the presence of **papilledema**, with swelling of the optic disc in the eye, caused by an increase in intracranial pressure. Treatment is directed at lowering the patient's blood pressure as quickly as possible. Blood pressure is usually in the 250/150 range.

Accelerated hypertension is a recent major increase over the patient's baseline blood pressure, not associated with target organ damage. Fundoscopic examination often

> **DEFINITIONS**
>
> **papilledema.** Swelling of the optic disc that is caused by intracranial pressure.

reveals flame-shaped hemorrhages or soft exudates, but without papilledema. Blood pressure is usually in the 220/120 range.

Over a period of time, hypertension damages the brain, cardiovascular system, and the kidneys, increasing the risk of coronary artery disease (CAD), myocardial infarction (MI), renal failure, and cerebrovascular accidents, particularly the hemorrhagic type. As generalized arteriolosclerosis develops, **atheromatous** plaques form more rapidly in the arteries. Arteriolosclerosis, typified by medial hypertrophy, hyperplasia, and hyalinization, is most readily evident in small arterioles, particularly in the eyes and kidneys. In the kidneys, as these changes continue to constrict the arterial flow, total peripheral vascular resistance increases, and hypertension worsens.

Left ventricular hypertrophy may occur, with resulting diastolic dysfunction. Ultimately, the ventricle dilates, causing dilated cardiomyopathy and heart failure secondary to systolic dysfunction. Nearly all patients with abdominal aortic aneurysms also have hypertension, and thoracic aortic dissection is often an effect of hypertension.

Other complications may include:

- Blood vessel damage (arteriosclerosis)
- Brain damage
- Congestive heart failure
- Chronic kidney disease
- Heart attack
- Hypertensive heart disease
- Loss of vision
- Peripheral artery disease
- Pregnancy complications

Fortunately, in the majority of cases, hypertension can be controlled with medications and lifestyle changes.

There are a wide variety of causes, types, and conditions associated with hypertension, which can make hypertension a challenge from the coding perspective.

The ICD-10-CM classification system, however, has streamlined the hypertension classification and related comorbid conditions. Rather than having separate subcategories for "benign" and "malignant" hypertension, these terms have been integrated into an inclusion note under category I10 Essential hypertension. The following table demonstrates how some of these same codes appear in ICD-10-CM. In many cases, multiple codes are required to fully report the condition accurately. Please review the coding guidelines as found in the *ICD-10-CM Official Guidelines for Coding and Reporting* or the instructional notes found at the code categories themselves to make accurate code selections.

Coding for Hypertension

ICD-9-CM		ICD-10-CM	
401.0	Essential hypertension, malignant	I10	Essential (primary) hypertension
401.1	Essential hypertension, benign		
401.9	Essential hypertension, unspecified		
402.01	Hypertensive heart disease, malignant, with heart failure	I11.0	Hypertensive heart disease with heart failure
402.11	Hypertensive heart disease, benign, with heart failure		
402.91	Hypertensive heart disease, unspecified, with heart failure		

> **DEFINITIONS**
>
> **atheroma.** Also referred to as plaque, atherosclerotic plaque, and arterial plaque, it is the buildup of fatty deposit in the innermost lining (intima) of an artery, caused by atherosclerosis.

> **CODING AXIOM**
>
> ICD-10-CM Official Coding Guideline I.C.9.a.7. provides instruction on code assignments for transient hypertension. This guideline states, "assign code R03.0 Elevated blood pressure reading without diagnosis of hypertension, unless the patient has an established diagnosis of hypertension. Assign code O13.- Gestational [pregnancy-induced] hypertension without significant proteinuria, or O14.- Pre-eclampsia, for transient hypertension of pregnancy."

ICD-9-CM		ICD-10-CM	
402.00	Hypertensive heart disease, malignant, without heart failure	I11.9	Hypertensive heart disease without heart failure
402.10	Hypertensive heart disease, benign, without heart failure		
402.90	Unspecified hypertensive heart disease without heart failure		
403.01	Hypertensive chronic kidney disease, malignant, with chronic kidney disease stage V or end stage renal disease	I12.0	Hypertensive heart and chronic kidney disease with stage 5 chronic kidney disease or end-stage renal disease
403.11	Hypertensive chronic kidney disease, benign, with chronic kidney disease stage V or end-stage renal disease		
403.91	Hypertensive chronic kidney disease, unspecified, with chronic kidney disease stage V or end-stage renal disease		

Cerebrovascular Disease

Atherosclerosis of the Precerebral and Cerebral Arteries

The precerebral arteries include the basilar, carotid, and vertebral arteries. The carotid emerges from the aorta as the common carotid artery and bifurcates into the internal and external carotid arteries. This bifurcation is a common site for atherosclerosis, which causes 90 percent of all extracranial carotid lesions. Atherosclerosis may result in narrowing of the common or internal artery. It may become a source of embolization where some of the plaque breaks off and travels to smaller blood vessels in the brain. Once lodged in the small vessel, it can inhibit the flow of blood to the brain temporarily (e.g., transient ischemic attack, or TIA) or permanently (e.g., stroke).

Additional causes of carotid lesions include:

- Aneurysms
- Arteritis
- Bends and twists of the vessel
- Carotid dissection
- Fibromuscular dysplasia
- Radiation
- Vasospasm

ICD-9-CM classifies occlusion and stenosis of the precerebral arteries to category 433, with a fourth digit designating the specific artery involved and a fifth digit indicating if a cerebral infarction occurred.

ICD-10-CM breaks this down even more to indicate if the stenosis or occlusion occurs in the artery on the left side or the right side, and even the specific portion of the artery involved (e.g., left anterior cerebral artery, right middle cerebral artery). It also specifies the arteries involved when pathology is present in bilateral arteries.

When discussing these types of infarcts, it is important to understand the terminology that describes the different mechanisms of vessel blockage. **Thrombosis** occurs when a blood clot forms within a vessel. An **embolism** occurs when an embolus travels through the bloodstream and becomes lodged in a blood vessel, blocking blood flow. Some types of embolism include air emboli, gas emboli, or fat emboli.

ICD-9-CM classifies infarction due to occlusion of one of the precerebral arteries by a thrombosis or embolism to category 433, with includes notes guiding the right code

---

DEFINITIONS

embolism. Obstruction of a blood vessel resulting from an embolus traveling through the bloodstream. Types of emboli include air, gas, and fat.

thrombosis. Condition arising from the presence or formation of blood clots within a blood vessel that may cause vascular obstruction and insufficient oxygenation.

choice. In ICD-10-CM, however, codes differentiate between an infarction of a specific artery due to one of these conditions, as demonstrated in the following table.

Coding for Infarction of the Carotid Artery

ICD-9-CM		ICD-10-CM	
433.11	Occlusion and stenosis of carotid artery with infarction	I63.031	Cerebral infarction due to thrombosis of right carotid artery
		I63.032	Cerebral infarction due to thrombosis of left carotid artery
		I63.039	Cerebral infarction due to thrombosis of unspecified carotid artery
		I63.131	Cerebral infarction due to embolism of right carotid artery
		I63.132	Cerebral infarction due to embolism of left carotid artery
		I63.139	Cerebral infarction due to embolism of unspecified carotid artery
		I63.231	Cerebral infarction due to unspecified occlusion or stenosis of right carotid arteries
		I63.232	Cerebral infarction due to unspecified occlusion or stenosis of left carotid arteries
		I63.239	Cerebral infarction due to unspecified occlusion or stenosis of unspecified carotid arteries

Intracranial Hemorrhage

An intracranial hemorrhage, which may occur at any age and can be due to a wide variety of conditions, is always a medical emergency that requires quick resolution to minimize severe disability due to brain damage or death. The specific location of the bleed and the underlying cause determine the patient's symptoms, the severity of the brain damage, and resulting debility, if any.

Most often due to abnormal arteries found at the base of the brain (cerebral aneurysms), subarachnoid hemorrhage refers to bleeding that occurs due to the rupture of a blood vessel just on the outside of the brain tissue itself and within the skull. Symptoms include a sudden headache, very intense neck pain, and nausea and vomiting. The headache is frequently described as the worst headache of one's life or a thunderclap headache. The rising pressure can quickly result in coma or death. The underlying cause of the hemorrhaging may be traumatic or nontraumatic, with the nontraumatic type being the less common of the two.

ICD-9-CM classifies subarachnoid hemorrhage, nontraumatic, to category 430 and traumatic subarachnoid hemorrhage to category 852. ICD-10-CM, however, goes beyond the traumatic versus nontraumatic classification by identifying the specific vessel that ruptures, as seen in the following table.

Coding for Subarachnoid Hemorrhage

ICD-9-CM		ICD-10-CM	
430	Subarachnoid hemorrhage	I60.00	Nontraumatic subarachnoid hemorrhage from unspecified carotid siphon and bifurcation
		I60.01	Nontraumatic subarachnoid hemorrhage from right carotid siphon and bifurcation
		I60.02	Nontraumatic subarachnoid hemorrhage from left carotid siphon and bifurcation
		I60.10	Nontraumatic subarachnoid hemorrhage from unspecified middle cerebral artery
		I60.11	Nontraumatic subarachnoid hemorrhage from right middle cerebral artery
		I60.12	Nontraumatic subarachnoid hemorrhage from left middle cerebral artery
		I60.20	Nontraumatic subarachnoid hemorrhage from unspecified anterior communicating artery
		I60.21	Nontraumatic subarachnoid hemorrhage from right anterior communicating artery
		I60.22	Nontraumatic subarachnoid hemorrhage from left anterior communicating artery
		I60.30	Nontraumatic subarachnoid hemorrhage from unspecified posterior communicating artery
		I60.31	Nontraumatic subarachnoid hemorrhage from right posterior communicating artery
		I60.32	Nontraumatic subarachnoid hemorrhage from left posterior communicating artery
		I60.50	Nontraumatic subarachnoid hemorrhage from unspecified vertebral artery
		I60.51	Nontraumatic subarachnoid hemorrhage from right vertebral artery
		I60.52	Nontraumatic subarachnoid hemorrhage from left vertebral artery
		I60.6	Nontraumatic subarachnoid hemorrhage from other intracranial arteries
		I60.7	Nontraumatic subarachnoid hemorrhage from unspecified intracranial artery
		I60.8	Other nontraumatic subarachnoid hemorrhage
		I60.9	Nontraumatic subarachnoid hemorrhage, unspecified

> **DEFINITIONS**
>
> **basal ganglia.** Area found at the base of the brain comprising clusters of neurons (nerve cells) that control movement and coordination.
>
> **brainstem.** Area of the brain that connects the spinal cord to the forebrain and cerebrum; comprises the medulla oblongata, pons Varolii, and midbrain.
>
> **cerebellum.** Portion of the brain in the rear cranial fossa behind the brainstem responsible for movement coordination.
>
> **cerebral cortex.** Outermost layer of gray matter of the brain, made up of a collection of nerve cell bodies responsible for higher functions of the brain, such as sensation, thought, reasoning, and memory, and the movement of voluntary muscle.

An intracerebral hemorrhage, also referred to as an intraparenchymal hemorrhage, intracranial hematoma, or simply ICH, occurs when a blood vessel that is weak or diseased erupts in the brain. The resulting pressure from the blood damages brain cells, and coma or death may occur. This happens most often in the **basal ganglia**, **brainstem**, **cerebellum**, or **cortex**. Although this condition is most frequently caused by hypertension, other causes include:

- Aberrant blood vessels, such as arteriovenous malformations (AVM)
- Blood-clotting deficiencies
- Infection
- Traumatic injury
- Tumors

Intracerebral hemorrhage accounts for 10 to 15 percent of all strokes. This type of stroke is associated with a much higher rate of mortality than that of the more common acute ischemic stroke, caused by thrombosis or embolism.

Intracerebral hemorrhages (nontraumatic) are classified to category 431 in ICD-9-CM, and traumatic hemorrhages are classified to category 851, regardless of where the bleeding occurs in the brain. ICD-10-CM classifies intracerebral hemorrhages according to whether the bleed was traumatic or nontraumatic, but also designates the specific part of the brain in which the bleed occurred for nontraumatic bleeds.

Coding for Intracerebral Hemorrhage

ICD-9-CM		ICD-10-CM	
431	Intracerebral hemorrhage	I61.0	Nontraumatic intracerebral hemorrhage in hemisphere, **subcortical**
		I61.1	Nontraumatic intracerebral hemorrhage in hemisphere, **cortical**
		I61.2	Nontraumatic intracerebral hemorrhage in hemisphere, unspecified
		I61.3	Nontraumatic intracerebral hemorrhage in brain stem
		I61.4	Nontraumatic intracerebral hemorrhage in cerebellum
		I61.5	Nontraumatic intracerebral hemorrhage, intraventricular
		I61.6	Nontraumatic intracerebral hemorrhage, multiple localized
		I61.8	Other nontraumatic intracerebral hemorrhage
		I61.9	Nontraumatic intracerebral hemorrhage, unspecified

Residual Effects of Cerebrovascular Disease

When a brain injury occurs due to a stroke or other type of cerebrovascular disease or due to a traumatic injury to the brain, residual effects can occur according to the severity and the site of the brain injury. This includes paralysis; speech and language problems, such as **aphasia**, **dysarthria**, and **dysphasia**; and **cognitive** defects. For both coding classification systems, these residual neurological deficits are reported in addition to the underlying brain injury code regardless of when the deficit occurs. Once again, ICD-10-CM classifies these conditions with greater specificity, including **hemiplegia** and **monoplegia** for which ICD-10-CM indicates if the left or right side or limb is dominant. ICD-9-CM simply refers to the dominant side, with no distinction between right and left. Speech deficits are also classified in much more detail in ICD-10-CM, specifying the underlying cause of the condition, as indicated in the following table.

Coding for Speech and Language Deficits

ICD-9-CM		ICD-10-CM	
438.13	Dysarthria	I69.022	Dysarthria following nontraumatic subarachnoid hemorrhage
		I69.122	Dysarthria following nontraumatic intracerebral hemorrhage
		I69.222	Dysarthria following other nontraumatic intracranial hemorrhage
		I69.322	Dysarthria following cerebral infarction
		I69.822	Dysarthria following other cerebrovascular disease
		I69.922	Dysarthria following unspecified cerebrovascular disease

---

DEFINITIONS

aphasia. Partial or total loss of the ability to comprehend language or communicate through speaking, the written word, or sign language. Aphasia may result from stroke, injury, Alzheimer's disease, or other disorder. Common types of aphasia include expressive, receptive, anomic, global, and conduction.

cognitive. Having to do with being aware by drawing from knowledge, such as judgment, reason, perception, and memory.

cortical. Pertaining to the cortex, which is the outer portion of an organ. In the brain it refers to the outer part of the *cerebrum*.

dysarthria. Difficulty pronouncing words.

dysphasia. Speech impairment manifested by incoordination and the inability to arrange words in their proper order.

hemiplegia. Paralysis of one side of the body.

monoplegia. Loss or impairment of motor function in one arm or one leg.

subcortical. Pertaining to the part of the brain below the *cerebral cortex*.

Definitions

fluency disorder. Interruption in the flow of speech, including stuttering, due to CVA that impedes communication. Fluency is typified by repetitious sounds and syllables, and anomalous protraction of sounds of speech.

ICD-9-CM		ICD-10-CM	
438.14	*Fluency disorder*	I69.023	Fluency disorder following nontraumatic subarachnoid hemorrhage
		I69.123	Fluency disorder following nontraumatic intracerebral hemorrhage
		I69.223	Fluency disorder following other nontraumatic intracranial hemorrhage
		I69.323	Fluency disorder following cerebral infarction
		I69.823	Fluency disorder following other cerebrovascular disease
		I69.923	Fluency disorder following unspecified cerebrovascular disease

Summary

The cardiovascular system houses some of the most important components needed for day-to-day survival. The heart and blood vessels in the circulatory system provide oxygen-rich blood, nutrients such as amino acids and electrolytes, and important hormones to all of the body's cells and carry off carbon dioxide and other waste products of metabolism. In addition, the cardiovascular system stabilizes body temperature and pH. It makes sense that a system so important to day-to-day survival would be complex, and it is critical that coders understand the function of various parts of the circulatory system in order to code efficiently and effectively under the ICD-10-CM classification system.

Chapter 8.
ICD-10-CM: Blood and Blood-Forming Organs

Anatomic Overview

Blood is a *viscous* liquid that the heart pumps through the blood vessels as described in the cardiovascular chapter. It is unique in that it is the only fluid-type tissue in the human body. Its many purposes can be divided into three main functions:

- Transportation
- Regulation
- Protection

The blood travels throughout the body and serves as the transport mechanism for the distribution of oxygen, nutrients, and hormones to the cells and tissues of the entire body. It also carries away the metabolic waste from these structures to the appropriate organ or system for disposal. By doing this, the blood regulates the pH and fluid volumes of the body. Moving throughout the body constantly, it also helps to maintain the body's temperature. There are also multiple types of individual cells within the blood that provide protective functions, such as fighting infection and *hemostasis*.

Due to its many functions, blood has many unique parts. There are formed elements, consisting of red blood cells, white blood cells, and platelets, and plasma, in which the formed elements "float." The formed elements all originate from stem cells in the bone marrow. These stem cells, or hemocytoblasts, can grow into a variety of specialized cell types. Two types of hemocytoblasts that evolve into blood cells: myeloid and lymphoid. Myeloid stem cells eventually form into red blood cells, platelets, and some white blood cells. Lymphoid stem cells become a highly-specialized type of white blood cell known as a lymphocyte, which is discussed in further detail later in this chapter. It is important to note that most blood cells do not divide but are destroyed and replaced by new cells that are formed in the bone marrow.

The composition of blood is obvious in a sample that is left sitting—clotting is prevented as the blood separates, leaving the red blood cells at the bottom, the white bloods cells and platelets in the middle, also called the buffy coat, and the plasma on top. For laboratory blood work, this separation is performed much quicker via *centrifuge*. Being able to separate blood is important in detecting disease and overall health, as each of these blood constituents is unique in structure, function, and life cycle, and a variance in any of these can reveal a disease or disorder. Recognizing and understanding the functions of each of the blood constituents is important to the proper coding of abnormalities that affect the blood and associated organs.

Red Blood Cells

Red blood cells (RBC), or erythrocytes, make up more than 99 percent of the formed elements. These cells travel throughout the body delivering oxygen and removing some of the carbon dioxide cells release. Normal RBCs are dish-shaped—round with a concave depression in the center. Because of its dome shape, RBCs can squeeze into even the smallest capillary to perform its function. The depression serves two

DEFINITIONS

centrifuge. Machine used to simulate gravitational effects or centrifugal force to separate substances of different densities.

hemostasis. Interruption of blood flow or the cessation or arrest of bleeding.

viscous. Pertaining to something thick, sticky, or glutinous.

INTERESTING A & P FACT

Bone marrow produces an average of an ounce of blood every day, which is approximately 100 billion new cells every day.

functions: it increases the surface area in which the diffusion of gases can take place and places the surface closer to the protein molecules that carry oxygen. The protein molecules, known as **hemoglobin**, are responsible for the blood's color. When the RBCs are carrying oxygen, the blood appears bright red; when the hemoglobin is de-oxygenated, the blood appears blue when viewed through blood vessel walls.

Figure 8.1: Red Blood Cells

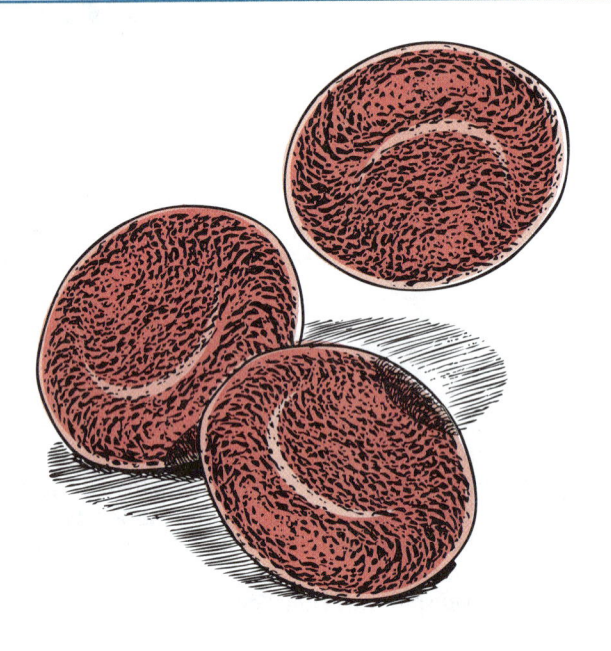

After about 100 to 120 days in circulation, a red blood cell begins to break down. The cell becomes fragile and brittle, and the hemoglobin becomes less effective. As they move throughout the smaller vessels, the cells begin to fragment. This happens most often in the extremely small vessels of the spleen, which is why the spleen is sometimes referred to as the "red blood cell graveyard." The fragments and ruptured RBCs are then destroyed by **macrophages**. Hemoglobin goes through multiple decomposition phases, resulting in iron that is transported back to the liver for storage and to the bone marrow for later use in producing new hemoglobin. Other byproducts are eventually converted into bilirubin.

RBCs also have surface molecules called antigens and antibodies. Two of these molecules are Rh group and blood type group. These are important in medicine today as they are responsible for determining blood compatibility. If blood is not compatible during a transfusion, the blood could clump, causing **agglutination**.

The blood type group is determined by identifying up to two antigens on the surface of an erythrocyte. These antigens are known as antigen A and antigen B. The absence or presence of these determine the four blood types:

- **A:** Antigen A is present.
- **B:** Antigen B is present.
- **AB:** Both antigens are present.
- **O:** Neither antigen is present.

> **DEFINITIONS**
>
> **agglutination.** Clumping together of cells due to the binding of agglutinin (a protein) molecules on the surface of each cell.
>
> **hemoglobin.** Oxygen-carrying component of the red blood cell.
>
> **macrophage.** Type of white blood cell.

Figure 8.2: Blood Types

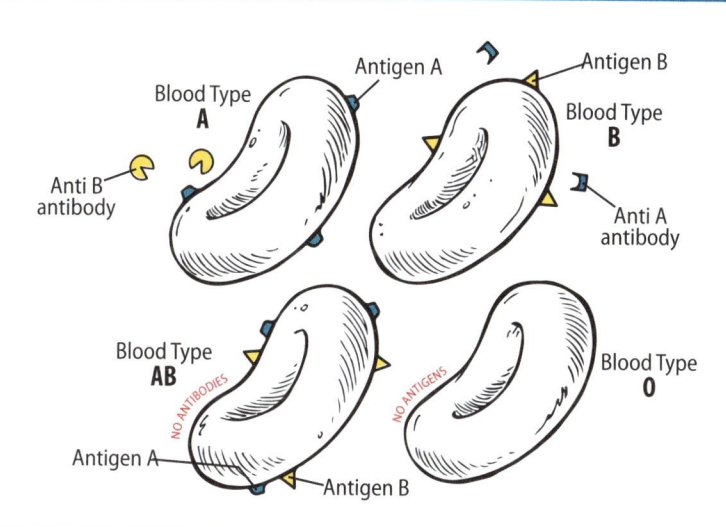

Babies are born without any of these antigens, but two to eight months after birth, the body develops its blood type and, in response, also develops antibodies that float in the plasma that correspond with the antigen. These antibodies attack whichever antigen the body did *not* produce. If the patient develops antigen A, antibody or anti-B is formed; if antigen B is developed, anti-A is formed. When antigens A and B are present, no antibodies are produced. When neither antigen is present, both anti-A and anti-B are formed. These antibodies cause blood to react when an antigen comes into contact with an antibody of the same type (e.g., anti-A attacks antigen A-covered RBCs). These combinations allow only certain blood types to be transfused to other blood types, as is demonstrated in the following table.

Blood Type	Acceptable Blood Type for Transfusion
A	A, O
B	B, O
AB	A, B, AB, O
O	O

CLINICAL NOTE

Blood type O is a universal donor because it is accepted by any blood type. Blood type AB is a universal recipient as it can accept any type of blood.

Rh factor is not as straightforward as blood type. There are many types of Rh antigens attached to the erythrocyte and if any of these are present, the blood is considered Rh-positive. If none are present, it is considered Rh-negative. The main difference between these types of antigens and the blood type is that Rh-negative blood does not automatically develop Rh antibodies (anti-Rh). An Rh-negative patient develops anti-Rh only when exposed to Rh-positive blood, therefore making a reaction unlikely the first time the patient is exposed. However, once the body develops the anti-Rh, the blood reacts if exposed again. An example of this occurs during pregnancy. If an Rh-negative mother carries an Rh-positive baby, the mother's body develops anti-Rh. This may not impact the first pregnancy, but if the Rh-negative mother carries a second Rh-positive baby, the mother's anti-Rh attacks the Rh-positive red blood cells of the fetus.

White Blood Cells

Unlike red blood cells, there is more than one type of white blood cell (WBC), but they all share the same basic function, to fight infection. Also known as leukocytes, most of their work is performed outside of the bloodstream via *diapedesis*, but they are transported in the blood. Leukocytes are drawn together en masse by chemicals released by damaged tissue or other WBCs, to destroy foreign bodies such as

DEFINITIONS

diapedesis. Passage of blood cells through the walls of blood vessels without damage to the cell or vessel.

infectious organisms, toxins, or tumor cells. The body then speeds up production of these cells, resulting in excessive amounts of leukocytes in the bloodstream, one of the first indications of active infections. Although these blood cells play a very important role, they make up less than 1 percent of whole blood in a healthy person.

Figure 8.3: White Blood Cells

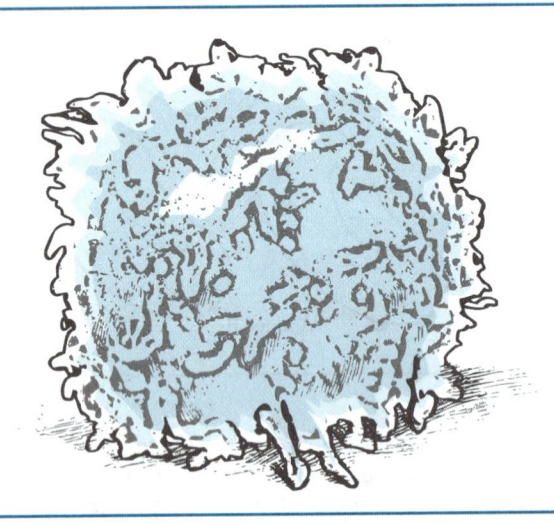

> **DEFINITIONS**
>
> **cytoplasm.** All of the substances of a cell except the nucleus.
>
> **granular.** Microscopically appearing to have particles resembling sand on its surface.
>
> **phagocytosis.** Engulfing and ingesting bacteria or other foreign bodies.

There are five types of WBCs that are first classified by the nature of the cell's *cytoplasm*. Some cells have a *granular* cytoplasm and are known as granulocytes. These cells are usually spherical and twice the size of a red blood cell. They have a short lifespan of approximately 12 hours. There are three types of granulocytes: neutrophils, eosinophils, and basophils.

Neutrophils are the "bacteria slayers," being able to ingest and destroy many types of bacteria and some fungi. These types of cells are chemically attracted to inflammation and are usually the first of the leukocytes to arrive at an infection site. Note that immature neutrophils are commonly found in a blood sample, known as *bands*. Bands increase in number during an active infection as the body is producing and releasing as many WBCs as it can to fight off the infection. When the number of aggregate WBCs, neutrophils, and bands all increase significantly, it is known as a "shift to the left" and is highly indicative of an active infection.

Eosinophils make up only 1 to 3 percent of circulating white blood cells. These cells are responsible for moderating allergic reactions by deactivating inflammatory chemicals released and decreasing the immune response by *phagocytosis* of antigen-antibody reactions. They defend against parasites that are too large for phagocytosis. They surround and chemically attack these organisms, dissolving them.

The least type of granulocyte is called a basophil. This type of cell is actively involved in the inflammatory process. Basophils gather at sites of damaged tissues where they release histamine, a chemical that opens the blood vessels to promote blood flow and attract other leukocytes. They also excrete heparin, a naturally occurring chemical that inhibits blood clotting. [*prevents*]

Cells that do not have a visibly granular cytoplasm are called agranulocytes. Lymphocytes and monocytes are the two classifications of agranulocytes. Although similar in structure, their functions are completely different.

Lymphocytes are the second most numerous type of leukocyte in the body; however, most of them are not found in the bloodstream. These cells can live for years in the body's lymphoid tissue (e.g., lymph nodes, spleen, etc.), hence the name lymphocyte. There are two types: T-cells and B-cells. T-cells specifically target virus-infected and tumor cells. B-cells eventually become plasma cells, which produce antibodies. More information on lymphocytes can be found in the lymphatic system chapter.

Monocytes are the largest of the blood cells. They are extremely active in the phagocytosis of bacteria, dead cells, and other foreign bodies. When a monocyte leaves the bloodstream, it becomes known as a *macrophage*.

When infectious organisms, dead cells, and leukocytes gather together at an inflamed area, a white viscous fluid, called pus, results. The pus remains while the organisms are present and is eventually absorbed into surrounding tissues if not expelled otherwise.

Platelets

Platelets, also known as thrombocytes, are different from the other formed elements found in the blood in that they are not cells in the strict sense, as they lack a nucleus. A platelet is a fragment of cytoplasm that has chipped off a large cell, called a megakaryocyte, found in the red bone marrow. The fragments that are too large to be considered platelets are diminished in size when they pass through the blood vessels of the lungs. When a blood vessel is damaged, platelets stick to the compromised area, forming a temporary barrier, and release serotonin, a vasoconstrictor that contracts the blood vessel and reduces blood flow to the area.

Figure 8.4: Platelets

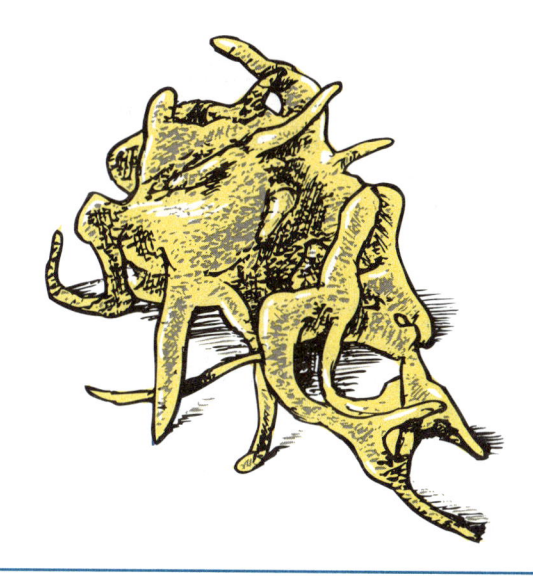

Plasma

Plasma is a straw-colored fluid in which the formed elements are suspended. The plasma carries the formed elements throughout the body. The liquid consists of electrolytes, water, wastes, nutrients, vitamins, hormones, gases, and proteins. The constant adjusting of the different components of the plasma maintains an acceptable pH of blood. The organs secrete and absorb the different substances. For example, the plasma picks up glucose at the small intestine and drops it off at the liver, where it is stored or converted to fat.

Hemostasis

As discussed in the introduction, an important function of blood is hemostasis. This process is a complex reaction to damage to or a break in a blood vessel. There are three mechanisms that occur in quick succession to stop bleeding as quickly as possible. First, the vessel induces a local spasm of its smooth-muscle lining, constricting the flow of blood to the area to allow more time for the other two responses to occur. At this point, platelets flood the area and form a platelet plug, temporarily sealing it. To form the plug, the normally smooth platelet cells begin to swell and grow spike-like processes to stick to other platelets and the exposed collagen fibers of the endothelial lining of the vessel. The last step, referred to as coagulation, takes more than 30 substances, called factors, to complete. During this stage, the liquid blood forms a gel covering the wound, otherwise known as a clot. Clot-forming factors are known as procoagulants. These are numbered I–XIII (i.e., factor VIII, factor X) in the order they were discovered. Factors that inhibit clotting are known as anticoagulants. The formation of a clot and healing of a wound depend on a delicate balance between these two types of factors. As the chemical reactions progress, fibrin strands are produced that form a web to catch the platelets and trap the other formed elements to form a clot.

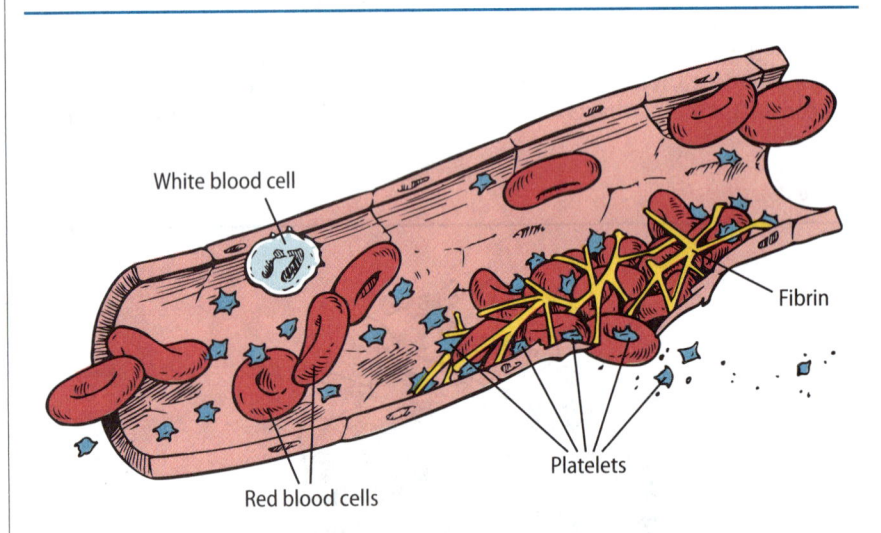

Figure 8.5: Blood Coagulation

Once a clot is established and the blood flow is stopped, the clot begins to retract, pulling the edges of the wound together. As the wound is being closed by this process, the platelets involved release a substance that stimulates regrowth of the surrounding original tissue. Because a blood clot is a temporary fix, the body also begins to dissolve it via a process called fibrinolysis. Eventually, the clot is completely absorbed and the wound is closed permanently by new tissue.

Spleen

The spleen is made up of lymphatic tissue, the splenic artery, the splenic vein, and efferent lymphatic vessels. The lymphatic tissue contains lymphocytes and microphages called white pulp. The white pulp surrounds central arteries that branch off the splenic artery. The spleen also contains areas termed red pulp, which is made up of splenic cords or tissue that contain microphages, lymphocytes, red blood cells, plasma cells, and granulocytes. Red pulp also has venous sinuses that are filled with blood.

Blood enters the venous sinuses via the splenic artery, where the surrounding white pulp contains the B and T-cells that provide the immune response and microphages that eradicate pathogens. The red pulp stores up to a third of the body's platelet supply, and eliminates worn-out or bad cells and platelets via the microphages.

Anatomy and Pathophysiology and the ICD-10-CM Code Set

Due to the overall diversity in the composition of the blood and its interaction with other organs and systems, there are many diseases that can affect the blood. Each of the formed blood elements has its own structure and function; each type of blood cell also has its own diseases and abnormalities. In many cases, ICD-9-CM and ICD-10-CM are similar to each other in the blood and blood forming organs chapters. In fact, there is a 69 percent one-to-one equivalent mapping between the synonymous chapters of the two classification systems.

Diseases of the Red Blood Cells

The major differences between the two classification systems regarding diseases of the red blood cells arise with the coding of **anemia**. There are many underlying causes of anemia, and ICD-9-CM effectively categorizes most general forms of anemia. There are, however, categories in which the underlying disease specified by ICD-9-CM is just another manifestation of a bigger underlying issue. For example, because vitamin B12 is used in red blood cell creation, if there is a deficiency in the vitamin, there is a decrease in the RBCs that can be produced. ICD-9-CM groups all B12 deficiency anemias together regardless of etiology, whereas ICD-10-CM takes the selection a step further by identifying the underlying cause of the B12 deficiency.

The most common underlying causes of B12 deficiency are nutritional deficiency and digestive malabsorption. Nutritional deficiency occurs from the lack of B12 in a person's diet but is actually quite rare because the body stores enough B12 to last at least a year, if not years. Dietary deficiency occurs most commonly in chronic alcoholics and elderly on a "tea and toast" diet; occasionally, this impacts people with strict vegan diets as the majority of dietary B12 comes from ingesting meat, poultry, and dairy products.

Digestive malabsorption can come from multiple sources. Vitamin B12 is extracted from ingested proteins once in the stomach. There it attaches to a protein called intrinsic factor (IF). The IF transports the B12 to the terminal ileum of the small intestine where it is absorbed into the bloodstream with the help of a molecule called transcobalamin II (TC II). Any disruption of this process can result in B12 deficiency. Frequent causes are HIV/AIDS, failure to release B12 from protein, IF deficiency, chronic pancreatic disease, competitive parasites, or lack of TC II.

The underlying cause of the B12 deficiency and subsequent anemia is an important piece of documentation needed when assigning codes for this condition in ICD-10-CM.

Coding for Vitamin B-12 Deficiency Anemia

ICD-9-CM		ICD-10-CM	
281.1	Other vitamin B12 deficiency anemia	D51.1	Vitamin B12 deficiency anemia due to selective vitamin B12 malabsorption with proteinuria
		D51.2	Transcobalamin II deficiency
		D51.3	Other dietary vitamin B12 deficiency anemia
		D51.8	Other vitamin B12 deficiency anemias
		D51.9	Vitamin B12 deficiency anemia, unspecified

Closely related to vitamin B12 deficiency is folate deficiency, which also causes anemia. Folate, or folic acid, is an enzyme that works with vitamin B12 in red blood cell production. Folate deficiency is commonly seen during pregnancy, infancy, and periods of stress. It is also frequently caused by pharmaceuticals, such as sulfa-based antibiotics and methotrexate. ICD-10-CM takes all of this into consideration within the folate deficiency anemia category.

DEFINITIONS

anemia. Deficiency in the blood whether in red blood cells, hemoglobin, or total blood count.

Coding for Folate Deficiency Anemia

ICD-9-CM		ICD-10-CM	
281.2	Folate-deficiency anemia	D52.0	Dietary folate deficiency anemia
		D52.1	Drug-induced folate deficiency anemia
		D52.8	Other folate deficiency anemias
		D52.9	Folate deficiency anemia, unspecified

Genetic anemias are also not uncommon in the American population. The two most significant types are sickle cell anemia and thalassemia. Sickle cell anemia and thalassemia are both inherited conditions that impact the red blood cells, but they are significantly different.

Thalassemia is a condition in which the body does not produce enough normal hemoglobin, resulting in severe anemia. An in-depth understanding of the genetic composition of the red blood cell is needed to distinguish between the different types of thalassemia. Hemoglobin is formed by two inherited proteins from both parents. These proteins are known as alpha globin and beta globin. There are four alpha (two from each parent) and two beta (one from each parent) globins that make up hemoglobin. When one or more of the globins are missing or deformed, the incomplete hemoglobin causes misshapen and fragile red blood cells. Due to their frail nature, the affected RBCs break apart and die quickly, resulting in a type of anemia specifically known as thalassemia.

Figure 8.6: Thalassemia

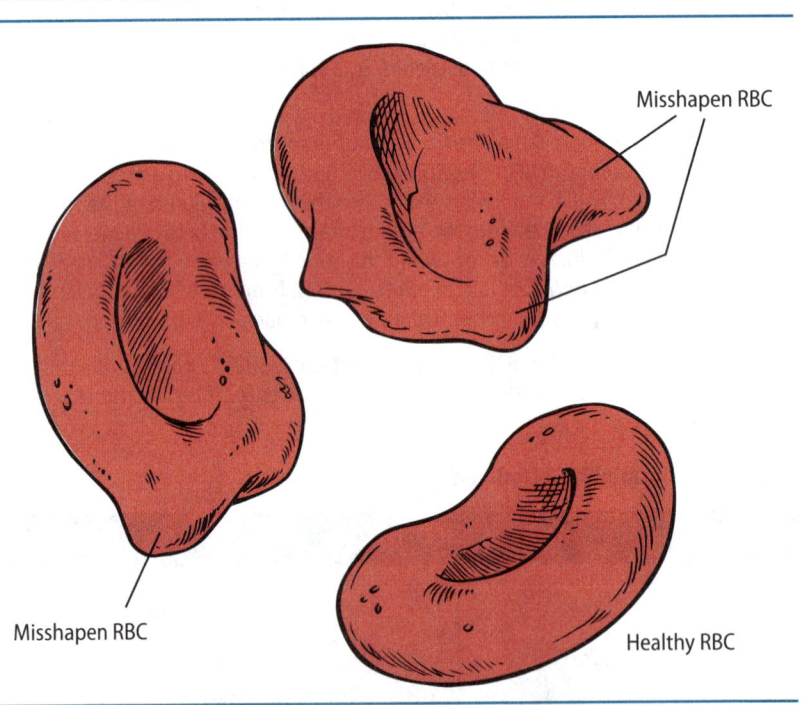

The different types of thalassemia are divided by the type and number of missing or deformed globins. The major categories are:

- **Alpha thalassemia:** Also called silent carrier, one alpha globin is missing.
- **Alpha thalassemia minor:** Also called alpha thalassemia trait, two alpha globins are missing.
- **Hemoglobin H disease:** Three alpha globins are missing.

- **Alpha thalassemia major:** Also called hydrops fetalis, four alpha globins are missing.
- **Beta thalassemia minor:** Also called beta thalassemia trait, there is one abnormal and one normal beta globin.
- **Beta thalassemia major:** Also called Cooley's anemia, both beta globins are abnormal.
- *Delta-Beta thalassemia*

ICD-10-CM requires documentation of the specific type of thalassemia in order to code correctly. Additional detail may be required in the provider documentation in order to make the most accurate code selections.

Coding for Thalassemia

ICD-9-CM	ICD-10-CM
282.49 Other thalassemia	D56.8 Other thalassemias

> **CLINICAL NOTE**
>
> **Delta-beta thalassemia.** About 3 percent of adult hemoglobin is made of alpha and delta globins rather than alpha and beta.

Another type of thalassemia not discussed above involves another red blood cell disorder called sickle cell disease or anemia. Sickle cell can occur with or without thalassemia, depending on the patient's genetics.

Sickle cell disease is characterized (and named) for the crescent or sickle-shaped deformity of the red blood cells caused by defective hemoglobin. The hemoglobin is abnormal due to an abnormal alpha globin, referred to as sickle globin. Because a person gets one alpha globin from each parent, both parents must carry sickle globin for sickle cell disease to occur; both alpha globins must be absent and replaced by sickle globins. If only one parent passes the genetic disposition to create sickle globin, the patient is considered to have sickle cell trait, an asymptomatic carrier status.

Figure 8.7: Normal and Sickle Red Blood Cells

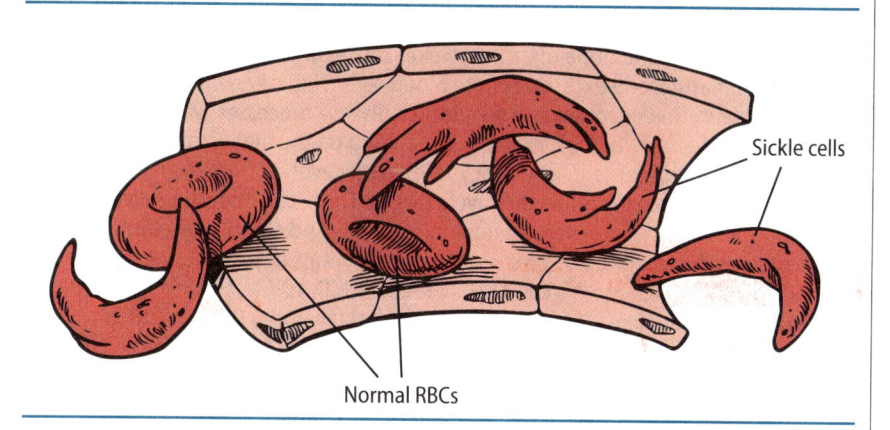

There are three main types of sickle cell disease:

- **Hemoglobin SS (Hb-SS):** Hemoglobin S gene is inherited from both parents.
- **Hemoglobin SC (Hb-C):** Hemoglobin S is inherited from one parent and hemoglobin C is inherited from the other parent.
- **Sickle beta thalassemia (thalassemia Hb-S):** Hemoglobin S is inherited from one parent, and the beta thalassemia gene is inherited from the other parent.

In sickle cell anemia, the hook-shape of the red blood cells not only makes the cells more fragile but also leads them to get trapped in blood vessels, causing blocked vessels. When this occurs, the blood flow is stopped, possibly leading to pain and tissue damage. Usually when a blockage episode occurs, the affected area is extremely painful. This is called a *crisis*. A sickle cell crisis can manifest in many ways but is commonly classified as vaso-occlusive pain in the bones, abdomen, or major joints; acute chest syndrome, in which blood is trapped in the small vessels of the lungs; and splenic sequestration, when blood cells clog the spleen, causing it to enlarge.

ICD-9-CM does distinguish between the main types of sickle cell disease and also provides codes for with and without crisis. However, the type of crisis is coded elsewhere. ICD-10-CM eliminates the need, in some cases, for an additional code to be reported as the categories are further expanded to include this information.

Coding for Sickle Cell Disease

ICD-9-CM		ICD-10-CM	
282.42	Sickle cell thalassemia with crisis	D57.411	Sickle-cell thalassemia with acute chest syndrome
		D57.412	Sickle-cell thalassemia with splenic sequestration
		D57.419	Sickle-cell thalassemia with crisis, unspecified
282.62	Hb-SS disease with crisis	D57.01	Hb-SS disease with acute chest syndrome
		D57.02	Hb-SS disease with splenic sequestration
		D57.00	Hb-SS disease with crisis, unspecified
282.64	Sickle-cell/Hb-C disease with crisis	D57.211	Sickle-cell/Hb-C disease with acute chest syndrome
		D57.212	Sickle-cell/Hb-C disease with splenic sequestration
		D57.219	Sickle-cell/Hb-C with crisis, unspecified

Diseases of White Blood Cells

As discussed in the anatomic overview of this chapter, all of the formed elements of the blood arise from myeloid or lymphoid stem cells in the red bone marrow. In some instances, the blood and bone marrow develop cancer and the stem cells produce abnormal, immature, and excessive white blood cells. This is known as leukemia, a generalized term that encompasses a variety of disease processes. Most leukemias can be classified as myeloid or lymphoid, depending on the malfunctioning stem cell producing the abnormal cells. Lymphocytic leukemia evolves from the lymphoid stem cells and myeloid leukemia the myeloid cells. These can be further divided into acute and chronic types—acute developing suddenly and chronic developing over a period of time. Knowing these generalizations is the most important piece of information needed to assign a code in ICD-9-CM or ICD-10-CM. However, ICD-10-CM further differentiates specific types of leukemia that fall under broader "other specified" categories in ICD-9-CM. The more specific types of lymphocytic leukemia featured in ICD-10-CM include:

- **Prolymphocytic leukemia of B-cell type:** Aggressive form of chronic lymphocytic leukemia involving mature B-cells.
- **Prolymphocytic leukemia of T-cell type:** Very rare form of chronic lymphoid leukemia involving mature T cells.
- **Mature B-cell leukemia, Burkitt type:** Form of acute lymphoid leukemia.

There is one additional type of lymphocytic leukemia that ICD-10-CM identifies. Occasionally leukemia is caused by a virus called the human T-lymphotropic virus (HTLV). In this type of disorder, the virus infects healthy T-cells and replicates within them.

Another important factor in choosing a code for any type of leukemia in either classification system is whether the cancer is active, in remission, or in relapse. The disease is considered active when it is first discovered and is current and causing signs and symptoms. Once treatment is rendered, usually in the form of chemotherapy or induction therapy, the abnormal blood cells disappear from the blood and the disease disappears. When this occurs, the patient is considered in remission. A relapse is when the disease returns after the patient has achieved remission. A patient can relapse multiple times.

Applying all of the above knowledge is the best way to assign the most appropriate code in ICD-9-CM or ICD-10-CM, but some additional understanding of the cell types is required for the new classification system.

Coding for Lymphocytic Leukemia

ICD-9-CM		ICD-10-CM	
204.80	Other lymphoid leukemia without achieved remission	C91.30	Prolymphocytic leukemia of B-cell type not having achieved remission
		C91.50	Adult T-cell lymphoma/leukemia (HTLV-1-associated) not having achieved remission
		C91.60	Prolymphocytic leukemia of T-cell type not having achieved remission
		C91.A0	Mature B-cell leukemia Burkitt-type not having achieved remission
		C91.Z0	Other lymphoid leukemia not having achieved remission
204.81	Other lymphoid leukemia in remission	C91.31	Prolymphocytic leukemia of B-cell type, in remission
		C91.51	Adult T-cell lymphoma/leukemia (HTLV-1-associated), in remission
		C91.61	Prolymphocytic leukemia of T-cell type, in remission
		C91.A1	Mature B-cell leukemia Burkitt-type, in remission
		C91.Z1	Other lymphoid leukemia, in remission
204.82	Other lymphoid leukemia in relapse	C91.32	Prolymphocytic leukemia of B-cell type, in relapse
		C91.52	Adult T-cell lymphoma/leukemia (HTLV-1-associated), in relapse
		C91.62	Prolymphocytic leukemia of T-cell type, in relapse
		C91.A2	Mature B-cell leukemia Burkitt-type in relapse
		C91.Z2	Other lymphoid leukemia, in relapse

Myeloid leukemia follows the same basic concepts as lymphocytic. But again, ICD-10-CM categorizes the more common types of specific acute myeloid leukemia. Those that are featured in the new classification system are:

- **Acute myeloblastic leukemia (AML):** Hemocytoblasts that form the myeloid stem cells are abnormal, causing immature and abnormal blood cells.
- **Acute promyelocytic leukemia (APL):** Blood cells are abnormal and there are excess promyelocytes or unevolved granulocytes found in the bloodstream.
- **Acute myelomonocytic leukemia (AMML):** Monocytes, as well as myeloid cells, are impacted.
- **Acute myeloid leukemia with 11q23-abnormality:** AML with a chromosomal abnormality.
- **Acute myeloid leukemia with multilineage dysplasia:** AML in patients who have previously been diagnosed with *myelodysplastic syndrome* or *myeloproliferative disease*.

CODING AXIOM

ICD-10-CM Official Coding Guideline I.C.2.n. states, "Leukemia, multiple myeloma, and malignant plasma cell neoplasms in remission versus personal history—The categories for leukemia, and category C90 Multiple myeloma and malignant plasma cell neoplasms, have codes indicating whether or not the leukemia has achieved remission. There are also codes Z85.6 Personal history of leukemia, and Z85.79 Personal history of malignant neoplasms of lymphoid, hematopoietic and related tissues. If the documentation is unclear as to whether the leukemia has achieved remission, the provider should be queried."

DEFINITIONS

myelodysplastic syndrome. Neoplasm of lymphatic and hematopoietic tissues, affecting the spinal cord.

myeloproliferative disease. Unusual proliferation of myelopoietic tissue.

Coding for Acute Myeloid Leukemia

ICD-9-CM		ICD-10-CM	
205.00	Acute myeloid leukemia without achieved remission	C92.00	Acute myeloblastic leukemia, not having achieved remission
		C92.40	Acute promyelocytic leukemia, not having achieved remission
		C92.50	Acute myelomonocytic leukemia, not having achieved remission
		C92.60	Acute myeloid leukemia w 11q23-abnormality, not having achieved remission
		C92.A0	Acute myeloid leukemia with multilineage dysplasia, not having achieved remission

Although there are many other types of diseases that impact the white blood cells, reporting for most of them is considerably similar between the two coding systems and does not require any additional knowledge.

Plasma Disorders

Most plasma disorders have a one-to-one crosswalk between ICD-9-CM and ICD-10-CM. However, because many plasma abnormalities can indicate other more serious diseases, specific classifications have been added to the newer coding system that identify abnormal findings in the plasma. Knowing the most commonly discussed plasma proteins is crucial to understanding the ICD-10-CM codes. The three protein abnormalities ICD-10-CM tracks are albumin, globulin, and alphafetoprotein. The differences are highlighted below.

Coding for Plasma Abnormalities

ICD-9-CM		ICD-10-CM	
790.99	Other nonspecific findings on examination of blood	R70.1	Abnormal plasma viscosity
		R77.0	Abnormality of albumin
		R77.1	Abnormality of globulin
		R77.2	Abnormality of alphafetoprotein
		R77.8	Other specified abnormalities of plasma proteins
		R77.9	Abnormality of plasma protein, unspecified

Abnormal Laboratory Blood Tests

Because blood transports substances to and from the organs and body systems, many abnormalities and diseases of different types can be diagnosed via a simple blood test that analyzes the constituents—not just the formed elements, but the electrolytes, chemicals, and variety of other substances. There are times when medical documentation specifies only that there was an abnormal blood test result. When using ICD-9-CM, these types of lab results were mostly classified as "other" abnormal chemistry.

ICD-10-CM has expanded this general code to capture a few more specific and common findings that can increase reporting capabilities for blood tests. The following table highlights a few of these new codes.

Chapter 9. ICD-10-CM: Lymphatic System

Anatomic Overview

The lymphatic system plays a key role in the movement and drainage of fluid in the tissues and the transporting of lipids, and is integral to the body's fight against infection and disease.

The lymphatic system comprises **lymphatic capillaries**, **lymphatic vessels**, and lymph nodes, as well as **lymph fluid** and lymphatic tissues such as the thymus, spleen, and lymphatic nodules.

This complex system begins at the cellular level. Lymphatic capillaries lie among the cells and are one-way structures that allow **interstitial fluid** to flow into but not out of the capillary. Once the interstitial fluid is in the lymphatic capillary, it is called lymph. The capillaries combine to become lymphatic vessels. Lymphatic nodes are found along the lymphatic vessels. These nodes are bean-shaped and contain masses of B and T-cells. Lymph fluid flows through nodes as it traverses the lymphatic system. In key areas of the lymphatic system there are a series, or "chain," of lymph nodes.

Figure 9.1: Lymphatic Capillaries

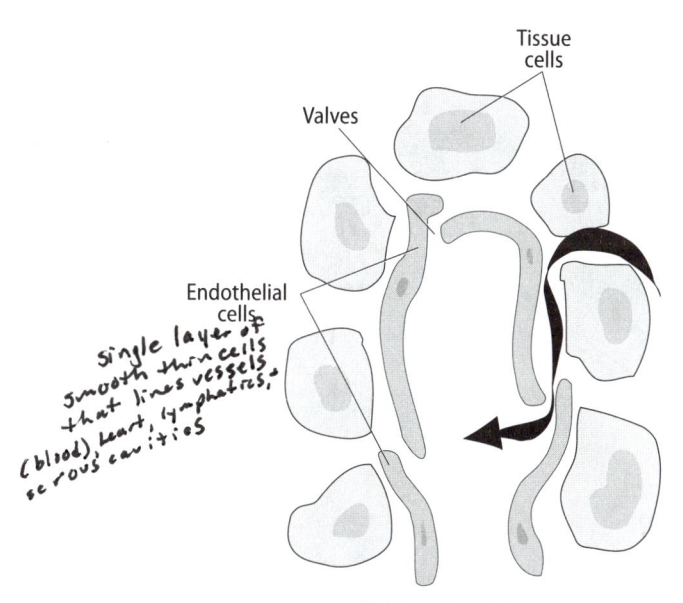

Fluids and particles can enter the capillary through overlapping valves

The subcutaneous lymphatic vessels generally follow the same route as blood veins, and the visceral lymphatic vessels generally follow the same route as arteries. Avascular tissues, such as cartilage, epidermis, and corneal tissue, do not have lymphatic vessels.

> **DEFINITIONS**
>
> **interstitial fluid.** Extracellular fluid filtered through capillaries and drained as lymph that surrounds most tissue outside of blood or lymph vessels.
>
> **lymphatic capillary.** Small tubular structure in the tissue that collects interstitial fluid using a one-way design; capillaries then combine into lymphatic vessels.
>
> **lymphatic fluid.** Clear, sometimes yellow fluid that flows through the tissues in the body, through the lymphatic system, and into the bloodstream.
>
> **lymphatic vessel.** Vessels with interspersed lymph nodes that transport lymph from the lymphatic capillaries to the lymph trunks.

Eventually the lymphatic vessels combine into lymph trunks. The trunks and the areas they drain include:

- **Lumbar trunk:** Abdominal wall, lower limbs, pelvis, kidneys, and adrenal glands
- **Intestinal trunk:** Intestines, stomach, pancreas, spleen, and liver
- **Bronchomediastinal trunk:** Heart, lung, and thoracic wall
- **Subclavian trunk:** Upper limbs
- **Jugular trunk:** Head and neck

The lymph flows from the *lymphatic trunk* into the *thoracic duct* or the *right lymphatic duct*. The entire left side of the body, lower abdomen and pelvic area, and lower extremities are drained by the thoracic duct. Only the right side of the head, right upper extremity, and right thoracic area are drained by the right lymphatic duct. The lymph from the thoracic duct is returned to the bloodstream.

DEFINITIONS

lymphatic trunk. Large vessel created when multiple lymphatic vessels combine.

right lymphatic duct. Large vessel that drains lymph from the lymphatic vessels and trunks of the head, right upper extremity, and right thoracic area.

thoracic duct. Large vessel that drains lymph from the lymphatic vessels and trunks of the left side of the body, lower abdomen and pelvic area, and lower extremities.

Figure 9.2: Lymphatic System

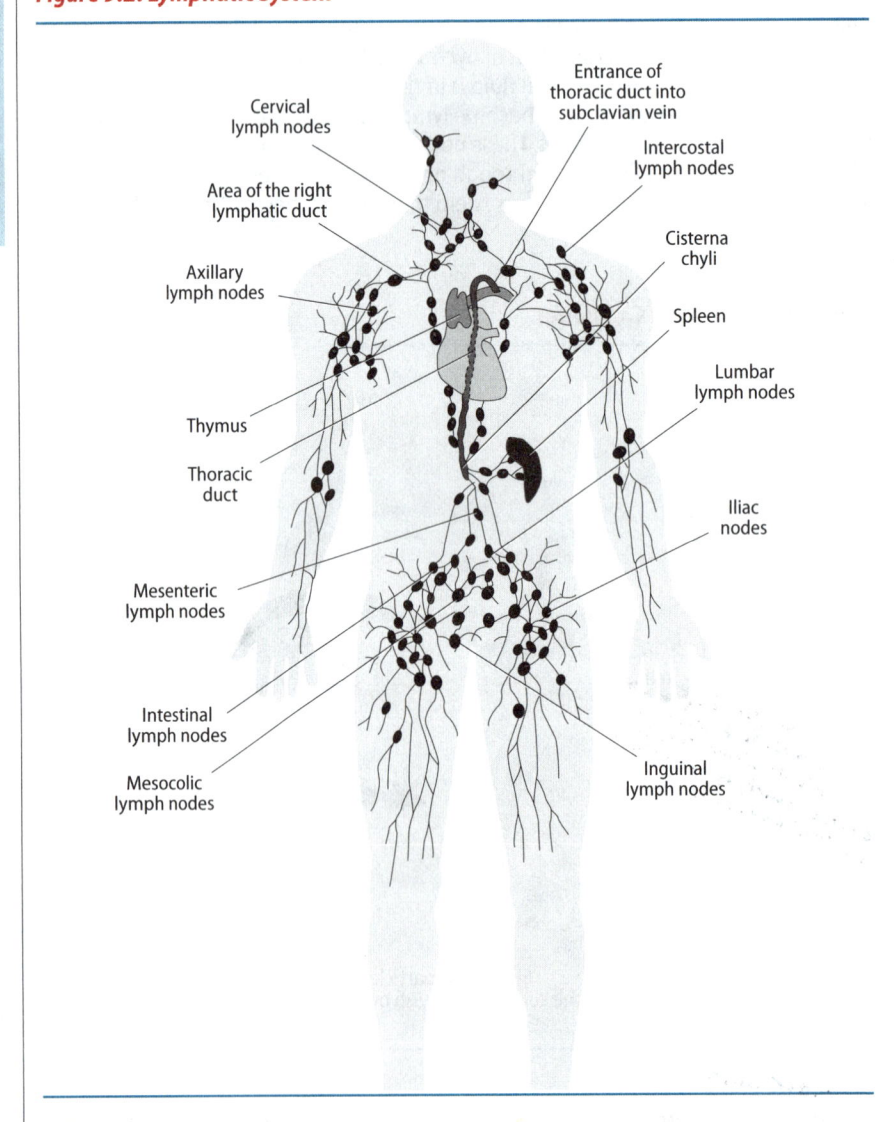

Immune response occurs primarily in the secondary lymphatic organs and tissues, lymph nodes, spleen, and lymphatic nodes. The primary lymphatic organs and tissues include red bone marrow production areas and the thymus.

Chapter 9. ICD-10-CM: Lymphatic System

Lymphatic Structures

Thymus

The thymus is located in the upper part of the chest, right beneath the sternum. The thymus contains large numbers of **T-cells** and is larger in infancy and childhood than in adulthood. Immature T-cells move from the red bone marrow to the thymus, where they multiply and mature. Epithelial cells in the thymus help the T-cells learn to differentiate between the body's cells and foreign matter. Mature T-cells can be found in the lymph nodes, spleen, and lymphatic tissue. **Dendritic cells**, also contained in the thymus, are important to immune response. **Microphages** within the thymus help to remove dead and dying cells.

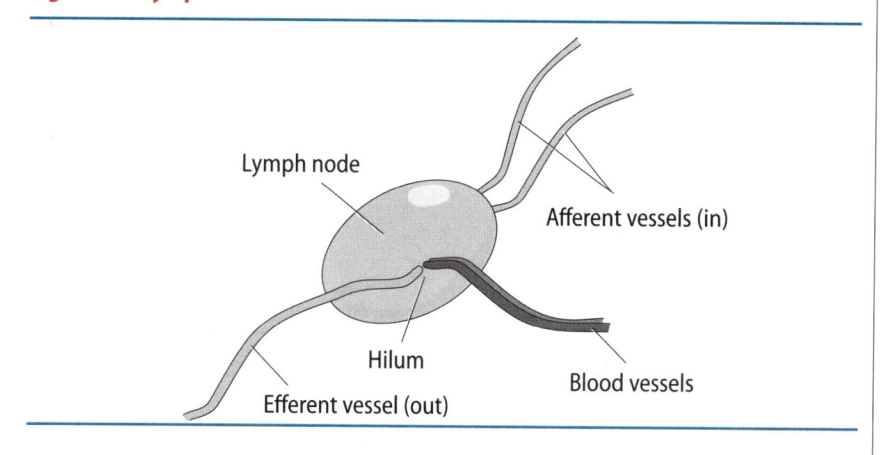

> **INTERESTING A & P FACT**
>
> The thymus is quite large in infancy and childhood; however, after puberty the thymus begins to shrink.

Figure 9.3: Thyroid Gland

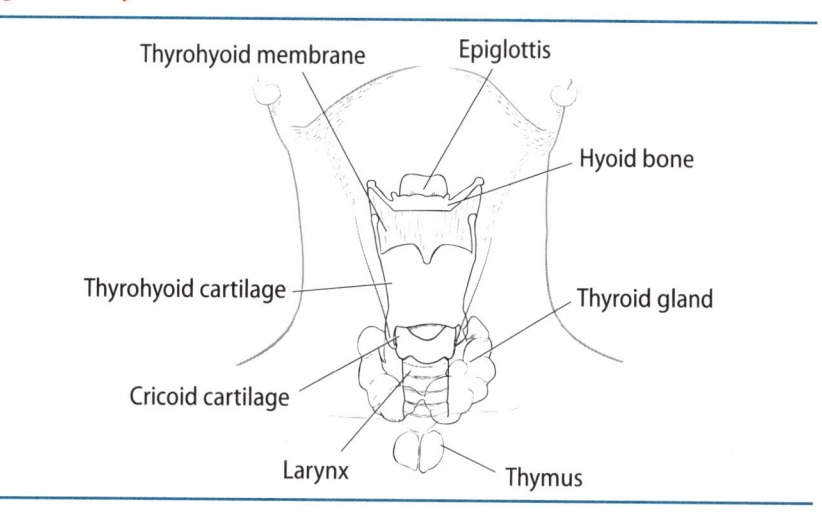

Thyrohyoid membrane
Epiglottis
Hyoid bone
Thyrohyoid cartilage
Thyroid gland
Cricoid cartilage
Larynx
Thymus

> **DEFINITIONS**
>
> **dendritic cells.** Antigen-presenting cells (APC) that activate T-cells, capture antigens, and help to create immunological memory with B-cells.
>
> **microphage.** Small phagocyte that ingests foreign matter and other small things like dead tissue and cells.
>
> **T-cells.** Type of lymphocyte that matures in the thymus and aids in adaptive immunity by destroying infected cells or activating an immune response. T-cell levels are an indicator of health for HIV/AIDS, some types of leukemia, and other diseases.

Lymph Nodes

There are approximately 600 lymph nodes in the body with greater groupings occurring in the axillae, near the mammary glands, and groin. It is important to realize that lymph nodes may be superficial or deep and that the lymph fluid flows one way only through the node. Foreign substances are trapped as they enter the lymph node. Macrocytes destroy some of the foreign material, and lymphocytes destroy other material through the immune response. Multiple lymphatic vessels may feed into a single lymph node that may terminate in one or more vessels.

Figure 9.4: Lymph Node

Lymph node
Afferent vessels (in)
Hilum
Efferent vessel (out)
Blood vessels

© 2015 Optum360, LLC

245

Figure 9.5: Axillary Lymph Nodes

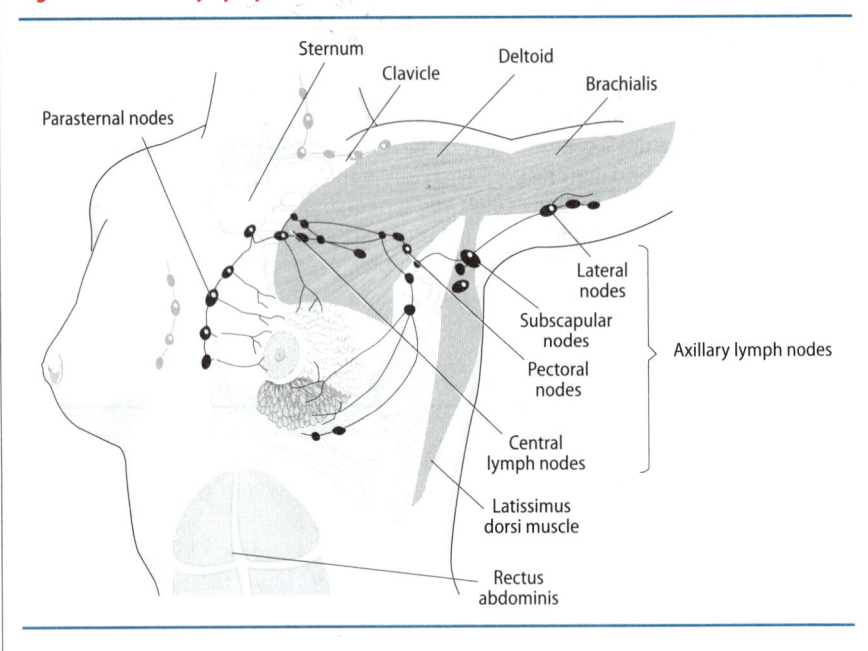

Spleen

The spleen is made up of lymphatic tissue, the splenic artery, the splenic vein, and efferent lymphatic vessels. The lymphatic tissue contains lymphocytes and microphages called white pulp. The white pulp surrounds central arteries that branch off the splenic artery. The spleen also contains areas termed red pulp, which is made up of splenic cords or tissue that contains microphages, lymphocytes, red blood cells, plasma cells, and granulocytes. Red pulp also has venous sinuses that are filled with blood.

Blood enters the venous sinuses via the splenic artery, where the surrounding white pulp contains the B and T-cells that provide the immune response and microphages that eradicate pathogens. The red pulp stores up to a third of the body's platelet supply and eliminates worn-out or bad cells and platelets by microphages.

Figure 9.6: Lymph Nodes of Trunk

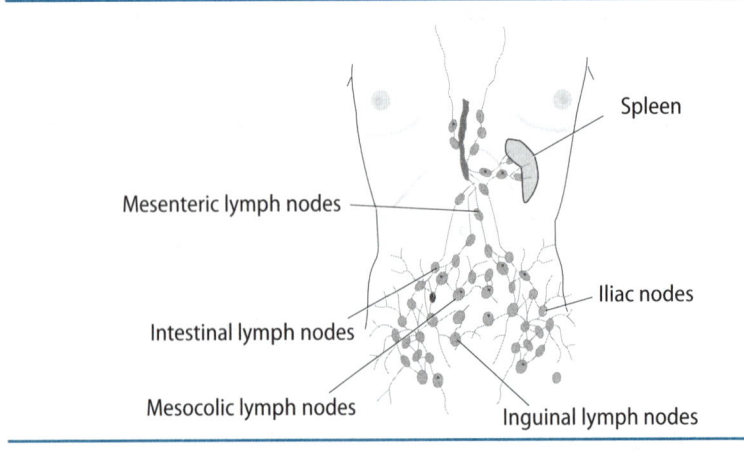

Lymphatic Nodules

Lymph nodes are encapsulated, whereas nodules are not encapsulated. Lymphatic nodules are found in connective tissue such as:

- Gastrointestinal lining
- Reproductive tract
- Respiratory airway
- Urinary tract

In the gastrointestinal lining, lymphatic nodules begin the process of transporting dietary lipids within the lymphatic system. These lipids are transported to the venous blood system.

Figure 9.7: Lymphatic Drainage

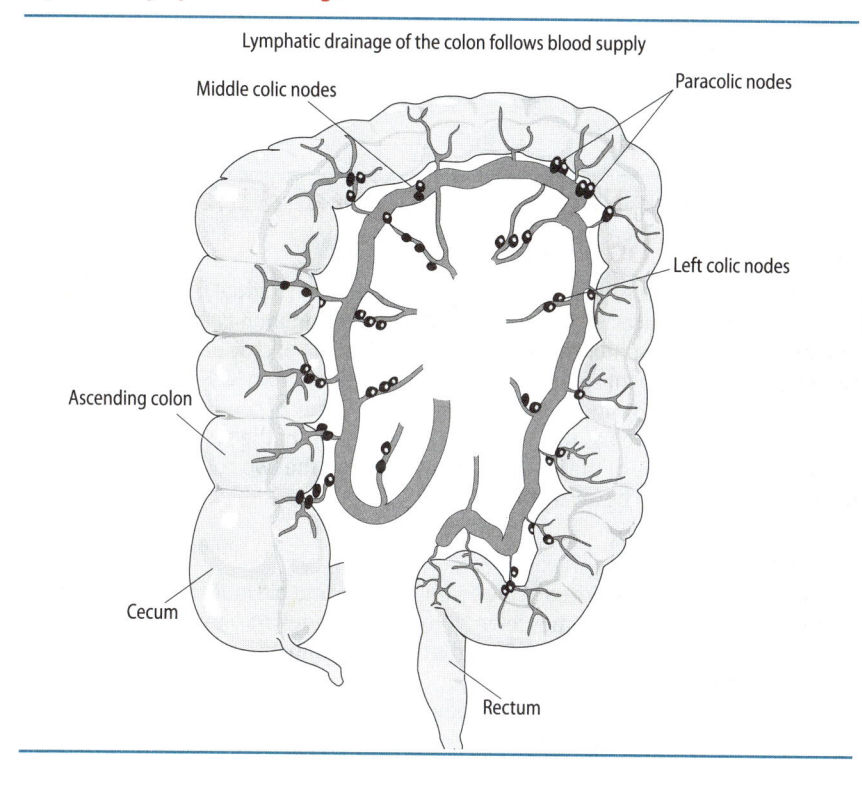

Lymphatic drainage of the colon follows blood supply
- Middle colic nodes
- Paracolic nodes
- Left colic nodes
- Ascending colon
- Cecum
- Rectum

Lymphatic nodules may be solitary or they may be larger masses of nodules. Most notable among the lymphatic nodules are:

- Adenoids
- Lingual tonsils
- Palatine tonsils
- Peyer's patches (in the ileum)
- Pharyngeal tonsil

Lymphatic nodules help the immune system fight foreign substances that are inhaled or ingested.

> ✓ **QUICK TIP**
>
> Diseases of the tonsils are found in the Respiratory chapter.

Figure 9.8: Tongue

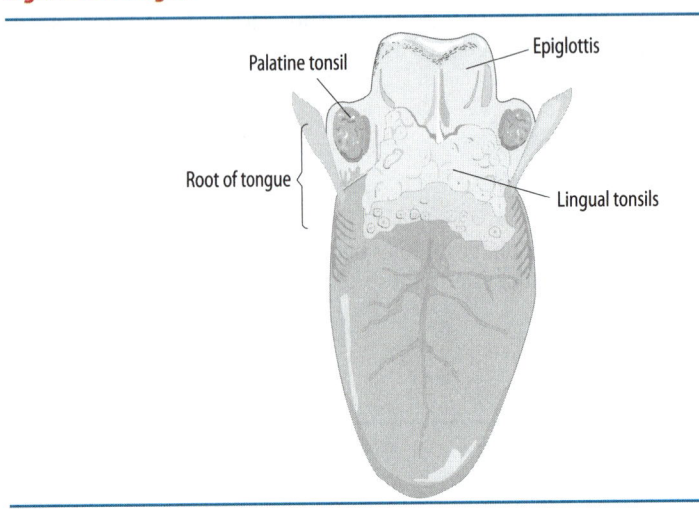

Anatomy and Pathophysiology and the ICD-10-CM Code Set

The primary goals of the lymphatic system are to move interstitial fluid throughout the body to help maintain fluid balance, and to provide immunity from foreign matter that may try to enter the body and cause damage and disease. The lymphatic system also helps prevent some cancers. In the transition from ICD-9-CM to ICD-10-CM, coders must understand the pathophysiology of conditions affecting the lymphatic system, as well as the anatomy and pathology of the system itself. This section discusses some of the key differences between the two code sets and points out important items to be aware of.

Lymphatic Cancer

Lymphatic cancer is categorized as **Hodgkin's lymphoma** or Hodgkin's disease and all other **lymphomas**, sometimes referred to as non-Hodgkin's lymphomas. Reticulosarcoma, lymphosarcoma, Burkitt's tumor, marginal zone lymphoma, mantle cell, and large cell lymphoma have a direct crosswalk to ICD-10-CM codes, although some descriptors use different terminology to describe the disease than was used in ICD-9-CM. ICD-10-CM tends to use the cell type, as opposed to the "disease name," to describe the malignancy. Primary central nervous system, anaplastic large cell, and other variants of lymphoma may require additional information in the medical record, as well as require the coder to understand additional information about the patient's disease process, to appropriately report these services under ICD-10-CM.

To code primary central nervous system lymphomas in ICD-10-CM, the lymphoma must be specified as diffuse large B-cell or nonfollicular lymphoma.

Hodgkin's lymphoma is a malignancy of the lymphatic system that may initially present with localized swelling of the lymph nodes. As the disease progresses, the swelling may become more generalized, spread to the spleen, and even involve the liver. Hodgkin's lymphoma is differentiated by the presence of a specific cell type, Reed-Sternberg. Hodgkin's lymphoma is further divided into lymphocyte-rich classical and nodular lymphocyte predominant types, as is demonstrated in the table below. Code selection is based upon the site and type of lymphatic cells.

DEFINITIONS

Hodgkin's lymphoma. Malignant disorder of lymphoid cells, characterized by the presence of progressively swollen lymph nodes and spleen; may also involve the liver.

lymphoma. Tumors occurring in the lymphoid tissues that are most commonly malignant.

CODING AXIOM

As with other neoplasms, the correct diagnosis code for all lymphomas depends on the affected sites.

Coding for Hodgkin's Disease

ICD-9-CM		ICD-10-CM	
201.40	Hodgkin's disease, lymphocytic-histiocytic predominance, unspecified site, extranodal and solid organ sites	C81.00	Nodular lymphocyte predominant Hodgkin lymphoma, unspecified site
		C81.09	Nodular lymphocyte predominant Hodgkin lymphoma, extranodal and solid organ sites
		C81.40	Lymphocyte-rich classical Hodgkin lymphoma, unspecified site
		C81.49	Lymphocyte-rich classical Hodgkin lymphoma, extranodal and solid organ sites
201.41	Hodgkin's disease, lymphocytic-histiocytic predominance of lymph nodes of head, face, and neck	C81.01	Nodular lymphocyte predominant Hodgkin lymphoma, lymph nodes of head, face, and neck
		C81.41	Lymphocyte-rich classical Hodgkin lymphoma, lymph nodes of head, face, and neck
201.42	Hodgkin's disease, lymphocytic-histiocytic predominance of intrathoracic lymph nodes	C81.02	Nodular lymphocyte predominant Hodgkin lymphoma, intrathoracic lymph nodes
		C81.42	Lymphocyte-rich classical Hodgkin lymphoma, intrathoracic lymph nodes
201.43	Hodgkin's disease, lymphocytic-histiocytic predominance of intra-abdominal lymph nodes	C81.03	Nodular lymphocyte predominant Hodgkin lymphoma, intra-abdominal lymph nodes
		C81.43	Lymphocyte-rich classical Hodgkin lymphoma, intra-abdominal lymph nodes
201.44	Hodgkin's disease, lymphocytic-histiocytic predominance of lymph nodes of axilla and upper limb	C81.04	Nodular lymphocyte predominant Hodgkin lymphoma, lymph nodes of axilla and upper limb
		C81.44	Lymphocyte-rich classical Hodgkin lymphoma, lymph nodes of axilla and upper limb
201.45	Hodgkin's disease, lymphocytic-histiocytic predominance of lymph nodes of inguinal region and lower limb	C81.05	Nodular lymphocyte predominant Hodgkin lymphoma, lymph nodes of inguinal region and lower limb
		C81.45	Lymphocyte-rich classical Hodgkin lymphoma, lymph nodes of inguinal region and lower limb
201.46	Hodgkin's disease, lymphocytic-histiocytic predominance of intrapelvic lymph nodes	C81.06	Nodular lymphocyte predominant Hodgkin lymphoma, intrapelvic lymph nodes
		C81.46	Lymphocyte-rich classical Hodgkin lymphoma, intrapelvic lymph nodes
201.47	Hodgkin's disease, lymphocytic-histiocytic predominance of spleen	C81.07	Nodular lymphocyte predominant Hodgkin lymphoma, spleen
		C81.47	Lymphocyte-rich classical Hodgkin lymphoma, spleen
201.48	Hodgkin's disease, lymphocytic-histiocytic predominance of lymph nodes of multiple sites	C81.08	Nodular lymphocyte predominant Hodgkin lymphoma, lymph nodes of multiple sites
		C81.48	Lymphocyte-rich classical Hodgkin lymphoma, lymph nodes of multiple sites

As previously discussed, lymphoma is reported as either Hodgkin's lymphoma or all other lymphomas. In ICD-10-CM, many of the lymphoma codes require additional information for reporting. However, there are exceptions, such as classical Hodgkin's lymphoma. These codes are separated in ICD-9-CM and reported according to the Hodgkin's lymphoma type: paragranuloma, granuloma, or sarcoma. In ICD-10-CM, they are grouped together as "classical Hodgkin's lymphoma" and are reported by site. Below is an example of this collapse of ICD-9-CM codes into a single ICD-10-CM code occurring in the head, face, and neck area.

> **KEY POINT**
>
> In ICD-10-CM, classical Hodgkin's lymphoma includes paragranuloma, granuloma, and sarcoma types.

Coding for Hodgkin's Paragranuloma

ICD-9-CM		ICD-10-CM	
201.01	Hodgkin's paragranuloma of lymph nodes of head, face, and neck	C81.71	Other classical Hodgkin lymphoma, lymph nodes of head, face, and neck
201.11	Hodgkin's granuloma of lymph nodes of head, face, and neck		
201.21	Hodgkin's sarcoma of lymph nodes of head, face, and neck		

Non-Hodgkin's lymphoma codes are selected based on the site of the affected cells and by cell type: large B-cell and other nonfollicular cell. **Diffuse large B-cell lymphoma is one of the most common of the lymphomas and is quite aggressive.** Standard therapy for this type of lymphoma includes one of several types of chemotherapy treatments.

Coding for Primary Central Nervous System Lymphoma

ICD-9-CM		ICD-10-CM	
200.50	Primary central nervous system lymphoma, unspecified site, extranodal and solid organ sites	C83.39	Diffuse large B-cell lymphoma, extranodal and solid organ sites
		C83.80	Other nonfollicular lymphoma, unspecified site
		C83.89	Other nonfollicular lymphoma, extranodal and solid organ sites
200.51	Primary central nervous system lymphoma, lymph nodes of head, face, and neck	C83.31	Diffuse large B-cell lymphoma, lymph nodes of head, face, and neck
		C83.81	Other nonfollicular lymphoma, lymph nodes of head, face, and neck
200.52	Primary central nervous system lymphoma, intrathoracic lymph nodes	C83.32	Diffuse large B-cell lymphoma, intrathoracic lymph nodes
		C83.82	Other nonfollicular lymphoma, intrathoracic lymph nodes
200.53	Primary central nervous system lymphoma, intra-abdominal lymph nodes	C83.33	Diffuse large B-cell lymphoma, intra-abdominal lymph nodes
		C83.83	Other nonfollicular lymphoma, intra-abdominal lymph nodes
200.54	Primary central nervous system lymphoma, lymph nodes of axilla and upper limb	C83.34	Diffuse large B-cell lymphoma, lymph nodes of axilla and upper limb
		C83.84	Other nonfollicular lymphoma, lymph nodes of axilla and upper limb
200.55	Primary central nervous system lymphoma, lymph nodes of inguinal region and lower limb	C83.35	Diffuse large B-cell lymphoma, lymph nodes of inguinal region and lower limb
		C83.85	Other nonfollicular lymphoma, lymph nodes of inguinal region and lower limb
200.56	Primary central nervous system lymphoma, intrapelvic lymph nodes	C83.36	Diffuse large B-cell lymphoma, intrapelvic lymph nodes
		C83.86	Other nonfollicular lymphoma, intrapelvic lymph nodes
200.57	Primary central nervous system lymphoma, spleen	C83.37	Diffuse large B-cell lymphoma, spleen
		C83.87	Other nonfollicular lymphoma, spleen
200.58	Primary central nervous system lymphoma, lymph nodes of multiple sites	C83.38	Diffuse large B-cell lymphoma, lymph nodes of multiple sites
		C83.88	Other nonfollicular lymphoma, lymph nodes of multiple sites

When reporting anaplastic large cell lymphoma in ICD-10-CM, it is necessary to identify whether the cells are anaplastic lymphoma kinase (ALK) positive or ALK negative. Those identified as ALK positive are believed to have a more positive prognosis, although treatment for both is similar. ALK is an enzyme, but the ALK gene is shown to be an "oncogene," having a direct link to many large cell lymphomas. ALK-positive patients are positive for this specific oncogene, whereas ALK-negative patients do not have this specific gene but still have the anaplastic large cell lymphoma.

Coding for Anaplastic Large Cell Lymphoma

ICD-9-CM		ICD-10-CM	
200.60	Anaplastic large cell lymphoma, unspecified site, extranodal and solid organ sites	C84.60	Anaplastic large cell lymphoma, ALK-positive, unspecified site
		C84.69	Anaplastic large cell lymphoma, ALK-positive, extranodal and solid organ sites
		C84.70	Anaplastic large cell lymphoma, ALK-negative, unspecified site
		C84.79	Anaplastic large cell lymphoma, ALK-negative, extranodal and solid organ sites
200.61	Anaplastic large cell lymphoma, lymph nodes of head, face, and neck	C84.61	Anaplastic large cell lymphoma, ALK-positive, lymph nodes of head, face, and neck
		C84.71	Anaplastic large cell lymphoma, ALK-negative, lymph nodes of head, face, and neck
200.62	Anaplastic large cell lymphoma, intrathoracic lymph nodes	C84.62	Anaplastic large cell lymphoma, ALK-positive, intrathoracic lymph nodes
		C84.72	Anaplastic large cell lymphoma, ALK-negative, intrathoracic lymph nodes
200.63	Anaplastic large cell lymphoma, intra-abdominal lymph nodes	C84.63	Anaplastic large cell lymphoma, ALK-positive, intra-abdominal lymph nodes
		C84.73	Anaplastic large cell lymphoma, ALK-negative, intra-abdominal lymph nodes
200.64	Anaplastic large cell lymphoma, lymph nodes of axilla and upper limb	C84.64	Anaplastic large cell lymphoma, ALK-positive, lymph nodes of axilla and upper limb
		C84.74	Anaplastic large cell lymphoma, ALK-negative, lymph nodes of axilla and upper limb

Variants of lymphoma and reticulosarcoma of the lymph nodes require further definition in ICD-10-CM. It is important to note if it is small cell, B-cell lymphoma, or other nonfollicular lymphoma. In ICD-9-CM, only the lymphoma or reticulosarcoma site is required. Due to the increased specificity in ICD-10-CM, there may be a learning curve for providers. Coders can help their providers understand the new levels of specificity in the ICD-10-CM code set. In some instances, a provider query may be needed to gather the additional information needed to code the condition properly.

Coding for Other Nonfollicular Lymphoma

ICD-9-CM		ICD-10-CM	
200.80	Other named variants of lymphosarcoma and reticulosarcoma, unspecified site, extranodal and solid organ sites	C83.00	Small cell B-cell lymphoma, unspecified site
		C83.09	Small cell B-cell lymphoma, extranodal and solid organ sites
		C83.80	Other non-follicular lymphoma, unspecified site
		C83.89	Other non-follicular lymphoma, extranodal and solid organ sites
		C83.90	Non-follicular (diffuse) lymphoma, unspecified, unspecified site
		C83.99	Non-follicular (diffuse) lymphoma, unspecified, extranodal and solid organ sites
		C86.5	Angioimmunoblastic T-cell lymphoma
		C86.6	Primary cutaneous CD30-positive T-cell proliferations
200.81	Other named variants of lymphosarcoma and reticulosarcoma of lymph nodes of head, face, and neck	C83.01	Small cell B-cell lymphoma, lymph nodes of head, face, and neck
		C83.81	Other non-follicular lymphoma, lymph nodes of head, face, and neck
		C83.91	Non-follicular (diffuse) lymphoma, unspecified, lymph nodes of head, face, and neck
200.82	Other named variants of lymphosarcoma and reticulosarcoma of intrathoracic lymph nodes	C83.02	Small cell B-cell lymphoma, intrathoracic lymph nodes
		C83.82	Other non-follicular lymphoma, intrathoracic lymph nodes
		C83.92	Non-follicular (diffuse) lymphoma, unspecified, intrathoracic lymph nodes
200.83	Other named variants of lymphosarcoma and reticulosarcoma of intra-abdominal lymph nodes	C83.03	Small cell B-cell lymphoma, intra-abdominal lymph nodes
		C83.83	Other non-follicular (diffuse) lymphoma, intra-abdominal lymph nodes
		C83.93	Non-follicular (diffuse) lymphoma, unspecified, intra-abdominal lymph nodes
200.84	Other named variants of lymphosarcoma and reticulosarcoma of lymph nodes of axilla and upper limb	C83.04	Small cell B-cell lymphoma, lymph nodes of axilla and upper limb
		C83.84	Other non-follicular lymphoma, lymph nodes of axilla and upper limb
		C83.94	Non-follicular (diffuse) lymphoma, unspecified, lymph nodes of axilla and upper limb
200.85	Other named variants of lymphosarcoma and reticulosarcoma of lymph nodes of inguinal region and lower limb	C83.05	Small cell B-cell lymphoma, lymph nodes of inguinal region and lower limb
		C83.85	Other non-follicular lymphoma, lymph nodes of inguinal region and lower limb
		C83.95	Non-follicular (diffuse) lymphoma, unspecified, lymph nodes of inguinal region and lower limb
200.86	Other named variants of lymphosarcoma and reticulosarcoma of intrapelvic lymph nodes	C83.06	Small cell B-cell lymphoma, intrapelvic lymph nodes
		C83.86	Other non-follicular lymphoma, intrapelvic lymph nodes
		C83.96	Non-follicular (diffuse) lymphoma, unspecified, intrapelvic lymph nodes
200.87	Other named variants of lymphosarcoma and reticulosarcoma of spleen	C83.07	Small cell B-cell lymphoma, spleen
		C83.87	Other non-follicular lymphoma, spleen
		C83.97	Non-follicular (diffuse) lymphoma, unspecified, spleen

ICD-9-CM		ICD-10-CM	
200.88	Other named variants of lymphosarcoma and reticulosarcoma of lymph nodes of multiple sites	C83.08	Small cell B-cell lymphoma, lymph nodes of multiple sites
		C83.88	Other non-follicular lymphoma, lymph nodes of multiple sites
		C83.98	Non-follicular (diffuse) lymphoma, unspecified, lymph nodes of multiple sites

Follicular lymphoma is a form of non-Hodgkin's lymphoma characterized by specific types of tumors. These tumors are made up of follicles that contain cells called centroblasts and centrocytes. In ICD-10-CM, nodular lymphoma is specified by lymphoma type. Codes specify the grade of follicular lymphoma (I, II, III, IIIa, IIIb) and whether it is diffuse follicle, cutaneous follicle, other types of follicular lymphoma, or unspecified follicular lymphoma. Note that the term nodular is not included in these codes. Although there is some controversy over the grading system, the World Health Organization recommends the following:

- Grade I: < 5 centroblasts per high power field
- Grade II: 6–15 centroblasts per high power field
- Grade III: > 15 centroblasts per high power field
    - grade IIIa: centrocytes are still present
    - grade IIIb: follicles consist almost entirely of centroblasts

The following table illustrates how these codes are reported in ICD-10-CM. This table is not all-inclusive of the nodular lymphoma codes but gives the coder an idea of what to expect.

Coding for Nodular Lymphoma

ICD-9-CM		ICD-10-CM	
202.00	Nodular lymphoma, unspecified site, extranodal and solid organ sites	C82.00	Follicular lymphoma grade I, unspecified site
		C82.09	Follicular lymphoma grade I, extranodal and solid organ sites
		C82.10	Follicular lymphoma grade II, unspecified site
		C82.19	Follicular lymphoma grade II, extranodal and solid organ sites
		C82.20	Follicular lymphoma grade III, unspecified, unspecified site
		C82.29	Follicular lymphoma grade III, unspecified, extranodal and solid organ sites
		C82.30	Follicular lymphoma grade IIIa, unspecified site
		C82.39	Follicular lymphoma grade IIIa, extranodal and solid organ sites
		C82.40	Follicular lymphoma grade IIIb, unspecified site
		C82.49	Follicular lymphoma grade IIIb, extranodal and solid organ sites
		C82.60	Cutaneous follicle center lymphoma, unspecified site
		C82.69	Cutaneous follicle center lymphoma, extranodal and solid organ sites
		C82.80	Other types of follicular lymphoma, unspecified site
		C82.89	Other types of follicular lymphoma, extranodal and solid organ sites
		C82.90	Follicular lymphoma, unspecified, unspecified site
		C82.99	Follicular lymphoma, unspecified, extranodal and solid organ sites

> *[handwritten note: extranodal when lymphoma is believed to have originated the lymph nodes]*

Other malignant lymphomas are reported only by site in ICD-9-CM. However, in ICD-10-CM, the type of lymphoma needs to be indicated—B-cell, large B-cell, or non-Hodgkin's lymphoma—and the lymphoma site must be identified to select a final diagnosis code. The following table contains an example of a "generic" ICD-9-CM code that links to more specific ICD-10-CM codes. These types of examples are found throughout the ICD-10-CM manual.

Blastic NK-cell lymphoma is a very rare and aggressive form of lymphoma that affects the natural killer cells of the immune system. In the early stages, patients often present with skin lesions and lymphadenopathy, and this disease typically affects elderly patients. Unfortunately, the condition is resistant to most of the common lymphoma treatments: chemotherapy, radiation therapy, and bone marrow transplantation. Prognosis tends to be poor for most patients diagnosed with blastic NK-cell lymphoma.

Coding for Other Malignant Lymphomas

ICD-9-CM		ICD-10-CM	
202.80	Other malignant lymphomas, unspecified site, extranodal and solid organ sites	C85.10	Unspecified B-cell lymphoma, unspecified site
		C85.19	Unspecified B-cell lymphoma, extranodal and solid organ sites
		C85.20	Mediastinal (thymic) large B-cell lymphoma, unspecified site
		C85.29	Mediastinal (thymic) large B-cell lymphoma, extranodal and solid organ sites
		C85.80	Other specified types of non-Hodgkin lymphoma, unspecified site
		C85.89	Other specified types of non-Hodgkin lymphoma, extranodal and solid organ sites
		C85.90	Non-Hodgkin lymphoma, unspecified, unspecified site
		C85.99	Non-Hodgkin lymphoma, unspecified, extranodal and solid organ sites
		C86.4	Blastic NK-cell lymphoma
202.81	Other malignant lymphomas of lymph nodes of head, face, and neck	C85.11	Unspecified B-cell lymphoma, lymph nodes of head, face, and neck
		C85.21	Mediastinal (thymic) large B-cell lymphoma, lymph nodes of head, face, and neck
		C85.81	Other specified types of non-Hodgkin lymphoma, lymph nodes of head, face, and neck
		C85.91	Non-Hodgkin lymphoma, unspecified, lymph nodes of head, face, and neck
		C86.0	Extranodal NK/T-cell lymphoma, nasal type
202.82	Other malignant lymphomas of intrathoracic lymph nodes	C82.52	Diffuse follicle center lymphoma, intrathoracic lymph nodes
		C84.92	Mature T/NK-cell lymphomas, unspecified, intrathoracic lymph nodes
		C85.12	Unspecified B-cell lymphoma, intrathoracic lymph nodes
		C85.22	Mediastinal (thymic) large B-cell lymphoma, intrathoracic lymph nodes
		C85.82	Other specified types of non-Hodgkin lymphoma, intrathoracic lymph nodes
		C85.92	Non-Hodgkin lymphoma, unspecified, intrathoracic lymph nodes

ICD-9-CM		ICD-10-CM	
202.83	Other malignant lymphomas of intra-abdominal lymph nodes	C85.13	Unspecified B-cell lymphoma, intra-abdominal lymph nodes
		C85.23	Mediastinal (thymic) large B-cell lymphoma, intra-abdominal lymph nodes
		C85.83	Other specified types of non-Hodgkin lymphoma, intra-abdominal lymph nodes
		C85.93	Non-Hodgkin lymphoma, unspecified, intra-abdominal lymph nodes
		C86.2	Enteropathy-type (intestinal) T-cell lymphoma
		C86.3	Subcutaneous panniculitis-like T-cell lymphoma

Lymphatic Disease

Sarcoidosis begins as inflammation and progresses to clusters of cells referred to as granulomas. Granulomas in general are typically a collection of immune cells that have attempted to wall off substances they deem foreign. In sarcoidosis, granulomas typically contain star-shaped structures called Schaumann bodies. The most common sites for sarcoidosis are the lymph nodes of the chest, skin, or lungs; however, it can also be found in the eyes, liver, brain, and heart. Nearly 66 percent of all patients may be termed as in remission within 10 years. Löfgren's syndrome, a frequent symptom of sarcoidosis, is also reported with ICD-9-CM code 135; however, a specific index or tabular reference is not yet available in ICD-10-CM. Sarcoidosis is differentiated according to the specific site.

Coding for Sarcoidosis

ICD-9-CM		ICD-10-CM	
135	Sarcoidosis	D86.1	Sarcoidosis of lymph nodes
		D86.2	Sarcoidosis of lung with sarcoidosis of lymph nodes
		D86.89	Sarcoidosis of other sites
		D86.9	Sarcoidosis, unspecified

Lymphadenitis, inflammation of the lymph nodes, is often localized and changes in the ICD-10-CM code set require that the location be identified. Note that coding only for acute conditions, not chronic lymphadenitis, calls for this additional information. In ICD-9-CM, rubric 289 is used to report chronic disease, and I88.0 through I88.9 is used in ICD-10-CM.

When reporting acute lymphadenitis, the site of the inflamed lymph nodes is used to determine the correct ICD-10-CM code.

Coding for Acute Lymphadenitis

ICD-9-CM		ICD-10-CM	
683	Acute lymphadenitis	L04.0	Acute lymphadenitis of face, head and neck
		L04.1	Acute lymphadenitis of trunk
		L04.2	Acute lymphadenitis of upper limb
		L04.3	Acute lymphadenitis of lower limb
		L04.8	Acute lymphadenitis of other sites
		L04.9	Acute lymphadenitis, unspecified

Enlargement of the lymph nodes without inflammation is reported with ICD-9-CM code 785.6. ICD-10-CM requires additional information about the nature of the enlarged lymph nodes, however. The term lymphadenopathy may also be used in the provider's documentation to describe this condition. Although there is not an "official" standard to follow, commonly "localized" describes the enlargement of lymph nodes in a single area of the body. "Generalized" describes the enlargement of lymph nodes in two or more areas of the body.

Coding for Enlargement of Lymph Nodes

ICD-9-CM		ICD-10-CM	
785.6	Enlargement of lymph nodes	R59.0	Localized enlarged lymph nodes
		R59.1	Generalized enlarged lymph nodes
		R59.9	Enlarged lymph nodes, unspecified

Immunity

The lymphatic system is integral to the body's immunity. The specificity for ICD-10-CM includes more detail to further define the type of immunity deficiency disorders than does ICD-9-CM.

Severe combined immunodeficiency disease (SCID) is characterized by a complete lack of or a significant deficiency of B-cells and T-cells in the body, which results in a lack of humoral and cell-mediated immunity in the body. It is somewhat commonly known as "Bubble boy syndrome," as one of the more famous cases occurred in the 1970s and 1980s involving a young boy who lived for 12 years in a germ-free plastic bubble. This disease is typically diagnosed in the first 3 to 6 months of life, when the patient's susceptibility to infection becomes obvious.

Major histocompatibility complex class I and class II are the two primary classes of human leukocyte antigens in genetic makeup that code proteins to assist in our immune response. Class I antigens are found on the surface of all nucleated cells. Class II antigens are found only on immunocompetent T-cells, such as macrophages and B-cells. A deficiency of this antigen significantly affects our immune response.

Hyperimmunoglobulin E (IgE) syndrome is a rare immunodeficiency disease, characterized by several symptoms, including multiple recurrent skin abscesses, upper respiratory issues such as pneumonia, high serum levels of IgE, issues related to teeth, and various other concerns. It is sometimes called Job syndrome, as originally it was thought that these patients were reminiscent of the biblical character Job, whose body was covered with boils by Satan. Treatment usually involves control of infections, although there is no single treatment for this condition.

Immune reconstitution syndrome is a condition that typically affects patients with immunosuppression or AIDS, whereby the immune system begins to recover and during that recovery responds to some type of a previously acquired infection with an overwhelming inflammatory response, making the infection worse. In some cases, the resulting inflammation can be quite dangerous to the patient and needs treatment. However, in many cases, this response often means that the body has a better chance to fight the infection than it did previously. There is no best treatment known for this condition.

Coding for Immunity Deficiency

ICD-9-CM		ICD-10-CM	
279.2	Combined immunity deficiency	D81.0	Severe combined immunodeficiency [SCID] with reticular dysgenesis
		D81.1	Severe combined immunodeficiency [SCID] with low T- and B-cell numbers
		D81.2	Severe combined immunodeficiency [SCID] with low or normal B-cell numbers
		D81.6	Major histocompatibility complex class I deficiency
		D81.7	Major histocompatibility complex class II deficiency
		D81.89	Other combined immunodeficiencies
		D81.9	Combined immunodeficiency, unspecified

ICD-9-CM		ICD-10-CM	
279.8	Other specified disorders involving the immune mechanism	D82.2	Immunodeficiency with short-limbed stature
		D82.3	Immunodeficiency following hereditary defective response to Epstein-Barr virus
		D82.4	Hyperimmunoglobulin E [IgE] syndrome
		D82.8	Immunodeficiency associated with other specified major defects
		D82.9	Immunodeficiency associated with major defect, unspecified
		D84.0	Lymphocyte function antigen-1 [LFA-1] defect
		D84.1	Defects in the complement system
		D89.3	Immune reconstitution syndrome
		D89.89	Other specified disorders involving the immune mechanism, not elsewhere classified
		M35.9	Systemic involvement of connective tissue, unspecified

When using ICD-10-CM codes to report mononucleosis, another immune disorder, more information is required from the documentation, including the type of virus causing mononucleosis and the absence or presence of complications. This may require additional information from the laboratory, which may delay coding.

Coding for Infectious Mononucleosis

ICD-9-CM		ICD-10-CM	
075	Infectious mononucleosis	B27.00	Gammaherpesviral mononucleosis without complication
		B27.09	Gammaherpesviral mononucleosis with other complications
		B27.10	Cytomegaloviral mononucleosis without complications
		B27.19	Cytomegaloviral mononucleosis with other complication
		B27.80	Other infectious mononucleosis without complication
		B27.89	Other infectious mononucleosis with other complication
		B27.90	Infectious mononucleosis, unspecified without complication
		B27.99	Infectious mononucleosis, unspecified with other complication

Spleen

Splenic sequestration and other diseases of the spleen are more detailed in ICD-10-CM than in ICD-9-CM. In ICD-10-CM, splenic sequestration codes depend on the type of sickle cell disorder and other splenic diseases depend on the type of disease.

Splenic sequestration is caused when the red blood cells become trapped in the spleen, which causes a significant decrease in the hemoglobin level in the body. This can cause the patient to go into hypovolemic shock and is a leading cause of death in children with sickle cell disease.

Coding for Splenic Sequestration

ICD-9-CM		ICD-10-CM	
289.52	Splenic sequestration	D57.02	Hb-SS disease with splenic sequestration
		D57.212	Sickle-cell/Hb-C disease with splenic sequestration
		D57.412	Sickle-cell thalassemia with splenic sequestration
		D57.812	Other sickle-cell disorders with splenic sequestration

Hyposplenism describes a reduction in the spleen function. An <u>infarction</u> of the spleen occurs when the oxygen supply to the spleen is interrupted in some way, typically due to the splenic artery's being occluded. This interruption in the oxygen supply causes tissue death in various areas of the spleen.

[Handwritten note: obstruction of blood supply to an organ or region of tissue]

Coding for Other Diseases of the Spleen

ICD-9-CM		ICD-10-CM	
289.59	Other diseases of spleen	D73.0	Hyposplenism
		D73.3	Abscess of spleen
		D73.4	Cyst of spleen
		D73.5	Infarction of spleen
		D73.89	Other diseases of spleen

Summary

The lymphatic system moves interstitial fluid throughout the body to help maintain fluid balance, transport lipids, and help the body fight off disease. The lymphatic system does not have a specific section in the ICD-9-CM or ICD-10-CM manual; codes are spread throughout the various sections. Coders and providers must increase their knowledge of lymphatic system diseases to correctly report the lymphatic conditions described in the ICD-10-CM manual.

Chapter 10. ICD-10-CM: Respiratory System

Anatomic Overview

The respiratory system comprises all the organs and structures involved in breathing. Oxygen is inhaled and carbon dioxide is expelled. Any malfunction within this process can lead to cell death within the tissues of the various organs of the body by reducing the amount of oxygen distributed to these organs or causing excess waste within the body's tissues. The *capillary* blood vessels enable the body to balance the fluid within every cell of the body. The respiratory system also helps regulate pH in the blood, as well as playing a vital role in our sense of smell and ability to vocalize sounds.

Function of the Respiratory System

When air enters the body through the nose or mouth, the *diaphragm* tightens, allowing more room within the chest cavity for the lungs to expand and take in the air. The *intercostal muscles* also contract, lifting the rib cage and helping to enlarge the area. The air moves into the lungs and *bronchial tubes*, reaching the *alveoli*. Running by these alveoli are capillaries carrying blood that has traveled through the body and been pumped from the right side of the heart through the pulmonary artery and then into capillaries. The alveoli transport the oxygen to the capillaries where hemoglobin helps it flow into the bloodstream. As the oxygen is absorbed, the carbon dioxide is extracted from the capillaries into the alveoli and is exhaled as a waste gas. The oxygenated blood then travels through the pulmonary vein to the left side of the heart, which pumps it to the rest of the body.

When the diaphragm and intercostal muscles relax, they minimize the space within the chest cavity. This causes air rich in carbon dioxide to leave the body.

The respiratory center in the brain stem sends signals via the spinal cord and nerves to the muscles responsible for breathing, allowing for regular function. This is not to say that a person cannot change his or her own breathing pattern voluntarily, such as during exercise, holding of breath, or when outside emotional factors warrant an increase or decrease in airflow. The body is also built with internal sensors that may adjust breathing as needed. For example, the brain works with the *carotid artery* and *aorta* to determine adequate levels of oxygen and carbon dioxide within the bloodstream. In addition, air passages can detect the presence of foreign matter that can cause problems, thus promoting a cough or sneeze to eliminate the foreign matter.

Functional Anatomy of the Respiratory System

There are two main parts to the respiratory system. The upper respiratory tract, situated above the chest, contains the nose, pharynx, and larynx. The lower respiratory tract, located within the chest, contains the trachea, bronchial tree, and the lungs.

DEFINITIONS

alveoli. Last structure within the lung and the primary spot for gas exchange between the lungs and capillaries.

aorta. Largest artery in the body. It is connected to the left ventricle of the heart and progresses through the thorax, leading to the abdomen, and divides into smaller branches to reach other parts of the body.

bronchial tubes. Part of the respiratory structure connecting the lungs to the trachea, allowing for air exchange within the lungs.

capillary. Tiny, minute blood vessel that connects the arterioles (smallest arteries) and the venules (smallest veins) and acts as a semipermeable membrane between the blood and the tissue fluid.

carotid arteries. Two blood vessels on either side of the neck just below the jaw that supply blood to the brain.

diaphragm. Muscular wall separating the thorax and its structures from the abdomen.

intercostal muscles. Muscles within the rib cage responsible for movement when breathing.

Comprehensive Anatomy and Physiology for ICD-10-CM and ICD-10-PCS Coding

> **INTERESTING A & P FACT**
>
> The respiratory system has two operational parts: The conducting zone filters the air we take in and distributes it to the lungs; the respiratory zone is responsible for the gas exchange between the air and bloodstream.

Figure 10.1: Lower Respiratory System

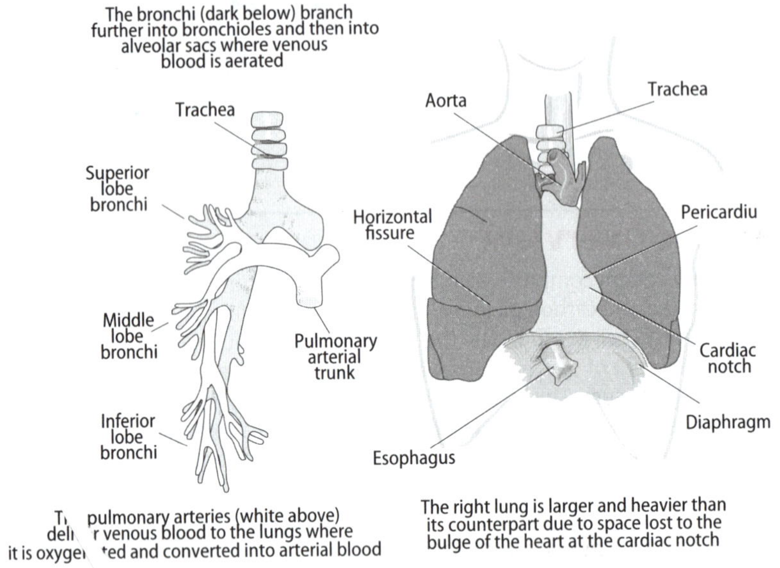

The bronchi (dark below) branch further into bronchioles and then into alveolar sacs where venous blood is aerated

Labels: Trachea, Superior lobe bronchi, Middle lobe bronchi, Inferior lobe bronchi, Pulmonary arterial trunk, Horizontal fissure, Aorta, Trachea, Pericardium, Cardiac notch, Diaphragm, Esophagus

The pulmonary arteries (white above) deliver venous blood to the lungs where it is oxygenated and converted into arterial blood

The right lung is larger and heavier than its counterpart due to space lost to the bulge of the heart at the cardiac notch

---

> **DEFINITIONS**
>
> **cartilage.** Nonvascular, fibrous, connective tissue that supports body tissues. Cartilage is less solid than bone.
>
> **hyoid bone.** Single, U-shaped bone palpable in the neck above the larynx and below the mandible (lower jaw) with various muscles attached but not articulating with any other bone.
>
> **lingual tonsils.** Tonsils positioned at the base of the tongue that house lymph nodes and become inflamed from bacterial or viral infections.
>
> **palatine tonsils.** Tonsils seen at the back of the mouth and considered one of the body's primary defenses against infections of the respiratory and digestive systems.
>
> **turbinates.** Shell-shaped elevations along the wall of the nasal cavity. The inferior turbinate is a separate bone, while the superior and middle turbinates are part of the ethmoid bone.

The nose is made up of bone and **cartilage** covered with skin on the outside and mucous membrane on the inside. Within the nose there are hairs known as cilia that catch germs and other particles inhaled with air. The internal nose comprises the paranasal sinuses and nasolacrimal ducts located over the roof of the mouth separated by the palatine bones. The nasal cavity is split by the septum and opens inside the nostrils, leading to the **turbinate** and then to the pharynx.

The paranasal sinuses are lined with mucous membranes that help produce secretions that drain into the nasal cavity. The sinuses provide a means to produce sound by serving as resonating chambers.

The pharynx, or throat, sends food into the esophagus and air into the larynx. This structure is positioned posterior to the oral cavity and runs between the nasal cavities and larynx. The pharynx is broken down into three parts: nasopharynx, oropharynx, and laryngopharynx. The oropharynx and laryngopharynx are considered part of the respiratory system, as well as the digestive system. The nasopharynx is situated just above the pharynx behind the nasal cavity leading to the soft palate. The soft palate is a moveable muscular structure at the back of the mouth that closes the nasal cavity when swallowing occurs.

There are five structures running off the nasopharynx:

- Two internal nares
- Two openings into auditory canals
- The opening leading to the oropharynx

The back wall of the nasopharynx is where the adenoids are positioned. The oropharynx is the middle portion of the pharynx at the back of the mouth starting at the soft palate and running to the **hyoid bone**. The hyoid bone is a single, u-shaped bone located in the neck just below the jaw but above the larynx. The **palatine** and **lingual tonsils** are positioned within the oropharynx.

The adenoids and tonsils are the first structures to encounter bacteria and viruses that enter the body and are considered the initial step in the body's immune response system. They can also be the site of recurrent bacterial infections and potentially lead to air passage obstructions or swallowing problems due to inflammation from these infections. Various symptoms indicate infection, but the most common are:

- Sore throat
- Difficulty/painful swallowing
- Fever
- White spots at the back of the throat
- Bad breath
- Swollen neck glands

Although typically such conditions are treated with antibiotics, in chronic cases, surgical removal of the adenoids or tonsils may be necessary. Surgery may also be a form of treatment in children with recurrent ear infections that could lead to hearing loss. In adults, tumors or other masses may require tonsil and/or adenoid removal.

The last section of the pharynx is the laryngopharynx that starts at the hyoid bone and connects to the esophagus and larynx. It is considered part of both the respiratory and the digestive systems, as it is both a pathway for air as well as a pathway for the digestive tract.

The larynx, or voice box, is the tubular structure between the laryngopharynx and the trachea and is responsible for speech. At the entrance of the larynx is the epiglottis, which closes when food is swallowed to prevent it from entering the respiratory tract. If foreign material enters the larynx, a reflex cough forces the glottis to open, sending air through the upper respiratory channels and typically expelling the foreign matter.

The larynx houses two pairs of vocal cords: false vocal cords positioned superior to the true vocal cords. Ligaments within the vocal cords stretch into the airway, constricting the glottis. When air hits this area, vibration occurs, producing sound. The pharynx, mouth, nasal cavity, and sinuses provide a type of echo chamber so that understandable speech can be produced.

Figure 10.2: Larynx

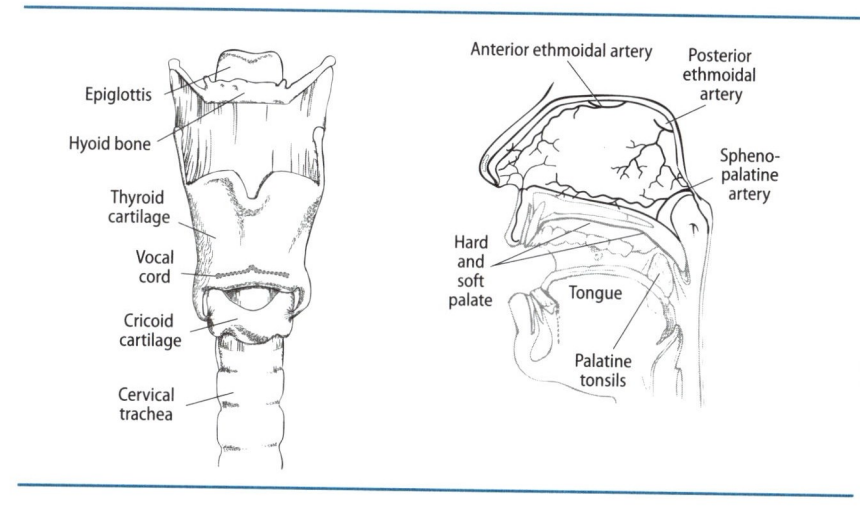

The trachea, or windpipe, begins at the larynx and divides into two branches within the chest: the left and right primary bronchi. The trachea is 12 centimeters in length and 2½ centimeters wide and is made up of C-shaped rings of hyaline cartilage within the **smooth muscle**.

The walls of the trachea are lined with mucous membranes that get more complex structurally as they travel deeper within the bronchial tree. Further within the respiratory tract, the epithelial tissue that lines the trachea begins to contain cilia that help move mucus and any potential foreign matter up and out of the respiratory tract to keep the lungs and respiratory channels clear. An area known as the *carina* is an internal ridge formed by a portion of the last hyaline tracheal cartilage where the

> **DEFINITIONS**
>
> **smooth muscle.** Thin layers of muscle tissue that function involuntarily as part of the body's natural processes; no conscious thought is required for such a muscle to function.

Comprehensive Anatomy and Physiology for ICD-10-CM and ICD-10-PCS Coding

📖 DEFINITIONS

arterioles. Very small arteries that deliver oxygenated blood from the lungs to other areas of the body.

connective tissue. Body tissue made from fibroblasts, collagen, and elastic fibrils that connects, supports, and holds together other tissues and cells and includes cartilage, collagenous, fibrous, elastic, and osseous tissue.

lymphatic vessels. Vessels that collect lymph from various tissues and deliver it to the bloodstream. See the section on the lymphatic system in this publication for more detailed information on these vessels.

terminal bronchiole. Last portion of the conducting zone where respiratory bronchioles are formed.

venules. Very small veins that take the used, or unoxygenated, blood back to the heart where it is pumped to the lungs to exchange carbon dioxide for oxygen.

👉 INTERESTING A & P FACT

The right lung handles 55 percent of the gas exchange within the body.

---

trachea divides into the right and left bronchi. The membrane in this area is the most sensitive to foreign matter and is primarily responsible for the reflex to expel any irritants in the respiratory tract.

The right bronchus enters the right lung and is shorter and wider than the left bronchus, which enters the left lung. The bronchi inside the lungs split into secondary bronchi, one for each lobe within the lung. This branching continues to progress into tertiary bronchi, bronchioles, and finally terminal bronchioles. The end result is a structure resembling an upside down tree, referred to as the bronchial tree.

The lungs are situated within the thoracic cavity, separated by the heart and other anatomic structures, and held in place by ligaments. Fissures, or deep grooves, divide each lung into lobes. The left lung contains two lobes while the right lung contains three. This division is further subdivided into bronchopulmonary segments, each supplied by a tertiary bronchus. The left lung contains eight such segments while the right lung contains 10. Disorders or anomalies in these segments can be removed and/or corrected with little upset to the neighboring lung tissues. The bronchopulmonary segments within the lungs include smaller subdivisions referred to as lobules. The lobules are protected by **connective tissue** each made up of a **lymphatic vessel**, an **arteriole**, a **venule**, and a **terminal bronchiole**. The terminal bronchioles divide further to establish very small respiratory bronchioles, which finally branch further to form the alveolar ducts.

Figure 10.3: Lungs

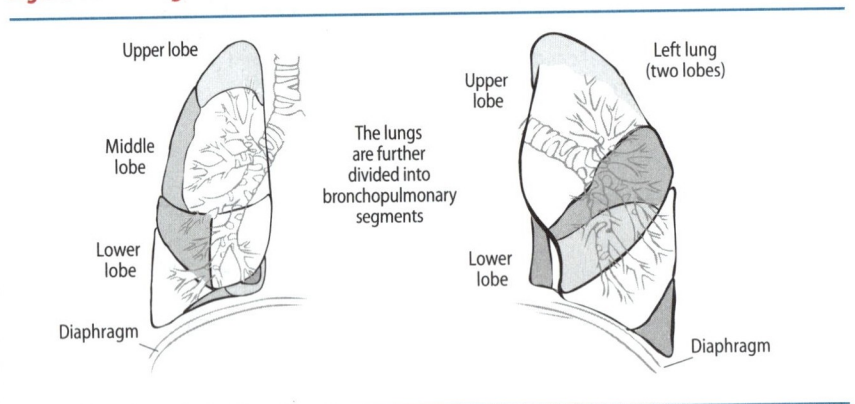

The mediastinum is the area between the right and left lungs that contains the heart, thoracic aorta, pulmonary vessels, vena cava, thymus, trachea, esophagus, and various nerves.

The primary bronchi, pulmonary blood vessels, and pleural tissue are contained within the mediastinum and form the root of the lung, entering through the triangular depression known as the hilum that is above and behind the cardiac impression. Once this network enters the lung, the bronchus and pulmonary veins and arteries divide, making up a vast network of capillaries and alveoli covering an area of 85 square meters. This area is referred to as the respiratory membrane with the primary function of providing gas exchange between air and blood.

The pleura are thin membranes covering the lungs and lining the inside of the chest wall. The pleura surround the lungs and are divided into the visceral and parietal layers. The visceral layer encapsulates the lung surface and the area between the lobes, while the parietal layer covers the inside surface of the chest wall. The area between these layers is the pleural cavity, which contains pleural fluid produced by the membranes. That fluid functions as a lubricant to decrease friction during respiration.

Figure 10.4: Upper Respiratory System

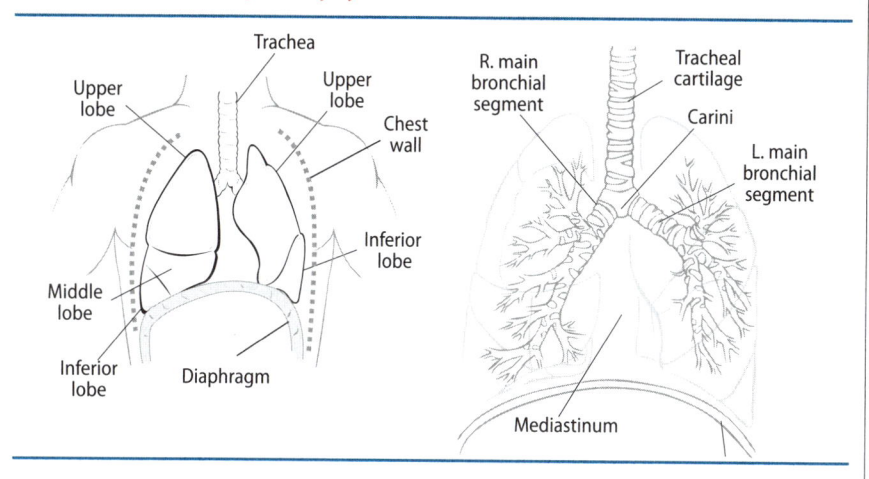

For the respiratory system to function properly, there must be adequate gas exchange within the lungs, as well as within the body's tissues. Gas exchange that takes place within the lungs is referred to as external respiration, and exchange within body tissues is referred to as internal respiration. Internal respiration can occur only via the diffusion process, meaning that gas exchange occurs through membranes, typically from a systemic capillary to the systemic tissue cells. Gases diffuse from an area of higher partial pressure or larger volume area to lower partial pressure or smaller volume area.

External respiration happens through three processes:

- **Ventilation:** Gas exchange within the pulmonary air passages.
- **Pulmonary perfusion:** Blood flow from the right side of the heart to the left side of the heart by way of pulmonary vessels.
- **Diffusion:** As discussed above in internal respiration, gas exchange through membranes where movement occurs from higher partial pressure or larger volume area to lower partial pressure or smaller volume area.

In addition to the breathing functions within the respiratory system, there is an acid-base (pH) balance function. The respiratory system helps regulate pH but not to the extent of the urinary system. When carbon dioxide increases within the body fluids, hydrogen ion levels increase, causing a decrease in blood pH. The respiratory system provides a natural buffer for this process. The rate and depth of breathing can have a major effect on the pH of body fluids, as the amount of carbon dioxide exhaled truly affects the overall acid-base balance in the body.

Anatomy and Pathophysiology and the ICD-10-CM Code Set

The respiratory system can be affected by many disease states, as well as injury and other underlying factors. It is important to remember that breathing requires the use of several muscles within the neck, chest, and abdomen, including the diaphragm, in addition to the nerves that control these movements. An injury to the spinal cord may damage the nerves that signal the brain to control independent breathing. It is important to understand the terminology surrounding many of these disease states and underlying factors as the ICD-10-CM code set describes them in a much more detailed way.

Streptococcal Sore Throat

Streptococcus is the most common bacterium that infects the throat. The bacteria are spread by personal contact with an infected person, most often with a sneeze or cough, and are very contagious. There are many forms of this condition, some leading to scarlet fever and, in more severe cases, to rheumatic fever if left undiagnosed and untreated. Diagnosis is made by throat culture with a rapid strep test or culture growth to determine infection. It is important to note that many sore throats are not a result of the strep infection and only those with these bacteria should be treated with antibiotics.

Tonsillitis and pharyngitis are nonspecific terms referring to inflammation in the tonsils or pharynx that can cause a sore throat. As you can see from the table below, it is important in ICD-10-CM coding to know whether the sore throat pain is originating from the pharynx or the tonsils, and also whether this is a recurrent problem if the patient has a tonsillitis.

Coding for Streptococcal Sore Throat

ICD-9-CM		ICD-10-CM	
034.0	Streptococcal sore throat	J02.0	Streptococcal pharyngitis
		J03.00	Acute streptococcal tonsillitis, unspecified
		J03.01	Acute recurrent streptococcal tonsillitis

Common symptoms for strep throat include fever, swollen neck glands, and white spots on the tonsils. However, these symptoms do not always indicate strep infection and may accompany several symptoms displayed in tonsillitis and pharyngitis, such as:

- Sore throat
- Headache
- Difficulty swallowing
- Muscle aches
- Weakness

Many symptoms are similar to the common cold or any number of viral infections, and strep throat infection must be determined by lab testing for proper diagnosis and prescription antibiotic treatment.

In order to report strep throat, the diagnosis needs to be documented in the medical record. Lab results may be needed before assigning the streptococcal codes if a rapid strep culture isn't available.

Aspergillosis

Aspergillosis is a fungal infection, growth, or allergic response that typically does not affect people with a normal immune system. This fungus grows in stored grain, compost, and other vegetation during the decay process. This condition presents as pneumonia or a fungal growth in the location of a previous lung disorder, such as tuberculosis or a lung abscess.

Allergic bronchopulmonary aspergillosis is an allergic reaction to this fungus that usually affects people who suffer from asthma or cystic fibrosis. Symptoms common to this form of aspergillosis include:

- Productive cough
- Fever
- Malaise
- Wheezing
- Weight loss
- Repeated airway obstruction

Additional symptoms may be seen that are specific to the body area affected, such as shortness of breath if the reaction is within the lung or sinusitis if the condition involves the nasal passages. Blood tests and a chest x-ray may help diagnose the condition, and in some cases a bronchoscopy may be performed to obtain a tissue sample from the trachea. Allergic bronchopulmonary aspergillosis is normally treated with prednisone to address the symptoms, in conjunction with an antifungal medication to attempt to eradicate the fungus.

Figure 10.5: Bronchoscopy

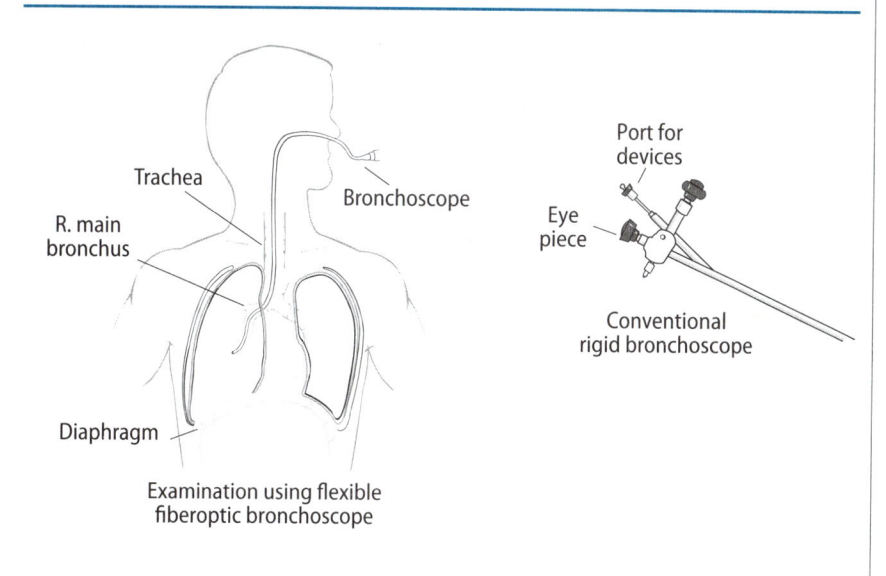

Invasive pulmonary aspergillosis is a more serious condition, as it spreads to other parts of the body and, like the allergic form, it is seen primarily in people with decreased white blood cell counts with disorders such as AIDS, cancer, and leukemia. This condition is treated with antifungal medications; however, significant fungal growth within the lung tissue may require surgical removal.

Aspergilloma is a fungal growth that can invade previously healthy tissue to form an abscess within the lungs. The growth may also spread to the brain, as well as other organs. Symptoms may never develop, and treatment may not be necessary except when coughing produces blood, in which case the bleeding needs to be controlled. Surgical intervention is a last resort due to complexity and high risk but may be necessary when excessive bleeding occurs within the lungs and/or breathing difficulties escalate.

> **DEFINITIONS**
>
> **mycosis.** Fungal disease in any organ of the body.
>
> **necropsy.** Postmortem examination performed to ascertain the cause of death or the changes caused by disease.

Tonsillar aspergillosis is much like other forms of aspergillosis but occurs specifically within the tonsil region. It is treated much like other forms of aspergillosis—with steroid and antifungal therapies.

Disseminated aspergillosis is seen throughout various areas of the body, indicating a compromised immune system. This condition is often quite difficult to diagnose and can be fatal, to be discovered only at **necropsy**.

Penicilliosis is a fungal pulmonary infection caused by *Penicillium marneffei*, and tends to be an opportunistic infection affecting HIV-positive individuals.

Geotrichosis is an uncommon fungal infection that causes lesions in various areas of the body with the initial attack on the lungs. This condition commonly occurs in immunosuppressed individuals with diabetes. The patients may deal with oral lesions, abdominal pain, diarrhea, rectal bleeding, cough with a thick, bloody sputum, and pulmonary lesions. Each of these symptoms is treated differently, depending on the severity.

Coding for Aspergillosis

ICD-9-CM		ICD-10-CM	
117.3	Aspergillosis	B44.0	Invasive pulmonary aspergillosis
		B44.1	Other pulmonary aspergillosis
		B44.2	Tonsillar aspergillosis
		B44.7	Disseminated aspergillosis
		B44.89	Other forms of aspergillosis
		B44.9	Aspergillosis unspecified
		B48.4	Penicillosis
117.9	Other and unspecified *mycoses*	B48.3	Geotrichosis
		B48.8	Other specified mycoses
		B49	Unspecified mycosis

Acute Bronchitis and Bronchiolitis

Bronchitis is a common condition that typically results from an upper respiratory infection or virus affecting the respiratory system. This condition affects the bronchial tubes, causing inflammation within the lining. Bronchiolitis is a similar condition, also common, affecting the bronchioles within the lung. Both conditions typically have a rapid onset and short duration in their acute form, typically resolving within a week or two.

Figure 10.6: Bronchioli and Alveoli

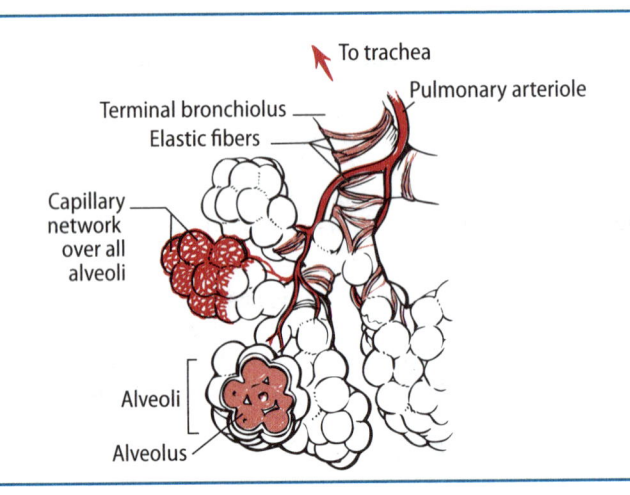

These conditions may be caused by a number of infective agents.

Mycoplasma pneumoniae is a bacterium often acquired when a person is exposed to someone with pneumonia. It typically is a mild form of pneumonia and is often referred to as atypical or walking pneumonia. The condition is characterized by a nine- to 12-day incubation period in most instances, and typically results in symptoms of an upper respiratory infection, dry cough, and fever.

Hemophilus influenzae is a bacterium that can lead to infections within the respiratory tract, which may progress and infect other organs. This bacterium is spread through sneezing, coughing, and touching. The symptoms vary depending on the organ affected and is usually detected by laboratory analysis of body tissue. It is important to note that children are immunized against type B (Hib) to prevent more serious and even deadly infections caused by these bacteria.

Streptococcus is a bacterium, commonly referred to as "strep," that causes infections such as strep throat, pneumonia, and rheumatic and scarlet fevers. It is a gram-positive bacterium, and there are many forms of streptococcal bacteria that grow in humans.

Coxsackie virus appears in the human digestive tract and is spread by unwashed hands and contaminated surfaces. This virus can show signs of mild flu-like symptoms that resolve on their own. However, the virus can also lead to more severe conditions, such as hand, foot, and mouth disease. Due to the transmission method, this virus tends to spread amongst children quickly, especially during warm weather months.

Parainfluenza virus is one of many viruses leading to respiratory infections, most often mild in older children and adults since they have been exposed and the body has built up an immunity to the virus. However, infants and people with a weakened immune system experience more severe symptoms with bronchiolitis caused by parainfluenza.

Respiratory syncytial virus, commonly known as RSV, is a large contributor to respiratory infections among children. Adults may experience this type of infection with mild cold-type symptoms, while children with underlying conditions that affect the lungs and immune systems can experience more serious symptoms and illness. RSV is highly contagious and is spread through contaminated surfaces and coughing, sneezing, and touching.

Rhinovirus is one of 200 viruses that contribute to the common cold. It can survive about three hours on the skin and other surfaces. There is no treatment for the virus, only management of the symptoms until the virus has run its course.

Echovirus, or enteric cytopathic human orphan virus, can cause gastrointestinal, skin, and respiratory infections spread by contaminated feces or particles in the air from infected people. This type of infection is common and is often mild, although in one in five cases the infection leads to viral meningitis. This type of infection often resolves itself; however, in more severe cases, immune system therapy may help people with weak immune systems.

Human metapneumovirus (hMPV) was discovered in 2001 but has no doubt been contributing to respiratory infections for more than 50 years. While most people experience mild symptoms, more severe cases have been reported in people younger than age 1 and within the elderly population or those with weak immune systems. Infection often occurs three to five days after exposure by close contact with an infected person or surface containing the virus. Transplant patients are among those at highest risk for acquiring this type of infection.

> **INTERESTING A & P FACT**
>
> Rhinovirus causes a cold in adults approximately 30 to 35 percent of the time. There are more than 110 types of rhinoviruses currently identified.

Coding for Acute Bronchitis

ICD-9-CM		ICD-10-CM	
466.0	Acute bronchitis	J20.0	Acute bronchitis due to Mycoplasma pneumoniae
		J20.1	Acute bronchitis due to Hemophilus influenzae
		J20.2	Acute bronchitis due to streptococcus
		J20.3	Acute bronchitis due to coxsackievirus
		J20.4	Acute bronchitis due to parainfluenza virus
		J20.5	Acute bronchitis due to respiratory syncytial virus
		J20.6	Acute bronchitis due to rhinovirus
		J20.7	Acute bronchitis due to echovirus
		J20.8	Acute bronchitis due to other specified organisms
		J20.9	Acute bronchitis, unspecified

Coding for these types of bronchitis and bronchiolitis will be more complicated under the ICD-10-CM code set due to the new codes established identifying the cause of the infection. In ICD-9-CM, acute bronchitis and bronchiolitis are coded with 466.xx. As illustrated in the tables above and below, understanding the various types of infectious agents is the key to correct code assignment under the ICD-10-CM system.

Coding for Acute Bronchiolitis

ICD-9-CM		ICD-10-CM	
466.19	Acute bronchiolitis due to other infectious organisms	J21.1	Acute bronchiolitis due to human metapneumovirus
		J21.8	Acute bronchiolitis due to other specified organisms
		J21.9	Acute bronchiolitis, unspecified

To code for bronchitis and bronchiolitis under ICD-10-CM, the coder needs to determine from the documentation which organism contributed to the condition—it is not enough to understand whether the patient presents with acute bronchitis or acute bronchiolitis. To code the encounter to the highest level of specificity, the coder may need to query the provider for additional information on the type of infectious agent.

Pneumonia in Whooping Cough and Other Infectious Diseases

Pneumonia is a lung infection caused by bacteria or viruses. When bacteria are the cause, the infection presents quickly with symptoms such as cough, fever, shortness of breath, chills, weakness, and nausea. When a virus is the cause, the infection presents more slowly and, while symptoms are similar, they may not be as easy to identify.

Whooping cough is a common name for a condition sometimes associated with pneumonia called pertussis, named after the bacterium *Bordetella pertussis,* its causative agent. Pertussis is a highly contagious respiratory disease and has been known as whooping cough due to its symptoms: severe coughing, followed by a loud "whooping" inspiration. Children in the United States generally receive vaccines for pertussis.

Parapertussis is similar to whooping cough in etiology and symptoms and can occur at any age, although it primarily affects children ages 3 to 5. Parapertussis occurs less frequently than pertussis and has a shorter duration as well. Vaccination against whooping cough does not provide immunity to parapertussis, and most people recover completely with extremely rare complications due to this infection.

CODING AXIOM

When pneumonia and hemoptysis are both documented, code the hemoptysis, R04.2, separately and sequenced after the appropriate pneumonia code. It is no longer a nonessential modifier in the index, as it is not always included with pneumonia.

Coding Clinic, 4Q, 13, 118

INTERESTING A & P FACT

Prior to widespread vaccination for *Bordetella pertussis,* which began in the 1940s, whooping cough killed 5,000 to 10,000 people in the United States every year. With vaccination, that number has dropped to fewer than 30 per year.

Ascariasis is an intestinal infection caused by roundworms and is most prevalent in unsanitary or overcrowded populations of the world. The symptoms, though rare in many cases, depend on the volume of worms and the site of infestation. Ascariasis pneumonia is caused by the roundworm larvae that travel through the bloodstream or lymph system into the lungs, causing coughing, shortness of breath, and wheezing lasting about six days before the larvae are expelled through a cough or reingested.

Coding for Pneumonia in Whooping Cough and Other Infectious Diseases

ICD-9-CM		ICD-10-CM	
484.3	Pneumonia in whooping cough	A37.01	Whooping cough due to Bordetella pertussis with pneumonia
		A37.11	Whooping cough due to Bordetella parapertussis with pneumonia
		A37.81	Whooping cough due to other Bordetella species with pneumonia
		A37.91	Whooping cough, unspecified species with pneumonia
484.8	Pneumonia in other infectious diseases classified elsewhere	B77.81	Ascariasis pneumonia
		J17	Pneumonia in diseases classified elsewhere

What was previously reported as pneumonia in whooping cough within the ICD-9-CM code set is broken down even further within ICD-10-CM to allow for specific causal agents to be reported that contribute to the condition. As has been the case with other conditions, it is important to understand how these causal agents relate. Coders need this information at the time of code selection, as it is not yet certain how payers will react to unlisted codes in the ICD-10-CM code set. Using the highest level of specificity at all times will be key to accurate payment for providers.

Emphysematous Bleb and Other Emphysema

Emphysema is a condition of the respiratory system that restricts the air flow during exhalation because the bronchioles and alveoli deteriorate gradually. This causes a loss of lung elasticity, which can result in significant breathing difficulty. As this condition progresses, the spherical air sacs within the lungs become irregular and contain holes, reducing not only the number of air sacs but also the amount of oxygen that can circulate into the blood from the lungs (a decrease in the gas exchange). As the air sacs deteriorate, the openings collapse, trapping air within the lungs. Treatment for this condition can slow down the deterioration; however, once the damage is done, it cannot be reversed or cured. Smoking and air pollution are main contributors to emphysema.

☛ INTERESTING A & P FACT

In addition to smoking and air pollution, some patients with emphysema, especially those that are diagnosed early in life, acquire the disease due to a rare genetic deficiency of serum alpha-1 antitrypsin (AAT). AAT protects the elasticity of the lungs and due to deficiency enzymes in the body cause damage resulting in emphysema.

Figure 10.7: Emphysema

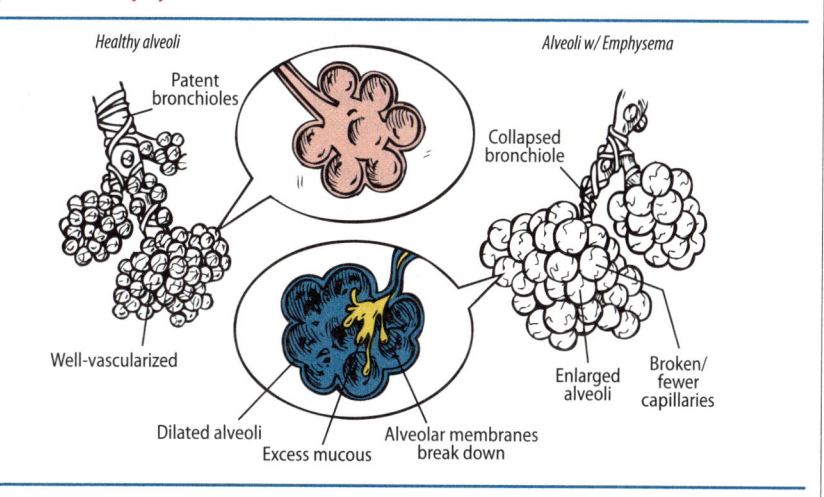

Healthy alveoli — Patent bronchioles — Well-vascularized

Alveoli w/ Emphysema — Collapsed bronchiole — Enlarged alveoli — Broken/fewer capillaries — Dilated alveoli — Excess mucous — Alveolar membranes break down

Comprehensive Anatomy and Physiology for ICD-10-CM and ICD-10-PCS Coding

Emphysematous bleb are blisters larger than 1 mm within an emphysematous lung that contain blood or serum. It is a fairly generic term, referring more to a symptom that occurs during emphysema than to a disease process itself.

Macleod's syndrome is a form of emphysema in which one lung becomes somewhat transparent in conjunction with the reduced oxygen and carbon dioxide exchange within the blood. Macleod's syndrome is also known as Swyer James syndrome or SJS.

Panlobular emphysema affects all parts of the lobes within the lungs. The right lung having three lobes and the left lung having two lobes, also further divides into hundreds of smaller lobules each containing a bronchiole and its own group of alveoli. A person with panlobular emphysema has a condition directly affecting all of these areas.

Centrilobular emphysema occurs mainly in the central part of the lobule and is the most common form of emphysema mostly in the upper lobe and more frequently seen in men than women. It is also associated with chronic bronchitis.

Coding for Emphysematous Bleb and other Emphysema

ICD-9-CM		ICD-10-CM	
492.0	Emphysematous bleb	J43.9	Emphysema, unspecified
492.8	Other emphysema	J43.0	Unilateral pulmonary emphysema [Macleod's syndrome]
		J43.1	Panlobular emphysema
		J43.2	Centrilobular emphysema
		J43.8	Other emphysema
		J43.9	Emphysema, unspecified

Although the ICD-10-CM code set allows for coding unspecified emphysema, it is clear the expansion of the terms narrows down the exact nature of the condition and tracks the variations of the disease. Keep in mind that unspecified codes may not be acceptable for payment purposes, so using the most specific code available based on the documentation will be important. In some instances, querying the provider may be an important part of the process.

Asthma

Asthma is a condition that affects the airways characterized by typically recurrent episodes of severe dyspnea, wheezing on inspiration and/or expiration, and sometimes coughing. This can also be accompanied by mucous secretions. Episodes of asthma can be brought on by infections, inhalation of cold air, allergens or pollutants, vigorous exercise, or emotional stress.

While asthma with specific levels of exacerbation is currently specified within the ICD-9-CM coding convention, the conversion to ICD-10-CM will give even more options applicable to the condition. It will be vitally important for the coder to understand the following terms when interpreting documentation and applying the appropriate ICD-10-CM codes.

- **Mild intermittent:** Classified based on the following indications:
    - symptom frequency twice a week or less
    - waking at night due to symptoms twice a month or less
    - necessary use of immediate relief inhaler twice a week
    - little or no interference with daily activities
    - normal peak flow readings between symptoms
    - not requiring the use of oral steroids to control or requiring them once per year
- **Mild persistent** Classified based on the following indications:
    - symptom frequency more than two days a week, but not every day

> **☞ INTERESTING A & P FACT**
>
> Recent reports from the Centers for Disease Control and Prevention show that more than 8 percent of Americans—or nearly 24.6 million people—have asthma.

- waking at night due to symptoms three to four times a month
- necessary use of immediate relief inhaler more than two times a week
- minor interference with daily activities
- peak flow readings equal to 80 percent of personal norm
- requiring the use of oral steroids twice a year
- **Moderate persistent:** Classified based on the following indications:
  - daily symptoms
  - waking at night due to symptoms more than one time a week
  - necessary use of immediate relief inhaler daily
  - some interference with daily activities
  - peak flow reading from 60 to 80 percent of personal norm
  - requiring the use of oral steroids twice a year
- **Severe persistent:** Classified based on the following indications:
  - frequent symptoms throughout the day
  - waking at night due to symptoms often every night
  - necessary use of immediate relief inhaler several times daily
  - symptoms that severely limit daily activities
  - peak flow readings less than 60 percent of personal norm
  - requiring the use of oral steroids two or more times a year

Currently, asthma is classified into groups: extrinsic and intrinsic. Asthma caused by allergies is known as extrinsic or allergic asthma. This form of asthma is a response to an irritant inhaled or ingested. Intrinsic asthma is typically seen in people aged 30 or older and is typically chronic and persistent rather than episodic in nature. Intrinsic asthma is often related to respiratory infections, inhaled chemicals, and/or pollution.

Coding for Extrinsic Asthma

ICD-9-CM		ICD-10-CM	
493.00	Extrinsic asthma, unspecified	J45.20	Mild intermittent asthma, uncomplicated
		J45.30	Mild persistent asthma, uncomplicated
		J45.40	Moderate persistent asthma, uncomplicated
		J45.50	Severe persistent asthma, uncomplicated
493.01	Extrinsic asthma with status asthmaticus	J45.22	Mild intermittent asthma with status asthmaticus
		J45.32	Mild persistent asthma with status asthmaticus
		J45.42	Moderate persistent asthma with status asthmaticus
		J45.52	Severe persistent asthma with status asthmaticus
493.02	Extrinsic asthma with exacerbation	J45.21	Mild intermittent asthma with (acute) exacerbation
		J45.31	Mild persistent asthma with (acute) exacerbation
		J45.41	Moderate persistent asthma with (acute) exacerbation
		J45.51	Severe persistent asthma with (acute) exacerbation

An exacerbation of a patient's condition is simply an increase in the seriousness of his or her disease, typically marked by a greater intensity of signs and symptoms. In the case of asthma, this often means an asthma attack, prompting the patient to seek medical assistance to receive medication to clear his or her airway to assist in breathing.

Status asthmaticus is classified as an acute and severe asthma attack that does not respond to the typical treatment with bronchodilators and can lead to respiratory

> **CODING AXIOM**
>
> When status asthmaticus and asthma in exacerbation are both documented, code only the most severe condition, which would be the status asthmaticus.
>
> *Coding Clinic*, 4Q, 12, 99

failure. Because this type of an attack requires immediate medical intervention, it is important to recognize the early symptoms, such as shortness of breath and difficulty talking in complete sentences.

Coding for Intrinsic Asthma

ICD-9-CM		ICD-10-CM	
493.10	Intrinsic asthma, unspecified	J45.20	Mild intermittent asthma, uncomplicated
		J45.30	Mild persistent asthma, uncomplicated
		J45.40	Moderate persistent asthma, uncomplicated
		J45.50	Severe persistent asthma, uncomplicated
493.11	Intrinsic asthma with status asthmaticus	J45.22	Mild intermittent asthma with status asthmaticus
		J45.32	Mild persistent asthma with status asthmaticus
		J45.42	Moderate persistent asthma with status asthmaticus
		J45.52	Severe persistent asthma with status asthmaticus
493.12	Intrinsic asthma with exacerbation	J45.21	Mild intermittent asthma with (acute) exacerbation
		J45.31	Mild persistent asthma with (acute) exacerbation
		J45.41	Moderate persistent asthma with (acute) exacerbation
		J45.51	Severe persistent asthma with (acute) exacerbation

Pneumoconiosis Due to Silica and Other Inorganic Dust

Pneumoconiosis is a condition caused by inhaling dust particles, typically associated with occupations that require regular exposure to mineral dusts. This condition is a form of interstitial lung disease that contributes to the inflammation of the air sacs, causing the lung tissue to harden. There is no cure for this disease, and treatment is focused on managing the patient's symptoms.

There are several common forms of pneumoconiosis in the United States:

- Asbestosis
- Silicosis
- Coal worker's pneumoconiosis
- Talc pneumoconiosis
- Kaolin pneumoconiosis
- Siderosis of the lung

Figure 10.8: Alveoli, Asbestoses, Air Sacs

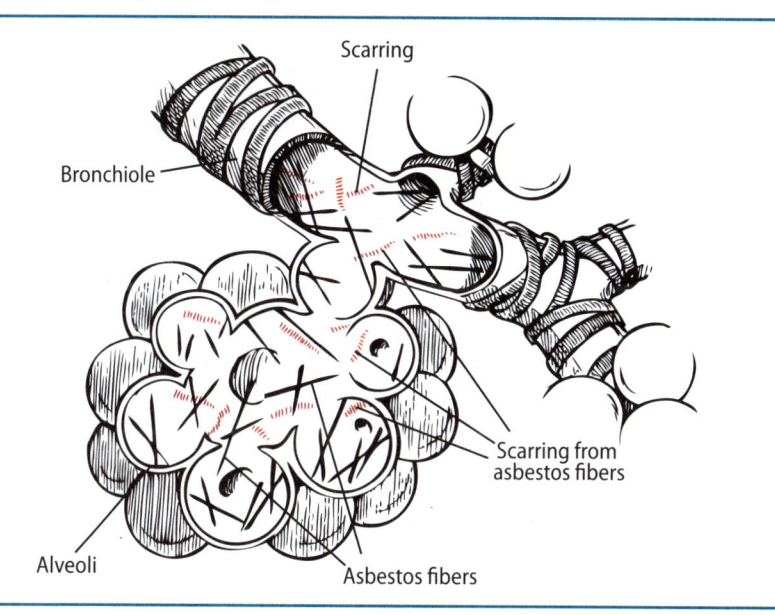

Definitions and Other Classifications of Pneumoconiosis

Asbestosis is a generic term for a group of minerals that cause this form of lung disease. These minerals are taken from underground deposits and have been historically used in insulation, tiles, and automobile parts. People who work in these industries are not the only groups that develop this condition. Those who live or work in structures that contain asbestos products that have begun to break down have also been known to acquire this condition; however, symptoms do not often occur until 20 years or more after exposure. In these patients, chest films often show small linear opacities distributed throughout the lung. This disease tends to be progressive, beginning with shortness of breath, progressing eventually to respiratory failure.

Silicosis is caused by regular exposure to white crystal compounds often associated with sand and quartz as seen in the manufacturing of glass and concrete products. This condition is often characterized by the development of nodular fibrosis in the lungs.

Coal worker's pneumoconiosis affects people who work in mines, manufacturing, or shipping of coal and graphite products with regular inhalation of these particles. It is characterized by the deposit of coal dust in the lungs and the formation of black nodules on the bronchioles, which results in focal emphysema. This condition is often referred to as black lung disease or anthracosis, and the progress can often be halted if further exposure to coal dust is prevented.

Talc pneumoconiosis is caused by regular exposure to talc dust often present in industries such as cosmetics, pharmaceutical, paper, ceramics, and electronics manufacturing. This stage of the disease is considered "simple pneumoconiosis;" continued overexposure leads to fibrosis.

Kaolin, or china clay, pneumoconiosis is named for the mineral that causes it (kaolin), which is used in the manufacturing of ceramics, paper, pharmaceuticals, and cosmetics.

Siderosis, also called welder's or silver polisher's lung, arises from exposure to iron particles or dust. A person with this condition may not display any symptoms, but a chest x-ray will show an abnormality in one or both of the lungs.

Aluminosis may also be referred to as aluminum lung. Typically, this condition afflicts those working in explosive or abrasive aluminum manufacturing, particularly aluminum welders or polishers. Recent studies show a small portion of these workers develops this condition over the course of 25 years or more of exposure.

Bauxite fibrosis of the lung is due to inhalation of bauxite dust, which can be found in combinations of hydrated aluminum oxides that include iron and silicon. Those who work with abrasive materials in spark plugs and furnaces are exposed to this type of dust.

Berylliosis is caused by the light-weight metallic element beryllium, which is used in aerospace, semiconductors, electrical industries, and copper alloy in springs. The most common use of this element is in electric light bulbs and fluorescent tubes. This condition was first recognized in the 1940s as an occupational lung disease. It remains very rare.

Graphite fibrosis of the lung is caused by the dust from graphite, which is one of many mineral forms of carbon with a wide variety of uses. Graphite can be mixed with clay as is done for making pencils and has uses in lubricants, polish, batteries, and nuclear reactor cores.

Stannosis results from overexposure to tin dust (stannic or tin oxide) and can be seen on a chest x-ray presenting as dense masses. These oxides are often used in the production of glass, enamels, and ceramic glazes.

Byssinosis, also referred to as brown lung disease, causes narrowing of air passages, like asthma. The primary cause of this condition is inhalation of cotton, which is frequently used in the textile industry.

Flax-dresser's disease is a form of byssinosis that is caused by inhaling remnants of flax, which is grown for the seed it produces and the oil component of that seed. The oil produced has many industrial, household, and animal uses, such as paint, varnish, ink, and protein meal for livestock. Recently flax seed has been recognized as a beneficial additive to human food due to the fatty acids in the oil.

Cannabinosis is another form of byssinosis specific to the inhalation of hemp and other unprocessed fibers within the textile manufacturing industry. People working in factories that produce yarn, thread, and fabric containing hemp are at increased risk of developing this condition.

As illustrated in the following table, it is important under ICD-10-CM to gather information from providers about the root of the patient's pneumoconiosis. What was previously a simple pneumoconiosis due to a type of inorganic dust is now a berylliosis or a siderosis. Coders must gather the most detailed information they can from the patient's history to code to the highest level of specificity.

Coding for Pneumoconiosis Due to Silica and Other Inorganic Dust

ICD-9-CM		ICD-10-CM	
502	Pneumoconiosis due to other silica or silicates	J62.0	Pneumoconiosis due to talc dust
		J62.8	Pneumoconiosis due to other dust containing silica
503	Pneumoconiosis due to other inorganic dust	J63.0	Aluminosis (of lung)
		J63.1	Bauxite fibrosis (of lung)
		J63.2	Berylliosis
		J63.3	Graphite fibrosis (of lung)
		J63.4	Siderosis
		J63.5	Stannosis
		J63.6	Pneumoconiosis due to other specified inorganic dusts
504	Pneumonopathy due to inhalation of other dust	J66.0	Byssinosis
		J66.1	Flax-dressers' disease
		J66.2	Cannabinosis
		J66.8	Airway disease due to other specified organic dusts

The pneumoconiosis group of diseases in particular is coded quite differently under the ICD-10-CM code set. It will take practice and physician education to ensure that the documentation specifies the form of the condition being tested for and treated so that ICD-10-CM coding is accurate. Accurate coding, in turn, is needed to determine the medical necessity of tests ordered to confirm diagnosis and determine the appropriate course of treatment, as well as to follow the progression of the disease.

Pleurisy

Pleurisy is a condition that is seen when the membrane lining the chest surrounding the lungs becomes inflamed. This condition may be in conjunction with pleural effusion, when fluid from the vessels or lymphatic system leak into the membrane lining. The typical symptoms associated with pleurisy are chest pain during inhale/exhale phases of breathing, shortness of breath, nonproductive cough, and fevers/chills. Chest pain increases with coughing, sneezing, and deep breathing and may radiate to the shoulder area. If pleurisy is accompanied by effusion, chest pain may subside due to the fluid accumulation that provides lubrication. However, excessive fluid retention adds pressure to the lungs, making it difficult to breathe. When this fluid becomes infected, additional symptoms occur. This condition is then known as empyema.

Pleural plaque is seen within the chest cavity as deposits of fibrous tissue, which may be attributed to asbestos exposure. These deposits often become calcified and can be viewed on a chest x-ray, depending on the density of the calcification. In recent studies, about 10 to 40 percent of these deposits appear on a standard chest radiograph. This plaque is typically benign in nature, and treatment focuses on symptoms, if any are present. Other studies indicate that 80 percent of patients with pleural plaque have been exposed to some form of asbestos. Patients with pleural plaque have an elevated risk of diffuse pleural fibrosis.

Fibrothorax is simply fibrosis within the pleural lining of the lungs. It is commonly seen as a stiff layer surrounding the lung and is attributed to traumatic hemothorax or pleural effusion.

Chylous pleural effusion is fluid within the pleural space that appears opaque and white, but the fluid is no longer opaque when combined with ether. This condition is due to the leaking of lymph contents into the space, usually as a result of thoracic duct damage or injury, as well as mediastinal lymphoma.

Hemothorax occurs when blood accumulates within the pleural cavity. While the most common contributor to this condition is trauma to the chest, it may also be observed in patients with the following conditions:

- Clotting defects
- Necrosis of lung tissue
- Cancer of the lung or within the pleura
- Central venous catheter placement
- Surgery within the chest cavity
- Tuberculosis

Hemothorax symptoms can range from anxiety and chest pain to shortness of breath and increased heart rate. Additionally, the physician may notice absence of breath sounds in the affected area, which requires further testing such as chest x-ray, computed tomography scan, or thoracentesis. Treatment centers on stopping the bleeding via a chest tube that may be left in place over the course of several days. If this is unsuccessful, a **thoracotomy** may be necessary.

> **DEFINITIONS**
>
> **thoracotomy.** Surgical procedure during which an incision is made into the chest to puncture the pleural space so that the blood and/or fluid from the area can be drained.

Figure 10.9: Pleural Effusion

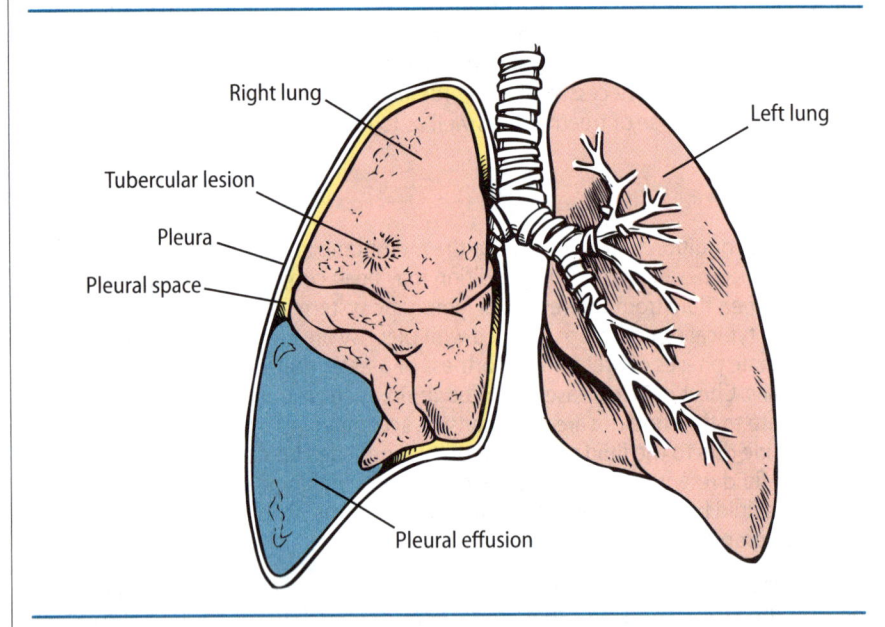

Coding for Pleurisy and Related Effusion

ICD-9-CM		ICD-10-CM	
511.0	Pleurisy without mention of effusion or current tuberculosis	J86.9	Pyothorax without fistula
		J92.0	Pleural plaque with presence of asbestos
		J92.9	Pleural plaque without asbestos
		J94.1	Fibrothorax
		J94.8	Other specified pleural conditions
		J94.9	Pleural condition, unspecified
		R09.1	Pleurisy
511.89	Other specified forms of effusion, except tuberculous	J90	Pleural effusion, not elsewhere classified
		J94.0	Chylous effusion
		J94.2	Hemothorax
		J94.8	Other specified pleural conditions

Understanding the differentiation between the forms of pleurisy is important for coders. Without the appropriate documentation, the coder may need to query the provider for additional information. In some instances, there may not be additional information and a simple diagnosis of pleurisy will be used.

Lung Abscess

An abscess within the lung is a growth often filled with pus and typically due to some kind of infection causing the surrounding tissue to become inflamed. Bacteria normally in the mouth may be inhaled into the lungs, leading to an infection as seen in some cases of periodontal disease. An abscess can also form in people with a weak immune system or airway obstruction. Symptoms that can indicate a lung abscess include productive cough, fever, loss of appetite, and fatigue mirroring pneumonia. A chest x-ray typically shows the presence of a lung abscess. In most cases, symptoms are slow to develop except when the infection is caused by *Staphylococcus aureus,* in which case they appear suddenly and can be fatal if not treated immediately. Most abscesses of the lung are treated with antibiotics. In some rare cases, a bronchoscopy is performed and a tube is inserted to drain the abscess.

Gangrene of the lung can occur when an area is cut off from regular blood supply. The lack of blood supply may be a result of an infection, injury, or disease.

Necrosis is the death of tissue and may occur in addition to gangrene.

Coding for Lung Abscess

ICD-9-CM		ICD-10-CM	
513.0	Abscess of lung	J85.0	Gangrene and necrosis of lung
		J85.1	Abscess of lung with pneumonia
		J85.2	Abscess of lung without pneumonia

There is only one applicable ICD-9-CM code for abscess of the lung; however, ICD-10-CM requires the coder to query the physician for more specific details if the documentation does not indicate gangrene or necrosis, or whether or not the abscess was somehow connected to pneumonia.

Pulmonary Congestion and Hypostasis

Pulmonary congestion is the build-up of fluid within the lungs, often as a result of an infection or congestive heart failure. Hypostasis is the accumulation of deposits of a specific substance in a body area because of lack of activity. With regard to the respiratory system, hypostasis typically occurs in the lungs of elderly and debilitated people because of lack of movement. Both conditions are coded in ICD-9-CM with code 514, but in ICD-10-CM, the specific type of congestion must be specified, as described below.

ICD-10-CM code J18.2 Hypostatic pneumonia, unspecified organism, is specifically associated with a lack of movement over a long period of time. Fluids settle in the patient's lung, causing the pneumonia. This condition often affects elderly, debilitated, or bedridden people. There may be an organism that is causing the pneumonia, but this particular code does not require that the organism be specifically identified.

ICD-10-CM code J81.1 Chronic pulmonary edema, is caused by excessive fluid within the lungs, causing inflammation. This is often a result of congestive heart failure.

Acute Chest Syndrome

Acute chest syndrome is associated with various forms of sickle-cell diseases. Coding for these conditions requires the use of more than one ICD-9-CM code, with acute chest syndrome code 517.3 as the secondary code. ICD-10-CM allows for more specific coding by using one primary code with the option of an additional code to specify any associated fever.

Hb-SS disease, also referred to as sickle cell anemia, is a hereditary deficiency within the red blood cells. This condition causes an irregular shape in the cells that decreases the amount of oxygen that can be carried throughout the body to the various organs. Symptoms, as well as episodes, can vary between patients. Some people have only one episode every few years, while others present with many episodes throughout a given year and still others require hospitalization. Typically symptoms are not seen until the patient is at least 4 months old. Common symptoms include:

- Abdominal pain
- Bone pain
- Developmental delay
- Fatigue
- Fever
- Increased heart rate
- Jaundice
- Chest pain
- Increased thirst

- Increased urination
- Skin ulcers

Ongoing treatment is frequently necessary to manage the condition outside of recurring episodes and may include folic acid supplements, as well as hydration.

Hb-C disease, or hemoglobin C disease, is a genetic blood disorder most often seen in those of African descent. This condition leads to anemia, in which the typical life span of the red blood cells is much shorter than normal. Most people with this condition do not display any symptoms but can develop jaundice, enlargement of the spleen, or gallstones that require treatment. Typically, this condition is managed with a folic acid supplement to assist in the production of normal red blood cells and control the anemia.

Thalassemia is another genetic blood disorder that reduces the number of red blood cells within the body. Mild cases require no treatment; however, more severe cases may require regular blood transfusions. Symptoms depend on the type and severity of the condition and can surface as early as newborn through age 2, while some people may never experience any symptoms.

Coding for Acute Chest Syndrome

ICD-9-CM		ICD-10-CM	
517.3	Acute chest syndrome	D57.01	Hb-SS disease with acute chest syndrome
		D57.211	Sickle-cell/Hb-C disease with acute chest syndrome
		D57.411	Sickle-cell thalassemia with acute chest syndrome
		D57.811	Other sickle-cell disorders with acute chest syndrome
		J99	Respiratory disorders in diseases classified elsewhere

Lung Involvement in Other Diseases

Coding in ICD-9-CM for lung involvement in diseases coded elsewhere obviously requires more than one code, with the secondary code 517.8 and instruction to code first the underlying condition. With ICD-10-CM, there is typically one specific code for the disease manifested within the lung.

Systemic lupus erythematosus (SLE) interferes with the body's normal immune response. This condition causes the body to attack normal, healthy cells, leading to inflammation in various parts of the body and, for this definition, specifically the lungs. It affects nine times more women than men, with symptoms occurring between the ages of 10 and 50. When the lungs are affected by SLE, symptoms include chest pain when breathing deeply, coughing up blood, and shortness of breath. A physician may hear a **pleural friction rub** when the patient is examined, and a chest x-ray may show **pleuritis** or pleurisy. Treatment might include nonsteroidal anti-inflammatory medications to control symptoms.

Dermatopolymyositis is a muscle disorder causing inflammation and weakness, as well as a skin rash. Symptoms of lung involvement reported, as in pulmonary fibrosis, are painful respiration and alveolitis and are often treated with corticosteroids.

Polymyositis is a muscle disorder causing inflammation and weakness in the skeletal muscles closest to the trunk of the body. This condition can occur at any age but is most common in adults ages 30 to 50 and is seen more in women than men. Symptoms develop slowly and progress over time, with lung involvement displayed in shortness of breath and speech deterioration. The overall cause cannot be pinpointed even though it is suggested the condition may be brought on by an infection. However, since symptoms at initial onset are slow to develop, it is almost impossible to determine the initial source.

DEFINITIONS

pleural friction rub. Low, grating sound heard when pleural surfaces rub against each other. This may be confused with a pericardial rub; cessation of the sound when the patient holds his or her breath indicates a pleural friction rub.

pleuritis. Inflammation of the lining surrounding the lungs and lining the inside of the chest.

Sicca syndrome, also referred to as Sjögren syndrome, is an autoimmune disease often displayed in conjunction with another condition such as polymyositis. Sicca syndrome is characterized by a significantly decreased fluid production within the body. Specific lung involvement relates to potential respiratory infections and pneumonias due to the dryness.

Coding for Lung Involvement in Other Diseases Classified Elsewhere

ICD-9-CM		ICD-10-CM	
517.8	Lung involvement in other diseases classified elsewhere	J99	Respiratory disorders in diseases classified elsewhere
		M32.13	Lung involvement in systemic lupus erythematosus
		M33.01	Juvenile dermatopolymyositis with respiratory involvement
		M33.11	Other dermatopolymyositis with respiratory involvement
		M33.21	Polymyositis with respiratory involvement
		M33.91	Dermatopolymyositis, unspecified with respiratory involvement
		M35.02	Sicca syndrome with lung involvement

Injuries

Many injuries can occur throughout the respiratory system. The ICD-10-CM code set allows the coder to more specifically describe the type and location of the injury, which in turn requires additional documentation and knowledge of terms. Here are some important terms to be aware of in defining injuries under the ICD-10-CM code set:

- **Unilateral:** Affecting one side of the body, or in the case of the lungs, affecting only one lung.
- **Bilateral:** Affecting both sides, or both lungs.
- **Initial encounter:** First visit to treat the injury.

Primary blast is an injury directly related to an explosive and the damage the shock wave's impact has on the body. Body organs that are filled with gas are typically the most affected by such an explosion, with the lungs often being the most severely affected and the most common fatality. The injury should be considered a primary blast if a person is exposed to an explosion and has symptoms of *bradycardia*, *apnea*, and *hypotension*. While usually present at initial evaluation, symptoms delayed as far out as 48 hours afterward are not uncommon. The effects can be seen on a chest x-ray and, in some cases, a *thoracostomy* may be necessary to avoid complications of anesthesia or air transport to a hospital.

A contusion is a superficial injury, often a bruise, as a result of trauma without a break in the skin. However, even this kind of injury can have serious complications when the contusion affects the respiratory system, particularly the lungs.

A laceration is a torn, ragged-edged wound. The initial concern is infection or damage to organs underneath the laceration. Deeper lacerations may require irrigation and/or stitches to close the affected area.

DEFINITIONS

apnea. Absence of breathing.

bradycardia. Slowed heart rate, usually defined as rate less than 60 beats per minute.

hypotension. Decreased blood pressure below the normal rate.

thoracostomy. Creation of an opening in the chest wall for drainage.

Coding for Injury Related to the Bronchus without Mention of Open Wound in Cavity

ICD-9-CM		ICD-10-CM	
862.21	Bronchus injury without mention of open wound in cavity	S27.401A	Unspecified injury of bronchus, unilateral, initial encounter
		S27.402A	Unspecified injury of bronchus, bilateral, initial encounter
		S27.409A	Unspecified injury of bronchus, unspecified, initial encounter
		S27.411A	Primary blast injury of bronchus, unilateral, initial encounter
		S27.412A	Primary blast injury of bronchus, bilateral, initial encounter
		S27.419A	Primary blast injury of bronchus, unspecified, initial encounter
		S27.421A	Contusion of bronchus, unilateral, initial encounter
		S27.422A	Contusion of bronchus, bilateral, initial encounter
		S27.429A	Contusion of bronchus, unspecified, initial encounter
		S27.431A	Laceration of bronchus, unilateral, initial encounter
		S27.432A	Laceration of bronchus, bilateral, initial encounter
		S27.439A	Laceration of bronchus, unspecified, initial encounter
		S27.491A	Other injury of bronchus, unilateral, initial encounter
		S27.492A	Other injury of bronchus, bilateral, initial encounter
		S27.499A	Other injury of bronchus, unspecified, initial encounter

A pulmonary contusion affects the lung tissue itself, leading to fluid and blood accumulation within the alveolar areas of the lung. About 20 percent of cases of blunt chest injuries also reported pulmonary contusions. In some cases, crackling noises known as rales can be heard in the chest through a stethoscope. If the contusion is left undiagnosed, complications such as *atelectasis*, pneumonia, and respiratory failure may occur. Once diagnosed, most lung contusions resolve in less than a week with fluid restriction and careful observation. Larger contusions may require more extensive treatment like oxygen or mechanical ventilation.

DEFINITIONS

atelectasis. Collapse of lung tissue, typically alveoli, affecting part or all of one lung, preventing normal oxygen absorption to healthy tissues.

Coding for Injury of Other Specified Intrathoracic Organ without Open Wound in Cavity

ICD-9-CM		ICD-10-CM	
862.29	Injury to other specified intrathoracic organs without mention of open wound into cavity	S27.50XA	Unspecified injury of thoracic trachea, initial encounter
		S27.51XA	Primary blast injury of thoracic trachea, initial encounter
		S27.52XA	Contusion of thoracic trachea, initial encounter
		S27.53XA	Laceration of thoracic trachea, initial encounter
		S27.59XA	Other injury of thoracic trachea, initial encounter
		S27.60XA	Unspecified injury of pleura, initial encounter
		S27.63XA	Laceration of pleura, initial encounter
		S27.69XA	Other injury of pleura, initial encounter
		S27.892A	Contusion of other specified intrathoracic organs, initial encounter
		S27.893A	Laceration of other specified intrathoracic organs, initial encounter
		S27.898A	Other injury of other specified intrathoracic organs, initial encounter
		S27.899A	Unspecified injury of other specified intrathoracic organs, initial encounter

Multiple and Unspecified Injuries to Intrathoracic Organs, with Open Wound into Cavity

Multiple injuries within the thoracic cavity have additional codes to capture various circumstances not covered elsewhere and when more than one injury, complication, or area might be affected.

Figure 10.10: Firearm Injury, X-ray

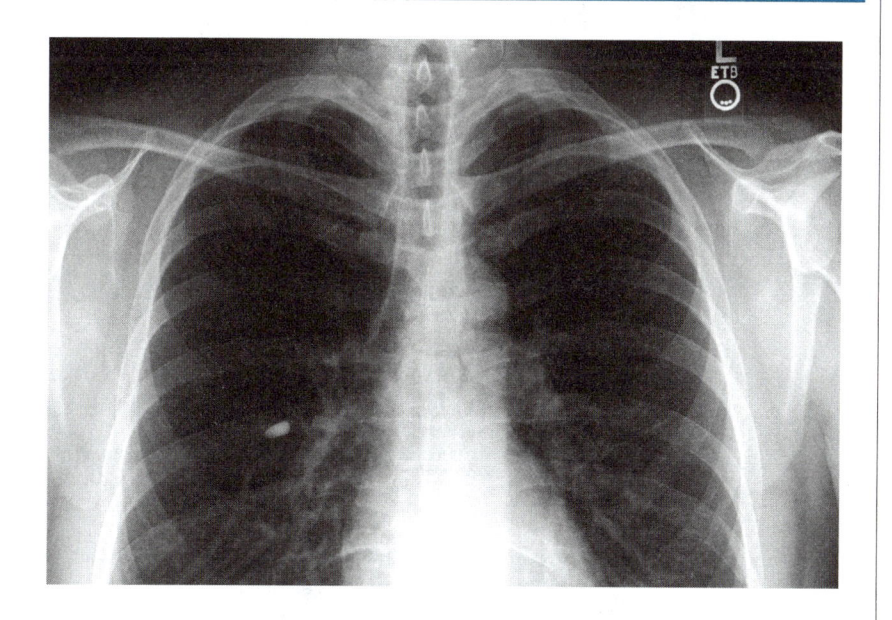

Comprehensive Anatomy and Physiology for ICD-10-CM and ICD-10-PCS Coding

A penetrating wound is one that pierces the skin and enters the body, possibly affecting underlying structures and organs.

A puncture is any injury that creates a hole in the skin and/or internal tissues or organs.

An open bite is a wound caused by teeth, human or animal.

A foreign body is an object or substance found in an organ or tissue that does not belong there under normal circumstances. The following table is an example of some of the many ICD-10-CM codes that ICD-9-CM code 862.9 maps to. For detailed information on ICD-9-CM to ICD-10-CM mapping, see Optum360's *ICD-10-CM Mappings*.

Coding for Multiple and Unspecified Injuries to the Intrathoracic Organs, with Open Wound into Cavity

ICD-9-CM		ICD-10-CM	
862.9	Injury to multiple and unspecified intrathoracic organs with open wound into cavity	S27.9XXA	Injury of unspecified intrathoracic organ, initial encounter
		AND	
		S21.311A	Laceration without foreign body of right front wall of thorax with penetration into thoracic cavity, initial encounter
		S21.312A	Laceration without foreign body of left front wall of thorax with penetration into thoracic cavity, initial encounter
		S21.321A	Laceration with foreign body of right front wall of thorax with penetration into thoracic cavity, initial encounter
		S21.322A	Laceration with foreign body of left front wall of thorax with penetration into thoracic cavity, initial encounter
		S21.331A	Puncture wound without foreign body of right front wall of thorax with penetration into thoracic cavity, initial encounter
		S21.332A	Puncture wound without foreign body of left front wall of thorax with penetration into thoracic cavity, initial encounter
		S21.341A	Puncture wound with foreign body of right front wall of thorax with penetration into thoracic cavity, initial encounter
		S21.342A	Puncture wound with foreign body of left front wall of thorax with penetration into thoracic cavity, initial encounter
		S21.351A	Open bite of right front wall of thorax with penetration into thoracic cavity, initial encounter
		S21.352A	Open bite of left front wall of thorax with penetration into thoracic cavity, initial encounter
		S21.401A	Unspecified open wound of right back wall of thorax with penetration into thoracic cavity, initial encounter
		S21.402A	Unspecified open wound of left back wall of thorax with penetration into thoracic cavity, initial encounter
		S21.411A	Laceration without foreign body of right back wall of thorax with penetration into thoracic cavity, initial encounter
		S21.412A	Laceration without foreign body of left back wall of thorax with penetration into thoracic cavity, initial encounter
		S21.421A	Laceration with foreign body of right back wall of thorax with penetration into thoracic cavity, initial encounter
(Continued on next page)			

ICD-9-CM		ICD-10-CM	
862.9	Injury to multiple and unspecified intrathoracic organs with open wound into cavity **(Continued)**	S21.422A	Laceration with foreign body of left back wall of thorax with penetration into thoracic cavity, initial encounter
		S21.431A	Puncture wound without foreign body of right back wall of thorax with penetration into thoracic cavity, initial encounter
		S21.432A	Puncture wound without foreign body of left back wall of thorax with penetration into thoracic cavity, initial encounter
		S21.441A	Puncture wound with foreign body of right back wall of thorax with penetration into thoracic cavity, initial encounter
		S21.442A	Puncture wound with foreign body of left back wall of thorax with penetration into thoracic cavity, initial encounter
		S21.451A	Open bite of right back wall of thorax with penetration into thoracic cavity, initial encounter
		S21.452A	Open bite of left back wall of thorax with penetration into thoracic cavity, initial encounter

The transition to ICD-10-CM requires that the coder be able to pinpoint more specifics within the documentation. There will no longer be just one applicable code for multiple thoracic injuries; instead, the definition of the type of injury, the general location of the wound, and whether or not a foreign body was present will all play a part in code selection. Physicians may need to be educated about the need to report these specifics in the documentation.

Injuries of the Face and Neck

The injuries of the face and neck are also much more detailed in ICD-10-CM than in ICD-9-CM, not unlike the injuries to the chest wall. The new code set zeroes in on the specific location of the injury, as well as the tissues and/or organs affected.

Figure 10.11: Upper Respiratory System

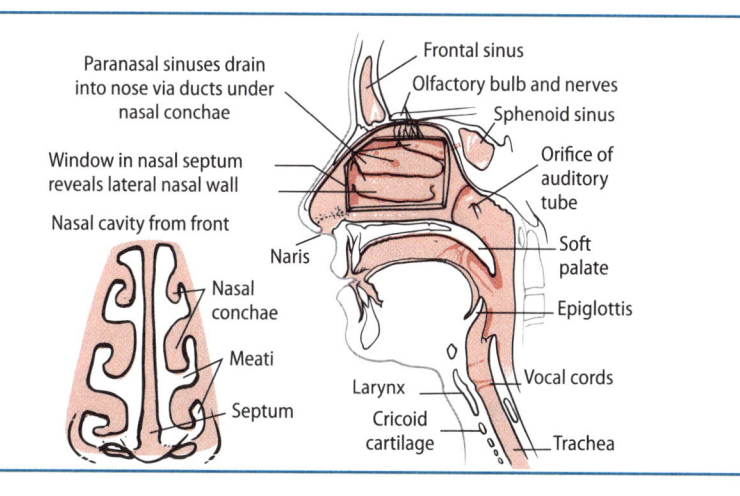

Fascia are fibrous sheets or bands of tissue that encase organs, muscles, and groups of muscles. The cervical trachea starts at the sixth cervical vertebra and extends to the sternum, where it divides into the bronchus. The vocal cords are a pair of strong bands of tissue located within the larynx. Their main purpose is to vibrate to produce sound for speaking or singing. They are also known as vocal folds, and injuries to these bands can obviously have a significant effect on a person's ability to communicate.

The thyroid gland is an endocrine gland located in the front of the lower neck composed of two lobes on either side of the trachea. The thyroid gland's main responsibility is secreting and storing the thyroid hormones that regulate metabolism.

The cervical esophagus connects the pharynx and stomach. This structure begins in the area of the fifth and sixth cervical vertebrae and runs to just above the sternum.

Coding for Other Injury of the Face and Neck

ICD-9-CM		ICD-10-CM	
959.09	Injury of face and neck, other and unspecified	S09.92XA	Unspecified injury of nose, initial encounter
		S09.93XA	Unspecified injury of face, initial encounter
		S16.8XXA	Other specified injury of muscle, fascia and tendon at neck level, initial encounter
		S16.9XXA	Unspecified injury of muscle, fascia and tendon at neck level, initial encounter
		S19.80XA	Other specified injuries of unspecified part of neck, initial encounter
		S19.81XA	Other specified injuries of larynx, initial encounter
		S19.82XA	Other specified injuries of cervical trachea, initial encounter
		S19.83XA	Other specified injuries of vocal cord, initial encounter
		S19.84XA	Other specified injuries of thyroid gland, initial encounter
		S19.85XA	Other specified injuries of pharynx and cervical esophagus, initial encounter
		S19.89XA	Other specified injuries of other specified part of neck, initial encounter
		S19.9XXA	Unspecified injury of neck, initial encounter

Summary

The human body uses oxygen in its cells to process nutrients. In return, these cells release carbon dioxide, a waste gas that needs to be released back into the atmosphere. The respiratory system manages these processes. Inspiration brings oxygen into the human body, and expiration releases the waste carbon dioxide back into the atmosphere. When these systems break down, there are many disease pathologies to understand.

ICD-9-CM had many specific codes for respiratory system related conditions, but ICD-10-CM has brought specificity to a new level. By learning more about the various areas of anatomy, pathology, and pathophysiology, coders will be better prepared to face the challenges of coding respiratory conditions under ICD-10-CM.

Chapter 11. ICD-10-CM: Digestive System

Anatomic Overview

The digestive system carries out the process of ***digestion*** and is composed of an alimentary canal, or the gastrointestinal tract, and accessory organs. The alimentary canal consists of the mouth, pharynx, esophagus, stomach, small intestine, large intestine, rectum, and anus. The accessory organs include the liver, gallbladder, and pancreas, as well as other structures such as the teeth, tongue, and salivary glands.

Digestion is a multistage process that can be divided into four main steps. The first—ingestion—involves placing food and liquids into the mouth. The second step—digestion—involves the breakdown of foods and can be divided into two subprocesses: chemical and mechanical. Mechanical digestion breaks larger pieces into smaller ones without altering their chemical composition, whereas chemical digestion breaks foods into simpler chemicals so that they can be absorbed into the bloodstream. The third step—absorption—involves the movement of nutrients from the digestive system to the circulatory and lymphatic systems through osmosis, active transport, or diffusion. The fourth and final step—excretion—involves removal of any undigested materials from the gastrointestinal tract through defecation.

> **DEFINITIONS**
>
> **digestion.** Mechanical, chemical, and enzymatic process whereby ingested food is converted into material suitable for assimilation for synthesis of tissues or liberation of energy.
>
> **mastication.** Process of chewing food to ready it for the digestive system.
>
> **peristalsis.** Smooth muscle action of automatic contractions that propel substances through the body, such as urine into the bladder and food through the digestive tract.

Figure 11.1: Digestive System

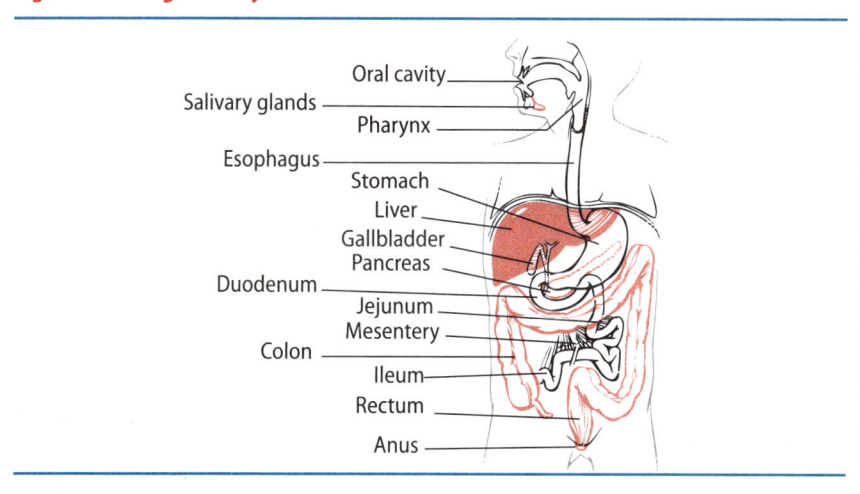

Digestion begins in the mouth where food is mechanically broken down in a process called ***mastication***. The mouth or oral cavity is the chamber behind the lips and between the tongue and palate. The narrow space between the teeth, cheeks, and lips is called the vestibule. During mastication, the teeth grind the food into smaller particles while the tongue mixes the food with saliva. Once the food has been thoroughly chewed and mixed with saliva, the bolus is ready to be passed into the esophagus.

The esophagus is a straight, collapsible tube approximately 25 centimeters in length. It begins at the base of the pharynx, descends behind the trachea, and passes through the diaphragm until it reaches the stomach. Food is moved down the esophagus by a process called ***peristalsis***. Peristalsis is a wavelike motion by which automatic smooth muscle contractions push the contents of tubular structures from one place in the tube to the place just ahead of it. No digestion occurs in the esophagus, as this tube merely functions as a passageway between the mouth and stomach.

The stomach is a small, J-shaped organ that hangs below the diaphragm in the upper portion of the abdominal cavity, mostly to the left of the median line. Its size and position are variable because an adult stomach is able to distend from a collapsed state to accommodate a volume of up to one liter or one and one-half liters, and it can be pushed up and down with inspiration and expiration.

There are three divisions of the stomach: the fundus, the body, and the pylorus. The fundus is the enlarged portion to the left above the cardiac sphincter. The body is the central part, and the pylorus is the lower narrowing portion. One of the primary critical functions of the stomach is to store partially digested food that is then churned, mixed, and moved into the duodenum. In addition, the stomach is a secretory organ that secretes gastric juices and an intrinsic factor to protect B12 before the vitamin's absorption. The stomach also absorbs some drugs, water, alcohol, and lactic fatty acids; produces gastrin hormone for digestive regulation; and helps destroy swallowed pathogenic bacteria.

Figure 11.2: Stomach and Pylorus

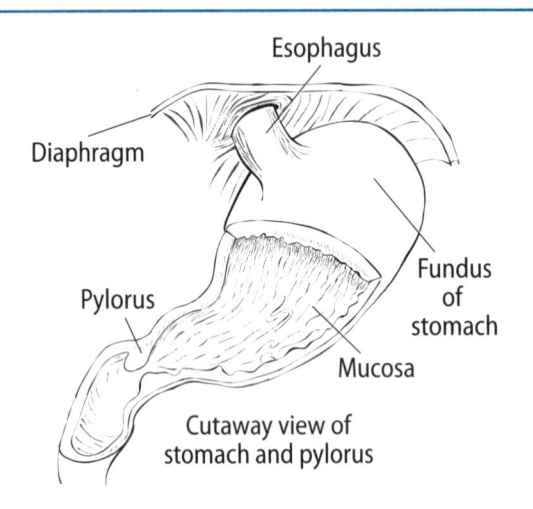

Cutaway view of stomach and pylorus

The small intestine, a tubular structure that extends from the pyloric region of the stomach to the beginning of the large intestine, consists of three distinct regions. The duodenum is about 25 centimeters long and is the portion of the small intestine that is the most immobile. The other two regions of the small intestine, the jejunum and the ileum, are mobile and lie freely within the peritoneal cavity. The jejunum, about 1 meter long, connects the duodenum to the final portion of the small intestine, the ileum. The ileum is about 2 meters long, and it connects the small intestine to the proximal end of the large intestine. Although the jejunum and the ileum are not distinctly separate parts, the diameter of the jejunum is greater than that of the ileum, and its wall is thicker, more vascular, and more active.

Figure 11.3: Duodenum

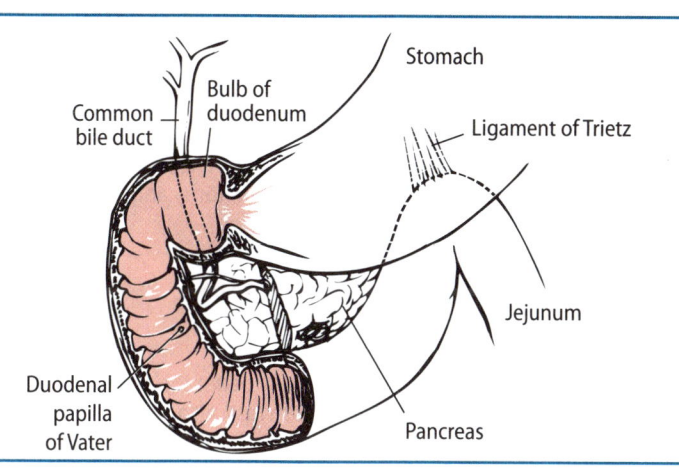

Labels: Stomach, Bulb of duodenum, Common bile duct, Ligament of Trietz, Jejunum, Pancreas, Duodenal papilla of Vater

---

The small intestine plays an important role in digestion. It secretes digestive enzymes that aid in the complete digestion of carbohydrates, proteins, lipids, and nucleic acids. Not only does the small intestine secrete digestive enzymes, but about 90 percent of all the products of digestion are absorbed in the small intestine.

The next portion along the gastrointestinal tract is the large intestine. It joins the small intestines at the ileocecal sphincter and is about 1.5 meters long. The large intestine consists of the cecum, colon, rectum, and anal canal. The colon is further subdivided into four portions: the ascending, transverse, descending, and sigmoid.

The main role of the large intestine is to pass waste material from the body, although water and some nutrients such as sodium are absorbed in the large intestine. Mucus is secreted to protect the intestinal wall against the material passing through, and it also binds to the fecal matter. The undigested food, or chyme, entering the large intestine contains materials the small intestine did not digest or absorb. It also contains water, electrolytes, mucus, and bacteria. After the large intestine absorbs the water and electrolytes, the substances remaining in the tube become feces and are stored in the distal portion of the large intestine until they are excreted from the rectum.

Digestion occurs along the various portions of the gastrointestinal tract, but without the help of various accessory organs, certain substances could not be digested. The pancreas, for instance, is a glandular organ that has both an endocrine and exocrine function. It is more commonly known for its role in glucose maintenance and the production of insulin (see the endocrine chapter for more information on this role of the pancreas), yet it also plays an important role in digestion by secreting a fluid called pancreatic juice. This juice contains enzymes that digest carbohydrates, fats, proteins, and nucleic acids. The pancreas also helps neutralize the acidic chyme that leaves the stomach and enters the intestine.

The liver is a large, reddish-brown, glandular organ in the upper right portion of the abdominal cavity. The liver is enclosed by a fibrous covering and is divided into lobes by a thick layer of connective tissue. The liver produces bile, which aids digestion by breaking fats into smaller droplets, a process called emulsification, so that enzymes can break them down even further. Also, the liver processes carbohydrates and proteins absorbed by the small intestine and acts as the detoxification center of the body by breaking down hormones and drugs and other foreign toxins.

The gallbladder is a pear-shaped sac on the liver's inferior surface. It connects to the cystic duct, which in turn is connected to the common hepatic duct. The gallbladder's role in digestion is to store **bile** between meals, reabsorb excess water to get more concentrated bile, and to contract so that the bile is released into the small intestine.

KEY POINT

- Peristalsis propels food content through the esophagus and the intestine.
- Mass peristalsis, which occurs only three to four times a day, moves the contents of the large intestine from one segment to the next.
- Reversed peristalsis occurs when the contractions occur in a direction that is opposite of normal, pushing the intestinal contents backwards.

CLINICAL NOTE

The pancreas is both an endocrine and exocrine gland.

- The endocrine function involves the secretion of insulin, the hormone that plays a major role in glucose maintenance and has a direct relationship to diabetes mellitus.
- The exocrine function is the secretion of pancreatic juices, which help break down carbohydrates, fats, nucleic acids, and proteins.

DEFINITIONS

bile. Yellowish-brown or green fluid secreted by the liver and discharged into the duodenum, where it aids in the emulsification of fats, increases peristalsis, and retards putrefaction.

Anatomy and Pathophysiology and the ICD-10-CM Code Set

Many diseases can affect the various parts of the digestive system. Some of them may have a direct effect on the gastrointestinal tract, and some affect the digestive accessory organs indirectly. This section outlines different diseases and highlights some of the areas where increased knowledge of anatomy and physiology is needed to understand the ICD-10-CM code set.

Diseases of the Accessory Digestive Organs

Tooth Loss

Teeth play a critical role in digestion because they begin the process of physically breaking down food into smaller particles. Tooth loss, also known as edentulism, signifies the loss of some or all natural teeth. Tooth loss is caused most commonly by periodontal disease and dental caries but can also be attributed to congenital conditions such as **Papillon–Lefèvre syndrome** (PLS), systemic conditions such as **Langerhans cell histiocytosis** (LCH), loss of supporting structures, and trauma.

Figure 11.4: Teeth

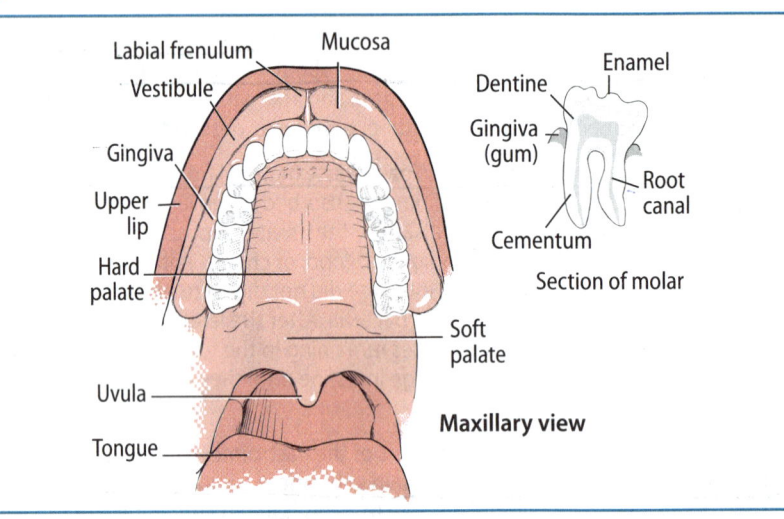

Edentulism can be classified as partial, the loss of one or multiple teeth, or complete, the loss of all teeth. Edentulism is divided into four classes that differ in the level of difficulty or complexity in treatment for complete edentulism and how compromised the presenting diagnostic criteria are in partial edentulism. Class IV is the most debilitating, requiring reconstructive surgery when all teeth are missing, and has the most severely compromised edentulous area in partial edentulism.

Coding for tooth loss in ICD-9-CM requires the use of two codes: a code from category 525.1X represents the cause of the edentulism and 525.4X or 525.5X represents the class of edentulism. However, due to the increased granularity in ICD-10-CM, coding for tooth loss no longer requires multiple codes. There are now combination codes that represent both the cause and the class of the edentulism.

DEFINITIONS

Langerhans cell histiocytosis. Set of closely related disorders unified by a common proliferation of Langerhans cells (epidermal dendritic cells). LCH has also been known as Hand-Schüller-Christian disease, Abt-Letterer-Siwe disease, and histiocytosis X.

Papillon–Lefèvre syndrome. Genetic disorder caused by a deficiency in the cathepsin C enzyme that is characterized by the severe destruction of periodontium, resulting in the loss of all primary and permanent teeth by age 14.

Coding for Edentulism

ICD-9-CM		ICD-10-CM	
525.11	Loss of teeth due to trauma	K08.111	Complete loss of teeth due to trauma, class I
		K08.112	Complete loss of teeth due to trauma, class II
		K08.113	Complete loss of teeth due to trauma, class III
		K08.114	Complete loss of teeth due to trauma, class IV
		K08.119	Complete loss of teeth due to trauma, unspecified class
		K08.411	Partial loss of teeth due to trauma, class I
		K08.412	Partial loss of teeth due to trauma, class II
		K08.413	Partial loss of teeth due to trauma, class III
		K08.414	Partial loss of teeth due to trauma, class IV
		K08.419	Partial loss of teeth due to trauma, unspecified class
525.12	Loss of teeth due to periodontal disease	K08.121	Complete loss of teeth due to periodontal disease, class I
		K08.122	Complete loss of teeth due to periodontal disease, class II
		K08.123	Complete loss of teeth due to periodontal disease, class III
		K08.124	Complete loss of teeth due to periodontal disease, class IV
		K08.129	Complete loss of teeth due to periodontal disease, unspecified class
		K08.421	Partial loss of teeth due to periodontal disease, class I
		K08.422	Partial loss of teeth due to periodontal disease, class II
		K08.423	Partial loss of teeth due to periodontal disease, class III
		K08.424	Partial loss of teeth due to periodontal disease, class IV
		K08.429	Partial loss of teeth due to periodontal disease, unspecified class
525.42	Complete edentulism, class II	K08.102	Complete loss of teeth, unspecified cause, class II
		K08.112	Complete loss of teeth due to trauma, class II
		K08.122	Complete loss of teeth due to periodontal disease, class II
		K08.132	Complete loss of teeth due to caries, class II
		K08.192	Complete loss of teeth due to other specified cause, class II
525.52	Partial edentulism, class II	K08.402	Partial loss of teeth, unspecified cause, class II
		K08.412	Partial loss of teeth due to trauma, class II
		K08.422	Partial loss of teeth due to periodontal disease, class II
		K08.432	Partial loss of teeth due to caries, class II
		K08.492	Partial loss of teeth due to other specified cause, class II

Sialoadenitis

The salivary glands secrete saliva, a predominantly alkaline fluid that moistens the mouth, softens food particles, and aids in chemical digestion. There are three pairs of major salivary glands. The first, and largest, pair is called the parotids, which secrete a clear, watery fluid rich in amylase, an enzyme that aids in breaking down carbohydrates. The second pair is the submandibular glands, which secrete a fluid containing a mixture of watery and mucus-type fluids that are slightly more viscous than the fluids secreted by the parotids. The third pair is the sublingual glands, which

> **INTERESTING A & P FACT**
>
> There are an additional 600 glands within the submucosa throughout the oral cavity, called minor salivary glands. They measure about 1 mm to 2 mm in diameter, are surrounded by connective tissue, have secretions made mostly of mucus, and serve to coat the oral cavity. Mucus secretions from these glands are generally the root cause of nonsticking denture problems.

secrete a thick, mucus-type fluid containing the enzyme lysozyme, which aids in the destruction of bacteria that may enter the oral cavity.

Figure 11.5: Saliva Glands

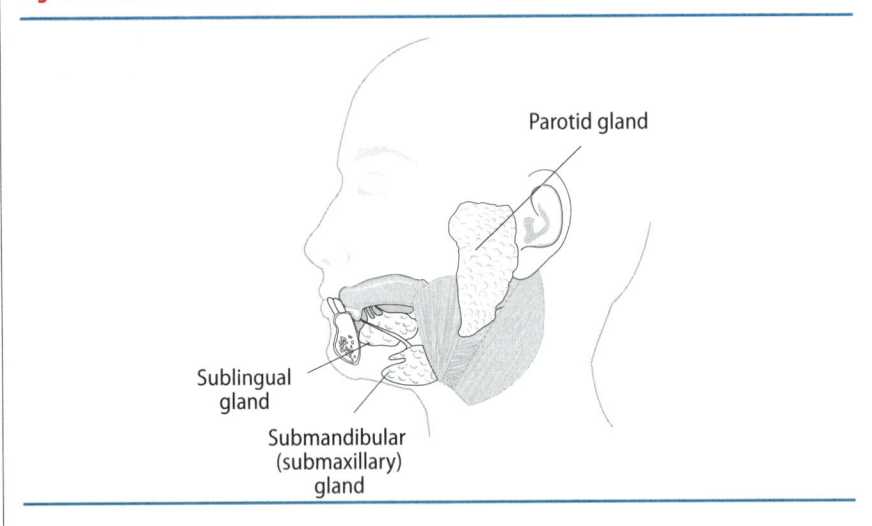

Sialoadenitis is a bacterial infection of one of the salivary glands, usually due to an obstruction or gland hyposecretion. It is characterized by swelling, pain, redness, and tenderness. The most common causal organism is **Staphylococcus aureus**, but sialoadenitis has also been known to be caused by streptococci, coliforms, and various other anaerobic bacteria.

Coding for sialoadenitis in ICD-9-CM is straightforward—there is only one code, 527.2, for this disease. However, in ICD-10-CM, coders need to know more than just that the disease is present.

Coding for Sialoadenitis in ICD-10-CM

K11.20   Sialoadenitis, unspecified

K11.21   Acute sialoadenitis

K11.22   Acute recurrent sialoadenitis

K11.23   Chronic sialoadenitis

To code this disease accurately in ICD-10-CM, coders need to know if it is acute, acute recurrent, chronic, or unspecified. Because this is a new concept for this disease, providers may not be documenting required information. For this reason, it may be a good idea to start reviewing those concepts that are new in ICD-10-CM now and begin educating providers on documentation needs.

Hepatitis and Cirrhosis of the Liver

Cirrhosis of the liver is a chronic, progressive disease characterized by damage to the hepatic parenchymal cells and nodular regeneration, fibrosis formation, and disturbance of the normal architecture. Two different types of cirrhosis have been described based on the amount of regenerative activity in the liver. There is chronic sclerosing cirrhosis, in which the liver is small and hard, and nodular cirrhosis, in which the liver may be quite large initially.

Chronic alcohol use can lead to both hepatitis and cirrhosis. The conditions may have similar features, and both can occur without the use of alcohol. However, alcoholic cirrhosis accounts for about 60 percent of all cirrhosis cases, and the risk appears to rise with the amount of alcohol consumed daily.

DEFINITIONS

staphylococcus aureus. Gram-positive bacteria that commonly resides on the skin and can cause a range of illnesses, from minor skin infections to life-threatening diseases like pneumonia, meningitis, endocarditis, bacteremia, and sepsis.

Figure 11.6: Liver

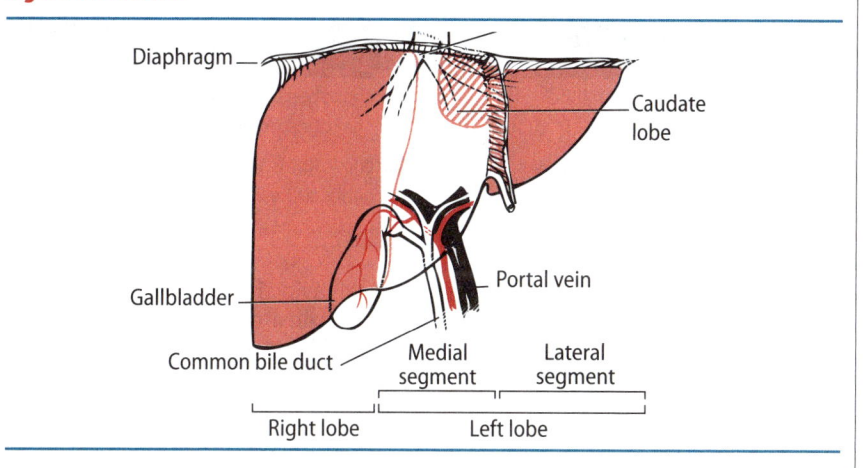

Hepatitis is the inflammation of the liver and may be caused by alcohol abuse or viruses. Alcoholic hepatitis is caused by prolonged excessive intake of alcohol and can be mild with only liver enzyme elevation or severe with symptoms that may include development of ascites or jaundice, prolonged prothrombin time, enlarged liver, and even liver failure. Many who consume excessive alcohol become malnourished due to the empty calories from alcohol, poor appetite, and poor absorption of nutrients. This condition is diagnosed by complete blood count (CBC), liver biopsy, and liver function test; and treatment includes alcohol cessation, rehabilitation and counseling programs, and vitamin B-complex and folic acid to help reverse the malnutrition.

Hepatitis due to viral infections, or viral hepatitis, is most commonly caused by one of the five unrelated hepatotropic viruses. Hepatitis A (HAV) is a picornavirus commonly found in children and young adults. It can be spread through person-to-person contact, consumption of raw shellfish, and drinking contaminated water. This form of hepatitis does not have a chronic stage and is the most common cause of acute viral hepatitis.

Hepatitis B (HBV) is a hepadnavirus that has both acute and chronic forms. HBV is the second most common cause of acute viral hepatitis, but its route of transmission is through contaminated blood, blood products, sexual contact, and via mother to child by breastfeeding. Routine screening for hepatitis B surface antigen (HbsAg) has nearly eliminated transmission via blood transfusion. However, needle sharing by drug users, sharing shaving accessories within closed institutions, and touching wounds of infected persons are still modes of transmission.

Hepatitis C (HCV) is a flavivirus that has six major subtypes. HCV infection is most often transferred through blood via needle sharing, tattoos, and body piercings. Transmission through sexual contact and from mother to baby is very rare, and HCV infection generally remains asymptomatic in patients for decades.

Hepatitis D (HDV), also called delta agent, has similar characteristics to a viroid as it can replicate only in the presence of HBV. HDV infection occurs as a coinfection with acute HBV or as a new infection in patients with chronic hepatitis B.

Hepatitis E (HEV) is an RNA virus that produces symptoms similar to HAV. Outbreaks of acute HEV infections have been linked to fecal contamination of the water supply and have occurred in China, India, Mexico, Pakistan, Peru, Russia, and central and northern Africa. Like hepatitis A, HEV does not have a chronic stage and does not produce chronic hepatitis or further develop into cirrhosis.

Codes for alcoholic cirrhosis and hepatitis in ICD-9-CM are in category 571 Chronic liver disease and cirrhosis. However, in ICD-10-CM coding for these conditions has been further specified as occurring with or without ascites.

Coding for Alcoholic Hepatitis and Cirrhosis

ICD-9-CM		ICD-10-CM	
571.1	Acute alcoholic hepatitis	K70.10	Alcoholic hepatitis without ascites
		K70.11	Alcoholic hepatitis with ascites
571.2	Alcoholic cirrhosis of the liver	K70.2	Alcoholic fibrosis and sclerosis of the liver
		K70.30	Alcoholic cirrhosis of liver without ascites
		K70.31	Alcoholic cirrhosis of liver with ascites

Ascites is an accumulation of fluid in the peritoneal cavity. The most common cause of ascites is advanced liver disease or cirrhosis. Approximately 81 percent of the ascites cases are thought to be due to cirrhosis and, of that number, 65 percent are attributed to alcohol use. Although the exact mechanism of ascites development is not completely understood, most theories suggest portal hypertension, which is an increased pressure in the liver blood flow, as the main contributor.

It is important to note that several conditions coded to 573.3 Unspecified hepatitis, in ICD-9-CM have their own codes in ICD-10-CM, as the list below indicates. Toxic liver disease refers to liver damage that is chemical- or drug-induced. Because this type of hepatitis is caused by a chemical, in ICD-10-CM instructional notes guide the coder to first code for the poisoning due to a drug or toxin, if applicable. The coder will use an additional code for adverse effect, if applicable, to identify the drug itself. Nonalcoholic steatohepatitis, or NASH, is a common, often "silent," liver disease. It resembles alcoholic liver disease but occurs in people who drink little or no alcohol. The major feature in NASH is fat in the liver, along with inflammation and damage. NASH can be severe and can lead to cirrhosis, in which the liver is permanently damaged and scarred and no longer able to work properly. Peliosis hepatitis is an uncommon condition characterized by randomly distributed multiple blood-filled cystic cavities throughout the liver. It is usually asymptomatic but has been known to develop into overt liver disease and can even cause rupture with hemorrhage. Mild cases are generally detected incidentally when liver function tests show abnormal results or when the cysts are seen on ultrasound.

Coding for Other Hepatitis Conditions in ICD-10-CM

- K71.0 Toxic liver disease with cholestasis
    - K71.10 Toxic liver disease with hepatic necrosis, without coma
    - K71.11 Toxic liver disease with hepatic necrosis, with coma
- K71.2 Toxic liver disease with acute hepatitis
- K71.3 Toxic liver disease with chronic persistent hepatitis
- K71.4 Toxic liver disease with chronic lobular hepatitis
    - K71.50 Toxic liver disease with chronic active hepatitis without ascites
    - K71.51 Toxic liver disease with chronic active hepatitis with ascites
- K71.6 Toxic liver disease with hepatitis, not elsewhere classified
- K71.7 Toxic liver disease with fibrosis and cirrhosis of liver
- K71.8 Toxic liver disease with other disorders of liver
- K71.9 Toxic liver disease, unspecified
- K75.2 Nonspecific reactive hepatitis
- K75.3 Granulomatous hepatitis, not elsewhere classified
    - K75.81 Nonalcoholic steatohepatitis (NASH)
    - K75.89 Other specified inflammatory liver diseases
- K75.9 Inflammatory liver disease, unspecified
- K76.4 Peliosis hepatis

The code descriptions include several manifestations with toxic liver disease. For instance, cholestasis refers to the impairment of bile flow, which has been known to be caused by many different drugs. Also mentioned is necrosis, the pathologic death of one or more cells, or of a portion of tissue or organ; in the liver this most commonly refers to the parenchymal cells. In toxic liver disease, necrosis is classified with or without coma. Lobular hepatitis is an inflammation localized to one of the lobes of the liver, and ascites is an accumulation of fluid in the peritoneal cavity and, as previously mentioned, is commonly caused by advanced liver disease or cirrhosis.

Acute or Chronic Pancreatitis

Pancreatitis is the inflammation of the pancreas and is classified as acute or chronic. The acute form is sudden, while chronic pancreatitis is recurring or persistent abdominal pain. Chronic pancreatitis is characterized by tissue changes that are irreversible and progressive and that result in a considerable amount of pancreatic function. Patients with chronic pancreatitis may have a flare-up of acute disease.

Figure 11.7: Pancreas

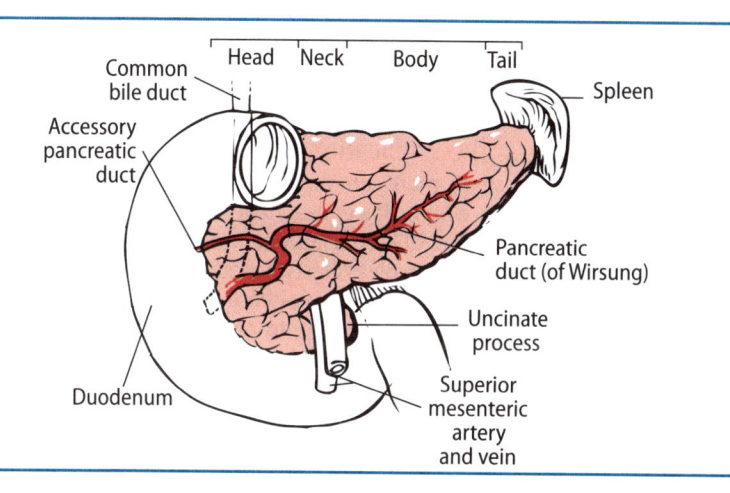

In ICD-9-CM, coding for pancreatitis is divided between two codes, 577.0 Acute pancreatitis, and 577.1 Chronic pancreatitis. ICD-10-CM still has two main categories of the disease, but the code range has been expanded to include the cause of the pancreatitis.

Patients who have had any type of procedure that requires cannulation or injection of the pancreatic ducts are at slightly higher risk for developing pancreatitis. The condition is also a major risk for patients who have undergone endoscopic retrograde cholangiopancreatography, which involves endoscopic and radiographic exam of the pancreatic and common bile ducts and is used to diagnose and treat conditions of the pancreatic and biliary ductal systems. During the procedure, the physician passes an endoscope through the oropharynx, esophagus, and small intestine where contrast material is injected through the ampulla of Vater in a direction opposite of normal flow. The common bile duct, biliary tract, and gallbladder are then visualized and imaged. Pancreatitis resulting from ERCP can be mild but can also require hospitalization and be life-threatening in rare cases.

Pancreatitis can also arise from **cytomegalovirus**, which can cause infections ranging widely in severity. Cytomegaloviral pancreatitis is coded from category B25 in ICD-10-CM.

> **DEFINITIONS**
>
> **cytomegalovirus.** Large herpesvirus, also known as *human herpesvirus 5*, that remains mostly latent in leukocytes and replicates very slowly. CMV is spread from direct person-to-person contact and is usually harmless but can cause severe disease in people with compromised immune systems.

The most common cause of acute pancreatitis is the presence of gallstones, small, pebble-like substances made of hardened bile that cause inflammation in the pancreas as they pass through the common bile duct. Excessive alcohol and drug use are two of the most common causes of chronic pancreatitis and can also be a contributing factor in acute pancreatitis.

Coding for Pancreatitis

ICD-9-CM		ICD-10-CM	
577.0	Acute pancreatitis	B25.2	Cytomegaloviral pancreatitis
		K85.0	Idiopathic acute pancreatitis
		K85.1	Biliary acute pancreatitis
		K85.2	Alcohol induced acute pancreatitis
		K85.3	Drug induced acute pancreatitis
		K85.8	Other acute pancreatitis
		K85.9	Acute pancreatitis, unspecified
577.1	Chronic pancreatitis	K86.0	Alcohol-induced chronic pancreatitis
		K86.1	Other chronic pancreatitis

Disease of the Gastrointestinal Tract

Esophageal Diseases and Complications

Gastroesophageal reflux disease, more commonly referred to as GERD, is characterized by incompetence of the lower esophageal sphincter that allows reflux of gastric acid into the esophagus. GERD is a fairly common disease, occurring in 30 to 40 percent of adults. Treatment involves lifestyle modification, acid suppression, and, in some instances, surgery. Coding for this disease in both ICD-9-CM and ICD-10-CM is straightforward, and there is a one-to-one mapping correlation between the two code sets. The only difference between the descriptions is that ICD-10-CM clarifies that no esophagitis is present.

Coding for Gastroesophageal Reflux Disease

ICD-9-CM		ICD-10-CM	
530.81	Esophageal reflux	K21.9	Gastro-esophageal reflux disease without esophagitis

Figure 11.8: Esophagus

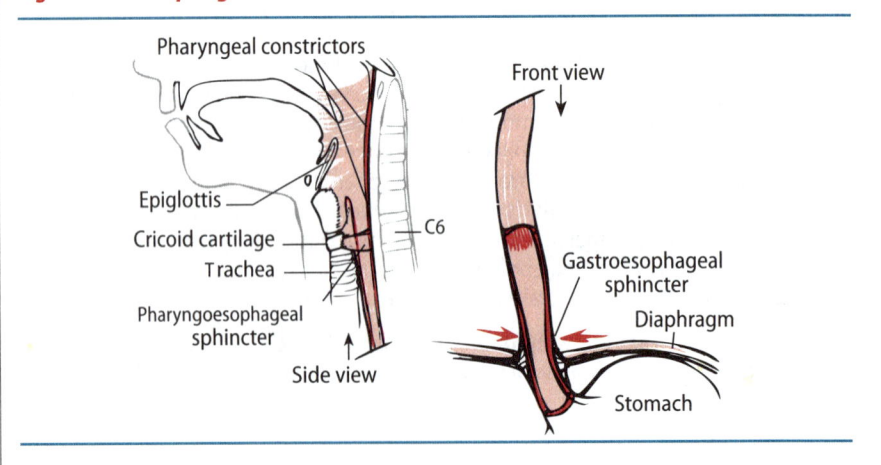

> **INTERESTING A & P FACT**
>
> Heartburn describes a burning sensation in the chest that is often found to be caused by an esophagus irritated by the reflux of stomach acid. This term is a misnomer, as the symptoms and cause of the condition are rarely related to any type of heart disease.

There may be an exact mapping relationship for GERD, but there are a few esophageal disorders with clinical differences in the code sets between ICD-9-CM and ICD-10-CM.

Barrett's esophagus refers to an abnormal change, known as **metaplasia**, in the cells of the inferior portion of the esophagus. The condition occurs due to chronic inflammation, usually caused by GERD. The chronic exposure of the cells in the lower esophagus to gastric acid damages those cells, resulting in the metaplasia. While there is no relationship between the severity of the reflux disease and the development of Barrett's esophagus, there is a relationship between chronic GERD and the development of Barrett's esophagus.

Coding for Barrett's Esophagus

ICD-9-CM	ICD-10-CM	
530.85 Barrett's esophagus	K22.70	Barrett's esophagus without dysplasia
	K22.710	Barrett's esophagus with low grade dysplasia
	K22.711	Barrett's esophagus with high grade dysplasia
	K22.719	Barrett's esophagus with dysplasia, unspecified

In addition to coding the Barrett's esophagus, coders need to familiarize themselves with the different grades of **dysplasia**. Dysplasia is defined as abnormal tissue development and is the earliest form of precancerous lesion recognizable in a biopsy. The cells of Barrett's esophagus can be classified into four general categories: nondysplastic, low-grade dysplasia, high-grade dysplasia, and frank carcinoma. High-grade dysplasia and frank carcinoma patients are generally advised to undergo surgical treatment. Nondysplastic and low-grade patients are generally advised to undergo annual observation with endoscopy. In high-grade dysplasia, the risk of developing cancer might be at 10 percent or greater per patient-year.

Ulcers

An ulcer is defined as a lesion through the skin or mucous membrane resulting from loss of tissue, usually with inflammation. Ulcers can occur in various places along the gastrointestinal tract, including within the oral cavity, esophagus, and gastrointestinal mucosa. A gastric ulcer is a condition formed by discreet tissue destruction within the lumen of the stomach. Duodenal ulcers form in the duodenum and typically occur about five times more frequently than gastric ulcers. Both conditions are a result of the increased activity of hydrochloric (gastric) acid and pepsin on the mucosal linings of the organs.

Nearly all ulcers are caused by *Helicobacter pylori* infection or use of nonsteroidal anti-inflammatory drugs (NSAID). Signs and symptoms of ulcers may include pain exacerbated by eating, weight loss, repeated vomiting of "coffee ground" material, hematemesis, black and tarry stools, burning, and epigastria tenderness. Treatments can include antacids, diet modifications, H_2 receptor agonist drugs, bismuth, subtotal gastrectomy, and vagotomy.

DEFINITIONS

dysplasia. Term used in pathology to refer to abnormal tissue development.

metaplasia. Transformation of one type of mature differentiated cell type into another mature differentiated cell type. Examples include squamous metaplasia of the columnar epithelial cells of salivary gland ducts when stones are present and squamous metaplasia of the transitional epithelium of the bladder when stones are present.

KEY POINT

NSAIDs are nonsteroidal anti-inflammatory drugs commonly used to treat the following:

- Inflammatory arthropathies
- Metastatic bone pain
- Mild-to-moderate pain due to inflammation and tissue injury
- Postoperative pain
- Pyrexia (fever)
- Rheumatoid arthritis

Figure 11.9: Stomach

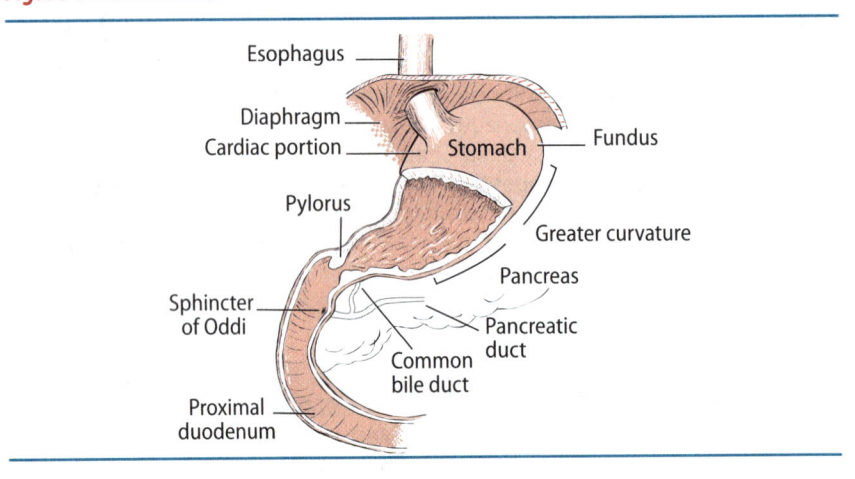

Illustration of the stomach showing: Esophagus, Diaphragm, Cardiac portion, Stomach, Fundus, Pylorus, Greater curvature, Pancreas, Sphincter of Oddi, Pancreatic duct, Common bile duct, Proximal duodenum.

The four categories of codes for gastrointestinal ulcers in ICD-9-CM are divided based on the specified site of the ulcer. Gastric ulcers are coded using category 531, duodenal ulcers are coded using category 532, gastrojejunal ulcers are coded using 534, and ulcers where the site is unspecified or documented as peptic ulcers are coded using category 533. In ICD-10-CM, there are still four distinct categories for the specified sites, but the coder no longer needs to indicate via a fifth character if an obstruction has occurred. Instead, two codes are required to report an ulcer with obstruction, one combination code for the ulcer identifying the site of the ulcer; whether the ulcer is acute, chronic or unspecified; and whether or not hemorrhage and/or perforation are present, along with an additional code for the obstruction.

Coding for Gastrointestinal Ulcers

ICD-9-CM		ICD-10-CM	
531.00	Acute gastric ulcer with hemorrhage, without mention of obstruction	K25.0	Acute gastric ulcer with hemorrhage
531.10	Acute gastric ulcer with perforation, without mention of obstruction	K25.1	Acute gastric ulcer with perforation
531.20	Acute gastric ulcer with hemorrhage and perforation, without mention of obstruction	K25.2	Acute gastric ulcer with both hemorrhage and perforation
531.30	Acute gastric ulcer without mention of hemorrhage, perforation, or obstruction	K25.3	Acute gastric ulcer without hemorrhage or perforation
531.40	Chronic or unspecified gastric ulcer with hemorrhage, without mention of obstruction	K25.4	Chronic or unspecified gastric ulcer with hemorrhage
531.50	Chronic or unspecified gastric ulcer with perforation, without mention of obstruction	K25.5	Chronic or unspecified gastric ulcer with perforation
531.60	Chronic or unspecified gastric ulcer with hemorrhage and perforation, without mention of obstruction	K25.6	Chronic or unspecified gastric ulcer with both hemorrhage and perforation
531.70	Chronic gastric ulcer without mention of hemorrhage, perforation, without mention of obstruction	K25.7	Chronic gastric ulcer without hemorrhage or perforation
531.90	Gastric ulcer, unspecified as acute or chronic, without mention of hemorrhage, perforation, or obstruction	K25.9	Gastric ulcer, unspecified as acute or chronic, without hemorrhage or perforation

The table above identifies the crosswalk for only category 531 Gastric ulcers. There are similar crosswalks for duodenal, peptic, and gastrojejunal ulcers.

When an ulcer causes scarring or swelling and this swelling prevents the contents of the stomach from properly entering into the duodenum, this condition is known as gastric outlet obstruction. In ICD-9-CM, unlike ICD-10-CM, code selection for ulcer is based on whether there was an obstruction. The only two complications of ulcers included in the code descriptions for ICD-10-CM are hemorrhage and perforation. The most common ulcer complication is gastrointestinal bleeding or hemorrhage, which occurs when the ulcerated tissue of the organ grows so thin that the gastric acids begin to erode the GI blood vessels. **Perforation** occurs when the ulcer erodes the wall of the GI organ, potentially spilling the stomach or intestinal contents into the abdominal cavity. Further complications from the spillage can lead to more serious conditions, such as peritonitis, pancreatitis, and penetration.

> **DEFINITIONS**
>
> **perforation.** Abnormal opening in a hollow organ or viscus.

Diverticular Disease

Diverticula are saclike out-pouchings of colonic mucosa and submucosa that protrude outward. Diverticulosis is the condition of having multiple diverticula in the colon. This disease can occur anywhere along the intestine but is most often found in the sigmoid colon. It has been suggested that diverticula are caused by increased intraluminal pressure, leading to mucosal extrusion through weaknesses in the muscle layer of the colon wall. About 70 percent of diverticula are asymptomatic, 15 to 25 percent are painful and become inflamed, and 10 to 15 percent bleed painlessly. The inflammation of diverticula is commonly referred to as diverticulitis.

Figure 11.10: Volvulus and Diverticulitis

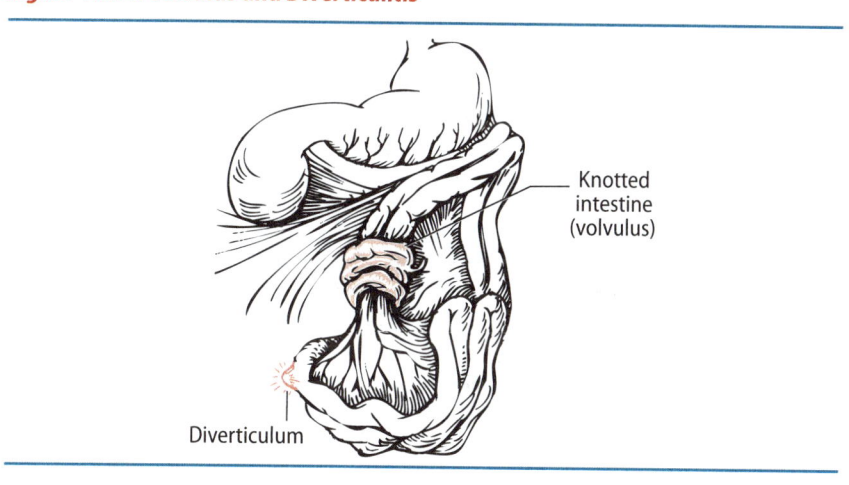

Diverticulitis occurs when a perforation occurs within a diverticulum and releases intestinal bacteria. For about 75 percent of the patients with this condition, the resultant inflammation remains localized. For the other 25 percent, this condition can progress and cause abscess, free intraperitoneal perforation, bowel obstruction, or fistulas.

Coding for diverticular disease is a bit more complex in ICD-10-CM than in ICD-9-CM. ICD-9-CM coders need to consider only the site of the diverticular disease and whether hemorrhage was present. In ICD-10-CM, coders also need to identify whether or not any additional complications exist.

Coding for Diverticular Disease

ICD-9-CM		ICD-10-CM	
562.00	Diverticulosis of small intestine (without mention of hemorrhage)	K57.10	Diverticulosis of small intestine without perforation or abscess without bleeding
		K57.50	Diverticulosis of both small and large intestine without perforation or abscess without bleeding
562.01	Diverticulitis of small intestine (without mention of hemorrhage)	K57.00	Diverticulitis of small intestine with perforation and abscess without bleeding
		K57.12	Diverticulitis of small intestine without perforation or abscess without bleeding
		K57.40	Diverticulitis of both small and large intestine with perforation and abscess without bleeding
		K57.52	Diverticulitis of both small and large intestine without perforation or abscess without bleeding
562.02	Diverticulosis of small intestine with hemorrhage	K57.11	Diverticulosis of small intestine without perforation or abscess with bleeding
		K57.51	Diverticulosis of both small and large intestine without perforation or abscess with bleeding
562.03	Diverticulitis of small intestine with hemorrhage	K57.01	Diverticulitis of small intestine with perforation and abscess with bleeding
		K57.13	Diverticulitis of small intestine without perforation or abscess with bleeding
		K57.41	Diverticulitis of both small and large intestine with perforation and abscess with bleeding
		K57.53	Diverticulitis of both small and large intestine without perforation or abscess with bleeding
562.10	Diverticulosis of colon (without mention of hemorrhage)	K57.30	Diverticulosis of large intestine without perforation or abscess without bleeding
		K57.50	Diverticulosis of both small and large intestine without perforation or abscess without bleeding
562.11	Diverticulitis of colon (without mention of hemorrhage)	K57.20	Diverticulitis of large intestine with perforation and abscess without bleeding
		K57.32	Diverticulitis of large intestine without perforation or abscess without bleeding
		K57.40	Diverticulitis of both small and large intestine with perforation and abscess without bleeding
		K57.52	Diverticulitis of both small and large intestine without perforation or abscess without bleeding
		K57.80	Diverticulitis of intestine, part unspecified, with perforation and abscess without bleeding
		K57.92	Diverticulitis of intestine, part unspecified, without perforation or abscess without bleeding
562.12	Diverticulosis of colon with hemorrhage	K57.31	Diverticulosis of large intestine without perforation or abscess with bleeding
		K57.51	Diverticulosis of both small and large intestine without perforation or abscess with bleeding
		K57.91	Diverticulosis of intestine, part unspecified, without perforation or abscess with bleeding

ICD-9-CM		ICD-10-CM	
562.13	Diverticulitis of colon with hemorrhage	K57.21	Diverticulitis of large intestine with perforation and abscess with bleeding
		K57.33	Diverticulitis of large intestine without perforation or abscess with bleeding
		K57.41	Diverticulitis of both small and large intestine with perforation and abscess with bleeding
		K57.53	Diverticulitis of both small and large intestine without perforation or abscess with bleeding
		K57.81	Diverticulitis of intestine, part unspecified, with perforation and abscess with bleeding
		K57.93	Diverticulitis of intestine, part unspecified, without perforation or abscess with bleeding

Code selection in ICD-10-CM begins the same as in ICD-9-CM. Coders need to first identify if the patient has diverticulosis or if the condition has progressed to diverticulitis. Unlike in ICD-9-CM, however, the coder needs not only to know whether there is a hemorrhage, but also to look for additional documentation on whether there is a perforation or abscess. These complications are what distinguish codes within each subcategory under category K57 Diverticular disease of the intestine.

Enteritis and Colitis

Regional enteritis is an inflammatory disease of the intestine characterized by a chronic **granulomatous** disease. It is chronic and can affect any part of the gastrointestinal tract but most commonly affects the ileum and colon. Also known as Crohn's disease, regional enteritis is identified by its characteristic cobblestone appearance where segments of diseased bowel are located between regions of healthy bowel tissue, hence the name regional enteritis.

There are five types of regional enteritis:

- Ileitis affects the ileum alone.
- Ileocolitis is the most common form and affects the lowest part of the small intestine (ileum) and the large intestine (colon).
- Jejunoileitis causes spotty patches of inflammation in the top half of the small intestine (jejunum).
- Crohn's (granulomatous) colitis affects only the large intestine.
- In some rare cases, gastroduodenal Crohn's disease causes inflammation in the stomach and first part of the small intestine, called the duodenum.

> **DEFINITIONS**
>
> **granulomatous.** Having to do with granuloma, which are nodular inflammatory lesions, usually small or granular, firm, persistent, and containing compactly grouped modified phagocytes.

Figure 11.11: Large Intestine

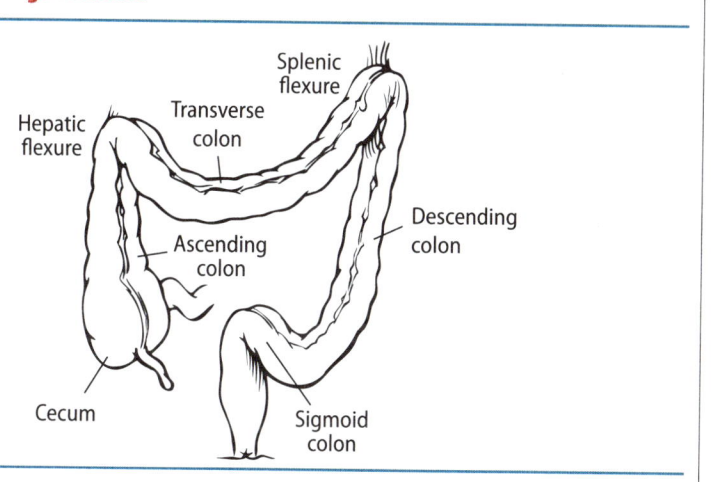

To code for this condition in ICD-10-CM, it is important to remember that the category title has changed. In ICD-9-CM, category 555 is entitled "Regional enteritis." The alphabetic index and the inclusion notes under the category title alert coders that this category also includes the coding for Crohn's disease and granulomatous enteritis. In ICD-10-CM, the opposite is true—the category title is Crohn's disease, and the alphabetic index and inclusion notes alert the coder that regional enteritis is coded under the category.

Another important difference between ICD-9-CM and ICD-10-CM is that coding for Crohn's disease and any of its complications no longer requires multiple codes. There is now one combination code that represents both conditions.

Coding for Regional Enteritis

ICD-9-CM		ICD-10-CM	
555.0	Regional enteritis of small intestine	K50.00	Crohn's disease of small intestine without complication
		K50.011	Crohn's disease of small intestine with rectal bleeding
		K50.012	Crohn's disease of small intestine with intestinal obstruction
		K50.013	Crohn's disease of small intestine with fistula
		K50.014	Crohn's disease of small intestine with abscess
		K50.018	Crohn's disease of small intestine with other complication
		K50.019	Crohn's disease of small intestine with unspecified complication
555.1	Regional enteritis of large intestine	K50.10	Crohn's disease of large intestine without complications
		K50.111	Crohn's disease of large intestine with rectal bleeding
		K50.112	Crohn's disease of large intestine with intestinal obstruction
		K50.113	Crohn's disease of large intestine with fistula
		K50.114	Crohn's disease of large intestine with abscess
		K50.118	Crohn's disease of large intestine with other complication
		K50.119	Crohn's disease of large intestine with unspecified complications
555.2	Regional enteritis of small intestine with large intestine	K50.80	Crohn's disease of both small and large intestine without complications
		K50.811	Crohn's disease of both small and large intestine with rectal bleeding
		K50.812	Crohn's disease of both small and large intestine with intestinal obstruction
		K50.813	Crohn's disease of both small and large intestine with fistula
		K50.814	Crohn's disease of both small and large intestine with abscess
		K50.818	Crohn's disease of both small and large intestine with other complication
		K50.819	Crohn's disease of both small and large intestine with unspecified complications

Chapter 11. ICD-10-CM: Digestive System

ICD-9-CM		ICD-10-CM	
555.9	Regional enteritis of unspecified site	K50.90	Crohn's disease, unspecified, without complications
		K50.911	Crohn's disease, unspecified, with rectal bleeding
		K50.912	Crohn's disease, unspecified, with intestinal obstruction
		K50.913	Crohn's disease, unspecified, with fistula
		K50.914	Crohn's disease, unspecified, with abscess
		K50.918	Crohn's disease, unspecified, with other complication
		K50.919	Crohn's disease, unspecified, with unspecified complications

Crohn's disease can lead to several complications, including obstruction, abscess, fistula, and hemorrhage. The formation of strictures and adhesions that narrow the lumen can block the passageway of intestinal contents and cause an intestinal obstruction. In Crohn's disease, fistulae, abnormal passages from one epithelial surface to another, can develop between two loops of bowel, between the bowel and bladder, between the bowel and vagina, and between the bowel and skin. Commonly found in the abdominal and perianal of Crohn's disease sufferers are abscesses, collections of pus that has accumulated in a cavity formed by the tissues containing the pus. Abscesses are frequently associated with swelling and other signs of inflammation

In ICD-9-CM, coders need to know only the specific site of the disease. Any documented Crohn's disease complication is reported with a separate code. However, coding for Crohn's disease and its complications in ICD-10-CM largely depends on selecting the appropriate fifth and sixth characters. The fifth character 0 (zero) indicates that there are no complications. The fifth character 1 indicates that there are complications, described by the sixth characters from the following list.

1. Rectal bleeding
2. Intestinal obstruction
3. Fistula
4. Abscess
8. Other complication
9. Unspecified complication

Regional enteritis is not the only intestinal disease that has been expanded in ICD-10-CM to include complications like abscess, obstruction, and fistulas. ICD-9-CM category 556 Ulcerative colitis has also undergone a similar expansion.

Ulcerative colitis causes inflammation and ulcers in the top layers of the lining of the large intestine. The inflammation usually occurs in the rectum and lower part of the colon but can affect other areas of the colon. Ulcerative colitis is a chronic, intermittent disease, with periods of exacerbated symptoms and periods that are relatively symptom-free. The symptoms of ulcerative colitis can sometimes diminish on their own, but they often require treatment to induce remission.

Coding for ulcerative colitis in ICD-10-CM is based on whether there is a complication and, if there is one, what it is. This is a new concept for this condition in ICD-10-CM. In ICD-9-CM, when a complication is documented, coders choose an additional code to represent it.

> **CODING AXIOM**
>
> When a patient presents with Crohn's disease of the small intestine with a rectal abscess, assign code K61.1 Rectal abscess, to report the specific site of the abscess, in addition to code K50.014 Crohn's disease of small intestine with abscess. Codes in category K50 do not capture the specificity necessary to report the site of the rectal abscess, as they describe intestinal abscess only.
>
> *Coding Clinic*, 4Q, 12, 104

Coding for Ulcerative Colitis

ICD-9-CM		ICD-10-CM	
556.3	Ulcerative (chronic) proctosigmoiditis	K51.30	Ulcerative (chronic) rectosigmoiditis without complications
		K51.311	Ulcerative (chronic) rectosigmoiditis with rectal bleeding
		K51.312	Ulcerative (chronic) rectosigmoiditis with intestinal obstruction
		K51.313	Ulcerative (chronic) rectosigmoiditis with fistula
		K51.314	Ulcerative (chronic) rectosigmoiditis with abscess
		K51.318	Ulcerative (chronic) rectosigmoiditis with other complication
		K51.319	Ulcerative (chronic) rectosigmoiditis with unspecified complications
556.4	Pseudopolyposis of colon	K51.40	Inflammatory polyps of colon without complications
		K51.411	Inflammatory polyps of colon with rectal bleeding
		K51.412	Inflammatory polyps of colon with intestinal obstruction
		K51.413	Inflammatory polyps of colon with fistula
		K51.414	Inflammatory polyps of colon with abscess
		K51.418	Inflammatory polyps of colon with other complication
		K51.419	Inflammatory polyps of colon with unspecified complications

Note that a few of the code descriptions in this category have been renamed. For example, ulcerative proctosigmoiditis in ICD-9-CM is now ulcerative chronic rectosigmoiditis. The terms recto and procto are sometimes used interchangeably, but both are considered medical terminology for the rectum.

Pseudopolyposis is a condition of numerous pseudopolyps in the colon and rectum, due to longstanding inflammation. In ICD-10-CM, the code description for this condition has been changed to "inflammatory polyps of colon." In fact, the term pseudopolyposis has been completely retired in ICD-10-CM. This term has been removed from both the code description and the alphabetic index. The only way to code this condition in ICD-10-CM is to be familiar with the new clinical concept of inflammatory polyps of the colon.

Colostomy and Enterostomy Complications

A colostomy is a procedure in which a portion of the large intestine is divided and the open end is secured to the skin to drain bowel contents outside the body. An enterostomy is similar to the colostomy but is performed to create a passageway into the patient's small intestine through the abdomen with an opening for drainage or to insert a tube for feeding. Enterostomies are often classified according to the part of the small intestine that is used to create the stoma. Documentation may reflect ileostomies, jejunostomies, and often physicians use the word "ostomy" to describe all types of enterostomies.

Figure 11.12: Colostomy

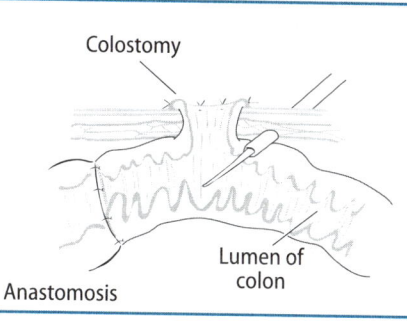

Formation of colostomies and enterostomies are surgical procedures and just as with any other surgical procedure, complications can occur. These can be both mechanical and other specified complications, such as infection or hemorrhage. Coding for the complications of colostomy and enterostomies in ICD-9-CM requires the coder to know only that a complication was present. However, in ICD-10-CM coders need to consider the anatomy of the intestine and be familiar with the names of the parts of the small and large intestines.

Coding for Colostomy and Enterostomy Complications

ICD-9-CM		ICD-10-CM	
569.60	Unspecified complication of colostomy or enterostomy	K94.00	Colostomy complication, unspecified
		K94.10	Enterostomy complication, unspecified
569.61	Infection of colostomy or enterostomy	K94.02	Colostomy infection
		K94.12	Enterostomy infection
569.62	Mechanical complication of colostomy and enterostomy	K94.03	Colostomy malfunction
		K94.13	Enterostomy malfunction
569.69	Other complication of colostomy or enterostomy	K94.01	Colostomy hemorrhage
		K94.09	Other complications of colostomy
		K94.11	Enterostomy hemorrhage
		K94.19	Other complications of enterostomy

Some of the common complications of colostomies and enterostomies include skin irritation or infection caused by stool that leaks under the bag, peristomal hernias, parastomal fistulas, narrowing bowel, and prolapse of the stoma. In ICD-9-CM, colostomy and enterostomy complications are grouped together under category 569.6. In ICD-10-CM, these are split into two separate categories. Coders need to pay close attention to the specific part of the intestine with the complication. Was the procedure documented as a colostomy, jejunostomy, ileostomy, or did the documentation just say ostomy?

Infectious Diseases of the Digestive System

The digestive system is a common and easily accessible portal of entry for microorganisms. As a result, microbes or their toxins that have entered the digestive system through the gastrointestinal tract can often cause infection, inflammation, or disease. Sources of GI infections may include an overgrowth of normal flora, contaminated food or water, contact with contaminated soil, or oral contact with fecal matter.

Typhoid fever is an acute generalized illness caused by the microorganism *Salmonella typhi*. Important clinical features include fever, headache, abdominal pain, cough, toxemia, **leucopenia**, abnormal pulse, rose spots on the skin, bacteremia, hyperplasia of the intestinal lymph nodes, and **Peyer's patches** in the intestines. Typhoid fever is generally transmitted through food or water that has

> **DEFINITIONS**
>
> **leukopenia.** Condition in which the total numbers of leukocytes circulating in the blood are less than normal.
>
> **Peyer's patches.** Aggregations of lymphoid tissue that are found in the ileum of humans and are used to visually differentiate the ileum from the jejunum and duodenum.

been contaminated with fecal matter but can also be contracted through close contact with an infected individual. Typhoid infections are treated with antimicrobial therapy, which shortens the clinical course of the infection and reduces the risk of death. However, one of the frequent complications of therapy is the development of antibiotic resistance.

Coding for typhoid fever infections in ICD-10-CM is a bit more complex than in ICD-9-CM due to the inclusion of various complications within the code descriptions. In ICD-9-CM, there is only one code option for typhoid fever, 002.0. The complications of the disease are coded elsewhere. However, in ICD-10-CM, there are seven possible code selections for this infection.

Coding for Typhoid Fever in ICD-10-CM

A01.00	Typhoid fever, unspecified
A01.01	Typhoid meningitis
A01.02	Typhoid fever with heart involvement
A01.03	Typhoid pneumonia
A01.04	Typhoid arthritis
A01.05	Typhoid osteomyelitis
A01.09	Typhoid fever with other complications

To select the appropriate code in ICD-10-CM, the coder must look for documentation that describes the associated typhoid complication. Documentation of meningitis, pneumonia, arthritis, osteomyelitis, and any cardiac condition that is due to *Salmonella typhi* or typhoid fever would be considered a complication of typhoid fever. For example, meningitis is an inflammation of the meninges, the covering over the brain and spinal cord. Documentation that this inflammation is due to *Salmonella typhi* or with typhoid fever would indicate typhoid meningitis. Coders need to understand the physiology behind the disease process and its complications to select the appropriate typhoid fever code in ICD-10-CM.

Amebiasis, ICD-9-CM code category 006, is defined as an infection of the large intestine caused by *Entamoeba histolytica*. In amebiasis, protozoa can live in the large intestine without causing symptoms or can invade the colon wall, causing severe colitis, acute dysentery, or chronic diarrhea. The infection may spread through the blood to the liver, lungs, brain, or other organs and often causes abscesses in the various organs.

There are many similarities between ICD-9-CM and ICD-10-CM when coding for amebiasis infections and the complications. All but one of the codes in ICD-9-CM has an exact mapping to a code in ICD-10-CM. The same amebiasis complications available in ICD-9-CM are also available in ICD-10-CM.

Coding for Amebiasis

ICD-9-CM		ICD-10-CM	
006.0	Acute amebic dysentery without mention of abscess	A06.0	Acute amebic dysentery
006.1	Chronic intestinal amebiasis without mention of abscess	A06.1	Chronic intestinal amebiasis
006.2	Amebic nondysenteric colitis	A06.2	Amebic nondysenteric colitis
006.3	Amebic liver abscess	A06.4	Amebic liver abscess
006.4	Amebic lung abscess	A06.5	Amebic lung abscess
006.5	Amebic brain abscess	A06.6	Amebic brain abscess
006.6	Amebic skin ulceration	A06.7	Cutaneous amebiasis
006.9	Unspecified amebiasis	A06.9	Amebiasis, unspecified

The one exception within this code category is for code 006.8 Other specified amebic infections. In ICD-10-CM this code has been expanded to identify some additional complications.

- **A06.3** Ameboma of intestine
- **A06.81** Amebic cystitis
- **A06.82** Other amebic genitourinary infections
- **A06.89** Other amebic infections

Amoebas usually remain in the host's gastrointestinal tract, but they can spread elsewhere. The expansion of the other specified category enables the coder to identify other specified sites where amebic infections may occur.

Intestinal trichomoniasis is characterized by colitis, diarrhea, or dysentery and is caused by the protozoan *Trichomonas*. A protozoan is a eukaryotic organism that is classified as parasitic to humans. Trichomoniasis is usually transmitted through sexual intercourse and is primarily an infection of the urogenital tract. The most common site of infection is the urethra and the vagina in women, but this protozoan may also colonize and infect the oropharynx, duodenum, and colon.

The ICD-9-CM code description for this infection is 007.3 Intestinal trichomoniasis. In ICD-10-CM, this condition does not have its own code but is coded using A07.8 Other specified protozoal intestinal diseases.

Coding for Intestinal Trichomoniasis

ICD-9-CM		ICD-10-CM	
007.3	Intestinal trichomoniasis	A07.8	Other specified protozoal intestinal diseases

To code this condition in ICD-10-CM, coders need to know that *Trichomonas* is classified as a protozoan. Intestinal trichomoniasis is listed as an includes term along with other protozoan intestinal diseases like microsporidiosis, sarcocystosis, and sarcosporidiosis.

Ascariasis is an intestinal infection that occurs when the eggs of the parasitic round worm, *Ascaris lumbricoides*, are ingested. Patients often remain asymptomatic, but the illness may cause visceral damage, peritonitis, enlargement of the liver and spleen, toxicity, and pneumonia. Infections are generally treated for one to three days with antiparasitic medications and, in cases of heavy infections, patients may require surgery to repair intestinal damage and remove the worms.

In ICD-9-CM, one code, 127.0, is used to report ascariasis and any complications must be coded separately. However in ICD-10-CM, the complications of the infection are also included in the code for infection.

Coding for Ascariasis in ICD-10-CM

- **B77.0** Ascariasis with intestinal complications
- **B77.81** Ascariasis pneumonia
- **B77.89** Ascariasis with other complications
- **B77.9** Ascariasis, unspecified

Another parasitic infection that has been expanded in ICD-10-CM is strongyloidiasis, caused by the roundworm *Strongyloides stercoralis*. Some common symptoms include gastric pain, vomiting, and diarrhea. Drug therapy for this condition includes ivermectin, but because the medication kills only the adult worm, repeat dosing is necessary to completely eradicate the infection.

Strongyloidiasis may infect a number of sites, including the skin and intestinal track, or may be disseminated throughout the body. In the ICD-10-CM coding system, correct code assignment is not only dependent on the infection, but also the infection site.

> **INTERESTING A & P FACT**
>
> The condition microsporidiosis is classified as a protozoal disease in ICD-10-CM, but microsporidia is in the fungi family.

Coding for Strongyloidiasis in ICD-10-CM

B78.0	Intestinal strongyloidiasis
B78.1	Cutaneous strongyloidiasis
B78.7	Disseminated strongyloidiasis
B78.9	Strongyloidiasis, unspecified

Pulmonary symptoms can occur when the larvae migrate into the lungs. Cutaneous symptoms may include urticarial rashes in the buttock and waist areas. If the infection becomes chronic and the patient becomes immunosuppressed, a potentially fatal condition called disseminated strongyloidiasis can occur. Symptoms include abdominal pain, distention, shock, pulmonary and neurologic complications, and septicemia.

Summary

The digestive system interacts closely with other organ systems to carry out the process of digestion. It is important to learn about the anatomy and physiology of the digestive tract, and the varied differences between ICD-9-CM and ICD-10-CM coding. Discovering areas where there are major anatomy, physiology, and disease pathology differences between the two code sets will help prepare coders for the ICD-10-CM transition.

Chapter 12. ICD-10-CM: Urinary System

Anatomic Overview

The urinary system is a collection of various organs, tubes, muscles, and nerves whose function is to create, store, and transport urine out of the body. It comprises two kidneys, two ureters, the bladder, two sphincter muscles, and the urethra.

Figure 12.1: Urinary System

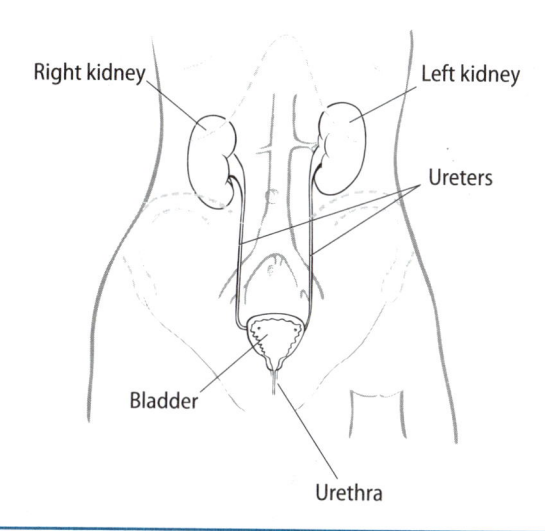

The body absorbs needed nutrients to maintain body function, including energy and self-repair from food. Once the body has the appropriate amount of nutrition, resulting waste products must be eliminated from the body. The urinary system, in conjunction with the lungs, skin, and intestines, excretes waste and keeps chemicals and water in the body in balance.

Specifically, the urinary system removes urea from the blood. Urea is generated when foods containing proteins (meat, poultry, and some vegetables) break down in the body.

The kidneys, bean-shaped organs approximately the size of a fist, perform the majority of the work within the urinary system, acting as a filter to remove waste and other foreign substances from the blood. The two main areas of the kidneys are the renal cortex and the renal medulla. The renal cortex is a superficial, light red, smooth-textured area that extends from the renal capsule to the base of the renal pyramids and into the spaces between them. The renal medulla is a darker reddish brown area made up of multiple cone-shaped renal pyramids; the base or wider end of each pyramid faces the renal cortex and its apex or narrower end points toward the renal hilum.

Figure 12.2: Kidney

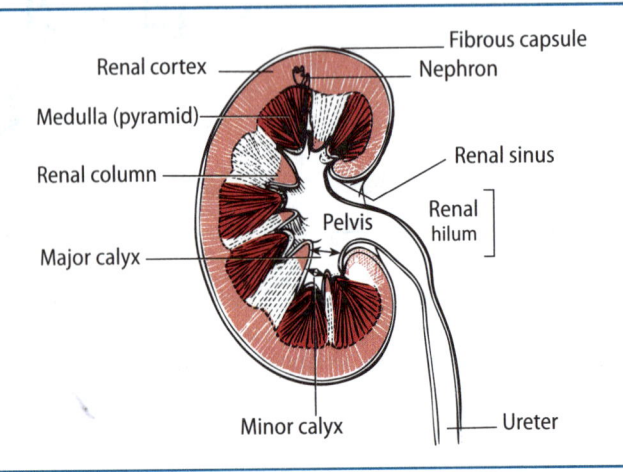

Blood comes into the kidneys by way of arteries that branch within the kidneys into small clusters of looping blood vessels. These clusters are called glomeruli, the tiny units in the kidney where blood is cleaned. Approximately 1 million glomeruli (filters) are in each kidney. Each glomerulus is attached to the opening of a small, fluid-collecting tube known as the tubule. Every glomerulus and tubule unit combined is called a nephron, or the functional unit of the kidneys. Each kidney contains approximately 1 million nephrons. The glomerulus functions as a filter keeping normal proteins and cells in the bloodstream while allowing extra fluid and wastes to pass through. Urea, combined with water, other waste materials, and excess salt, forms urine.

Figure 12.3: Nephron

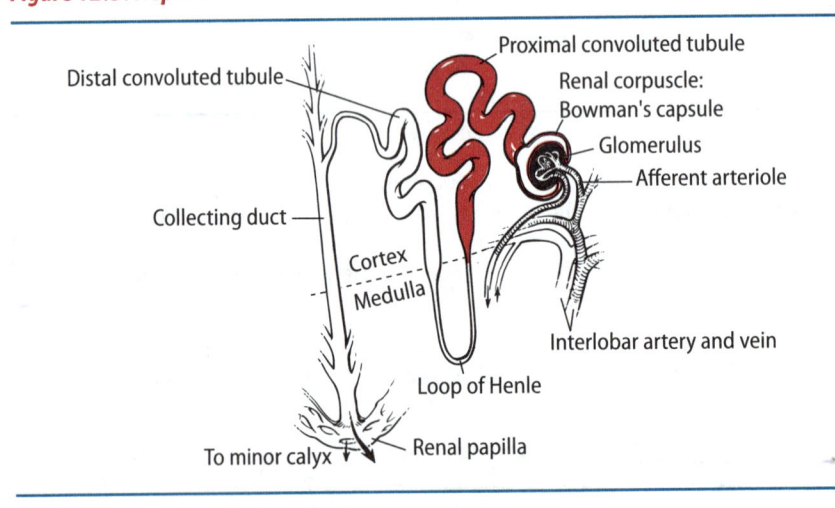

The kidneys also perform other necessary functions, including:

- Regulate:
    - blood ionic composition
    - blood pH
    - blood pressure
    - blood glucose level

- Produce three important hormones:
  - **erythropoietin (EPO):** Stimulates bone marrow to produce red blood cells.
  - **renin:** Regulates blood pressure.
  - **calcitriol:** An active form of vitamin D, this hormone helps to maintain calcium for bones and normal chemical balance in the body.

Once the urine is formed, it passes through the nephrons and down the renal tubules of the kidney and is subsequently funneled from the renal pelvis, the area at the center of the kidney, into the ureters, which then transport the urine to the bladder. The ureters are tube-shaped structures approximately 8 to 10 inches long that connect the kidney to the urinary bladder. Muscles within the ureters continually contract and relax in order to force urine downward into the urinary bladder. The glomerular membrane separates the blood vessel from the tubule, allowing waste products and extra water to pass into the tubule while at the same time keeping blood cells and protein in the bloodstream.

The urinary bladder is a triangular or pear-shaped, expandable hollow organ located in the pelvic area, held in place by ligaments that bind to the pelvic bones. It is the organ in the urinary system that stores urine and allows urination to be infrequent and voluntary. The urinary bladder muscles relax in order to allow urine to enter from the ureters and contract to excrete urine from the body by way of the urethra. Layers of muscle tissue stretch to house urine, with a capacity of 400 to 600 mL being considered normal. Note that in the average healthy adult, approximately two cups, or 400 to 500 mL, of urine can be stored in the bladder for approximately two to five hours. Once the urinary bladder is full, nerves within the bladder signal the brain the need to urinate. To release urine, the muscles in the urinary bladder contract.

> **CLINICAL NOTE**
>
> Urine is excreted from the kidneys every 10 to 15 seconds and collected in the bladder.

Figure 12.4: Bladder

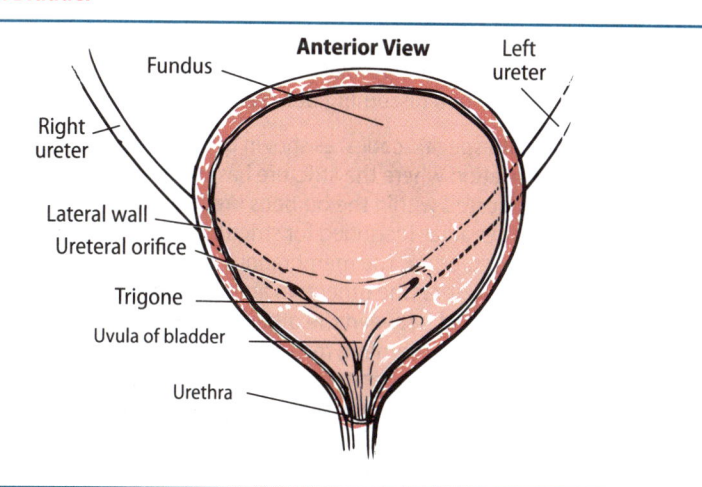

Anterior View — Fundus, Left ureter, Right ureter, Lateral wall, Ureteral orifice, Trigone, Uvula of bladder, Urethra

The urethra is the tube through which urine is drained from the bladder. In men, the urethra is approximately 20 cm long. In women, the urethra is approximately 4 cm long. There are two sphincters associated with the urethra: the internal sphincter, which surrounds the urethra at the top where it meets the bladder, and the external sphincter, which surrounds the urethra at the pelvic floor. These two sphincters control urinary voiding, allowing the flow of urine through the urethra.

> **INTERESTING A & P FACT**
>
> Approximately 440 gallons of blood passes through the kidneys of a healthy adult on a daily basis, resulting in about 1.5 liters of urine.

Anatomy and Pathophysiology and the ICD-10-CM Code Set

The urinary system can be affected by many disease states, including aging, illness, and injury. Aging, in particular, can affect the structure of the kidneys and thereby cause a loss of ability to remove wastes from the blood. Furthermore, the muscles within the ureters, bladder, and urethra often tend to lose some of the elasticity or strength, which can lead to an increase in urinary infections due to the bladder's inability to empty completely. This lack of elasticity and strength in the muscles can also cause incontinence, an unwanted leakage of urine. Injuries such as blunt force trauma or penetrating wounds or illness can also lead to the kidneys being unable to filter blood completely or even blocking the passage of urine. Additionally, in the case of injuries, other complications can occur such as bleeding or the leakage of urine to surrounding tissues, which can cause infection.

The ICD-10-CM coding system offers more detail in code selection pertaining to the urinary system. In this section, a number of common conditions or disease processes that afflict the urinary system will be discussed. Attention is focused on conditions that have notable coding distinctions or differences from ICD-9-CM to ICD-10-CM.

Urethral Strictures

ICD-9-CM code 598.00 reports a urethral stricture as the result of an unspecified infection. A urethral stricture is a narrowing of the urethra, the tube that allows urine to exit the body. As indicated in the aforementioned code, this condition can be attributed to infection; however, it can also be caused by inflammation, injury, disease, or even scar tissue from prior surgeries. ICD-10-CM identifies where the stricture occurs within the urethra, such as the meatus, the external opening where urine passes out of the body, and also details the stricture as postinfective or occurring after the infection, which was not previously specified in ICD-9-CM. Other subcategories describing urethral strictures, such as posttraumatic strictures, make the same anatomical distinctions. A solid grasp of anatomical terms related to the urinary system is useful when discerning between the various codes.

In the grouping of male-specific codes, as shown below, a number of terms identify the exact anatomic location where the stricture has occurred. In code N35.112, the particular stricture is located within the bulbous urethra, which is the widest area within the urethra. Other areas identified for strictures include the membranous urethra and the anterior urethra. The membranous urethra is one of three sections that make up the male urethra (the other two areas include the prostatic urethra and the spongy urethra). Located between the other two areas, the membranous urethra is the shortest and narrowest segment, measuring approximately 0.5 to 0.75 inches long, and passes through the urogenital diaphragm. Controlling the passage of urine along the urethra through the urogenital diaphragm is the external urethral sphincter. This circular muscle is under voluntary control, meaning that urine can be stopped in midstream at this passageway. An anterior urethral stricture describes a narrowing of the portion of the urethra that is the furthest from (distal) the urogenital diaphragm.

Coding for Urethral Strictures Due to Unspecified Infection

ICD-9-CM		ICD-10-CM	
598.00	Urethral stricture due to unspecified infection	N35.111	Postinfective urethral stricture, not elsewhere classified, male, meatal
		N35.112	Postinfective bulbous urethral stricture, not elsewhere classified
		N35.113	Postinfective membranous urethral stricture, not elsewhere classified
		N35.114	Postinfective anterior urethral stricture, not elsewhere classified
		N35.119	Postinfective urethral stricture, not elsewhere classified, male, unspecified
		N35.12	Postinfective urethral stricture, not elsewhere classified, female

Other categories of urethral strictures in ICD-10-CM include traumatic and postoperative; the distinctions noted and described above include the same anatomical terms and descriptions and are divided into the male and female categories as well.

Glomerular Diseases

A large number of conditions within the urinary system affect the **glomeruli** and hinder the filtering efficacy of the kidneys. The two most common conditions that affect the glomeruli are nephritic and nephrotic syndromes.

Nephritic syndrome is a type of glomerulonephritis or an inflammation of the glomeruli. It is often associated with an immune response that resulted from an infection or other disease process but, in rare cases, can be hereditary in origin. Basically antibodies attach directly to the kidney cells or to antigens outside of the kidney and are then carried to the kidney through the bloodstream. The antigens get trapped in the glomeruli, causing inflammation. When enough of the glomeruli are damaged, blood filtering is decreased and waste products build up in the blood. Scarring may develop, which also impairs filtering.

In nephrotic syndrome, damage to the glomeruli allows large amounts of protein to be lost from the blood into the urine, which results in a blood protein deficiency. The condition arises when, instead of circulating, fluid begins to accumulate in the tissues of the body, causing swelling and puffiness. When nephritic syndrome is due to an inflammatory process, there are large numbers of red blood cells in the urine, whereas in noninflammatory nephrotic syndrome, there are no red blood cells present in the urine. In severe cases of nephrotic syndrome, the glomeruli become scarred and kidney damage can occur.

Glomerular diseases include a number of conditions with a myriad of genetic and environmental causes. However, they can be separated into two major categories:

- **Glomerulonephritis:** Inflammation of the membrane tissue in the kidney that acts as a filter, separating wastes and extra fluid from the blood.
- **Glomerulosclerosis:** Scarring or hardening of the tiny blood vessels within the kidneys.

Both conditions can lead to kidney failure.

These conditions are assigned to categories 580 to 583 in ICD-9-CM. Differentiation is often made between acute and chronic versions of these conditions. However, it should be noted that ICD-10-CM categories for these conditions refer to a number of terms not noted as relevant in ICD-9-CM.

For example, ICD-10-CM codes N00 to N08 describe glomerular diseases, N10 to N16 are assigned to renal tubulo-interstitial diseases, and N17 to N19 are assigned to acute kidney failure and chronic kidney disease. In ICD-10-CM, specificity is now

> **DEFINITIONS**
>
> **glomeruli.** Clusters of microscopic blood vessels located within the kidneys containing small pores through which blood is filtered; tuft of capillaries situated within a Bowman's capsule at the end of a renal tubule in the kidney that filters waste products from the blood and subsequently forms urine. A single glomeruli is called a glomerulus.

provided for the various *types* of glomerulonephritis and therefore a thorough understanding of the disease process is necessary to distinguish between the various code choices and to differentiate between acute, chronic, or recurrent and persistent conditions. In fact, codes within the section for glomerular diseases are first classified according to whether the condition is described as acute, rapid progressive, recurrent and persistent, chronic, or unspecified and then subsequently catalogued according to the specific type of glomerulonephritis (GN).

Acute glomerulonephritis (AGN), ICD-10-CM category N00, is a grouping of renal diseases caused by a number of immunologic reactions that cause inflammation and proliferation of glomerular tissue. Proliferation is defined as a rapid reproduction of tissue. This condition often presents with the sudden onset of blood or protein in the urine, known as hematuria or proteinuria, respectively, along with red blood cells. Hypertension, edema (swelling due to fluid retention), and impaired renal function may likely accompany these symptoms.

In AGN, the basic disease process involves deposits or in situ deposits of **immune complexes** in the glomeruli. As a result of this, the kidneys become enlarged and may increase to twice the size of normal kidneys.

AGN is often categorized based on whether it is proliferative or nonproliferative. Nonproliferative AGN is not associated with a large number of cells and consists of minimal change GN, membranous GN, and focal segmental glomerulosclerosis.

In contrast, proliferative AGN is significantly more cellular in nature, and conditions related to proliferative AGN often lead to renal failure. Conditions associated with proliferative AGN include IgA disease, commonly referred to as Berger's nephropathy, Henoch-Schönlein purpura (HSP), postinfectious GN, mesangiocapillary GN, and rapidly progressive or crescentic GN. Note that in ICD-10-CM, greater detail is provided as to the types of cells identified histologically as the result of biopsies (e.g., crescentic, etc.).

Types of Glomerulonephritis

Focal Segmental Glomerulonephritis

Focal segmental glomerulosclerosis (FSGS) presents as a nephrotic syndrome. Nephrotic syndrome is, essentially, a collection of symptoms, including proteinuria, swelling, and low blood protein levels, and is caused by damage to the kidneys as the result of infection (e.g., strep throat, hepatitis, or mononucleosis), use of certain drugs, cancer, genetic disorders, immune disorders, or diseases that affect multiple body systems such as diabetes, systemic lupus erythematous (SLE), multiple myeloma, and amyloidosis. Often, nephrotic syndrome accompanies kidney disorders such as GN, focal and segmental glomerulosclerosis, and mesangiocapillary glomerulonephritis.

FSGS refers to scar tissue that has formed in the glomeruli. The term "focal" describes the part of the glomeruli that has become scarred while the rest remains normal. "Segmental" indicates that only a part of an individual glomerulus has been damaged.

It is estimated that FSGS contributes to approximately 10 to 15 percent of all nephrotic syndrome cases.

Membranous Glomerulonephritis

Membranous glomerulonephritis also presents as a nephrotic syndrome and is said to be the leading cause of nephrotic syndrome in adults. Typically, this specific type of GN is associated with cancer, yet most of the time it arises spontaneously without any known cause. No significant cellularity or growth in cells is noted in this specific type of GN despite the basement membrane thickening. As this condition progresses, the kidneys degenerate (waste away).

DEFINITIONS

immune complexes. Clusters of antigens and antibodies that are locked together. Under normal circumstances, the spleen removes these immune complexes from the blood; however, on occasion, they can continue to circulate and may become trapped in various body tissues, which causes inflammation and tissue damage.

IgA (Berger's Nephropathy)
IgA (Berger's nephropathy) is the most common form of proliferative GN and the most common form of GN worldwide. It often presents with blood in the urine and can progress to nephrotic syndrome.

Henoch-Schönlein Purpura (HSP) is a variation of IgA, and its pathology, or origin, is a vasculitis of the small vessels.

Postinfectious GN
As indicated by its name, postinfectious GN is the type of AGN associated with streptococcal infections.

Mesangiocapillary GN
Mesangiocapillary GN is associated with systemic lupus erythematous (SLE), viral hepatitis, and hypocomplementemia, a condition in which one or another component of complement is lacking or reduced in amount. It is associated with immune complex diseases and cases of membranoproliferative glomerulonephritis in which nephritic factor is present. Complement is a group of proteins that move throughout the bloodstream freely, work with the immune system, and contribute to the development of inflammation within the body.

Rapidly Progressive GN (Crescentic GN)
As the name implies, rapidly progressive GN is characterized by a rapid decrease in the glomerular filtration rate (GFR) of 50 percent or more over a relatively short period of time; typically, anywhere from a few days to three months. The crescentic adjective in the name is attributed to pathological findings, after biopsy, of extensive glomerular crescent formation. Goodpasture's syndrome, Wegener's granulomatosis, and polyarteritis are all conditions categorized to this type of GN.

In the following table, note the use of the following terms to differentiate the various types of glomerulonephritis: focal, segmental, and crescentic. These terms are used to describe scattered variations of renal disease identified by histologic study.

Endocapillary Glomerulonephritis
Endocapillary glomerulonephritis is usually referred to as "diffuse" endocapillary GN but in some instances can be segmental or focal. It is described as a cellular proliferation affecting mesangial areas and capillary lumens. In other words, the number of cells increases due to cell growth and division, specifically mesangials, endothelials, and circulating inflammatory cells that have migrated to the capillary tuft. As a result of the cellular proliferation and subsequent endothelial cells edema, there is often an occlusion, or blockage, of capillary lumens. Sometimes, this can be accompanied by extracapillary proliferation (crescents).

Mesangial Proliferative Glomerulonephritis
Mesangial proliferative glomerulonephritis is a rare form of GN that typically presents as nephrotic syndrome and upon biopsy is identified histologically by the appearance of diffuse glomerular increases in endocapillary and mesangial cells and in mesangial matrix. Also called diffuse mesangial proliferation, characteristics of this disease process include blood in the urine caused by a particular type of inflammation inside the kidneys. Abnormalities within the immune system can lead to abnormal immune deposits in the mesangial cells (part of the capillaries inside the kidneys) of the kidneys. As a result, the mesangial cells become bigger and their numbers increase.

Dense Versus Diffuse
In addition to the particular descriptive types of GN described above, references to the terms "dense" and "diffuse" are also noted throughout this section in ICD-10-CM. The word "dense" is generally used when a thick or closely packed group of cells is noted on histologic examination; likewise, the term "diffuse" represents a more dispersed or scattered group of cells.

Codes are also subdivided into conditions described as acute, chronic, recurrent or persistent, and rapidly progressive. When a condition is defined as "acute," it refers to the rapid onset and/or worsening of that condition, whereas a "chronic" condition develops and worsens over time.

The following table is an example of the increased code choices in ICD-10-CM for glomerulonephritis and demonstrates the use of many of the aforementioned terms. The increased specificity is a common theme throughout the section on glomerular diseases, which includes nephritic and nephrotic syndrome, as well as nephropathy.

Coding for Acute Glomerular Disease with Lesion of Proliferative GN

ICD-9-CM		ICD-10-CM	
580.0	Acute glomerulonephritis with lesion of proliferative glomerulonephritis	N00.0	Acute nephritic syndrome with minor glomerular abnormality
		N00.1	Acute nephritic syndrome with focal and segmental glomerular lesions
		N00.2	Acute nephritic syndrome with diffuse membranous glomerulonephritis
		N00.3	Acute nephritic syndrome with diffuse mesangial proliferative glomerulonephritis
		N00.4	Acute nephritic syndrome with diffuse endocapillary proliferative glomerulonephritis
		N00.5	Acute nephritic syndrome with diffuse mesangiocapillary glomerulonephritis
		N00.6	Acute nephritic syndrome with dense deposit disease
		N00.7	Acute nephritic syndrome with diffuse crescentic glomerulonephritis

Nephrotic Syndrome

Nephrotic syndrome results in excessive amounts of protein being excreted in the urine and typically leads to the accumulation of fluid in the body, as well as low levels of protein albumin and high levels of fats in the blood due to glomeruli damage.

Nephrotic syndrome can be congenital, primary (affecting only the kidneys), or secondary (caused by a disease process that affects other parts of the body such as diabetes mellitus or systemic lupus erythematosus). It may also be caused by viral infections or glomerulonephritis.

Primary or congenital nephrotic syndrome, once classified to category 581 Nephrotic syndrome, in the ICD-9-CM system, is now classified to category N04 Nephrotic syndrome, in ICD-10-CM.

Secondary nephrotic syndrome in ICD-9-CM coded to 581.81 Nephrotic syndrome, in diseases classified elsewhere. Due to the wide range of underlying causes to which secondary nephrotic syndrome can result, there are several codes in ICD-10-CM that may be appropriate when coding this condition and its underlying etiology, including N08 Glomerular disorders in diseases classified elsewhere, and combination codes in categories E08 Diabetes mellitus due to underlying condition, or E09 Drug or chemical induced diabetes mellitus.

Renal Tubulointerstitial Diseases

When diseases affecting the kidney involve structures outside the glomerulus, they are broadly referred to as tubulointerstitial, or involving the tubules and/or interstitium of the kidneys. A tubule is a small, fluid-filled collecting tube at the end of each glomerulus. The glomerulus and tubule unit combined is called a nephron, or the functional unit of the kidneys. Each kidney contains approximately 1 million nephrons.

Tubulointerstitial kidney diseases can present as acute or chronic and often involve a number of varied etiologies. Generally, acute tubulointerstitial nephritis (ATIN) involves allergic reactions to different types of medications, including antibiotics and nonsteroidal anti-inflammatory drugs (NSAID), immune system diseases such as lupus or Goodpasture's syndrome, organ transplant rejection, and infections (e.g., bacterial, viral, fungal, or parasitic).

Tubulointerstitial nephritis, also called interstitial nephritis, is caused by damage to the tubules of the kidneys and the tissues around them, called interstitial tissue. Essentially, kidney tubules help return filtered substances such as sodium and water to the blood. Drugs such as penicillin also move through the tubules and leave the body through the urine. Tubulointerstitial nephritis may be acute or chronic in nature and can cause kidney failure.

Acute tubulointerstitial nephritis (ATIN) is the sudden onset of the condition and is often triggered by certain types of drugs such as analgesics, lithium, diuretics, and cyclosporine; certain infections including bacterial (streptococcus, staphylococcus, and salmonella); and viruses such as Epstein Barr, cytomegalovirus (CMV), and human immunodeficiency virus (HIV); or it may be idiopathic.

Chronic tubulointerstitial nephritis (CTIN) arises when recurrent chronic tubular attacks cause gradual interstitial infiltration and fibrosis, tubular atrophy and dysfunction, and a gradual deterioration of renal function, usually over years. Glomerular involvement (glomerulosclerosis) is much more commonly noted when categorized as chronic rather than acute. CTIN can be attributed to a number of causes, including hereditary renal diseases, exogenous or metabolic toxins, autoimmune disorders, and neoplastic disorders.

There is no category specific to this condition in the ICD-9-CM coding system; however, the ICD-10-CM system is much more specific with three categories classifying the condition. Categories N10, N11, and N12 classify tubulointerstitial and tubular conditions according to acute or chronic. Note that when the documentation does not describe the condition as acute (rapid onset) or chronic (a more long-term condition), category N12 Tubulo-interstitial nephritis, not specified as acute or chronic, is used.

N10	Acute tubulo-interstitial nephritis
N11	Chronic tubulo-interstitial nephritis
N12	Tubulo-interstitial nephritis, not specified as acute or chronic

Uropathy

Types of Uropathy

Obstructive uropathy involves blocked urine flow and the inability to drain urine through a ureter, causing it to back up and injure one or both kidneys. Swelling can occur in the kidneys, referred to as hydronephrosis.

Reflux uropathy describes a condition in which urine backs up into the ureters with the remaining amount emptying through the urethra. This can occur for a few reasons, including:

- Sphincter muscle at the junction of the bladder and the ureter is abnormally tight
- Inability of the bladder muscles to close off the opening to the ureters due to weakness
- Bladder infection or irritation
- Ureteral congenital abnormality

DEFINITIONS

reflux. Return or backward flow.

Comprehensive Anatomy and Physiology for ICD-10-CM and ICD-10-PCS Coding

This condition can impact one or both ureters and can be classified as mild or severe. It is associated more commonly with children than adults and boys more so than girls.

Vesicoureteral-reflux (VUR) describes the abnormal flow of urine from the bladder back into the ureters. There are two types of VUR: primary and secondary.

Primary VUR usually occurs when a child is born with an impaired valve and the ureter connects to the bladder as the result of the ureters not growing long enough during development in utero. Because the valve does not close properly, urine backs up (refluxes) from the bladder to the ureters, and eventually to the kidneys. Primary VUR may improve or dissipate entirely as the child gets older because the ureter gets longer during the growth period and the function of the valve improves.

Secondary VUR is associated with a blockage anywhere within the urinary system. Blockages can be caused by a bladder infection that subsequently triggers swelling of the ureters and a reflux of urine to the kidneys.

Hydroureter is a term used with code N13.4 Hydroureter, and is also referenced in subcategory N13.7 Vesicoureteral-reflux.

> **DEFINITIONS**
>
> **hydroureter.** Distention (enlargement, swelling) of the ureter with urine due to blockage or obstruction.

Coding for Vesicoureteral Reflux

ICD-9-CM	ICD-10-CM
593.71 Vesicoureteral reflux with reflux nephropathy, unilateral	N13.721 Vesicoureteral-reflux with reflux nephropathy without hydroureter, unilateral
	N13.731 Vesicoureteral-reflux with reflux nephropathy with hydroureter, unilateral

Note that ICD-10-CM specifies whether a hydroureter is present, whereas ICD-9-CM does not.

Below is another example of the terms previously discussed and their use in ICD-10-CM to provide greater coding specificity.

Coding for Vesicoureteral Reflux with Reflux Nephropathy NOS

ICD-9-CM	ICD-10-CM
593.73 Vesicoureteral reflux with reflux nephropathy, NOS	N13.729 Vesicoureteral-reflux with reflux nephropathy without hydroureter, unspecified
	N13.739 Vesicoureteral-reflux with reflux nephropathy with hydroureter, unspecified
	N13.9 Obstructive and reflux uropathy, unspecified

A clear understanding and comprehension of these specific terms assist in appropriate code selection.

Pyelonephritis and Pyonephrosis

Pyelonephritis is a type of kidney infection caused by bacteria that primarily affects the interstitial area of the kidney, as well as the renal pelvis or, less often, the renal tubules. In ICD-9-CM, there is one code for unspecified pyelonephritis (590.80), which encompasses both pyelitis NOS and pyelonephritis NOS. ICD-10-CM uses three codes to describe the same condition.

Coding for Unspecified Pyelonephritis

ICD-9-CM	ICD-10-CM
590.80 Pyelonephritis, unspecified	N11.9 Chronic tubulo-interstitial nephritis, unspecified
	N12 Tubulo-interstitial nephritis, not specified as acute or chronic
	N13.6 Pyonephrosis

Pyonephrosis *enlarged swollen*

Pyonephrosis is <u>distention</u> of the kidney with infected pus-producing urine in an obstructed collecting system. Similar in nature to an abscess, pyonephrosis is typically associated with fever, chills, and flank pain; though patients can present as asymptomatic. This condition may be caused by a broad spectrum of pathologic conditions involving a urinary tract infection or the spread of a bacterial pathogen in the bloodstream.

Coding for Malignant Neoplasms of the Kidney and Other and Unspecified Urinary Organs

Unlike ICD-9-CM codes, ICD-10-CM codes indicate laterality for the right or left sides. Coders should therefore determine from the documentation which kidney or other urinary organ has been treated. When documentation does not specify the right or left side, an unspecified code is available in urinary malignant neoplasm category C64 for the kidney, C65 for the renal pelvis, and C66 for the ureters.

Coding for Neurogenic Bladder, NOS

Code 596.54 in ICD-9-CM is assigned for a nonspecific dysfunctional bladder due to a lesion in the central or peripheral nervous system that causes incontinence, residual urine retention, urinary infection, stones, and renal failure. ICD-10-CM describes three types of dysfunctional bladder.

An uninhibited neuropathic bladder is an abnormal condition that disrupts the normal inhibitory control of the detrusor muscle function by the central nervous system due to underdevelopment or impairment (usually by a lesion), resulting in urgency, frequent involuntary urination, uncontrolled urine leakage or **anuresis**. Simply put, a patient with this condition often does not realize the bladder has filled until urine begins to empty from it.

Reflex neuropathic (neurogenic) bladder is an interruption in both the sensory and motor bladder pathways in the spinal cord, just above the sacral segments. Bladder sensations are absent as the result of lesions above the lower thoracic cord. As a result, the detrusor muscle contracts spontaneously and the sphincter muscles may completely relax, resulting in incontinence. Reflex neuropathic bladder is often associated with spinal cord injuries. In such cases, patients can develop a condition called detrusor sphincter dyssynergia with detrusor hyperreflexia (DSD-DH), or the inability to completely empty the bladder due to overactivity in the bladder and sphincter muscles.

Neuromuscular dysfunction of the bladder is a general term that describes the loss of normal bladder function because of damage to an area of the nervous system. The ICD-10-CM code for this condition is assigned a fourth character of 9 and is the most generic code of the three. If documentation is not specific enough to assign one of the aforementioned codes, this code is the most likely choice.

Coding for Neuromuscular Dysfunction of Bladder, NEC

ICD-9-CM	ICD-10-CM	
596.54 Neurogenic bladder, NOS	N31.0	Uninhibited neuropathic bladder, not elsewhere classified
	N31.1	Reflex neuropathic bladder, not elsewhere classified
	N31.9	Neuromuscular dysfunction of bladder, unspecified

Urinary Incontinence

Urinary incontinence is a loss of bladder control resulting from weakened or overactive bladder muscles. The severity of incontinence can range from mild leaking of urine to uncontrollable wetting. While commonly associated with aging, urinary incontinence can be diagnosed in any age group. Weak bladder muscles can

---

DEFINITIONS

anuresis. Inability to urinate or the retention of urine in the bladder.

contribute to "accidents" when sneezing, laughing, or lifting heavy objects because the muscles are unable to keep the opening to the bladder closed. Bladder muscles that are too active give the strong urge to use the bathroom when, in fact, very little urine is actually in the bladder.

Urinary incontinence is not a disease; rather, it is a symptom. It is often caused by everyday habits, or an underlying medical condition. Some causes of temporary urinary incontinence include alcohol or caffeine consumption, overhydration, dehydration, bladder irritation, and certain medications. In addition, there are some easily treated medical conditions that may also cause urinary incontinence, such as a urinary tract infection. More chronic, persistent types of urinary incontinence are often attributed to pregnancy and childbirth, aging, hysterectomy, interstitial cystitis, prostate conditions (prostatitis, enlarged prostate, prostate cancer), bladder cancer or stones, neurological disorders, or obstructions.

Treatment for urinary incontinence are wide ranging, including behavioral techniques (bladder training, scheduled toilet trips, or fluid and diet management), physical therapy (pelvic floor exercises or electrical stimulation), medications (anticholinergics, topical estrogen, or Imipramine), special devices (urethral inserts, pessary), therapies (radiofrequency therapy, botulinum toxin type A, bulking material injections, or sacral nerve stimulation), or surgery (sling procedures, bladder neck suspension, artificial urinary sphincter).

Types of Urinary Incontinence

There are many types of urinary incontinence, such as:

- Stress incontinence
- Urge incontinence
- Overflow incontinence
- Mixed incontinence
- Functional incontinence
- Gross total incontinence

Stress Incontinence
Stress incontinence describes a loss of urine when the bladder is stressed by coughing, sneezing, laughing, exercising, or lifting something heavy. It is caused by weak sphincter muscles of the bladder due to physical changes from pregnancy and childbirth or menopause in women; in men, removal of the prostate gland can cause this type of incontinence.

Urge Incontinence
Urge incontinence is an unexpected, powerful urge to urinate followed by a small involuntary loss of urine. This type of incontinence is described as bladder muscle contractions that afford only a few seconds to a minute of warning before those afflicted need to use the bathroom. Patients with urge incontinence often indicate a frequent need to urinate, including throughout the night. This type of incontinence is often attributed to urinary tract infections (UTI), bladder irritants, bowel problems, Parkinson's or Alzheimer's disease, stroke, injury, or nervous system damage associated with multiple sclerosis (MS). When no known etiology can be identified, urge incontinence is also called overactive bladder.

Overflow Incontinence
Incontinence described as a frequent or constant dribble of urine is called overflow incontinence and is the inability to fully empty one's bladder. Patients with this type of incontinence often feel as though they can never completely empty their bladder, producing only a weak stream of urine. Often, overflow incontinence is associated with a damaged bladder, blocked urethra, or nerve damage from diabetes mellitus or, in men, prostate gland problems.

Mixed Incontinence
When symptoms from more than one type of urinary incontinence are present, such as stress and urge incontinence, a patient is described as having mixed incontinence. Mixed incontinence is most commonly found in women. The cause of the two forms may or may not be related.

Functional Incontinence
Functional incontinence is the inability to make it to the toilet in time due to a physical or mental impairment, such as in the case of a person with severe arthritis not being able to unbutton his or her pants quickly enough. This type of incontinence is commonly noted in older adults, especially those residing in nursing homes. It is the most common type of incontinence among older adults with arthritis, Parkinson's disease, or Alzheimer's disease. Patients with this type of incontinence are often unable to control their bladder before reaching the bathroom due to limitations in moving, thinking, or communicating.

Gross Total Incontinence
Gross total incontinence is continuous leaking of urine, both day and night, or periodic uncontrollable leaking of large volumes of urine. Essentially, this indicates the bladder is incapable of storing urine. This type of incontinence is typically seen in patients born with an anatomical defect with injuries to the spinal cord or urinary system, or with an abnormal opening (fistula) between the bladder and an adjacent structure, such as the vagina.

Male Urinary Incontinence

Urinary incontinence in men is typically limited to the following three types: stress, urge, and overflow incontinence, generally associated with nerve or prostate problems. In order for the urinary system to function, muscles and nerves must work together to contain urine in the bladder and release it at the appropriate time. Nerve problems are defined as any disease, condition, or injury that impairs the nerves, leading to problems with urination. For example, male patients with diabetes mellitus can develop nerve damage that affects bladder control. Strokes, Parkinson's disease, and multiple sclerosis can all affect the brain and nervous system, thereby impacting bladder function. Overactive bladder, or urge incontinence, can often be caused by nervous damage or it can occur with unknown etiology. Spinal cord injuries also can interrupt nerve signals required for bladder control.

As discussed in the male reproductive chapter, the prostate gland is approximately the size and shape of a walnut and surrounds the urethra just beneath the bladder. Its function is to add fluid to semen prior to ejaculation. One prostate condition that can contribute to urinary incontinence is benign prostatic hyperplasia (BPH), which is an enlarged prostate. When the prostate becomes enlarged, pressure is applied to the urethra, thereby affecting urine flow. The term for urinary symptoms associated with BPH is lower urinary tract symptoms (LUTS). BPH with LUTS typically occurs in men aged 60 to 80 years old. Note that while it is common to have hesitation, interrupted or weak urine stream, urgency, or leaking, as well as urge and frequency with urination, particularly at night, this does not necessarily mean an enlarged prostate is the cause.

Male patients who have undergone radical prostatectomy or external beam radiation for prostate cancer can also experience impotence and incontinence.

Female Urinary Incontinence

Incontinence occurs in females twice as often than in men, due largely in part to the anatomical structure of the female urinary tract, pregnancy and childbirth, as well as menopause. Additionally, older female patients tend to experience urinary tract-related problems more frequently than do younger female patients. Common types of incontinence associate with females include stress, urge (overactive bladder), functional, overflow, and mixed.

As previously stated, urinary incontinence is not a disease process but a symptom and as such, is coded to the signs, symptoms, and ill-defined conditions section in ICD-9-CM. Codes in this section are classified to category 788.3 with a fifth-digit subclassification assigned for the specific type of incontinence, including:

788.30	Urinary incontinence, unspecified
788.31	Urge incontinence
788.32	Stress incontinence, male
788.33	Mixed incontinence (male) (female)
788.34	Incontinence without sensory awareness
788.35	Post-void dribble
788.36	Nocturnal enuresis
788.37	Continuous leakage
788.38	Overflow incontinence
788.39	Other urinary incontinence

In ICD-10-CM, equivalent mapping is available for the ICD-9-CM codes. For example, 788.30 Urinary incontinence, unspecified, is mapped to R32 Unspecified urinary incontinence.

Urinary incontinence codes in ICD-10-CM are classified to category N39 Other disorders of urinary system, with stress incontinence assigned to N39.3 and the remaining types assigned to category N39.4 with a fifth character identifying the specific type. Other specified urinary incontinence is assigned to category N39.49 with a sixth character identifying the specific type as N39.490 Overflow incontinence, or N39.498 Other specified urinary incontinence. See the table below for equivalent mapping.

Coding for Urinary Incontinence

ICD-9-CM		ICD-10-CM	
788.31	Urge incontinence	N39.41	Urge incontinence
788.32	Stress incontinence, male	N39.3	Stress incontinence (female) (male)
788.33	Mixed incontinence (male) (female)	N39.46	Mixed incontinence
788.34	Incontinence without sensory awareness	N39.42	Incontinence without sensory awareness
788.35	Post-void dribble	N39.43	Post-void dribbling
788.36	Nocturnal enuresis	N39.44	Nocturnal enuresis
788.37	Continuous leakage	N39.45	Continuous leakage
788.38	Overflow incontinence	N39.490	Overflow incontinence
788.39	Other urinary incontinence	N39.498	Other specified urinary incontinence

Note that female stress urinary incontinence is coded in ICD-9-CM to category 625 Pain and other symptoms associated with female genital organs, with the fourth digit specifying stress incontinence, female. However, in ICD-10-CM, female stress urinary incontinence is not separately distinguished but rather is included in the same code as male stress urinary incontinence N39.3 Stress incontinence (female) (male).

Injury to the Kidneys and Pelvic Organs

An injury to the kidney can involve a laceration, contusion, hematoma, or an unspecified injury. ICD-9-CM category 866 Injury to kidney is further subdivided into two subcategories: injury to kidney without mention of open wound into cavity and injury to kidney with open wound into cavity. A fifth-digit subclassification is provided for use with this category to provide greater specificity as follows:

- Unspecified injury
- Hematoma without rupture of capsule
- Laceration
- Complete disruption of **kidney parenchyma**

ICD-10-CM provides laterality codes that permit coders to indicate *which* specific kidney has been injured and also allows coders to note the type of encounter. In the examples below, "A" indicates the initial encounter. However, other seventh-character codes are available, including "D" for subsequent encounter and "S" for sequela. *Consequence of a previous disease*

> **DEFINITIONS**
>
> **kidney parenchyma.** Primary, essential, and functional units of the kidney, specifically the nephrons.

Coding for Injury to the Kidney without Mention of Open Wound into the Cavity, Unspecified

ICD-9-CM	ICD-10-CM
866.00 Unspecified kidney injury without mention of open wound into cavity	S37.001A Unspecified injury of right kidney, initial encounter
	S37.002A Unspecified injury of left kidney, initial encounter
	S37.009A Unspecified injury of unspecified kidney, initial encounter

ICD-9-CM code 866.01 Kidney hematoma without rupture of capsule or mention of open wound into cavity, does not enable the coder to specify laterality; ICD-10-CM, however, does provide laterality choices, along with a seventh character noting the encounter. Additional terms are also used to describe the contusion (hematoma) as major or minor. No option is provided to the coder for a contusion not described as major or minor; therefore, documentation needs to indicate the severity of the hematoma.

Coding for Kidney Hematoma without Rupture of Capsule or Mention of Open Wound in Cavity

ICD-9-CM	ICD-10-CM
866.01 Kidney hematoma without rupture of capsule or mention of open wound into cavity	S37.011A Minor contusion of right kidney, initial encounter
	S37.012A Minor contusion of left kidney, initial encounter
	S37.019A Minor contusion of unspecified kidney, initial encounter
	S37.021A Major contusion of right kidney, initial encounter
	S37.022A Major contusion of left kidney, initial encounter
	S37.029A Major contusion of unspecified kidney, initial encounter

ICD-9-CM code 866.02 follows a similar mapping to ICD-10-CM codes as the tables above, with the ICD-10-CM code specifying both the laterality and type of encounter, as well as whether the laceration was considered minor or moderate, or was unspecified. Major lacerations involve a complete disruption of the kidney parenchyma (866.03).

There is an interesting difference in coding between ICD-9-CM and ICD-10-CM when it comes to injuries to the kidney that involve an *open wound* into the cavity. Note in the table below that *two* codes are necessary in ICD-10-CM to describe a condition assigned only one code in ICD-9-CM.

ICD-9-CM codes 866.11, 866.12, and 866.13 map to two ICD-10-CM codes: one that specifies laterality, encounter type, and whether the hematoma was minor or major, and a secondary code that more adequately describes the severity of the hematoma, laceration, or disruption of the kidney parenchyma, and the open wound into the cavity. Seventh characters in ICD-10-CM identify the type of encounter, with "A" indicating the initial encounter, "D" indicating subsequent encounters, and "S" used for sequela.

Coding for Kidney Hematoma without Rupture of Capsule, with Open Wound into Cavity

ICD-9-CM		ICD-10-CM	
866.11	Kidney hematoma, without rupture of capsule, with open wound into cavity	S37.019A	Minor contusion of unspecified kidney, initial encounter
		S37.029A	Major contusion of unspecified kidney, initial encounter
		AND	
		S31.001A	Unspecified open wound of lower back and pelvis with penetration into retroperitoneum, initial encounter

Another example is shown below.

Coding for Kidney Laceration with Open Wound into Cavity

ICD-9-CM		ICD-10-CM	
866.12	Kidney laceration with open wound into cavity	S37.039A	Laceration of unspecified kidney, unspecified degree, initial encounter
		S37.049A	Minor laceration of unspecified kidney, initial encounter
		S37.059A	Moderate laceration of unspecified kidney, initial encounter
		AND	
		S31.001A	Unspecified open wound of lower back and pelvis with penetration into retroperitoneum, initial encounter

ICD-9-CM code 866.13 maps to ICD-10-CM codes S37.069A Major laceration, unspecified kidney, initial encounter, and S31.001A Unspecified open wound of lower back and pelvis with penetration into the retroperitoneum, initial encounter.

ICD-9-CM category 867 Injury to pelvic organs, includes categories for other organs within the urinary system. For example, 867.0 and 867.1 describe an injury to the bladder and urethra, with or without mention of an open wound into the cavity, respectively. Likewise, categories are provided for an injury to the ureter with (867.3) and without (867.2) open wound into the cavity. No fifth-digit subclassification is provided for use with category 867. In ICD-10-CM, codes for injuries to the bladder or urethra without mention of an open wound include the specific type of injury (contusion, laceration, other, or unspecified) and a seventh character identifying the encounter type.

Chapter 13. ICD-10-CM: Reproductive Systems

Note: This chapter includes both the male and female reproductive systems, as well as a separate section on pregnancy, childbirth, and the puerperium. For ease of use, each section is discussed separately, beginning with the male reproductive system.

Anatomic Overview: Male Reproductive System

Three primary organs make up the external male reproductive system: the penis, scrotum, and testicles (testes). Internal organs, also referred to as accessory organs, include:

- Bulbourethral glands
- Ejaculatory ducts
- Epididymis
- Prostate gland
- Seminal vesicles
- Urethra
- Vas deferens

External Organs

The first primary external organ is the penis and it has three parts: the root, which attaches to the wall of the abdomen; the body (shaft); and the glans, the cone-shaped part at the end of the penis, often referred to as the head of the penis (glans penis). At birth, this area is covered with a loose layer of skin called the foreskin. The urethral opening is at the tip of the penis and, as discussed in the urinary section, is the tube that transports urine from the body. In the male reproductive system, semen is also transported through the urethra. In addition, the penis also contains a number of sensitive nerve endings.

Figure 13.1: Male Genitalia

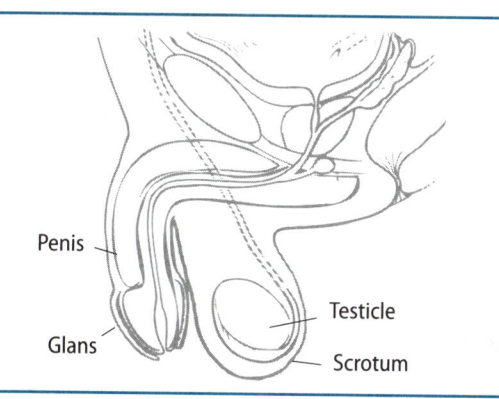

> **CLINICAL NOTE**
>
> Circumcision is a procedure involving the surgical removal of the foreskin, the tissue covering the head of the penis. The procedure involves the freeing of the foreskin, or prepuce, from the head of the penis (glans), and clipping the excess foreskin off. When performed on a newborn, the procedure takes approximately five to 10 minutes; adults may take one hour. Healing occurs usually within five to seven days.

© 2015 Optum360, LLC

> **INTERESTING A & P FACT**
>
> The scrotum is an external reproductive organ since temperatures inside the human body are too high for sperm to survive.

Figure 13.2: Glans Penis

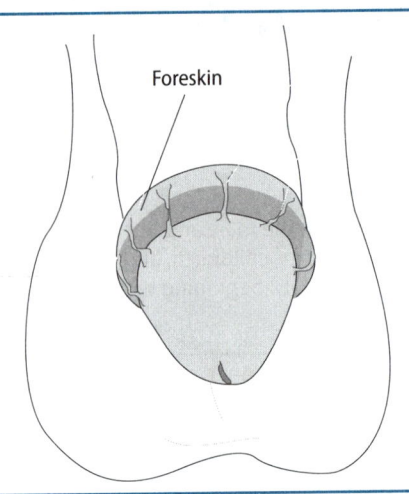

Behind and just below the penis lies a loose, pouch-like sac of skin known as the scrotum, which houses the testicles, commonly known as the testes. A number of nerves and blood vessels are located within the scrotum. The main function of the scrotum is to control the temperature of the testes to that of a slightly lower-than-normal body temperature in order to ensure healthy sperm development. The scrotum wall contains special muscles that contract and relax, thereby allowing the testicles to move closer to the body as necessary for warmth or further away in order to cool the temperature back down.

The last of the external male sex organs are the testicles (testes), which function to make the primary male sex hormone, testosterone, and to generate sperm. Most men have two testes. The testicles are oval in shape and approximately the size of large olives, protected at either end by the spermatic cord. Within the testes lie the *seminiferous tubules*, which produce sperm cells.

> **DEFINITIONS**
>
> **seminiferous tubules.** Small tubes found in the testes where the spermatozoa develop.

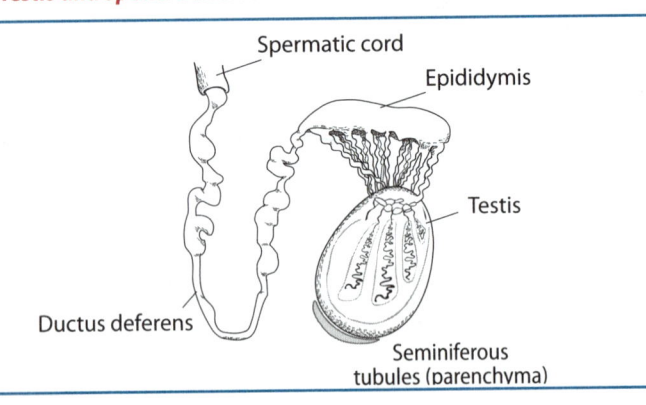

Figure 13.3: Testis and Sperm Generation

Internal Organs

The epididymis, a long, firm tube that lies on the backside of each testicle, coils in order to stay contained within its small space. It is approximately 20 feet in length and functions as a storage area for sperm, allowing room and time for sperm emerging from the testes to mature. The epididymis comprises three sections: the head or expanded upper end, the body, and the pointed tail. It is the task of the epididymis to nourish the sperm by absorbing fluid and adding substances that help the sperm reach maturity in order to be capable of fertilization. During sexual arousal, contractions of the epididymis force sperm into the vas deferens.

As the excretory duct of the testicles, the vas deferens is a continuation of the epididymis canal. Often referred to as the ductus deferens or the seminal duct, the vas deferens is a long, muscular tube that transports mature sperm to the urethra in preparation for ejaculation. Starting at the lower part of the epididymis tail, it moves into the pelvic cavity, located behind the bladder. The structure of the vas deferens, or ductus deferens, consists of three "coats": an external or areolar coat, a muscular coat, and an internal or mucous coat. In the larger part of the tube, the muscular coat is made up of two layers of unstriped muscular fiber: an outer layer, longitudinal in direction, and an inner, circular layer. At the beginning area of the ductus, a third layer is present, encompassing longitudinal fibers between the circular stratum and the mucous membrane. The internal or mucous coat is light in color and runs lengthwise.

There are two ejaculatory ducts, approximately 2 cm in length, formed by the fusing of the vas deferens and the seminal vesicles. The ducts begin at the base of the prostate, running both forward and downward between the middle and lateral lobes, as well as along the sides of the prostatic utricle and ending just within the utricle margins, diminishing in size as they do so. The coats of the ejaculatory ducts are extremely thin and consist of a fibrous outer layer, muscular fibers made up of a thin circular outer layer, and a longitudinal inner layer as well as mucous membrane.

As discussed in the urinary chapter, the tube that carries urine from the bladder is called the urethra. In males, the urethra has the additional responsibility of ejaculating semen upon orgasm. During intercourse, the penis is erect and the flow of urine is blocked from the urethra, thereby permitting only the release of semen upon orgasm.

A pair of small, tubular glands in the male genitourinary system, seminal vesicles appear as sac-like pouches attached to the vas deferens near the bladder's base. The seminal vesicles produce a fructose-rich seminal fluid that is a component of semen. This fluid is a source of energy, assisting the sperm to move, and makes up a significant amount of the volume of a man's ejaculate. The seminal vesicles can very often be an early location for metastasis from prostate cancer.

The prostate gland is comparable in size to a walnut and is located below the urinary bladder, in front of the rectum, surrounding the neck of the bladder and urethra. It has a muscular and glandular makeup and ducts that open into the prostatic portion of the urethra. It consists of three lobes: right, left, and middle. The primary function of the prostate gland is to secrete an additional fluid that makes up part of the ejaculate. Additionally, during orgasm, muscular glands of the prostate help force prostate fluid, including sperm produced in the testicles, into the urethra.

Figure 13.4: Prostate and Seminal Vesicles

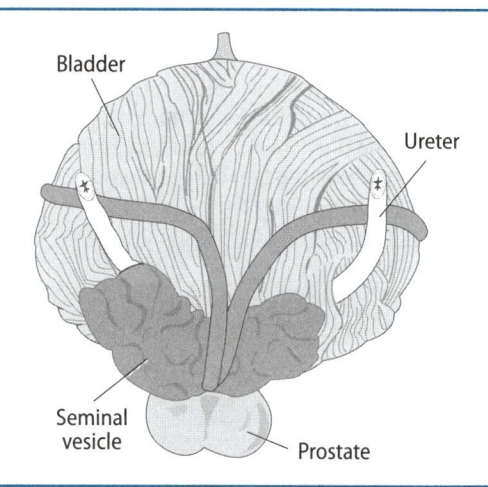

Bulbourethral glands, also known as Cowper's glands, are small, pea-sized, yellowish colored, lobular-like bodies located behind and to the sides of the urethra, below the prostate gland. These glands produce a transparent, slick fluid that serves as a lubricant to the urethra, as well as a neutralizing agent to any acid left behind by urine droplets in the urethra. Each gland contains an excretory duct, approximately 2.5 cm in length, that empties directly into the urethra.

The male reproductive system relies on hormones—chemicals produced by the body to help regulate the various functions of a myriad of different cell types or organs. Hormones primarily involved in regulating the male reproductive system include follicle-stimulating hormone (FSH), luteinizing hormone (LH), and testosterone. Each of the three hormones is necessary for sperm production, though testosterone is also responsible for developing many male characteristics, such as facial hair growth, voice changes, body muscle mass size and strength, fat distribution, and sex drive.

Anatomy and Pathophysiology and the ICD-10-CM Code Set: Male Reproductive System

The human reproductive system, like all complex organ systems, is affected by a number of disease processes that can be grouped into four main categories: congenital abnormalities, cancers, infections including sexually transmitted diseases (STD), and functional problems brought about by injury or physical damage, environmental factors, psychological issues, autoimmune disorders, or other causes. There are some reproductive diseases that often present as a sign or symptom of another disease or disorder or have multiple causes of unknown etiology, creating difficulty when trying to classify or categorize them.

The ICD-10-CM coding system allows for greater specificity when assigning codes related to the reproductive system, in part through the use of more descriptive terms within the code descriptors that ensure improved accuracy and significantly more detail in code selection. Throughout the ICD-10-CM coding system, there are minimal or minor distinctions, such as in the case of ICD-9-CM code 601.0 Acute prostatitis, listed under the category for inflammatory diseases of the prostate. In ICD-10-CM, there are now two codes to choose from: Acute prostatitis with or without hematuria (blood in the urine). In order to select the appropriate code, it is necessary to understand the meaning of the term "hematuria," as well as whether the documentation indicated that the patient had blood in his urine in addition to the acute prostatitis. This section focuses on disease processes identified as having an obvious and significant coding distinction or difference between the current ICD-9-CM coding system and ICD-10-CM.

Other Specified Disorders of the Prostate

Within the ICD-9-CM coding system, there is one code (602.8) designated for other specified disorders of the prostate; however, ICD-10-CM provides three code options under the same titled category: prostatodynia syndrome, prostatosis syndrome, and other specified disorders of the prostate. As a result, the coder must know and understand the difference between the two different syndromes before resorting to the least specific of the three codes.

Figure 13.5: Male Urinary and Reproductive Systems

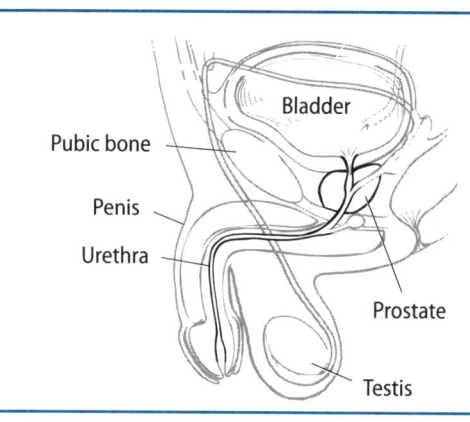

Prostatodynia syndrome describes a deep burning or aching type of pain that appears to originate from the prostate. Many times, prostate pain is diagnosed as prostatitis, an inflammatory condition often caused by infection. Patients with prostatodynia feel the prostate pain radiate into the rectum, which can sometimes lead to an incorrect clinical diagnosis of proctalgia, a term that refers to pain in the rectum. Difficulty urinating or pain during voiding may accompany prostatodynia. The term prostatosis is somewhat ambiguous, general in nature and means "a condition of the prostate." Pain emanating from the prostate without an accompanying infection is considered more of a symptom. The terms prostatosis and prostatodynia are often used interchangeably. While these two conditions are often characterized by many of the same symptoms associated with chronic bacterial prostatitis, no bacteria are identified in the patient's urine and prostatic fluid cultures are negative.

Coding for Other Specified Disorders of the Prostate

ICD-9-CM	ICD-10-CM
602.8 Other specified disorder of the prostate	N42.81 Prostatodynia syndrome
	N42.82 Prostatosis syndrome
	N42.89 Other specified disorders of prostate

Redundant Prepuce and Phimosis

Phimosis is a constriction, or tightening, of the prepuce (foreskin). In this condition, the foreskin contracts and is not able to be retracted or pulled back behind the glans or tip of the penis. Often, phimosis is caused from chronic infections of the foreskin. However, it may also be congenital, or present at birth. Circumcision is a common treatment for phimosis.

> **DEFINITIONS**
>
> **phimosis.** Condition in which the foreskin is contracted and cannot be drawn back behind the glans penis. Phimosis is a common medical reason for circumcision in the United States and the most common complication of balanitis.

Figure 13.6: Slitting of Prepuce

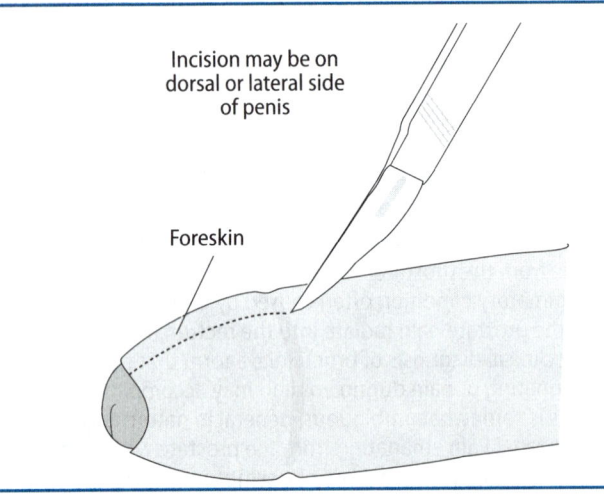

In contrast to phimosis, paraphimosis is considered a urological emergency requiring immediate treatment. In this condition, the foreskin retracts and tightens below the glans. As a result, lymphatic drainage is compromised, causing the glans to swell. If the condition is left untreated, blood flow within the penis is hindered by the ever-tightening band of foreskin, thereby causing increased swelling of the glans penis. The lack of oxygen associated with the decreased blood flow can lead to necrosis, or tissue death.

The term "adherent prepuce" describes a condition whereby a growth or adhesion blocks the foreskin from pulling back off the glans penis. This condition is considered an indication for circumcision. A "deficient" foreskin is one in which the prepuce is considered incomplete or inadequate. Finally, adhesions of the prepuce and penis may occur following circumcision if the residual skin is not pulled back after healing. During a circumcision, normal intact tissue is divided and, without proper care, it is possible for the tissue at the area of the removal to reattach to glans tissue, creating an adhesion or scar tissue. These adhesions can often be easily freed by simply cutting through the scar tissue. In some cases, however, the tissues have fused together in such a way that further intervention may be required.

Coding for Redundant Prepuce and Phimosis

ICD-9-CM		ICD-10-CM	
605	Redundant prepuce and phimosis	N47.0	Adherent prepuce, newborn
		N47.1	Phimosis
		N47.2	Paraphimosis
		N47.3	Deficient foreskin
		N47.4	Benign cyst of prepuce
		N47.5	Adhesions of prepuce and glans penis
		N47.7	Other inflammatory diseases of prepuce
		N47.8	Other disorders of prepuce

Male Infertility: Azoospermia and Oligospermia

Azoospermia is a condition in which there is total absence of sperm in the ejaculate fluid. Blockage within the testes or a missing duct can lead to a lack of sperm during ejaculation despite sperm being produced. In other cases, sperm may not be produced as the result of a hormonal issue or a **varicocele**.

Oligospermia, or low sperm count, occurs when semen contains fewer sperm than normal. Abnormal sperm count is defined as fewer than 15 million sperm per milliliter of semen. There are a number of medical conditions that can contribute to oligospermia, including but not limited to:

- Hormonal imbalance
- Infection
- Sperm duct defect
- Tumors
- Undescended testicle
- Varicocele

In addition, environmental and lifestyle factors can also lead to a low sperm count, including exposure to pesticides or radiation/x-rays, prolonged cycling, overheating of the testicles from excessive hot tub or sauna use, smoking, alcohol or drug abuse, age, weight, and emotional stress.

The need to understand the various causes and factors associated with male infertility becomes increasingly more important with the adoption of ICD-10-CM.

In the ICD-9-CM coding system, under category 606 Male infertility, four subcategories are provided: 606.0 Azoospermia, 606.1 Oligospermia, 606.8 Infertility due to extratesticular causes, and 606.9 Male infertility, unspecified.

However, in ICD-10-CM, under category N46 Male infertility, there are two main subcategories: azoospermia and oligospermia. Both subcategories are further divided into two classifications: organic and due to extratesticular causes. Additional characters are provided to indicate the "extratesticular causes" as shown in the following table.

Note that code N46.8 Other male infertility is mapped to ICD-9-CM code 606.8 Infertility due to extratesticular causes, despite also being incorporated into the new classifications for N46.0 Azoospermia, and N46.1 Oligospermia; however, N46.9 Male infertility, unspecified, directly corresponds to existing ICD-9-CM code 606.9.

Coding for Male Infertility: Azoospermia and Oligospermia

ICD-9-CM		ICD-10-CM	
606.0	Azoospermia	N46.01	Organic azoospermia
		N46.021	Azoospermia due to drug therapy
		N46.022	Azoospermia due to infection
		N46.023	Azoospermia due to obstruction of efferent ducts
		N46.024	Azoospermia due to radiation
		N46.025	Azoospermia due to systemic disease
606.1	Oligospermia	N46.11	Organic oligospermia
		N46.121	Oligospermia due to drug therapy
		N46.122	Oligospermia due to infection
		N46.123	Oligospermia due to obstruction of efferent ducts
		N46.124	Oligospermia due to radiation
		N46.125	Oligospermia due to systemic disease
		N46.129	Oligospermia due to other extratesticular causes
606.8	Infertility due to extratesticular causes	N46.029	Azoospermia due to other extratesticular causes
		N46.8	Other male infertility
606.9	Unspecified male infertility	N46.9	Male infertility, unspecified

---

DEFINITIONS

varicocele. Abnormal enlargement of the veins in the scrotum, most commonly seen on the left side, that prevents proper blood flow, leading to swelling and widening of the veins, essentially creating varicose veins. Varicoceles are slow to develop, typically seen in males between the ages of 15 to 25, and are often a cause of male infertility.

INTERESTING A & P FACT

In a healthy adult male, approximately 500 million sperm mature every day.

Other Specified Disorders of Penis: Impotence of Organic Origin/Male Erectile Dysfunction

Impotence, or as it is now more commonly termed, erectile dysfunction, is the failure to attain or maintain an erection when sexually aroused. It may be the result of psychological factors (e.g., guilt, anxiety, conflict, depression) or due to organic or physical causes. Since organic causes impede any erection, the occurrence of any normal erections would rule out impotence of organic origin.

In the current coding system, erectile dysfunction (ED) due to physiological causes is classified under the category 607.84 Impotence of organic origin. No further specificity is provided. In ICD-10-CM, category N52 Male erectile dysfunction, is further divided into six subcategories:

N52.0	Vasculogenic erectile dysfunction
N52.1	Erectile dysfunction due to diseases classified elsewhere
N52.2	Drug-induced erectile dysfunction
N52.3	Post-surgical erectile dysfunction
N52.8	Other male erectile dysfunction
N52.9	Male erectile dysfunction, unspecified

Furthermore, subcategories N52.0 Vasculogenic erectile dysfunction, and N52.3 Post-surgical erectile dysfunction, also contain additional classifications to allow for greater detail and specificity as to the exact type of vascular condition or surgery causing the impotence.

Vasculogenic Erectile Dysfunction

Three specific conditions are identified under category N52.0: ED due to arterial insufficiency, corporo-venous occlusive ED, and combined arterial insufficiency and corporo-venous occlusive ED. Correct code assignment necessitates a clear understanding of these conditions, as well as the differences between them. A discussion of each condition follows.

Simply put, arterial insufficiency means there is not enough blood flowing through the arteries to meet the needs of the tissue. When arterial flow to the penis is impeded, a decrease in venous pressure results that subsequently leads to an inadequate erection. A number of factors can contribute to a decline in arterial flow including, but not limited to, peripheral artery disease (PAD). Peripheral artery disease is often directly linked to common risk factors such as smoking, high blood pressure, diabetes mellitus, and high cholesterol. However, other environmental or outside causes do exist, as well, including injury or radiation to the pelvic region. A patient presenting with ED of organic origin would be evaluated to determine the risk and possibility of peripheral or coronary artery disease (CAD).

The corpora cavernosa are two compartments made of spongy tissue within the penis that run lengthwise against the organ. Blood flows into the space and fills the open areas in the spongy tissue, causing an erection. Corporal veno-occlusive dysfunction (CVOD) is one of the most common forms of erectile dysfunction and is noted to be associated with aging. Other disease processes can also be associated with the corpora cavernosa and contribute to venous *occlusive* ED. The term "venous occlusive" means blocked veins that impede circulation to the penis.

In addition to understanding the differences in these various conditions, it is also necessary for the medical record documentation to clearly identify the specific procedure performed when ED is considered a postoperative condition related to the prior surgery in order to ensure correct code assignment.

DEFINITIONS

occlusive. Having to do with constriction, closure, or blockage of a passage.

Figure 13.7: Penis

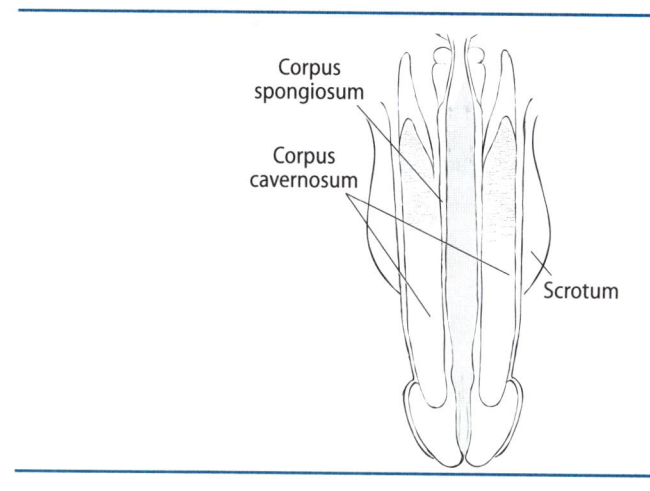

Coding for Male Erectile Dysfunction

ICD-9-CM		ICD-10-CM	
607.84	Impotence of organic origin	N52.01	Erectile dysfunction due to arterial insufficiency
		N52.02	Corporo-venous occlusive erectile dysfunction
		N52.03	Combined arterial insufficiency and corporo-venous occlusive erectile dysfunction
		N52.1	Erectile dysfunction due to diseases classified elsewhere
		N52.2	Drug-induced erectile dysfunction
		N52.31	Erectile dysfunction following radical prostatectomy
		N52.32	Erectile dysfunction following radical cystectomy
		N52.33	Erectile dysfunction following urethral surgery
		N52.34	Erectile dysfunction following simple prostatectomy
		N52.39	Other post-surgical erectile dysfunction
		N52.8	Other male erectile dysfunction
		N52.9	Male erectile dysfunction, unspecified

Summary: Male Reproductive System

The conditions discussed in this section were just a few of the common disease processes associated with the male reproductive system. As previously mentioned, being vigilant and prudent when reviewing and selecting codes within the ICD-10-CM coding system is vitally important to ensure accuracy. This requires a strong understanding of the specific terms and conditions detailed within ICD-10-CM as they relate to the anatomy and physiology of the male reproductive system, and certainly helps to facilitate a more straightforward and uncomplicated transition to the new coding system.

Anatomic Overview: Female Reproductive System

The female reproductive system comprises external and internal structures. External structures include the labia majora, labia minora, Bartholin's glands, and the clitoris. These organs allow sperm to enter the body, as well as to safeguard the internal genital organs from infection. The internal reproductive organs consist of the following:

- Fallopian tubes
- Ovaries
- Uterus
- Vagina

Several functions take place within the female reproductive system, including the production of egg cells, called ova or oocytes, the transport of the ova to the fallopian tubes for conception, and then the transport of the ova to the uterus for fetal development, all part of the menstrual cycle. In the event that egg fertilization does not occur, the system commences menstruation—the monthly shedding of the uterine lining. Other functions of the female reproductive system involve production of female sex hormones necessary for maintaining the reproductive cycle.

External Organs

The labia majora are two large, fleshy, longitudinal, cutaneous folds that extend downward and backward from the mons pubis to the perineum, and are the counterpart to the scrotum in a male. They contain sweat and oil-secreting glands. Pubic hair covers the labia majora after puberty begins. The smaller labia minora lie on the inside of the labia majora surrounding the opening to the vagina and urethra and are approximately 2 inches wide. The Bartholin's glands lie next to the vaginal opening and produce mucus. The clitoris, a collection of nerves approximately the size of a pea located where the two labia minora meet, is highly sensitive to stimulation and is responsible for feelings of sexual pleasure. Similar to foreskin on the glans penis, the clitoris is covered by a skin fold called the prepuce. The clitoris is the counterpart to the penis in the male reproductive system.

> **INTERESTING A & P FACT**
>
> During the course of fetal development, approximately 6 to 7 million eggs are generated with no further eggs to be produced; at birth only about 1 million eggs remain. By the time a woman reaches puberty, it is estimated that only 300,000 to 400,000 eggs remain. Of these, an average of 300 to 400 will be ovulated over the course of a woman's reproductive lifetime.

Figure 13.8: Female External Genitalia

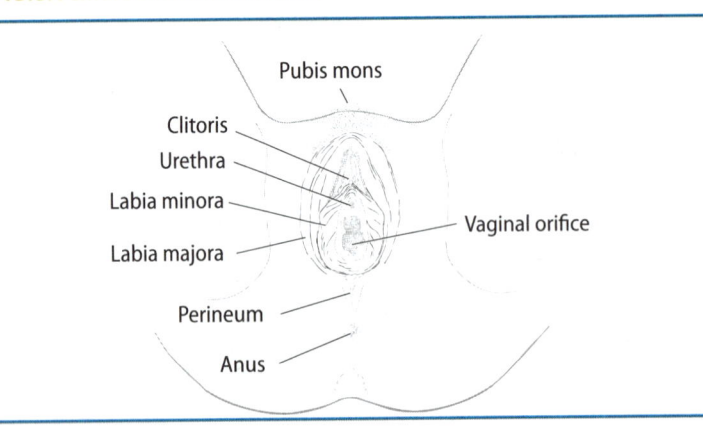

Internal Organs

The vagina or birth canal is a passageway that adjoins the lower part of the uterus, called the cervix, to the outside of the body. The hollow, pear-shaped organ, which houses the fetus during development, is called the uterus. It has two parts: the cervix or lower portion as described above and the corpus or main body. Naturally, the corpus is designed to expand to accommodate a developing baby. The cervix contains a channel that permits sperm to enter and menstrual blood to exit when fertilization does not occur. On either side of the uterus lie small, oval-shaped glands called ovaries that produce eggs and hormones. The fallopian tubes attach to the upper part of the uterus and are the means by which the egg cells travel from the ovaries to the uterus. Conception, fertilization of an egg by a sperm, typically occurs in the fallopian tubes, whereupon the egg continues down the tube to the uterus, where it implants in the uterine wall.

Figure 13.9: Female Reproductive System

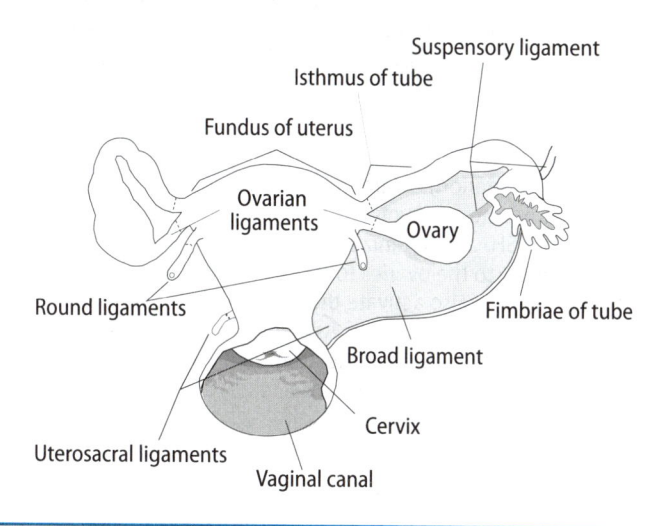

Breasts

Breasts are often considered a part of the female reproductive system in large part due to the role they play in providing nourishment to a newborn baby, as well as for the sexual stimulation generated during intercourse. The breast is also sometimes seen as part of the integumentary system. Breast development begins in puberty with the release of estrogen and later progesterone, triggering changes in the breast form, usually over a three- to four-year period and typically completed by age 16. Additional detail regarding the breast, its structure, and disorders related to breast tissue can be found in chapter 2.

A female breast is made up of four structures: lobules or glands, milk ducts, fat, and connective tissue. A grouping of lobules form a larger unit called a lobe. Approximately 15 to 20 lobes are in each breast, emanating from the nipple and areolar area, that appear to be arranged in a wheel-spoke pattern. Distribution of the lobes is not even, and there is a predominate amount of glandular tissue in the upper and outer portions of the breast. This accounts for the tenderness experienced by many women prior to the menstrual cycle. Note that this is the site of more than half of all diagnosed breast cancers.

Lobes empty into milk ducts that course through the breast towards the nipple/areolar region, converging into about 6 to 10 larger ducts called collecting ducts. These collecting ducts enter at the base of the nipple and connect to the outside of the body. During lactation, which is the production and secretion of milk by the mammary glands, the breast milk is emptied via this course on its way to the infant.

Of course, each woman is different; therefore, it makes sense that breast lobes would vary from woman to woman. However, as a general rule, glandular tissue has a firm, almost nodular feel to it, and fat surrounds the glandular portion of the breast. In contrast, fat is almost always soft. Ducts are not usually palpable unless engorged with milk, inflamed, or containing a tumor or mass. All components of the breast structure are affected by female hormones, though glandular tissue is the most sensitive.

There are a number of congenital abnormalities of the breast, with the most common being accessory nipples and/or breast tissue, which occurs in about 2 to 6 percent of the population. Severe underdevelopment or absence of one or both breasts is another congenital abnormality but is extremely rare.

Menstrual Cycle

The menstrual cycle is the process by which a woman's body prepares for the possibility of pregnancy. The term "menstru" means monthly; hence the word menstruation describes the monthly shedding of the uterine lining. On average, a menstrual cycle is 28-days long and takes place in three phases as described below.

Follicular Phase

The first day of the cycle (period) commences the follicular phase. During this phase, two of the four major hormones involved in the menstrual cycle are released: follicle stimulating hormone (FSH) and luteinizing hormone (LH). These hormones travel through the bloodstream to the ovaries to stimulate the development of several ovarian follicles. FSH and LH also activate the production of estrogen, a third hormone involved in the menstrual cycle. As levels of estrogen rise, it deactivates the FSH, thereby allowing the body to limit the number of follicles that reach maturity. Each follicle contains one egg. As FSH levels decrease, only one follicle in one ovary continues to develop. This dominant follicle stifles all other follicles within the group, causing them to cease growing and subsequently die. This dominant follicle continues producing estrogen.

Ovulation

The second phase in the menstrual cycle is called the ovulatory phase, or more commonly ovulation, which occurs approximately 14 days after the follicular phase began. This is considered the midpoint of the menstrual cycle. Typically, the next period starts within two weeks from this point. An increase in estrogen levels from the dominant follicle then generates a surge in luteinizing hormone. The increase in LH stimulates the release of an egg from the ovary (ovulation), which is then collected by the finger-like projections protruding from the ends of the fallopian tubes (fimbriae). The actions of the fimbriae sweep the egg into the fallopian tube. Estrogen levels peak during the surge, and the progesterone level starts to increase. An increase in the amount and thickness of mucus produced by the cervix also occurs so that if a woman were to engage in sexual intercourse during this phase, the thicker mucus would help to collect the male sperm, nourish it, and move it toward the egg for fertilization.

Luteal Phase

The third and final phase in the menstrual cycle begins after the release of the egg, when the empty follicle begins transforming into a new structure called the corpus luteum. The corpus luteum emits the hormones estrogen and progesterone. As the fourth hormone in the menstrual cycle, progesterone prepares the uterus for the possibility of receiving a fertilized egg to implant. Progesterone and estrogen stimulate the endometrium (lining of the uterus) to thicken, filling it with fluids and nutrients necessary to nourish the fetus. Progesterone also prompts the mucus in the cervix to thicken, making it less likely that sperm or bacteria can enter the uterus. Finally, it triggers the body temperature to slightly rise and remain elevated until the menstrual period begins. If an egg is not fertilized, it passes down through the uterus and, because the endometrium is no longer needed to support a pregnancy, it begins to break down and shed, beginning menstruation.

The consistency of the breasts is dramatically affected by the menstrual cycle as well, most notably just prior to menstruation when the levels of estrogen and progesterone are peaking. After menstruation, when hormone levels are at their lowest, breasts become softer and less tender, making it the recommended time to perform breast self-examination or to have a mammogram.

Anatomy and Pathophysiology and the ICD-10-CM Code Set: Female Reproductive System

As mentioned previously in the male reproductive section, the human reproductive system is affected by various disease processes, such as congenital abnormalities, cancers, infections including sexually transmitted diseases (STD), and functional problems brought about by injury or physical damage, environmental factors, psychological-related issues, autoimmune disorders, or other causes. Further complicating matters are reproductive diseases or disorders, such as endometriosis, with multiple or unknown causes that make classification difficult.

This section discusses conditions that afflict the female reproductive system with an emphasis on diagnoses that contain noteworthy coding distinctions and differences between ICD-9-CM and ICD-10-CM.

Inflammatory Disease of Ovary, Fallopian Tube, Pelvic Cellular Tissue, and Peritoneum

Infection and **inflammation** involving the fallopian tubes is called salpingitis; when the ovaries are involved, the term is oophoritis. In the current coding system, the two conditions are combined into single code categories to indicate acute, chronic, or unspecified. However, in ICD-10-CM, an individual code is available for salpingitis, oophoritis, or salpingitis and oophoritis combined; again, separate categories designate acute, chronic, or unspecified.

> **DEFINITIONS**
>
> **inflammation.** Cytologic and chemical reactions that occur in affected blood vessels and adjacent tissues in response to injury or abnormal stimulation from a physical, chemical, or biologic agent.

Figure 13.10: Ovary and Fallopian Tube

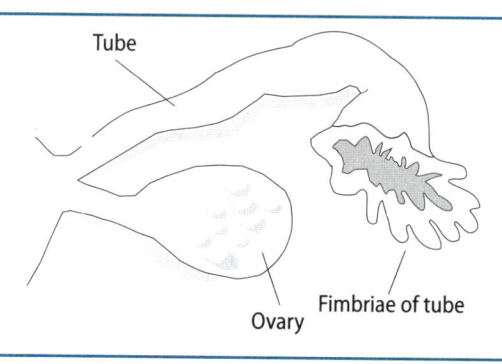

Coding for Inflammatory Diseases of Female Pelvic Organs

ICD-9-CM		ICD-10-CM	
614.0	Acute salpingitis and oophoritis	N70.01	Acute salpingitis
		N70.02	Acute oophoritis
		N70.03	Acute salpingitis and oophoritis
614.1	Chronic salpingitis and oophoritis	N70.11	Chronic salpingitis
		N70.12	Chronic oophoritis
		N70.13	Chronic salpingitis and oophoritis
614.2	Salpingitis and oophoritis not specified as acute, subacute, or chronic	N70.91	Salpingitis, unspecified
		N70.92	Oophoritis, unspecified
		N70.93	Salpingitis and oophoritis, unspecified

Other codes under category 614 Inflammatory disease of ovary, fallopian tube, pelvic cellular tissue, and peritoneum, generally show a one-to-one coding designation with ICD-10-CM with the exception of code 614.9 Unspecified inflammatory disease of female pelvic organs and tissues. In this example, ICD-10-CM contains three options: A56.11 Chlamydial female pelvic inflammatory disease, N73.5 Female pelvic peritonitis, unspecified, and N73.9 Female pelvic inflammatory disease, unspecified.

Inflammatory Disease of Cervix, Vagina, and Vulva

Similar to the codes for salpingitis and oophoritis, the codes for vaginitis and vulvovaginitis are also assigned ICD-10-CM codes that separate the two conditions into distinct categories, as well as individual codes to indicate whether the condition is acute or subacute and chronic.

Vaginitis is a condition that encompasses symptoms such as swelling, itching, and burning in the vagina, often accompanied by an abnormal discharge that can be caused by several different kinds of germs. The term vaginitis is often used to describe any infection or inflammation of the vagina. When the infection or inflammation also involves the vulva, the term used is vulvovaginitis.

Coding for Inflammatory Diseases of Female Pelvic Organs

ICD-9-CM		ICD-10-CM	
616.10	Unspecified vaginitis and vulvovaginitis	N76.0	Acute vaginitis
		N76.1	Subacute and chronic vaginitis
		N76.2	Acute vulvitis
		N76.3	Subacute and chronic vulvitis

Noninflammatory Disorders of Ovary, Fallopian Tube, and Broad Ligament

ICD-9-CM category 620.3 Acquired atrophy of ovary and fallopian tube, describes a condition that was not present at birth but developed over time. From a medical standpoint, the word "acquired" describes something recent or new. An acquired condition is considered to be new in the sense that it was not inherited and that it may have arisen sometime later in the patient's life as opposed to the patient being born with it.

Atrophy is defined as the reduction in size or activity in an anatomic structure, due to wasting away from disease or other factors. Thus, acquired atrophy of the ovary or fallopian tube describes a condition that developed over time and that has caused a decrease or decline in the size or function of that structure.

As with previously discussed codes, the ICD-10-CM coding system divides the conditions into distinct code categories for ovary, fallopian tube, and a combination of both anatomical sites.

Coding for Acquired Atrophy of Ovary and Fallopian Tube

ICD-9-CM		ICD-10-CM	
620.3	Acquired atrophy of ovary and fallopian tube	N83.31	Acquired atrophy of ovary
		N83.32	Acquired atrophy of fallopian tube
		N83.33	Acquired atrophy of ovary and fallopian tube

Torsion of Ovary, Ovarian Pedicle, or Fallopian Tube

As the fifth most common gynecologic emergency, torsion, or twisting of the ovary, affects females of all age ranges. However, most cases tend to present in patients in their early reproductive years. Children younger than age 15 have an increased risk for this condition. Most often, an ovarian torsion occurs on one side, with 60 percent of cases occurring on the right side. Delay in diagnosing and treating ovarian torsion can lead to the torsion worsening and cutting off arterial blood flow into and venous blood flow out of the ovary. When this happens, the result is necrosis (death) of the ovarian tissue. The ovarian (vascular) pedicle is the area of the ovary containing the ovarian artery and vein. Cysts and neoplasms often cause the ovary to swing on its vascular pedicle much more easily than normal, and the larger the cyst or mass, the greater the potential for torsion unless the mass develops to such a size that movement is hindered.

Torsion of the fallopian tube is a much rarer event but has been reported in both normal and pathological fallopian tubes. A number of possible causes can be attributed to this condition, such as tubal ligation, hematosalpinx (bleeding into the tubes), congenital hydrosalpinx (blockage at the end of the tube with fluid that causes swelling), and neoplasms, as well as trauma, pregnancy, adhesions, and ovarian tumors.

Torsion of the fallopian tube is usually accompanied by torsion of the ovary with an ovarian mass being present in approximately 50 to 60 percent of fallopian tube torsion cases. As in the case with an ovarian torsion, the right side is more commonly affected than the left.

ICD-9-CM currently encompasses torsion involving the ovary, ovarian pedicle, and fallopian tube under one code, 620.5, but as evidenced with other code sets, ICD-10-CM provides for greater specificity by splitting ovarian and ovarian pedicle torsion into one code and torsion of the fallopian tube into its own code category. A third code category has been developed to describe cases in which the torsion occurs in all three areas

Coding for Torsion of Ovary, Ovarian Pedicle, and Fallopian Tube

ICD-9-CM		ICD-10-CM	
620.5	Torsion of ovary, ovarian pedicle, or fallopian tube	N83.51	Torsion of ovary and ovarian pedicle
		N83.52	Torsion of fallopian tube
		N83.53	Torsion of ovary, ovarian pedicle and fallopian tube

Dysplasia of Vagina

Dysplasia describes abnormal changes in the cells found on the surface of the vagina. It is categorized by three stages: mild, moderate, and severe. The most common form of dysplasia is mild, and more than 65 percent of cases diagnosed as mild tend to return to a normal state of tissue without any intervention. Mild dysplasia is defined as only involving approximately 25 percent of the thickness of the cell layer overlying the vagina. Unfortunately, moderate and severe forms of dysplasia rarely resolve without intervention and have an increased chance of developing into cancer. Moderate dysplasia is defined as having 50 percent involvement of the cell layer, and severe dysplasia generally means that most, if not all, of the full-thickness of the cell layer covering the vagina have abnormal cells present.

ICD-9-CM describes only the mild and moderate forms of this condition, whereas ICD-10-CM identifies whether the dysplasia is classified as mild, moderate, or unspecified. Severe dysplasia is coded in ICD-9-CM to code 233.31 Carcinoma in situ of breast and genitourinary system, other and unspecified female genital organs, vagina, and is mapped to ICD-10-CM code D07.2 Carcinoma in situ of other and unspecified genital organs, carcinoma in situ of vagina.

Coding for Other Noninflammatory Disorders of the Vagina

ICD-9-CM		ICD-10-CM	
623.0	Dysplasia of vagina	N89.0	Mild vaginal dysplasia
		N89.1	Moderate vaginal dysplasia
		N89.3	Dysplasia of vagina, unspecified

Summary: Female Reproductive System

Careful review of the terms and descriptions used in the ICD-10-CM coding system helps ensure accurate code assignment. Not all conditions associated with the female reproductive system have been addressed; however, many of the common disease processes within the female reproductive system with notable distinctions between the two coding systems were discussed to demonstrate the areas coders should focus on during the transition to ICD-10-CM.

Anatomic Overview: Pregnancy, Childbirth, and the Puerperium

This section represents only those conditions that relate to, or are aggravated by, pregnancy, childbirth, and the puerperium. Many coding concepts in ICD-9-CM remain consistent in ICD-10-CM. For example, guidelines state that codes from this chapter (15) in ICD-10-CM continue to take precedence over codes from other chapters. However, additional codes can be used in conjunction with codes from this chapter to add further specificity to the reporting of conditions.

Providers must state whether any condition the patient is being treated for affects the pregnancy; when this information is not stated, it is presumed that the condition does impact pregnancy and is reported with a code from chapter 15 in ICD-10-CM.

> **CODING AXIOM**
>
> Chapter 15 codes should be reported only on the maternal record, never on the newborn record.

Anatomy and Pathophysiology and the ICD-10-CM Code Set: Pregnancy, Childbirth, and the Puerperium

Delivery Status

In ICD-9-CM, delivery status is reported with a fifth-character classification system that is not used in ICD-10-CM. Instead, most codes in chapter 15 require the assignment of a final character to indicate the pregnancy trimester **at the time of the encounter**.

The three trimesters include:

- First: Less than 14 weeks, 0 days
- Second: 14 weeks, 0 days to less than 28 weeks, 0 days
- Third: 28 weeks, 0 days until delivery

Example:

    O26.0   Excessive weight gain in pregnancy

Fifth-character choices:

    O26.00   Excessive weight gain in pregnancy, unspecified trimester
    O26.01   Excessive weight gain in pregnancy, first trimester
    O26.02   Excessive weight gain in pregnancy, second trimester
    O26.03   Excessive weight gain in pregnancy, third trimester

A number of coding categories are affected by this particular change, including but not limited to 641.01 Placenta previa without hemorrhage, 641.11 Hemorrhage from placenta previa, and 641.21 Premature separation of the placenta. Note that ICD-9-CM codes with a fifth-digit subclassification of 1 or 3 indicate the codes within ICD-10-CM with the greater specificity by trimester. This is explained by the fact that in ICD-9-CM, the number one (1) describes a subclassification for "delivered, with or without mention of antepartum condition" and the number three (3) describes an "antepartum condition or complication" episode of care. The other two fifth-digit subclassifications are already encompassed in the trimester definitions shown above.

Additional Categories Designating Trimesters and Conditions During Childbirth or Affecting the Puerperium

ICD-10-CM guidelines also differ from those for ICD-9-CM in that they have categories that designate trimesters, as well as specific codes for conditions that occur during childbirth or that affect the puerperium.

Example:

    O99.3   **Mental disorders and disease of the nervous system complicating pregnancy, childbirth, and the puerperium**

Additional character choices:

    O99.31   Alcohol use complicating pregnancy, childbirth, and the puerperium
        Use additional code(s) from F10 to identify the manifestations of the alcohol use

        O99.310   Alcohol use complicating pregnancy, unspecified trimester
        O99.311   Alcohol use complicating pregnancy, first trimester
        O99.312   Alcohol use complicating pregnancy, second trimester
        O99.313   Alcohol use complicating pregnancy, third trimester
        O99.314   Alcohol use complicating childbirth
        O99.315   Alcohol use complicating the puerperium

> **CODING AXIOM**
>
> ICD-10-CM Official Coding Guideline I.C.15.a.4. provides assistance in selecting the appropriate trimester for patients whose stay in the hospital spans more than one trimester. This guideline states, "In instances when a patient is admitted to a hospital for complications of pregnancy during one trimester and remains in the hospital into a subsequent trimester, the trimester character for the antepartum complication code should be assigned on the basis of the trimester when the complications developed, not the trimester of the discharge. If the condition developed prior to the current admission/encounter or represents a pre-existing condition, the trimester character for the trimester at the time of the admission/encounter should be assigned."

Coding for Trimester

Trimester is not always a component of a code, either because the trimester is not applicable or because the condition always occurs in a specific trimester. For example, for O32 Maternal care for malpresentation of fetus, malpresentation is a condition associated with delivery and, therefore, would not apply to the first and second trimesters.

Seventh-Character Extensions for Multiple Gestations

A seventh-character extension for multiple gestations in categories that designate maternal care for a fetal anomaly, damage, or other problem is required in order to indicate the affected fetus. Using the aforementioned example, category O32 Maternal care for malpresentation of fetus, states that a seventh character is to be assigned to each code under this category with "0," indicating a single gestation or a multiple gestation where the fetus is unspecified. Characters 1 through 9 are used for multiple gestations to identify the fetus to which the code applies. In addition, a code from category O30 Multiple gestation, must also be assigned if a code is reported from category O32 with a seventh character of 1 through 9.

Character	Fetus
1	1
2	2
3	3
4	4
5	5
9	Other fetus

Gestational Diabetes

In ICD-10-CM, gestational diabetes (GD) is divided into three subcategories: pregnancy, childbirth, and the puerperium, with final subdivision of these codes specifying whether the GD is diet controlled, insulin controlled, or unspecified control. Trimester is not applicable to these codes but does apply where preexisting Type 1 or Type 2 diabetes in pregnancy is noted and would be subdivided by trimester.

ICD-9-CM code 648.8 Abnormal glucose tolerance, is the category under which gestational diabetes is located. A fifth-digit subclassification denotes the episode of care. Under ICD-10-CM, codes are classified to category O24.4 Gestational diabetes mellitus, with the three aforementioned subcategories, O24.41 Gestational diabetes in pregnancy, O24.42 Gestational diabetes in childbirth, and O24.43 Gestational diabetes in the puerperium. Under each subcategory, three subclassifications are denoted by characters 0, 4, or 9, indicating whether the gestational diabetes is diet controlled, insulin controlled, or unspecified, respectively.

Chapter 13. ICD-10-CM: Reproductive Systems

Coding for Abnormal Glucose Tolerance: Gestational Diabetes

ICD-9-CM	ICD-10-CM	
648.8[0-4] Abnormal maternal glucose tolerance, complicating pregnancy, childbirth, or the puerperium **5th Character meanings for codes as indicated** 0 unspecified as to episode of care 1 delivered, with or without mention of antepartum condition 2 delivered, with current postpartum complication 3 antepartum condition or complication 4 postpartum condition or complication	O24.410	Gestational diabetes mellitus in pregnancy, diet controlled
	O24.414	Gestational diabetes mellitus in pregnancy, insulin controlled
	O24.419	Gestational diabetes mellitus in pregnancy, unspecified control
	O24.420	Gestational diabetes mellitus in childbirth, diet controlled
	O24.424	Gestational diabetes mellitus in childbirth, insulin controlled
	O24.429	Gestational diabetes mellitus in childbirth, unspecified control
	O24.430	Gestational diabetes mellitus in the puerperium, diet controlled
	O24.434	Gestational diabetes mellitus in the puerperium, insulin controlled
	O24.439	Gestational diabetes mellitus in the puerperium, unspecified control
	O99.810	Abnormal glucose complicating pregnancy
	O99.814	Abnormal glucose complicating childbirth
	O99.815	Abnormal glucose complicating the puerperium

Spontaneous Abortion

A spontaneous abortion is the premature expulsion or removal of the products of conception from the uterus, often referred to as a miscarriage. In ICD-9-CM, this condition is coded to category 634 with a fourth digit identifying the subcategory and a fifth digit identifying the stage, such as complete, incomplete, or unspecified. For the most part, these subcategories have a one-to-one mapping in ICD-10-CM; however, code 634.7 Spontaneous abortion with other specified complications, unspecified (0), incomplete (1), and complete (2) are combined differently in ICD-10-CM. The unspecified spontaneous abortion and complete abortion codes are described by a single set of codes: O03.8 Other and unspecified complications following complete or unspecified spontaneous abortion.

Coding for Other and Unspecified Complications Following Complete or Unspecified Spontaneous Abortion

ICD-9-CM	ICD-10-CM	
634.7[0, 2] Spontaneous abortion with other specified complications **5th Character meanings for codes as indicated** 0 unspecified 2 complete	O03.85	Other venous complications following complete or unspecified spontaneous abortion
	O03.86	Cardiac arrest following complete or unspecified spontaneous abortion
	O03.88	Urinary tract infection following complete or unspecified spontaneous abortion
	O03.89	Complete or unspecified spontaneous abortion with other complications

ICD-9-CM code 634.71 Incomplete spontaneous abortion with other specified complications has its own category in ICD-10-CM, O03.3 Other and unspecified complications following incomplete spontaneous abortion, with a fifth character identifying the specific type of complication.

© 2015 Optum360, LLC

Coding for Other and Unspecified Complications Following Incomplete Spontaneous Abortion

ICD-9-CM		ICD-10-CM	
634.71	Incomplete spontaneous abortion with other specified complications	O03.35	Other venous complications following incomplete spontaneous abortion
		O03.36	Cardiac arrest following incomplete spontaneous abortion
		O03.38	Urinary tract infection following incomplete spontaneous abortion
		O03.39	Incomplete spontaneous abortion with other complications

Legally Induced Abortion

A legally induced abortion is the intentional expulsion of the products of conception from the uterus performed by a medical professional within the boundaries of the law. This often occurs by the patient's choice (elective), through a court order or other mandated action (legal), or for reasons such as the mother's health or life is at risk (therapeutic). These codes are categorized similarly to the spontaneous abortion codes. In ICD-9-CM, this condition is coded to category 635 with a fourth digit identifying the subcategory and a fifth digit identifying the stage, such as complete, incomplete, or unspecified. For the most part, these subcategories have a one-to-one mapping in ICD-10-CM; however, ICD-9-CM code 635.7 Legally induced abortion with other specified complications, unspecified (0), incomplete (1), and complete (2) is now described by a single set of codes in ICD-10-CM under category O04.8 (Induced) termination of pregnancy with other and unspecified complications.

Coding for Legally Induced Abortion With Other Specified Complications

ICD-9-CM		ICD-10-CM	
635.7[0, 2]	Legally induced abortion with other specified complications	O04.85	Other venous complications following (induced) termination of pregnancy
5th Character meanings for codes as indicated 0 unspecified 2 complete		O04.86	Cardiac arrest following (induced) termination of pregnancy
		O04.88	Urinary tract infection following (induced) termination of pregnancy
		O04.89	(Induced) termination of pregnancy with other complications

Antepartum Hemorrhage Associated with Coagulation Defects

Antepartum hemorrhage associated with coagulation defects describes a condition in which the uterine hemorrhages prior to delivery. Coagulation defect is a general term for various conditions that disrupt the body's ability to control blood clotting.

Afibrinogenemia is an uncommon, inherited blood disorder that affects the blood's ability to clot by causing a serious deficiency in fibrinogen, a protein produced by the liver. This protein is required to stop bleeding by forming clots. In this condition, an abnormal gene is typically passed from both parents.

Disseminated intravascular coagulation (DIC) is a serious disorder in which the proteins that control blood clotting become abnormally active. It is normal for certain proteins in the blood to become active and travel in the bloodstream, such as when an injury occurs in order to stop bleeding. But for patients with DIC, the proteins become abnormally active and can result in the development of clots and more often severe bleeding. When small blood clots are formed within the blood vessels, blood supply can be cut off to the liver, brain, or kidneys. Once this happens, the organs cease to function. Additionally, clotting proteins in the blood can be exhausted, placing the patient at risk for severe bleeding from even a minor cut. The blood clots also have the potential to destroy healthy red blood cells. Some of the risk factors for this condition include cancer, especially certain types of leukemia (cancer of the blood); bacterial or fungal blood infections; complications of pregnancy, such as retained placenta after delivery; surgery/anesthesia; sepsis; and severe liver disease.

ICD-9-CM code 641.3 Antepartum hemorrhage associated with coagulation defects, is subdivided into categories by the episode of care. In ICD-10-CM, categories O46.00 Antepartum hemorrhage with coagulation defect, unspecified, O46.01 Antepartum hemorrhage with afibrinogenemia, O46.02 Antepartum hemorrhage with disseminated intravascular coagulation, and O46.09 Antepartum hemorrhage with other coagulation defects, enable coders to assign a code specific to the condition rather than to a general term such as coagulation defects. Understanding the specific terms referenced by ICD-10-CM is the key to assigning and reporting the correct code within this category.

Coding for Antepartum Hemorrhage, Associated with Coagulation Defects

ICD-9-CM		ICD-10-CM	
641.30	Antepartum hemorrhage associated with coagulation defects, unspecified as to episode of care	O46.009	Antepartum hemorrhage with coagulation defect, unspecified, unspecified trimester
		O46.019	Antepartum hemorrhage with afibrinogenemia, unspecified trimester
		O46.029	Antepartum hemorrhage with disseminated intravascular coagulation, unspecified trimester
		O46.099	Antepartum hemorrhage with other coagulation defect, unspecified trimester
641.3[1, 3]	Antepartum hemorrhage associated with coagulation defects *5th Character meanings for codes as indicated* *1 with delivery* *3 antepartum*	O46.001	Antepartum hemorrhage with coagulation defect, unspecified, first trimester
		O46.002	Antepartum hemorrhage with coagulation defect, unspecified, second trimester
		O46.003	Antepartum hemorrhage with coagulation defect, unspecified, third trimester
		O46.011	Antepartum hemorrhage with afibrinogenemia, first trimester
		O46.012	Antepartum hemorrhage with afibrinogenemia, second trimester
		O46.013	Antepartum hemorrhage with afibrinogenemia, third trimester
		O46.021	Antepartum hemorrhage with disseminated intravascular coagulation, first trimester
		O46.022	Antepartum hemorrhage with disseminated intravascular coagulation, second trimester
		O46.023	Antepartum hemorrhage with disseminated intravascular coagulation, third trimester
		O46.091	Antepartum hemorrhage with other coagulation defect, first trimester
		O46.092	Antepartum hemorrhage with other coagulation defect, second trimester
		O46.093	Antepartum hemorrhage with other coagulation defect, third trimester

Postpartum Hemorrhage: Third Stage

A postpartum hemorrhage is defined as a blood loss of greater than 500 ml after the birth of a baby, and a severe postpartum hemorrhage constitutes blood loss of more than 1,000 ml after delivery.

The third stage of labor is the period of time between the birth of the baby and the expulsion of the placenta. It is during this time frame when the uterine muscles contract downward and the placenta begins to separate from the uterine walls. Blood loss depends on how long it takes the placenta to come apart from the uterine wall. When the uterus fails to begin normal contractions, known as uterine atony, blood vessels in the placenta stay open and can result in severe bleeding.

This condition is categorized to ICD-9-CM code 666.0 Third-stage hemorrhage, with a fifth-digit subclassification to indicate the current episode of care; fifth-digit choices in this category are limited to the delivery characters 2 delivered, with mention of postpartum complication, or 4 postpartum condition or complication.

In ICD-10-CM, two codes are required to accurately and correctly report this condition: O72.0 Third-stage hemorrhage, and O43.21 Placenta accrete, O43.22 Placenta increta, or O43.23 Placenta percreta. In addition, a sixth character for each of the three categories is necessary to identify the trimester in which the hemorrhage occurred.

> **CODING AXIOM**
>
> ICD-10-CM Official Coding Guideline I.C.15.o.1. states that "the postpartum period begins immediately after delivery and continues for six weeks following delivery. The peripartum period is defined as the last month of pregnancy to five months postpartum."

Coding for Third Stage Hemorrhage with Morbidly Adherent Placenta

ICD-9-CM	ICD-10-CM		
666.0[2,4] Third-stage postpartum hemorrhage	O72.0	Third-stage Hemorrhage	AND
	O43.21[1–3]	Placenta accreta	OR
5th Character meanings for codes as indicated	O43.22[1–3]	Placenta increta	OR
2 with delivery	O43.23[1–3]	Placenta percreta	
4 postpartum			
	6th Character meanings for codes as indicated		
	1 first trimester		
	2 second trimester		
	3 third trimester		

Placenta accreta, increta, and percreta all describe a condition whereby the placenta attaches too deeply into the uterine wall; the difference between the three depends on the severity of the attachment. The least invasive and most common is placenta accreta and accounts for approximately 75 percent of all cases. Placenta increta is a moderate form of the condition with a deeper attachment, penetrating into the uterine muscle. Placenta percreta is the most severe where the attached placenta penetrates through the entire uterine wall and actually attaches to another nearby organ, such as the bladder. It is rare, accounting for approximately 5 percent of all cases.

Summary: Pregnancy, Childbirth, and the Puerperium

The chapter on pregnancy, childbirth, and the puerperium encompasses a significant number of disease processes and disorders. As demonstrated in some of the earlier examples, many ICD-9-CM code categories have been expanded in ICD-10-CM to include a character indicating the trimester at the time of the encounter. It is important and necessary to pay close attention to the distinctions and differences between the two coding systems. The additional detail and specificity afforded by the ICD-10-CM coding system is certainly a benefit, though it is clear that proper code selection rests on thoroughly understanding the new terms referenced and how certain ICD-9-CM categories break out in ICD-10-CM.

Chapter 14. ICD-10-PCS Introduction

Importance of Anatomy and Physiology in ICD-10-PCS

The anatomy and physiology of the human body has not changed with the advent of ICD-10-PCS; however, what has changed is how anatomy and physiology is defined and applied in the ICD-10-PCS code structure. The previous chapters have presented a great deal of detail about organ systems and body areas, as well as some specific physiology needed to understand and apply ICD-10-CM diagnosis codes. Although what was learned in the previous chapters is useful when using the ICD-10-PCS code set, it is important to know that the anatomy and physiology of the human body is represented in a slightly different way for ICD-10-PCS than it is for ICD-10-CM.

Coders must not only understand the intent and final objective of the procedure, but must also be familiar with anatomy and the definitions associated with each of the ICD-10-PCS character values. PCS codes are constructed from component parts found in tables. Many of these code elements, such as body system, root operation, body part, approach, device, and qualifier, require knowledge about anatomy, physiology, and disease pathology. Physicians and other providers will not necessarily use the same terminology in their documentation that is used in the ICD-10-PCS tables. A strong background in these clinical areas is needed to be able to "translate" the terminology, as well as to know when a physician query is needed to gather additional information.

In order to lay the foundation for the method that PCS uses to build codes, a brief overview of the seven characters that make up each code is provided in this chapter. This book focuses mainly on the characters involving the human anatomy—specifically characters (2) Body system and (4) Body part. Guidelines specific to body systems and body parts are included. For detailed instructions on the code characters (3) Root Operation, (5) Approach, (6) Device, and (7) Qualifier, refer to Optum360's *Detailed Instruction for Appropriate ICD-10-PCS Coding*.

Overview

Every PCS code is made up of seven characters, and each character represents a distinct value. An alphabetic index is used to direct the coder to a specific PCS table, where the rest of the code values are selected. By using a table format, exponentially more codes may be constructed in PCS than were available in ICD-9 CM Volume 3.

Characters

Each character in PCS can contain up to 34 character-value options. Each value represents a specific option for the general character definitions. The alphabetic characters A–H, J–N, and P–Z, along with numbers 0–9, are used as character values in any character position. In order to avoid confusion with numbers 0 and 1, the letters I and O are not used. The vast majority of PCS codes follow the format below, with a few exceptions related to slightly different character definitions for some of the ancillary-related types of services.

Character 1	Character 2	Character 3	Character 4	Character 5	Character 6	Character 7
Section	Body System	Root Operation	Body Part	Approach	Device	Qualifier

A code is constructed by choosing a specific value for each of the seven characters. Based on details about the procedure performed, values for each character specifying the section, body system, root operation, body part, approach, device, and qualifier are assigned. As the definition of each character is also a function of its physical position in the code, the same letter or number placed in a different position in the code has a different meaning. Codes are constructed using tables that are defined by the first three character values. Understanding anatomy and physiology is vitally important to choosing the appropriate options from the table.

Tables

Tables make up the largest section of the PCS system. The structure of the tables is always the same: the information related to the first three character values of a section of codes is found within the top section. For a majority of codes, the first character value is the section (e.g., medical and surgical), the second character is the body system (e.g., hepatobiliary system and pancreas), and the third character is the root operation (e.g., excision). The remainder of the table contains four columns that represent the remaining four character values for valid codes (body part, approach, device, and qualifier). When constructing codes, the values must be selected across a row. If one character value does not appear on the same row in the table, those character values may not be combined to form a valid code. For example, review table ØFB below:

Ø Medical and Surgical
F Hepatobiliary System and Pancreas
B Excision Cutting out or off, without replacement, a portion of a body part

Body Part Character 4	Approach Character 5	Device Character 6	Qualifier Character 7
Ø Liver 1 Liver, Right Lobe 2 Liver, Left Lobe 4 Gallbladder G Pancreas	Ø Open 3 Percutaneous 4 Percutaneous Endoscopic	Z No Device	X Diagnostic Z No Qualifier
5 Hepatic Duct, Right 6 Hepatic Duct, Left 8 Cystic Duct 9 Common Bile Duct C Ampulla of Vater D Pancreatic Duct F Pancreatic Duct, Accessory	Ø Open 3 Percutaneous 4 Percutaneous Endoscopic 7 Via Natural or Artificial Opening 8 Via Natural or Artificial Opening Endoscopic	Z No Device	X Diagnostic Z No Qualifier

Note that the first three character values are listed at the top of the table, along with the definition of the root operation (excision). There are only two rows in this particular table, but valid codes may only be constructed moving across one row. For example, ØFBØ4ZX is a valid code from this table that represents a laparoscopic excisional liver biopsy.

Section	Body System	Root Operation	Body Part	Approach	Device	Qualifier
Ø	F	B	Ø	4	Z	X
Medical & Surgical	Hepatobiliary System and Pancreas	Excision	Liver	Percutaneous Endoscopic	No Device	Diagnostic

Referring back to table ØFB above, code ØFBØ7ZX is not a valid code because the approach value 7 Via Natural or Artificial Opening, is not in the same row with the body part Ø Liver. Typically, it is not anatomically possible to access the liver through a natural or artificial opening in the body. Coders must review the tables carefully to ensure that the values selected are all contained within the same row. Be aware that some of the PCS tables are very lengthy; if using an ICD-10-PCS book, be sure to review rows that may be found on subsequent pages in the book.

Character 1: Section

The procedures are divided into 17 sections that identify the general type of the procedural service (e.g., medical and surgical, obstetrics, and imaging). Ten of the sections are designated as medical- and surgical-related sections and six are considered ancillary sections.

Effective October 1, 2015, The Centers for Medicare and Medicaid Services (CMS) introduced a new 17th section for ICD-10-PCS, Section X (New Technology). Section X provides a place for codes that uniquely identify procedures requested via the New Technology Application Process such as infusion of new technology drugs or other new technologies not currently classified in ICD-10-PCS.

Section X does not introduce any new coding concepts or unusual guidelines, and uses the same root operation and body part values as their closest equivalents in other sections of ICD-10-PCS.

Characters can have different definitions in different sections. The focus of this publication is the medical and surgical section (0) because it constitutes the vast majority of procedures reported in an inpatient setting. For more detail on the remaining sections, refer to Optum360's *Detailed Instruction for Appropriate ICD-10-PCS Coding*. The 17 sections in ICD-10-PCS are listed in the following table.

Section	Title
0	Medical and Surgical section
1	Obstetrics
2	Placement
3	Administration
4	Measurement and Monitoring
5	Extracorporeal Assistance and Performance
6	Extracorporeal Therapies
7	Osteopathic
8	Other Procedures
9	Chiropractic
B	Imaging
C	Nuclear Medicine
D	Radiation Therapy
F	Physical Rehabilitation and Diagnostic Audiology
G	Mental Health
H	Substance Abuse Treatment
X	New Technology

Character 2: Body System

The second character (body system) in each PCS code from the medical and surgical section defines the general physiological system or anatomical region on which the procedure is performed. There are 31 body system character values contained in the medical/surgical section, including systems such as the respiratory system (B), gastrointestinal system (D), and endocrine system (G). For some body systems represented in ICD-10-CM, there is a corresponding body system character value in ICD-10-PCS, as is the case in the respiratory system. Other ICD-10-CM body systems have several body system character values in ICD-10-PCS. In the example below, notice that the breakdown of the circulatory system in ICD-10-PCS includes five separate body system character values. These PCS body systems are still general in nature and do not identify the specific body part within that body system.

ICD-10-CM	ICD-10-PCS
Circulatory System	Heart and Great Vessels
	Upper Arteries
	Lower Arteries
	Upper Veins
	Lower Veins

Three of the 31 body systems are titled Anatomical Regions, which are only assigned in certain circumstances such as when a procedure is performed on an anatomical region rather than on a specific body part. Do not use a character from these three regions if the procedure is being performed on a location with a more specific body part value. The root operations control and detachment are offered as choices only in the anatomical regions tables. ICD-10-PCS also provides guidelines that will assist in the appropriate body system selection.

Body System—ICD-10-PCS Official Coding Guidelines

Body System: B2.1

The procedure codes in the general anatomical regions body systems should only be used when the procedure is performed on an anatomical region rather than a specific body part (e.g., root operations control, detachment, or drainage of a body cavity) or on the rare occasion when no information is available to support assignment of a code to a specific body part.

Example:

Control of postoperative hemorrhage is coded to the root operation control, found in the general anatomical regions body systems.

Additional examples of this guideline:

- Drainage of the pleural cavity is found in the general anatomical system; however, drainage of the left lower lung is found in the more specific respiratory system
- Control of a postoperative tonsillectomy hemorrhage is coded to the root operation control found only in the general anatomical system
- Amputation of the right thumb, which is the root operation detachment, is found in the body system anatomical regions, upper extremities

Body System: B2.1b

Body systems designated as upper or lower contain body parts located above or below the diaphragm, respectively.

Example:

Vein body parts above the diaphragm are found in the upper veins body system; vein body parts below the diaphragm are found in the lower veins body system.

Additional examples of this guideline:

- Thoracic vertebra and right clavicle are found in upper bones
- Lumbar vertebra and right acetabulum are found in lower bones
- Azygos vein and right subclavian vein are found in upper veins
- Inferior vena cava and right hypogastric vein are found in lower veins

---

KEY POINT

When coding detachment of a body part, many layers of body systems are involved in the procedure—skin, subcutaneous tissue, muscle, vessels, bone, etc. Anatomical Regions Body System: Upper or Lower Extremities encompasses all of the many body systems and provides more efficiency with one code rather than six or more codes.

INTERESTING A & P FACT

The Diaphragm is a sheet of fiber and muscle that rises and falls as we breathe. It neatly bisects the human body into upper and lower halves, which is why the PCS definitions indicate that body parts above the diaphragm are to be classified as "upper" and those below it are classified as "lower."

Chapter 14. ICD-10-PCS Introduction

Character Meaning Table

It may be difficult to ascertain at times which specific body system is the correct choice. To assist with this task, tables called Character Meanings have been provided at the beginning of each body system in the PCS section of this book to use as a tool to determine the body parts that code to a specific body system.

For instance ICD-10-PCS has split the nervous system into Character 0 Central Nervous System and Character 1, Peripheral Nervous System. If a procedure is being performed on the cervical nerve or the phrenic nerve, a quick check of the following Peripheral Nervous System Character Meaning Table shows that both nerves are listed in this table and therefore the peripheral nervous system (1) would be the correct body system to build the rest of the code. If the procedure was performed on the cervical spinal cord, a review of the Peripheral Nervous System Character Meaning Table would show that this body site is not represented in this table. The user would then refer to the Central Nervous System Character Meaning Table to determine if the cervical spinal cord is represented there.

Each table also defines what root operation, body part, approach, device, and qualifier can be used in a particular body system. These tables should not be used to build the full seven character code; they are simply a resource that will assist the user in finding the correct body system needed to begin building the code. The Character Meaning tables in this book are a great resource to use alongside an ICD-10-PCS coding book and can be found as an appendix in Optum360's *ICD-10-PCS Complete Official Code Set* coding book.

> **DEFINITIONS**
>
> **sacral nerves.** Five nerves (S1-S5) on each side of the sacrum that pass from the sacral canal through the sacral foramina and form the sacral and coccygeal plexus.

Character Meaning Table: Peripheral Nervous System

Operation–Character 3	Body Part–Character 4	Approach–Character 5	Device–Character 6	Qualifier–Character 7
2 Change	0 Cervical Plexus	0 Open	0 Drainage Device	1 Cervical Nerve
5 Destruction	1 Cervical Nerve	3 Percutaneous	2 Monitoring Device	2 Phrenic Nerve
8 Division	2 Phrenic Nerve	4 Percutaneous Endoscopic	7 Autologous Tissue Substitute	4 Ulnar Nerve
9 Drainage	3 Brachial Plexus	X External	M Neurostimulator Lead	5 Median Nerve
B Excision	4 Ulnar Nerve		Y Other Device	6 Radial Nerve
C Extirpation	5 Median Nerve		Z No Device	8 Thoracic Nerve
D Extraction	6 Radial Nerve			B Lumbar Nerve
H Insertion	8 Thoracic Nerve			C Perineal Nerve
J Inspection	9 Lumbar Plexus			D Femoral Nerve
N Release	A Lumbosacral Plexus			F Sciatic Nerve
P Removal	B Lumbar Nerve			G Tibial Nerve
Q Repair	C Pudendal Nerve			H Peroneal Nerve
S Reposition	D Femoral Nerve			X Diagnostic
U Supplement	F Sciatic Nerve			Z No Qualifier
W Revision	G Tibial Nerve			

(Continued on next page)

© 2015 Optum360, LLC

365

Character Meaning Table: Peripheral Nervous System (Continued)

Operation–Character 3	Body Part–Character 4	Approach–Character 5	Device–Character 6	Qualifier–Character 7
X Transfer	H Peroneal Nerve			
	K Head and Neck Sympathetic Nerve			
	L Thoracic Sympathetic Nerve			
	M Abdominal Sympathetic Nerve			
	N Lumbar Sympathetic Nerve			
	P Sacral Sympathetic Nerve			
	Q Sacral Plexus			
	R *Sacral Nerve*			

Character 3: Root Operation

The root operation is the third character and identifies the objective of the procedure. There is a clear distinction between each root operation with precise code values defined in the system. PCS provides definitions, explanations, and examples of each root operation. The 31 root operations found in the medical and surgical section (0) with definitions and explanations are listed in the following table. Some root operations may only be assigned with procedures involving devices and are indicated in the table with the Optum360 DVC icon **DVC**.

Each root operation character in the medical and surgical section is the same regardless of the body system in which it's found. For example, if repair was performed on a body site in the endocrine system, the root operation of repair is represented by the character Q. This same character (Q) is also used if the repair was performed on a body site in the subcutaneous tissue and fascia body system. However, please note that not every root operation character is used in every body system table. For example, the root operation transfer (X) is not an option in the head and facial bones body system. Refer to appendix C in the back of this book for a complete list of all the root operations with definitions, explanations, and examples.

Alteration (0)	**Definition:** Modifying the anatomic structure of a body part without affecting the function of the body part **Explanation:** Principal purpose is to improve appearance
Bypass (1)	**Definition:** Altering the route of passage of the contents of a tubular body part **Explanation:** Rerouting contents of a body part to a downstream area of the normal route, to a similar route and body part, or to an abnormal route and dissimilar body part. Includes one or more anastomoses, with or without the use of a device
Change (2) DVC	**Definition:** Taking out or off a device from a body part and putting back an identical or similar device in or on the same body part without cutting or puncturing the skin or a mucous membrane **Explanation:** All CHANGE procedures are coded using the approach EXTERNAL
Control (3)	**Definition:** Stopping, or attempting to stop, postprocedural bleeding **Explanation:** The site of the bleeding is coded as an anatomical region and not to a specific body part

DVC Root operation for procedures that always involve a device.

Chapter 14. ICD-10-PCS Introduction

Creation (4)	**Definition:** Making a new genital structure that does not take over the function of a body part **Explanation:** Used only for sex change operations
Destruction (5)	**Definition:** Physical eradication of all or a portion of a body part by the direct use of energy, force, or a destructive agent **Explanation:** None of the body part is physically taken out
Detachment (6)	**Definition:** Cutting off all or a portion of the upper or lower extremities **Explanation:** The body part value is the site of the detachment, with a qualifier if applicable to further specify the level where the extremity was detached
Dilation (7)	**Definition:** Expanding an orifice or the lumen of a tubular body part **Explanation:** The orifice can be a natural orifice or an artificially created orifice. Accomplished by stretching a tubular body part using intraluminal pressure or by cutting part of the orifice or wall of the tubular body part
Division (8)	**Definition:** Cutting into a body part, without draining fluids and/or gases from the body part, in order to separate or transect a body part **Explanation:** All or a portion of the body part is separated into two or more portions
Drainage (9)	**Definition:** Taking or letting out fluids and/or gases from a body part **Explanation:** The qualifier DIAGNOSTIC is used to identify drainage procedures that are biopsies
Excision (B)	**Definition:** Cutting out or off, without replacement, a portion of a body part **Explanation:** The qualifier DIAGNOSTIC is used to identify excision procedures that are biopsies
Extirpation (C)	**Definition:** Taking or cutting out solid matter from a body part **Explanation:** The solid matter may be an abnormal byproduct of a biological function or a foreign body; it may be imbedded in a body part or in the lumen of a tubular body part. The solid matter may or may not have been previously broken into pieces
Extraction (D)	**Definition:** Pulling or stripping out or off all or a portion of a body part by the use of force **Explanation:** The qualifier DIAGNOSTIC is used to identify extraction procedures that are biopsies
Fragmentation (F)	**Definition:** Breaking solid matter in a body part into pieces **Explanation:** Physical force (e.g., manual, ultrasonic) applied directly or indirectly is used to break the solid matter into pieces. The solid matter may be an abnormal byproduct of a biological function or a foreign body. The pieces of solid matter are not taken out
Fusion (G)	**Definition:** Joining together portions of an articular body part rendering the articular body part immobile **Explanation:** The body part is joined together by fixation device, bone graft, or other means
Insertion (H) DVC	**Definition:** Putting in a nonbiological appliance that monitors, assists, performs, or prevents a physiological function but does not physically take the place of a body part
Inspection (J)	**Definition:** Visually and/or manually exploring a body part **Explanation:** Visual exploration may be performed with or without optical instrumentation. Manual exploration may be performed directly or through intervening body layers
Map (K)	**Definition:** Locating the route of passage of electrical impulses and/or locating functional areas in a body part **Explanation:** Applicable only to the cardiac conduction mechanism and the central nervous system

DVC   Root operation for procedures that always involve a device.

Occlusion (L)	**Definition:** Completely closing an orifice or the lumen of a tubular body part **Explanation:** The orifice can be a natural orifice or an artificially created orifice
Reattachment (M)	**Definition:** Putting back in or on all or a portion of a separated body part to its normal location or other suitable location **Explanation:** Vascular circulation and nervous pathways may or may not be reestablished
Release (N)	**Definition:** Freeing a body part from an abnormal physical constraint by cutting or use of force **Explanation:** Some of the restraining tissue may be taken out but none of the body part is taken out
Removal (P) DVC	**Definition:** Taking out or off a device from a body part **Explanation:** If a device is taken out and a similar device put in without cutting or puncturing the skin or mucous membrane, the procedure is coded to the root operation CHANGE. Otherwise, the procedure for taking out a device is coded to the root operation REMOVAL
Repair (Q)	**Definition:** Restoring, to the extent possible, a body part to its normal anatomic structure and function **Explanation:** Used only when the method to accomplish the repair is not one of the other root operations
Replacement (R) DVC	**Definition:** Putting in or on biological or synthetic material that physically takes the place and/or function of all or a portion of a body part **Explanation:** The body part may have been taken out or replaced, or may be taken out, physically eradicated, or rendered nonfunctional during the REPLACEMENT procedure. A REMOVAL procedure is coded for taking out the device used in a previous replacement procedure
Reposition (S)	**Definition:** Moving to its normal location, or other suitable location, all or a portion of a body part **Explanation:** The body part is moved to a new location from an abnormal location, or from a normal location where it is not functioning correctly. The body part may or may not be cut out or off to be moved to the new location
Resection (T)	**Definition:** Cutting out or off, without replacement, all of a body part
Restriction (V)	**Definition:** Partially closing an orifice or the lumen of a tubular body part **Explanation:** The orifice can be a natural orifice or an artificially created orifice
Revision (W) DVC	**Definition:** Correcting, to the extent possible, a portion of a malfunctioning device or the position of a displaced device **Explanation:** Revision can include correcting a malfunctioning or displaced device by taking out or putting in components of the device such as a screw or pin
Supplement (U) DVC	**Definition:** Putting in or on biological or synthetic material that physically reinforces and/or augments the function of a portion of a body part **Explanation:** The biological material is nonliving, or is living and from the same individual. The body part may have been previously replaced, and the SUPPLEMENT procedure is performed to physically reinforce and/or augment the function of the replaced body part
Transfer (X)	**Definition:** Moving, without taking out, all or a portion of a body part to another location to take over the function of all or a portion of a body part **Explanation:** The body part transferred remains connected to its vascular and nervous supply

DVC Root operation for procedures that always involve a device.

Transplantation (Y)	**Definition:** Putting in or on all or a portion of a living body part taken from another individual or animal to physically take the place and/or function of all or a portion of a similar body part
	Explanation: The native body part may or may not be taken out, and the transplanted body part may take over all or a portion of its function

DVC Root operation for procedures that always involve a device.

All of the root operation definitions and explanations contained in ICD-10-PCS are unique to PCS and may not match definitions commonly found in medical dictionaries. A good example is extirpation, a term not familiar to many coders:

Extirpation is defined in *Stedman's Medical Dictionary 28th Edition* as "Partial or complete removal of an organ or diseased tissue."

Extirpation is defined by ICD-10-PCS as "Taking or cutting out solid matter from a body part."

These two definitions describe completely different procedures. It is extremely important for the coder to know and understand the definitions and explanations of the root operations *as defined by ICD-10-PCS* in order to assign the appropriate root operation character. Physicians rarely document using terms like extirpation in the context that PCS defines, so it is up to the coder to accurately translate these terms when enough information is given, rather than query the physician.

There are many official guidelines provided by ICD-10-PCS, including several in the root operation section. For a complete listing refer to Optum360's *ICD-10-PCS Complete Official Code Set* coding book or CMS website http://www.cms.gov/Medicare/Coding/ICD10/2016-ICD-10-PCS-and-GEMs.html.

Even though common procedure terminology is not used in ICD-10-PCS, many commonly used terms such as adenoidectomy can be found in the alphabetic index. These entries will then refer the user to specific PCS root operations and corresponding tables for which the code can be compiled; the user will choose the correct code based on the objective of the procedure.

Examples:

- Adenoidectomy
  - See Excision, Adenoids 0CBQ
  - See Resection, Adenoids 0CTQ
- Bursotomy
  - See Division, Bursae and Ligaments 0M8
  - See Drainage, Bursae and Ligaments 0M9
- Lithotripsy
  - See Fragmentation
  - With removal of fragments—see Extirpation
- Marsupialization
  - See Drainage
  - See Excision

Optum360's exclusive *Root Operation Definitions table* has been provided in appendix D. This table includes a comprehensive listing of common procedures with their related PCS root operation characters, including helpful tips for appropriate code selection.

Character 4: Body Part

The body part is specified in the fourth character and indicates the specific part of the body system on which the procedure was performed. Many of the body parts specify laterality: left, right, or bilateral. If a procedure is done on both sides of a body part

---

CODING AXIOM

ICD-10-PCS Official Coding Guideline Convention A11: Many of the terms used to construct PCS codes are defined within the system. It is the coder's responsibility to determine what the documentation in the medical record equates to in the PCS definitions. The physician is not expected to use the terms used in PCS code descriptions, nor is the coder required to query the physician when the correlation between the documentation and the defined PCS terms is clear.

Example: When the physician documents "partial resection," the coder can independently correlate "partial resection" to the root operation excision without querying the physician for clarification.

CODING AXIOM

ICD-10-PCS Official Coding Guideline: Root Operation B3.5: If the root operations excision, repair, or inspection are performed on overlapping layers of the musculoskeletal system, the body part specifying the deepest layer is coded.

Example: Excisional debridement that includes skin, subcutaneous tissue, and muscle is coded to the muscle body part.

that does not have laterality choices, the procedure should be coded twice to indicate both sides.

One new concept for coders related to body part characters involves tubular body parts. Tubular body parts are hollow tubes that transport solids, liquids, or gases through the body. These tubular parts can be found in many parts of the body, including the gastrointestinal system, cardiovascular system, genitourinary system, biliary tract, and respiratory system. The body part value works in combination with the body system value (character 2) to define the precise location of the procedure.

PCS provides information and tools to assist in appropriate body part selection, including body part keys, alphabetical index, and guidelines and conventions.

Body Part Key and Body Part Definitions

CMS has provided a Body Part Key and a Body Part Definitions Table for ICD-10-PCS to aid in the selection of the correct anatomical body part that corresponds to a PCS definition. The Body Part Definitions table contains the same information as the Body Part Key but is organized in a different format. These are not just optional resources but vital references to check in order to select the appropriate body part character according to the official ICD-10-PCS definition. It is assumed that CMS will continue to update these keys periodically, so be sure to replace them yearly when the new code sets are released. These keys can be found in appendixes B and C in this book.

Body Part Key—Anatomical Term to PCS Character Description

There are many anatomical terms that are not represented by a more general PCS body part character. The Body Part Key lists those terms in alpha order and maps them to the appropriate PCS body part value.

Examples:

- For accessory obturator nerve   Use lumbar plexus
- For bony vestibule   Use inner ear, right or left
- For fibular artery   Use peroneal artery
- For orbicularis oculi mucle   Use upper eyelid, right or left

Body Part Definitions—PCS Character Description to Anatomical Term

Body Part Definitions Table lists the PCS defined body part with the anatomical terms/parts that are represented by that body part character.

Examples:

- Ampulla of Vater   Includes duodenal ampulla, hepatopancreatic ampulla
- Cerebral hemisphere   Includes frontal lobe, occipital lobe, parietal and temporal lobe
- Lumbar spinal cord   Includes cauda equina, conus medullaris
- Skin   Includes dermis, epidermis, sebaceous gland, sweat gland

ICD-10-PCS Alphabetic Index

Similar to the Body Part Key and Body Part Definitions table, the alphabetical index in PCS provides assistance in determining the correct body part character. This can be accomplished in two ways: by accessing the index by anatomical site or by root operation.

When referencing the index by anatomical site, the index entry directs the user to an alternate anatomical site. The alternate anatomical site represents an official PCS body part contained in one or more of the PCS code tables; however, it does not identify the specific character value associated with that site. In order to build the

---

✓ QUICK TIP

When coding multiple procedures, referring to the Body Part Definitions table can efficiently show if the procedures are being performed on body parts with the same body value. For example, the Body Part Definitions table shows that the frontal, parietal, and temporal lobe of the brain are all included in the body part value cerebral hemisphere. If an open excision of a lesion is performed on all three lobes, code 00B70ZZ (open excision of cerebral hemisphere lesion) would be reported three times to signify that lesions in three separate areas in the cerebral hemisphere were excised.

ICD-10-PCS Official Coding Guideline—Root Operation B3.2b: During the same operative episode, multiple procedures are coded if the same root operation is repeated in multiple body parts, and those body parts are separate and distinct body parts classified to a single ICD-10-PCS body part value.

correct code, the user has to locate the alternate term in the table being used to construct the code and apply the appropriate fourth character.

Examples:

- For abdominal aortic plexus   Use nerve, abdominal sympathetic
- For buccinator muscle   Use muscle, facial
- For obturator vein   Use vein, hypogastric, left/right

When accessing the index by root operation, the user will be directed to both the appropriate table and the correct body part, providing the user with the first four characters needed to build the code.

Examples:

Occlusion
    Artery
        Anterior Tibial
            Left 04LQ

Extirpation
    Nerve
        Pudendal 01CC

Dilation
    Vein
        Azygos 0570

Although coders are allowed to build PCS codes directly from the tables without reviewing the alphabetical index first, it may prove helpful to consult the index until acquainted with PCS body part definitions. Note that some entries in the index may provide a full seven character code; however, regardless of how many characters provided, it is important to *always* consult the tables to confirm the code was constructed correctly and the most appropriate for the situation. The consistent use of the Body Part Key and Body Part Definitions table assists the coder in building codes directly from the tables.

Body Part—ICD-10-CM Official Coding Guidelines

General: B4.1a

If a procedure is performed on a portion of a body part that does not have a separate body part value, code the body part value corresponding to the whole body part.

Example:

A procedure performed on the alveolar process of the mandible is coded to the mandible body part.

Additional examples of this guideline:

- A procedure on the anterior cruciate ligament (ACL) is coded to knee bursa and ligament
- A procedure performed on the occipital lymph node is coded to lymphatic neck, right/left
- A procedure performed on the talocalcaneal joint is coded to the tarsal joint, right/left
- A procedure performed on the capitate or lunate bone is coded to carpal, right/left

General: B4.1b

If the prefix "peri" is combined with a body part to identify the site of the procedure, and the site of the procedure is not further specified, then the procedure is coded to

> **CODING AXIOM**
>
> **ICD-10-PCS Official Coding Guideline—Convention A7:** Consulting the index first is not required before proceeding to the table to complete the code. A valid code may be chosen directly from the tables.

the body part named. This guideline applies only when a more specific body part value is not available.

Example:

A procedure site identified as perirenal is coded to the kidney body part.

Additional examples of this guideline:

- Perianal = anus
- Perisplenic = spleen
- Periesophageal = esophagus

Branches of Body Parts: B4.2

Where a specific branch of a body part does not have its own body part value in PCS, the body part is coded to the closest proximal branch that has a specific body part value.

Example:

A procedure performed on the mandibular branch of the trigeminal nerve is coded to the trigeminal nerve body part value.

Additional examples of this guideline include:

- For deep branch of ulnar nerve — Use ulnar nerve
- For superficial epigastric artery — Use femoral artery, right/left
- For pectoral and deltoid branch — Both are branches of the thoracoacromial artery, which code to axillary artery right/left

Some of these branches can be found in the Body Part Key but for others it will help to have a good anatomy reference. In addition, some physicians document a certain portion of a body part using terminology related to another nearby body part. For example, prostatic urethra is the portion of the urethra that is near/through the prostate, not a portion of the prostate itself. Prostatic urethra in the Body Part Key will refer the user to urethra.

Bilateral Body Part Values: B4.3

Bilateral body part values are available for a limited number of body parts. If the identical procedure is performed on contralateral body parts, and a bilateral body part value exists for that body part, a single procedure is coded using the bilateral body part value. If no bilateral body part value exists, each procedure is coded separately using the appropriate body part value.

Example:

The identical procedure performed on both fallopian tubes is coded once using the body part value fallopian tube, bilateral. The identical procedure performed on both knee joints is coded twice using the body part values knee joint, right and knee joint, left.

Coronary Arteries: B4.4

The coronary arteries are classified as a single body part further specified by number of sites treated and not by name or number of arteries. Separate body part values are used to specify the number of sites treated when the same procedure is performed on multiple sites in the coronary arteries.

Example:

Angioplasty of two distinct sites in the left anterior descending coronary artery with placement of two stents is coded as dilation of coronary arteries, two sites, with intraluminal device.

Angioplasty of two distinct sites in the left anterior descending coronary artery, one with stent placed and one without, is coded separately as dilation of coronary artery, one site with intraluminal device, and dilation of coronary artery, one site with no device.

Tendons, Ligaments, Bursae, and Fascia Near a Joint: B4.5

Procedures performed on tendons, ligaments, bursae, and fascia supporting a joint are coded to the body part in the respective body system *that is the focus of the procedure*. Procedures performed on *joint structures* themselves are coded to the body part in the joint body systems.

Example:

Repair of the anterior cruciate ligament of the knee is coded to the knee bursae and ligament body part in the bursae and ligaments body system. Knee arthroscopy with shaving of articular cartilage is coded to the knee joint body part in the lower joints body system.

Additional examples of this guideline:

- For division of Achilles tendon   Use lower leg tendon right/left
- For excision of subacromial bursa   Use shoulder bursa and ligament right/left
- For repair of abductor hallucis tendon   Use foot tendon right/left

Knowing the body part that is the focus of the procedure is critical for code selection. Remember to refer to the Body Part Key, Body Part Definitions table, and/or alphabetical index for assistance.

Skin, Subcutaneous Tissue, and Fascia Overlying a Joint: B4.6

If a procedure is performed on the skin, subcutaneous tissue, or fascia overlying a joint, the procedure is coded to the following body part:

- Shoulder is coded to upper arm
- Elbow is coded to lower arm
- Wrist is coded to lower arm
- Hip is coded to upper leg
- Knee is coded to lower leg
- Ankle is coded to foot

The initial instinct of a coder upon seeing one of the listed body sites in an operative report is to code the procedure to a body part representing the joint. However, when a procedure is performed on the surrounding tissue of the joint (e.g., skin, subcutaneous tissue) and not on the actual joint structure, based on this guideline, a more general anatomical site should be used instead of the specific joint site.

Examples:

- For extirpation of foreign body of subcutaneous tissue of left knee   Use subcutaneous tissue of left lower leg
- For excision of lesion of skin of right elbow   Use skin of right lower arm
- For drainage of subcutaneous abscess of left hip   Use left upper leg

> ✓ **QUICK TIP**
>
> Tendons are named for their muscles. This information can aid in the selection of the correct body part value. For example, the extensor digitorum longus tendon cannot be found in the Body Part Key or the alphabetical index. However, the extensor digitorum longus muscle *is* listed in the Body Part Key and the alphabetical index, both of which instruct the user to apply the lower leg muscle body part value. Therefore, code the tendon to the lower leg tendon body part value.

Fingers and Toes: B4.7

If a body system does not contain a separate body part value for fingers, procedures performed on the fingers are coded to the body part value for the hand. If a body system does not contain a separate body part value for toes, procedures performed on the toes are coded to the body part value for the foot.

Example:

Excision of finger muscle is coded to one of the hand muscle body part values in the muscles body system.

This guideline includes muscles, tendons, ligaments, subcutaneous tissue, fascia, and skin. However, bones of fingers and toes have their own body part values in the upper and lower bone body systems.

Upper and Lower Intestinal Tract: B4.8

In the gastrointestinal body system, the general body part values upper intestinal tract and lower intestinal tract are provided as an option for the root operations change, inspection, removal, and revision. Upper intestinal tract includes the portion of the gastrointestinal tract from the esophagus down to and including the duodenum. The lower intestinal tract includes the portion of the gastrointestinal tract from the jejunum down to and including the rectum and anus.

Example:

In the root operation Change table, change of a device in the jejunum is coded using the body part Lower Intestinal Tract.

Additional examples include:

- EGD is coded to inspection of the upper intestinal tract
- Colonoscopy is coded to inspection of the lower intestinal tract

Character 5: Approach

The fifth character is the approach, which is the method used to reach the site of the procedure. There are seven approach values made of three distinct components: the access location, the method, and the type of instrumentation. The same procedure performed with a different approach will result in a different code. PCS has provided detailed definitions in addition to guidelines to assist in the selection of the appropriate approach value. For example, ICD-10-PCS Official Coding Guideline B5.2 explains that procedures performed using an open approach, with percutaneous endoscopic assistance, are coded to the open approach.

The character meaning tables that introduce each body system in this book display the approach values that are valid with each particular body system. The following table illustrates the seven different types of approaches as described by PCS, as well as the definition, access location, method, instrumentation, and some examples. For detailed information regarding the approach characters and the guidelines that pertain to the approach, see Optum360's *ICD-10-PCS Complete Official Code Set* coding book or CMS website: http://www.cms.gov/Medicare/Coding/ICD10/2016-ICD-10-PCS-and-GEMs.html.

Approach	Definition	Access Location	Method	Type of Instrumentation	Example
Open (0)	Cutting through the skin or mucous membrane and any other body layers necessary to expose the site of the procedure	Skin or mucous membrane and any other body layers	Cutting	None	Abdominal hysterectomy
Percutaneous (3)	Entry, by puncture or minor incision, of instrumentation through the skin or mucous membrane and any other body layers necessary to reach the site of the procedure	Skin or mucous membrane and any other body layers	Puncture or minor incision	Without visualization	Needle biopsy of liver, Liposuction
Percutaneous Endoscopic (4)	Entry, by puncture or minor incision, of instrumentation through the skin or mucous membrane and any other body layers necessary to reach and visualize the site of the procedure	Skin or mucous membrane and any other body layers	Puncture or minor incision	With visualization	Arthroscopy, Laparoscopic cholecystectomy
Via Natural or Artificial Opening with Percutaneous Endoscopic Assistance (F)	Entry of instrumentation through a natural or artificial external opening and entry, by puncture or minor incision, of instrumentation through the skin or mucous membrane and any other body layers necessary to aid in the performance of the procedure	Skin or mucous membrane and any other body layers	Direct entry with puncture or minor incision for instrumentation only	With visualization	Laparoscopic-assisted vaginal hysterectomy
Via Natural or Artificial Opening (7)	Entry of instrumentation through a natural or artificial external opening to reach the site of the procedure	Natural or artificial external opening	Direct entry	Without visualization	Endotracheal tube insertion, Foley catheter placement
Via Natural or Artificial Opening Endoscopic (8)	Entry of instrumentation through a natural or artificial external opening to reach and visualize the site of the procedure	Natural or artificial external opening	Direct entry	With visualization	Sigmoidoscopy, EGD, ERCP
External (X)	Procedures performed directly on the skin or mucous membrane and procedures performed indirectly by the application of external force through the skin or mucous membrane	Skin or mucous membrane	Direct or indirect application	None	Closed fracture reduction, Resection of tonsils

Character 6: Device

Devices are reported by the sixth character of the PCS code in the medical surgical section and should only be assigned for devices that remain in the patient at the conclusion of the procedure. No device value should be assigned for small devices that are considered integral to the performance of the procedure, such as sutures, clips, ligatures, radiological markers, and postop wound drains. There are four major types of devices:

- Biological or synthetic material that takes the place of all or a portion of a body part (e.g., skin graft, joint prosthesis)
- Biological or synthetic material that assists or prevents a physiological function (e.g., IUD)
- Therapeutic material not absorbed by, eliminated by, or incorporated into a body part (e.g., radioactive implant)
- Mechanical or electronic appliances used to assist, monitor, take the place of, or prevent a physiological function (e.g., cardiac pacemaker, orthopedic pin)

Device characters may be assigned with many various root operation characters. When no device is used or left in the body after the procedure, the appropriate value for the sixth character position is Z— No device. The specific root operations listed below can *only* be assigned when performed in conjunction with a procedure involving a device.

- Insertion
- Replacement
- Supplement
- Change
- Removal
- Revision

The character meaning tables that introduce each body system in this book display the device values that are valid with each particular body system. Be aware that the sixth character may have different meanings in sections other than the medical/surgical section. For example, in the chiropractic section, the sixth character defines the method.

Device Key and Device Aggregation Table

The Device Key is a resource for the PCS code set that maps a specific device, by brand or common name, to a valid PCS character (see the following table). As new devices are developed, the key will be updated. Often these device names can also be found in the Alphabetical Index.

Device	PCS Description
3f (Aortic) Bioprosthesis valve	Zooplastic Tissue in Heart and Great Vessels
AbioCor® Total Replacement Heart	Synthetic Substitute
Absolute Pro Vascular (OTW) Self-Expanding Stent System	Intraluminal Device
Acculink (RX) Carotid Stent System	Intraluminal Device
Acellular Hydrated Dermis	Nonautologous Tissue Substitute
Acetabular cup	Liner in Lower Joints
Activa PC neurostimulator	Stimulator Generator, Multiple Array for Insertion in Subcutaneous Tissue and Fascia

Device	PCS Description
Activa RC neurostimulator	Stimulator Generator, Multiple Array Rechargeable for Insertion in Subcutaneous Tissue and Fascia
Activa SC neurostimulator	Stimulator Generator, Single Array for Insertion in Subcutaneous Tissue and Fascia

In some cases, PCS groups devices into a general "catch all" device value. What can be difficult for coders is deciding what specific devices are included in the more general device value; this is where the Device Aggregation Table can be helpful. For example, the following excerpt from the Device Aggregation Table illustrates that for the body system heart and great vessels, the general device character of M Cardiac lead, should be used for all procedures involving a cardiac lead **EXCEPT** when the root operation is insertion. If the objective of the procedure is insertion of a cardiac lead for a pacemaker or a defibrillator, the more specific device value K Cardiac lead, defibrillator, or J Cardiac lead, pacemaker, should be used.

Specific Device	for Operation	in Body System	General Device	
Cardiac Lead, Defibrillator (K)	Insertion	Heart and Great Vessels	M	Cardiac Lead
Cardiac Lead, Pacemaker (J)	Insertion	Heart and Great Vessels	M	Cardiac Lead
Cardiac Resynchronization Defibrillator Pulse Generator (9)	Insertion	Subcutaneous Tissue and Fascia	P	Cardiac Rhythm Related Device
Cardiac Resynchronization Pacemaker Pulse Generator (7)	Insertion	Subcutaneous Tissue and Fascia	P	Cardiac Rhythm Related Device

> **KEY POINT**
>
> Always be aware of the specific body system site of the device insertion. For example, the insertion of a pacemaker or defibrillator generator is not inserted into the heart chambers (the leads are) or the general anatomical region of the chest wall. It is inserted into the subcutaneous tissue of the chest and is found in the subcutaneous tissue and fascia body system table.

The full Device Key, Device Aggregation Table, as well as official guidelines pertaining to the selection of an appropriate device value can be found in Optum360's *Detailed Instruction for Appropriate ICD-10-PCS Coding,* Optum360's *ICD-10-PCS Complete Official Code Set,* or CMS website http://www.cms.gov/Medicare/Coding/ICD10/2016-ICD-10-PCS-and-GEMs.html.

Character 7: Qualifier

The qualifier is specified in the seventh character and contains unique values essential in portraying the complete objective of a procedure. Some qualifiers may even identify another part of the human anatomy. The most common qualifier is diagnostic (X), which is used to indicate that a biopsy procedure was performed. Some other examples of the use of a qualifier include:

- To indicate the destination body part site of a bypass procedure, which is the body part that something is bypassed "to"
- To indicate whether an orthopedic implant was cemented or not cemented
- To indicate the approach site and column of a spinal fusion (e.g., anterior approach, anterior column)
- To indicate the type of transplant tissue (e.g., allogenic, syngenic, or zooplastic)
- To indicate type of cesarean section
- To indicate extent of a detachment procedure (e.g., complete, partial, high, mid, low). Detachment or amputations use the qualifier to describe the extent of the detachment of the body part. There are specific definitions for each of the qualifier values that are described in the following table.

Qualifier Definition	Arm	Leg
1 **High:** Amputation at the proximal portion of the shaft of the:	Humerus	Femur
2 **Mid:** Amputation at the middle portion of the shaft of the:	Humerus	Femur
3 **Low:** Amputation at the distal portion of the shaft of the:	Humerus	Femur

Qualifier Definition	Hand	Foot
Ø Complete 1st through 5th Rays Ray: digit of hand or foot with corresponding metacarpus or metatarsus	Through carpo-metacarpal joint, **Wrist**	Through tarso-metatarsal Joint, **Ankle**
4 Complete 1st Ray	Through carpo-metacarpal joint, **Thumb**	Through tarso-metatarsal joint, **Great Toe**
5 Complete 2nd Ray	Through carpo-metacarpal joint, **Index Finger**	Through tarso-metatarsal joint, **2nd Toe**
6 Complete 3rd Ray	Through carpo-metacarpal joint, **Middle Finger**	Through tarso-metatarsal joint, **3rd Toe**
7 Complete 4th Ray	Through carpo-metacarpal joint, **Ring Finger**	Through tarso-metatarsal joint, **4th Toe**
8 Complete 5th Ray	Through carpo-metacarpal joint, **Little Finger**	Through tarso-metatarsal joint, **Little Toe**
9 Partial 1st Ray	Anywhere along shaft or head of metacarpal bone, **Thumb**	Anywhere along shaft or head of metatarsal bone, **Great Toe**
B Partial 2nd Ray	Anywhere along shaft or head of metacarpal bone, **Index Finger**	Anywhere along shaft or head of metatarsal bone, **2nd Toe**
C Partial 3rd Ray	Anywhere along shaft or head of metacarpal bone, **Middle Finger**	Anywhere along shaft or head of metatarsal bone, **3rd Toe**
D Partial 4th Ray	Anywhere along shaft or head of metacarpal bone, **Ring Finger**	Anywhere along shaft or head of metatarsal bone, **4th Toe**
F Partial 5th Ray	Anywhere along shaft or head of metacarpal bone, **Little Finger**	Anywhere along shaft or head of metatarsal bone, **Little Toe**

Qualifier Definition	Finger or Thumb	Toe
Ø **Complete:** Amputation at the metacarpophalangeal/metatarsal-phalangeal joint	Finger or Thumb, any one 1st -5th	Toe, any one 1st -5th
1 **High:** Amputation anywhere along the proximal phalanx	Finger or Thumb, any one 1st -5th	Toe, any one 1st -5th
2 **Mid:** Amputation through the proximal intraphalangeal joint or anywhere along the middle phalanx	Finger or Thumb, any one 1st -5th	Toe, any one 1st -5th
3 **Low:** Amputation through the distal interphalangeal joint or anywhere along the distal phalanx	Finger or Thumb, any one 1st -5th	Toe, any one 1st -5th

Some of the sections outside of medical and surgical (Ø), including OB, administration, and measuring and monitoring, utilize many more values for the qualifier character. However, the majority of tables only offer one choice (e.g., character Z for no qualifier). There are currently no guidelines pertaining specifically to the use of the qualifier character (7). The available, valid qualifier values are listed in each of the upcoming body system character meaning tables.

Summary

The move to ICD-10-PCS coding is a valuable one from a variety of perspectives, not only from the reimbursement side but also in the areas of research, quality measures, and other data related areas. The ICD-10-PCS code set, like the ICD-10-CM code set, is much more precise, detailing the anatomy of the human body and the surgical approaches and devices used in a code set that can be updated more easily and be extrapolated for specific data elements.

ICD-10-PCS has developed better tools to assist in building more detailed codes. The challenge now is to learn how to correctly use the tools provided to aid in the selection of appropriate codes. Coders must be prepared to understand this information and learning about anatomy and physiology is a great first step to ICD-10-PCS preparation.

The following sections discuss various terms used throughout the ICD-10-PCS tables, most specifically within the body part key. Although some information discussed in the ICD-10-CM chapters may be duplicated, the intent of the next few chapters is to solely focus on how anatomy and physiology is broken out in the PCS code set. For more details on general anatomy and physiology in these areas, please refer back to the organ system primers at the beginning of the ICD-10-CM chapters.

Knowledge Assessment Questions

1. There are _____ (number) body systems in the medical/surgical section (0).

2. When coding an amputation, the appropriate root operation value is _____ and is only offered in which two body systems?
   a. Upper and lower bones
   b. Subcutaneous tissue and fascia
   c. Anatomical regions, lower extremities
   d. Anatomical regions, upper extremities

3. Label the following arteries as located in the upper or lower artery body system.
   a. Innominate artery_____
   b. Superior mesenteric artery_____
   c. Subclavian artery, left_____
   d. Colic artery, right_____

4. Match the root operations with the correct ICD-10-PCS definitions.

   a. Excision   ___ 1. Partially closing off an orifice or the lumen of a tubular body part.
   b. Resection   ___ 2. Completely closing an orifice or lumen of a tubular body part.
   c. Bypass   ___ 3. Cutting out or off, without replacement, all of a body part.
   d. Drainage   ___ 4. Taking or cutting out solid matter from a body part.
   e. Occlusion   ___ 5. Taking or letting out fluids and/or gases from a body part.
   f. Restriction   ___ 6. Cutting out or off, without replacement, a portion of a body part.
   g. Extirpation   ___ 7. Altering the route of passage of the contents of a tubular body part.

5. What PCS body parts do the following terms correspond to?
   a. Abdominal aortic plexus   Use _____
   b. Biceps femoris muscle   Use _____
   c. Choana   Use _____
   d. Gastric lymph node   Use _____
   e. Infundibulopelvic ligament   Use _____
   f. Mitral annulus   Use _____
   g. Pancreatic vein   Use _____
   h. Rima glottidis   Use _____
   i. Sinus venosus   Use _____
   j. Sweat gland   Use _____

6. What other body terms are included with each of the following PCS body part characters?

   a. Auditory ossicle, right/left
      Includes _____

   b. Brain
      Includes _____

   c. Esophagus, upper
      Includes _____

   d. Optic nerve
      Includes _____

   e. Tibia, right/left
      Includes _____

7. Using the Alphabetical Index of ICD-10-PCS, what appropriate PCS body part does the index lead to for the following specific body part terms?

   a. Anterior crural nerve   Use _____
   b. Brachiocephalic artery   Use _____
   c. Hepatic flexure   Use _____
   d. Jugular body   Use _____
   e. Sacral lymph node   Use _____

8. Shaving of the cartilage of a joint is coded in the bursae and ligament body system because it supports the joint.

   a. True
   b. False

9. Which root operation *always* needs a device?

   a. Reposition
   b. Restriction
   c. Replacement
   d. Repair

10. When a laparoscope is used to aid an open procedure, the fifth character assigned for the approach would never be Ø for open.

    a. True
    b. False

Chapter 15. ICD-10-PCS: Nervous and Circulatory Systems

Central Nervous System (Ø)

Procedures involving the central nervous system can cover a variety of body parts, such as the brain, nerves, and spinal cord, and a number of types of procedures. Some procedures performed may include nerve transfers, mapping procedures, and insertion of neurostimulator leads. A compiled table for body system character 0 Central nervous system, shows all of the valid characters for that system under ICD-10-PCS.

Operation–Character 3	Body Part–Character 4	Approach–Character 5	Device–Character 6	Qualifier–Character 7
1 Bypass	Ø Brain	Ø Open	Ø Drainage Device	Ø Nasopharynx
2 Change	1 Cerebral Meninges	3 Percutaneous	2 Monitoring Device	1 Mastoid Sinus
5 Destruction	2 Dura Mater	4 Percutaneous Endoscopic	3 Infusion Device	2 Atrium
8 Division	3 Epidural Space	X External	7 Autologous Tissue Substitute	3 Blood Vessel
9 Drainage	4 Subdural Space		J Synthetic Substitute	4 Pleural Cavity
B Excision	5 Subarachnoid Space		K Nonautologous Tissue Substitute	5 Intestine
C Extirpation	6 Cerebral Ventricle		M Neurostimulator Lead	6 Peritoneal Cavity
D Extraction	7 Cerebral Hemisphere		Y Other Device	7 Urinary Tract
F Fragmentation	8 Basal Ganglia		Z No Device	8 Bone Marrow
H Insertion	9 Thalamus			9 Fallopian Tube
J Inspection	A Hypothalamus			B Cerebral Cisterns
K Map	B Pons			F Olfactory Nerve
N Release	C Cerebellum			G Optic Nerve
P Removal	D Medulla Oblongata			H Oculomotor Nerve
Q Repair	E Cranial Nerve			J Trochlear Nerve
S Reposition	F Olfactory Nerve			K Trigeminal Nerve
T Resection	G Optic Nerve			L Abducens Nerve
U Supplement	H Oculomotor Nerve			M Facial Nerve
W Revision	J Trochlear Nerve			N Acoustic Nerve
X Transfer	K Trigeminal Nerve			P Glossopharyngeal Nerve
	L Abducens Nerve			Q Vagus Nerve
	M Facial Nerve			R Accessory Nerve
	N Acoustic Nerve			S Hypoglossal Nerve
	P Glossopharyngeal Nerve			X Diagnostic
	Q Vagus Nerve			Z No Qualifier
	R Accessory Nerve			
	S Hypoglossal Nerve			
	T Spinal Meninges			
	U Spinal Canal			
	V Spinal Cord			
	W Cervical Spinal Cord			
	X Thoracic Spinal Cord			
	Y Lumbar Spinal Cord			

© 2015 Optum360, LLC

> **KEY POINT**
>
> Most of the *associated terms* listed under each body part character on the following pages correspond to what can be found in the Body Part Key or the Body Part Definitions table located in appendix B and C, respectively. However, some terms listed may not be found in the body part keys but are included in that body part because they have no separate body part value of their own. Since they are anatomically located in this body part, guideline B4.1a would apply.

This table provides a great basis from which to study important terminology concerning the central nervous system, as well as terms used throughout ICD-10-PCS in general.

Body Part — Character 4

The body part characters in ICD-10-PCS detail the specific site where the procedure was performed. Again, the physician may use different terminology than is used in the table, so it is vital to understand not only the term as given in the table but also associated terms and body parts that are included in each PCS character. Refer to the following pages and/or the Body Part Key and Body Part Definitions for this important information.

Figure 15.1: Brain Sections

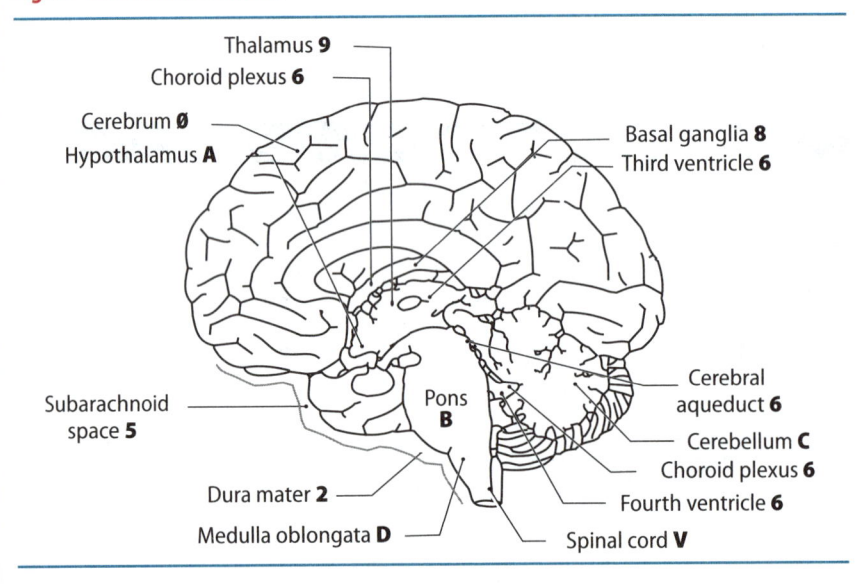

Character Value — 0, Brain

Associated Terms: Cerebrum, corpus callosum, encephalon

The cerebrum is the large uppermost section of the brain, which is divided into two hemispheres. The corpus callosum is the band of nerve fibers that joins the two cerebral hemispheres together. Encephalon refers to all of the contents of the cranium, such as the cerebrum, the cerebellum, and the other structures of the brain.

Character Value — 1, Cerebral Meninges

Associated Terms: Arachnoid mater—intracranial, leptomeninges—intracranial, pia mater—intracranial

The meninges are the membranes that enclose the brain and the spinal cord, and the cerebral meninges are those that specifically enclose the cerebrum. The arachnoid membrane or mater/sheath lies between the dura mater and the pia mater to help protect the brain. The pia mater is the inner most layer of membrane helping to protect the brain. This membrane layer is rich in blood vessels to help supply the nervous tissue. The leptomeninges is a term used to describe both the pia mater and the arachnoid membrane in combination with one another.

Character Value — 2, Dura Mater

Associated Terms: Diaphragma sellae, dura mater—intracranial, falx cerebri, tentorium cerebelli

The dura mater is the outermost membrane of those that enclose the brain and spinal cord. The denticulate ligaments are "tooth-like" portions of ligament that attach the pia mater to the dura mater and arachnoid membranes, and are known to give some stability to the spinal cord with the vertebral column. Several of these terms are different types of dura mater. The diaphragma sellae is the portion of the dura mater that creates a partition between the pituitary gland and the brain above. The falx cerebri is a sickle-shaped fold of the dura mater that extends into the fissure between the two hemispheres of the cerebrum. The tentorium cerebelli is a horizontal projection of the meningeal dura mater that separates the cerebellum in the posterior cranial fossa from the posterior portion of the cerebral hemispheres.

Character Value — 3, Epidural Space

Associated Terms: Epidural space—intracranial, extradural space—intracranial

The epidural space surrounds the dura mater of the brain or the spinal cord, beneath the endosteum of the cranium or the spinal column. The extradural space is the space between the outermost layer of dura mater and the cranial cavity.

Character Value — 4, Subdural Space

Associated Terms: Subdural space—intracranial

The subdural space is the potential space that results from the separation of the arachnoid mater from the dura mater as a result of trauma, pathologic process, or the absence of cerebrospinal fluid. This can exist at the cranial level, as well as at the spinal level.

Figure 15.2: Skull Layers

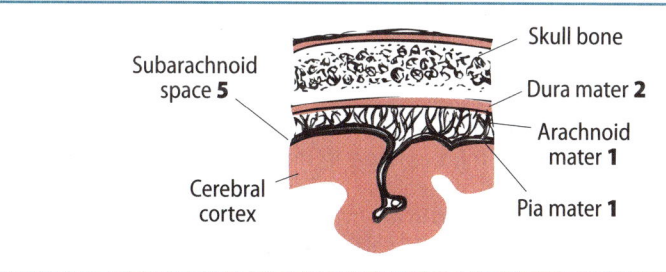

Character Value — 5, Subarachnoid Space

Associated Terms: Subarachnoid space—intracranial

The subarachnoid space is the space between the arachnoid membranes and the pia mater membranes. This space contains cerebrospinal fluid and can exist in both the cranial and spinal levels.

Character Value — 6, Cerebral Ventricle

Associated Terms: Aqueduct of Sylvius, cerebral aqueduct (Sylvius), choroid plexus, ependyma, foramen of Monro (intraventricle), fourth ventricle, interventricular foramen (Monro), left lateral ventricle, right lateral ventricle, third ventricle

There is a set of four structures in the brain that contain cerebrospinal fluid, known as the ventricles. These four structures include the left and right lateral ventricles, the third ventricle, and the fourth ventricle. The cerebral aqueduct (Sylvius), also known as the aqueduct of Sylvius, is a channel between the third and fourth ventricle through which cerebrospinal fluid is passed. The choroid plexus is the structure in the ventricles responsible for the production of the cerebrospinal fluid. The interventricular foramen (Monro), also known as the ependymal foramen of Monro, is a channel between the left and right lateral ventricles and the third ventricle.

Character Value — 7, Cerebral Hemisphere

Associated Terms: Frontal lobe, occipital lobe, parietal lobe, temporal lobe

The cerebral hemispheres are the two halves of the cerebrum. The hemispheres are divided into four main lobes: the frontal lobe, the occipital lobe, the parietal lobe, and the temporal lobe. The lobes are responsible for various brain functions.

Character Value — 8, Basal Ganglia

Associated Terms: Basal nuclei, claustrum, corpus striatum, globus pallidus, substantia nigra, subthalamic nucleus

The basal ganglia, or basal nuclei, are located within each cerebral hemisphere and are mainly responsible for voluntary motor control. Claustrum describes a sheet-like structure of neurons that can be found in the area of the basal ganglia, but can also be found in other areas of the brain. The corpus striatum, the globus pallidus, the substantia nigra, and the subthalamic nucleus are all additional components of the basal ganglia system of the brain.

Character Value — 9, Thalamus

Associated Terms: Epithalamus, geniculate nucleus, metathalamus, pulvinar

The thalamus is a pair of large oval structures in the brain that are part of the diencephalon. Two other portions of the diencephalon are the epithalamus and the metathalamus, which have different functions than the thalamus. The geniculate nucleus is a structure found within the thalamus that involves hearing and vision. The term pulvinar refers to the posterior portion of the thalamus, and is involved in visual attention, the suppression of irrelevant stimuli, and the utilization of various types of information to initiate eye movements.

Character Value — A, Hypothalamus

Associated Terms: Mammillary body

The hypothalamus is a portion of the diencephalon of the brain that forms the floor and part of the lateral wall of the third ventricle. Its main role is to activate and control the autonomic nervous system. A mammillary body is either of the two small round masses of gray matter that are located in the hypothalamus. They are involved with the processing of recognition memory and are believed to add the element of smell to memories.

Character Value — B, Pons

Associated Terms: Apneustic center, basis pontis, locus ceruleus, pneumotaxic center, pontine tegmentum, superior olivary nucleus

The pons is a prominence on the brain stem that serves as a "bridge" between the cerebral cortex and the medulla oblongata. There are various areas on the pons that control body functions or assist in different sensory areas. The apneustic center works with the dorsal respiratory center to control the intensity of breathing. The basis pontis is the anterior part of the pons and works to control motor function. The locus ceruleus helps to create physiological responses to panic and stress. The pneumotaxic center works with the pontine respiratory group to regulate the respiratory rate. The pontine tegmentum is involved in the regulation of REM sleep. Superior olivary nuclei are involved in hearing.

Character Value — C, Cerebellum

Associated Terms: Culmen

The cerebellum is located in the posterior cranial fossa, behind the brain stem, and is mainly responsible for coordinating voluntary muscular activity. It is made up of two lateral hemispheres and a middle section called the vermis. The term culmen is used to describe the upper ridge of the vermis section.

Character Value — D, Medulla Oblongata

Associated Terms: Myelencephalon

The medulla oblongata is one of the three parts of the brain stem, and is separated from the pons by a horizontal groove. The main functions of the medulla oblongata are to control the cardiac, vasomotor, and respiratory functions for the body. The myelencephalon is the lower portion of the embryonic hindbrain, from which the medulla oblongata develops.

Figure 15.3: Cranial Nerves

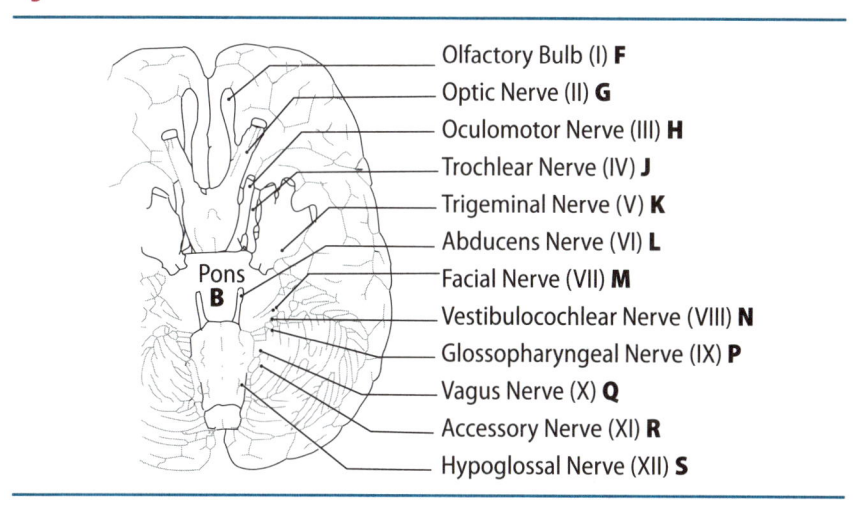

- Olfactory Bulb (I) **F**
- Optic Nerve (II) **G**
- Oculomotor Nerve (III) **H**
- Trochlear Nerve (IV) **J**
- Trigeminal Nerve (V) **K**
- Abducens Nerve (VI) **L**
- Pons **B**
- Facial Nerve (VII) **M**
- Vestibulocochlear Nerve (VIII) **N**
- Glossopharyngeal Nerve (IX) **P**
- Vagus Nerve (X) **Q**
- Accessory Nerve (XI) **R**
- Hypoglossal Nerve (XII) **S**

Character Value — F, Olfactory Nerve

Associated Terms: First cranial nerve, olfactory bulb

The olfactory nerve is the first cranial nerve, and is one of a pair of nerves associated with the sense of smell. The olfactory bulb is the area of the brain where the olfactory nerves end and the olfactory tracts begin.

Character Value — G, Optic Nerve

Associated Terms: Optic chiasm, second cranial nerve

Optic nerves, also known as the second cranial nerves, transmit visual impulses. There is a point in the brain near the thalamus and hypothalamus known as the optic chiasm where parts of each optic nerve cross over one another.

Character Value — H, Oculomotor Nerve

Associated Terms: Third cranial nerve

Oculomotor nerves, also known as the third cranial nerves, are essential for eye movements, allowing specific intrinsic and extrinsic eye muscles to move.

Character Value — J, Trochlear Nerve

Associated Terms: Fourth cranial nerve

Trochlear nerves, also known as the fourth cranial nerves, are also essential for eye movements, as well as for stability and sensibility in the eye muscles.

Character Value — K, Trigeminal Nerve

Associated Terms: Fifth cranial nerve, gasserian ganglion, mandibular nerve, maxillary nerve, ophthalmic nerve, trifacial nerve

Trigeminal nerves, also known as the fifth cranial nerve or the trifacial nerve, are the largest pair of cranial nerves, and are essential to both the ability to chew, as well as the general muscle sensibility of the face. Some of the branches of this nerve include the mandibular nerve, the maxillary nerve, and the ophthalmic nerve. The gasserian ganglion is a bundle of interconnected nerve fibers, specifically of the trigeminal nerves.

Character Value — L, Abducens Nerve

Associated Terms: Sixth cranial nerve

Abducens nerves, or the sixth cranial nerves, arise in the pons and end in the orbit, with the specific task of controlling the lateral rectus muscle to turn the eye outward.

Character Value — M, Facial Nerve

Associated Terms: Chorda tympani, geniculate ganglion, greater superficial petrosal nerve, nerve to the stapedius, parotid plexus, posterior auricular nerve, seventh cranial nerve, submandibular ganglion

Facial nerves, or the seventh cranial nerve, innervate the scalp, forehead, eyelids, facial muscles, cheeks, and jaw. The facial nerve divides into several branches, such as the chorda tympani, the greater superficial petrosal nerve, and the posterior auricular nerve. The branch point and grouping of vessels in the facial nerves is called the parotid plexus. There are two important ganglia involving the facial nerves: the geniculate ganglion and the submandibular ganglion.

Character Value — N, Acoustic Nerve

Associated Terms: Cochlear nerve, eighth cranial nerve, Scarpa's (vestibular) ganglion, spiral ganglion, vestibular nerve, vestibular (Scarpa's) ganglion, vestibulocochlear nerve

Acoustic nerves, also known as vestibular nerves, cochlear nerves, vestibulocochlear nerves, or the eighth cranial nerves, are the pair of cranial nerves that provide the sense of hearing, as well as the sense of balance. Two important ganglia involving the acoustic nerves are Scarpa's (or vestibular) ganglion and the spiral ganglion.

Character Value — P, Glossopharyngeal Nerve

Associated Terms: Carotid sinus nerve, ninth cranial nerve, tympanic nerve

Glossopharyngeal nerves, also known as the ninth cranial nerves, are essential to the sensation of taste. They branch off into the carotid sinus nerve and the tympanic nerve.

Character Value — Q, Vagus Nerve

Associated Terms: Anterior vagal trunk, pharyngeal plexus, pneumogastric nerve, posterior vagal trunk, pulmonary plexus, recurrent laryngeal nerve, superior laryngeal nerve, tenth cranial nerve

Vagus nerves are the longest cranial nerves, also known as the pneumogastric nerves and the tenth cranial nerves. Branches of the vagus nerve include the posterior vagal trunk, the recurrent laryngeal nerve, and the superior laryngeal nerve. There are two plexus points involving the vagus nerve: the pharyngeal plexus and the pulmonary plexus.

Character Value — R, Accessory Nerve

Associated Terms: Eleventh cranial nerve

Accessory nerves, also known as the eleventh cranial nerves, are vital for speech, swallowing, and specific types of movements of the head and shoulders.

Character Value — S, Hypoglossal Nerve

Associated Terms: Twelfth cranial nerve

Hypoglossal nerves, also known as the twelfth cranial nerves, are essential for tongue movement and for swallowing.

Character Value — T, Spinal Meninges

Associated Terms: Arachnoid mater—spinal, denticulate (dentate) ligament, dura mater—spinal, leptomeninges—spinal, pia mater—spinal

The meninges are the membranes that enclose the brain and the spinal cord. The spinal meninges are those that specifically enclose the spinal cord or the brain and spinal cord. The arachnoid membrane or mater/sheath lies between the dura mater and the pia mater to help protect the brain. The pia mater is the innermost layer of membrane helping to protect the brain. This membrane layer is rich in blood vessels to help supply the nervous tissue. The denticulate ligament is a lateral extension of the pia mater from the spinal cord. There is one on each side of the body, and it attaches to the dura mater to help anchor the spinal cord. Leptomeninges is a term used to describe the pia mater and the arachnoid membrane in combination with one another.

Character Value — U, Spinal Canal

Associated Terms: Epidural space—spinal, extradural space—spinal, subarachnoid space—spinal, subdural space—spinal, vertebral canal

The spinal canal is the space in vertebrae through which the spinal cord passes.

Character Value — V, Spinal Cord

Character Value — W, Cervical Spinal Cord

Character Value — X, Thoracic Spinal Cord

Character Value — Y, Lumbar Spinal Cord

Associated Terms: Cauda equina, conus medullaris

The spinal cord is a cylindrical bundle of nervous tissue that extends from the brain down the spinal column to the level of the first or second lumbar vertebrae. It provides a vital link between the brain and body and vice versa. Based on its location within the vertebral canal, different portions of the spinal cord can be referred to as cervical, thoracic, lumbar, or sacral. ICD-10-PCS coding has specific body part characters for the cervical, thoracic, and lumber spinal cord sections. The cauda equina is the section of the spinal cord that contains the second through fifth lumbar nerve pairs, the first through fifth sacral nerve pairs, and the coccygeal nerve. The conus medullaris is just above the cauda equina, typically found at the first or second lumbar vertebrae. It is the tapered lower end of the spinal cord, just before it branches out into the cauda equina.

> **CLINICAL NOTE**
>
> It is important to remember that the spinal cord is part of the central nervous system. Body part characters V, W, X, and Y all represent elements of the spinal cord.

Qualifier — Character 7

In the central nervous system, there are character values for the 7th character for three types of procedures: ventricular and spinal canal shunt procedures and nerve transfer procedures. The body part found in the qualifier character represents the destination of the bypass/shunt procedure or the site transferred to in the nerve grafting services. The 7th character values for the bypass (shunting) procedures include such sites as blood vessel, pleural cavity, intestine, peritoneal cavity, urinary tract, and cerebral cisterns. Nerve transfer characters are provided for nerves such as olfactory, optic, trigeminal, facial, vagus, and hypoglossal. It is important for coders to understand the location of these body sites and how they relate to the corresponding body part values in character 4.

Representative ICD-10-PCS Code Examples

1. **Percutaneous placement of ventriculoperitoneal shunt, Medtronic adjustable pressure valve**

    00163J6   Bypass cerebral ventricle to peritoneal cavity with synthetic substitute, percutaneous approach

    Note: Providing an alternative route of passage between two body parts meets the definition of root operation bypass. The body part being bypassed from is the cerebral ventricle and the site bypassed to (7th character) is the peritoneal cavity. The approach is specified as percutaneous.

2. **Lumbar puncture, percutaneous, therapeutic**

    009U3ZZ   Drainage of spinal canal, percutaneous approach

3. **Open removal of a lesion of the frontal lobe**

    00B70ZZ   Excision of cerebral hemisphere, open approach

    Note: According to the body part key, the frontal lobe is included in body part cerebral hemisphere. Excision rather than resection is used, since only the lesion was removed and not the entire cerebral hemisphere.

4. **Trigeminal to seventh cranial nerve transfer, percutaneous endoscopically**

    00XK4ZM   Transfer trigeminal nerve to facial nerve, percutaneous endoscopic approach

    Note: The trigeminal nerve is the body part transferred "from." According to the body part key, the seventh cranial nerve is coded as facial nerve. The facial nerve would then be the seventh character—the qualifier—indicating the body part that is transferred "to."

CODING AXIOM

A ventriculoperitoneal shunt placed percutaneously with laparoscopic assistance can be coded with two codes as long as the laparoscope was used for inspection of the peritoneal cavity and not the actual placement of the device.

00163J6   Bypass cerebral ventricle to peritoneal cavity with synthetic substitute, percutaneous approach

0WJG4ZZ   Inspection of peritoneal cavity, percutaneous endoscopic approach

Coding Clinic, 2Q, 13, 36

CODING AXIOM

Spinal canal, not spinal cord, is the most appropriate body part from table 009 to code a diagnostic lumbar spinal tap.

Coding Clinic, 1Q, 14, 8

Peripheral Nervous System (1)

The peripheral nervous system includes all nerves outside of the central nervous system, and procedures can include nerve grafts, repairs, excisions, or other various procedures. A compiled table for body system character 1 Peripheral nervous system, provides all of the valid characters for that system in ICD-10-PCS.

> **DEFINITIONS**
>
> **sacral nerves.** Five nerves (S1-S5) on each side of the sacrum that pass from the sacral canal through the sacral foramina and form the sacral and coccygeal plexus.

Operation–Character 3	Body Part–Character 4	Approach–Character 5	Device–Character 6	Qualifier–Character 7
2 Change	0 Cervical Plexus	0 Open	0 Drainage Device	1 Cervical Nerve
5 Destruction	1 Cervical Nerve	3 Percutaneous	2 Monitoring Device	2 Phrenic Nerve
8 Division	2 Phrenic Nerve	4 Percutaneous Endoscopic	7 Autologous Tissue Substitute	4 Ulnar Nerve
9 Drainage	3 Brachial Plexus	X External	M Neurostimulator Lead	5 Median Nerve
B Excision	4 Ulnar Nerve		Y Other Device	6 Radial Nerve
C Extirpation	5 Median Nerve		Z No Device	8 Thoracic Nerve
D Extraction	6 Radial Nerve			B Lumbar Nerve
H Insertion	8 Thoracic Nerve			C Perineal Nerve
J Inspection	9 Lumbar Plexus			D Femoral Nerve
N Release	A Lumbosacral Plexus			F Sciatic Nerve
P Removal	B Lumbar Nerve			G Tibial Nerve
Q Repair	C Pudendal Nerve			H Peroneal Nerve
S Reposition	D Femoral Nerve			X Diagnostic
U Supplement	F Sciatic Nerve			Z No Qualifier
W Revision	G Tibial Nerve			
X Transfer	H Peroneal Nerve			
	K Head and Neck Sympathetic Nerve			
	L Thoracic Sympathetic Nerve			
	M Abdominal Sympathetic Nerve			
	N Lumbar Sympathetic Nerve			
	P Sacral Sympathetic Nerve			
	Q Sacral Plexus			
	R *Sacral Nerve*			
	Y Peripheral Nerve			

Body Part — Character 4

The body part characters detail the various nerves and structures in the peripheral nervous system.

Figure 15.4: Peripheral Nervous System

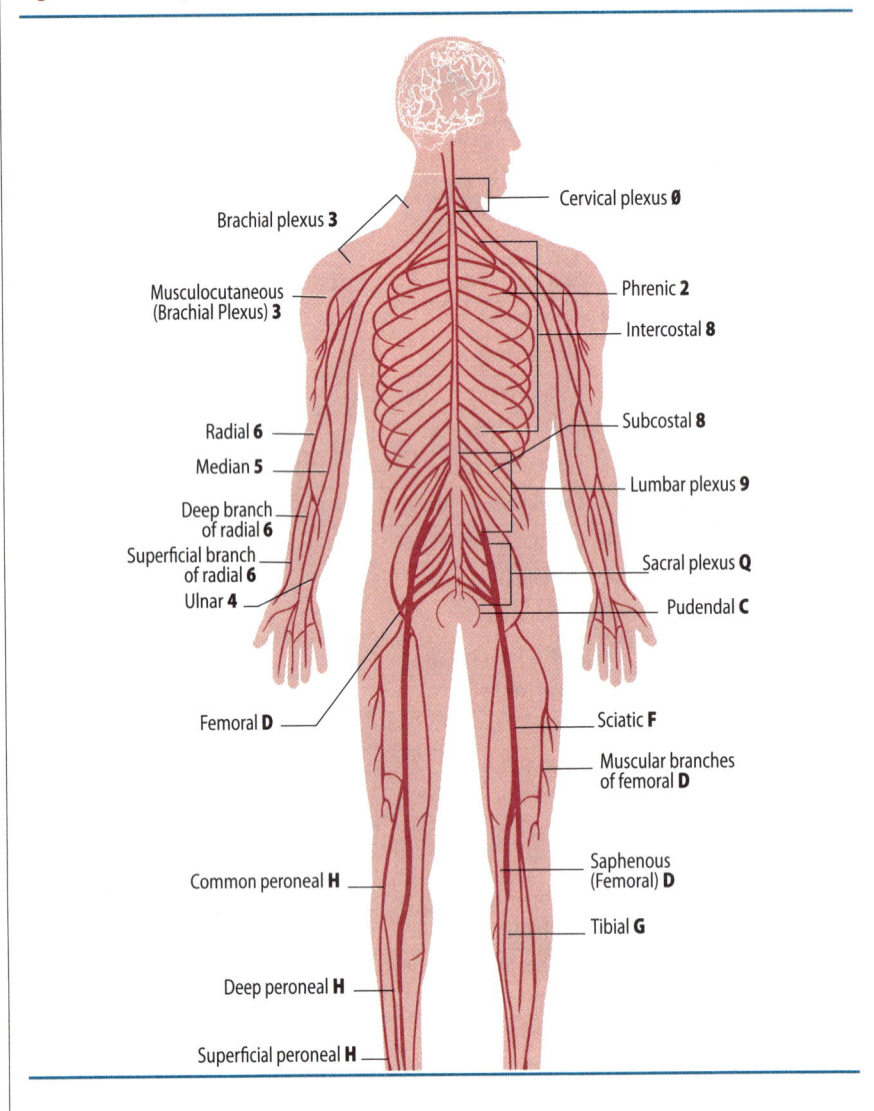

- Cervical plexus **0**
- Brachial plexus **3**
- Musculocutaneous (Brachial Plexus) **3**
- Phrenic **2**
- Intercostal **8**
- Radial **6**
- Median **5**
- Subcostal **8**
- Deep branch of radial **6**
- Lumbar plexus **9**
- Superficial branch of radial **6**
- Sacral plexus **Q**
- Ulnar **4**
- Pudendal **C**
- Femoral **D**
- Sciatic **F**
- Muscular branches of femoral **D**
- Saphenous (Femoral) **D**
- Common peroneal **H**
- Tibial **G**
- Deep peroneal **H**
- Superficial peroneal **H**

Character Value — 0, Cervical Plexus

Associated Terms: Ansa cervicalis, cutaneous (transverse) cervical nerve, great auricular nerve, lesser occipital nerve, supraclavicular nerve, transverse (cutaneous) cervical nerve

The cervical plexus is a network of nerves made up of the first four cervical spinal nerves. There are several branches of nerves that arise from the cervical plexus, including the ansa cervicalis, the cutaneous (transverse) cervical nerve, the great auricular nerve, the lesser occipital nerve, the supraclavicular nerve, and the transverse (cutaneous) cervical nerve.

Character Value — 1, Cervical Nerve

Associated Terms: Greater occipital nerve, spinal nerve—cervical, suboccipital nerve, third occipital nerve

Eight pairs of nerves originate from the spinal cord in the cervical region, known as the cervical nerves. The anterior distribution of nerves includes the greater occipital nerve, the suboccipital nerve, and the third occipital nerve. The posterior distribution includes the cervical and brachial plexuses, which are not considered part of this body part character.

Character Value — 2, Phrenic Nerve

Associated Terms: Accessory phrenic nerve

Phrenic nerves are a pair of branches of the cervical plexus, the main function of which is to serve as the motor nerve to the diaphragm. The accessory phrenic nerve is an additional nerve that may branch from the phrenic nerve itself or from the trigeminal nerve.

Figure 15.5: Brachial Plexus

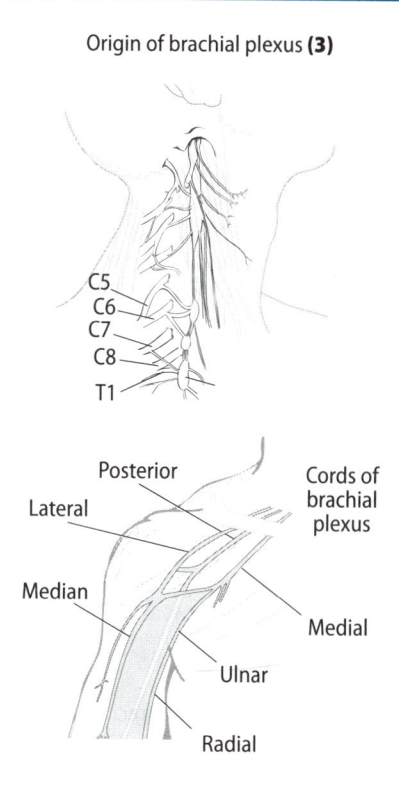

Character Value — 3, Brachial Plexus

Associated Terms: Axillary nerve, dorsal scapular nerve, first intercostal nerve, long thoracic nerve, musculocutaneous nerve, subclavius nerve, suprascapular nerve

The brachial plexus is a network of nerves made up of the cervical spinal nerves C5 through C8, as well as T1. It provides innervation to the upper limbs by breaking off into several different branches. Some of these branches include the axillary nerve, the dorsal scapular nerve, the first intercostal nerve, the long thoracic nerve, the musculocutaneous nerve, the subclavius nerve, and the suprascapular nerve.

Figure 15.6: Median and Ulnar Nerves

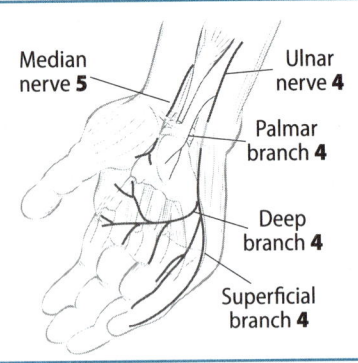

Character Value — 4, Ulnar Nerve

Associated Terms: Cubital nerve

One of the branches of the brachial plexus is the ulnar nerve, which is part of the medial cord of the brachial plexus and runs along the ulna in the forearm. This nerve is sometimes referred to as the cubital nerve because the channel it runs through to travel past the elbow is known as the cubital tunnel.

Character Value — 5, Median Nerve

Associated Terms: Anterior interosseous nerve, palmar cutaneous nerve

The median nerve is another branch of the brachial plexus, extending through the forearm along the radius and into the hand. The purpose of this nerve is to innervate the muscles and skin in these areas. As the median nerve moves through the arm and hand, it breaks into two branches: the anterior interosseous nerve and the palmar cutaneous nerve.

Character Value — 6, Radial Nerve

Associated Terms: Dorsal digital nerve, musculospiral nerve, palmar cutaneous nerve, posterior interosseous nerve

The largest branch of the brachial plexus, the radial nerve travels through the posterior portion of the arm innervating the skin of the arm and forearm, as well as the extensor muscles. The radial nerve has many branches that serve other portions of the upper extremity, such as the dorsal digital nerve, the musculospiral nerve, the palmar cutaneous nerve, and the posterior interosseous nerve.

Character Value — 8, Thoracic Nerve

Associated Terms: Intercostal nerve, intercostobrachial nerve, subcostal nerve, thoracic spinal nerve

Twelve pairs of nerves originate from the spinal cord in the thoracic region, known as thoracic nerves. There are 11 intercostal nerves (T1–T11) that run between the ribs. Some of these intercostal nerves further branch into the intercostal-brachial nerves. There is one subcostal nerve (T12) and it runs below the twelfth rib.

Character Value — 9, Lumbar Plexus

Associated Terms: Accessory obturator nerve, genitofemoral nerve, iliohypogastric nerve, ilioinguinal nerve, lateral femoral cutaneous nerve, obturator nerve, superior gluteal nerve

A large network of intersecting nerves in the abdominal wall, the lumbar plexus serves to innervate much of the lower abdominal area, the pelvic region, and the upper portion of the lower extremities. Nerves that originate in the lumbar plexus include the accessory obturator nerve, the genitofemoral nerve, the iliohypogastric nerve, the ilioinguinal nerve, the lateral femoral cutaneous nerve, and the obturator nerve.

Character Value — B, Lumbar Nerve

Associated Terms: Lumbosacral trunk, spinal nerve—lumbar, superior clunic (cluneal) nerve

Lumbar nerves arise from the lumbar region of the spinal cord. There are five pairs of lumbar nerves, corresponding with the five lumbar vertebrae. The superior cluneal nerves are the branches from L1, L2, and L3, which innervate the skin on the upper part of the buttocks. The smallest part of the nerve branch from L4 and the nerve from L5 combine to form the lumbosacral trunk. This joins the lumbar plexus and the sacral plexus together to create the **lumbosacral plexus.**

Character Value — C, Pudendal Nerve

Associated Terms: Posterior labial nerve, posterior scrotal nerve

Arising from the sacral plexus, the pudendal nerve provides innervation for the external genitalia, as well as many other muscles in the pelvic region. The posterior labial nerve and posterior scrotal nerves are branches that arise from the pudendal nerve.

Character Value — D, Femoral Nerve

Associated Terms: Anterior crural nerve, saphenous nerve

Starting from the lumbar plexus, the femoral nerve is the largest and main nerve in the anterior thigh. Also referred to as the anterior crural nerve, the femoral nerve does have branches, one of which is the saphenous nerve.

Character Value — F, Sciatic Nerve

Associated Terms: Ischiatic nerve

The sciatic nerve, also known as the ischiatic nerve, originates from the sacral plexus and extends through the entire lower extremity to the foot. It has numerous branches throughout the leg.

Character Value — G, Tibial Nerve

Associated Terms: Lateral plantar nerve, medial plantar nerve, medial popliteal nerve, medial sural cutaneous nerve

A branch of the sciatic nerve, the tibial nerve and its branches function to innervate much of the lower leg and foot. Some of the branches include the lateral plantar nerve, the medial plantar nerve, the medial popliteal nerve, and the medial sural cutaneous nerve.

Character Value — H, Peroneal Nerve

Associated Terms: Common fibular nerve, common peroneal nerve, external popliteal nerve, lateral sural cutaneous nerve

Originating from the sciatic nerve, the peroneal nerve, also known as the common fibular nerve, the common peroneal nerve, or the external popliteal nerve, provides innervation to the skin of leg through two of its branches. These branches are known as the lateral sural cutaneous nerve and the sural communicating nerve.

DEFINITIONS

lumbosacral plexus. Area where the anterior divisions of the lumbar, sacral, and coccygeal nerves meet.

Figure 15.7: Sympathetic Nervous System

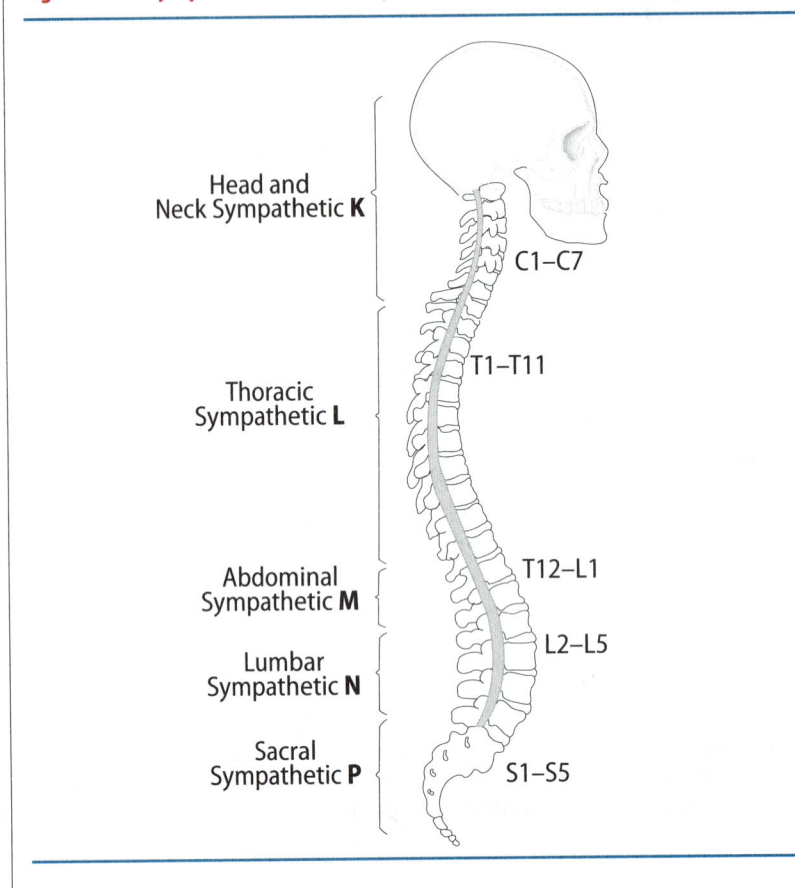

- Head and Neck Sympathetic **K** — C1–C7
- Thoracic Sympathetic **L** — T1–T11
- Abdominal Sympathetic **M** — T12–L1
- Lumbar Sympathetic **N** — L2–L5
- Sacral Sympathetic **P** — S1–S5

Character Value — K, Head and Neck Sympathetic Nerve

Associated Terms: Cavernous plexus, cervical ganglion, ciliary ganglion, internal carotid plexus, otic ganglion, pterygopalatine (sphenopalatine) ganglion, sphenopalatine (pterygopalatine) ganglion, stellate ganglion, submandibular ganglion, submaxillary ganglion

The autonomic nervous system is the part of the peripheral nervous system that controls the involuntary body systems, such as heart activity, the glands, and the smooth muscles. The cavernous plexus and internal carotid plexus, as well as the otic ganglion, the pterygopalatine (sphenopalatine) ganglion, the stellate ganglion, the submandibular ganglion, and the submaxillary ganglion, are part of the head and neck portion of the sympathetic nervous system.

Character Value — L, Thoracic Sympathetic Nerve

Associated Terms: Cardiac plexus, esophageal plexus, greater splanchnic nerve, inferior cardiac nerve, least splanchnic nerve, lesser splanchnic nerve, middle cardiac nerve, pulmonary plexus, superior cardiac nerve, thoracic aortic plexus, thoracic ganglion

Nerves that may be considered a part of the sympathetic nervous system at the thoracic level are the greater splanchnic nerve, the inferior cardiac nerve, the least splanchnic nerve, the lesser splanchnic nerve, the middle cardiac nerve, and the superior cardiac nerve. Important networks of intersecting nerves are the cardiac plexus, the pulmonary plexus, and the thoracic artery plexus. The thoracic ganglia are bundles of nerve fibers along the sympathetic trunk in the abdominal area.

Character Value — M, Abdominal Sympathetic Nerve

Associated Terms: Abdominal aortic plexus, Auerbach's (myenteric) plexus, celiac ganglion, celiac (solar) plexus, gastric plexus, hepatic plexus, inferior hypogastric plexus, inferior mesenteric ganglion, inferior mesenteric plexus, Meissner's (submucous) plexus, myenteric (Auerbach's) plexus, pancreatic plexus, pelvic splanchnic nerve, renal plexus, solar (celiac) plexus, splenic plexus, submucous (Meissner's) plexus, superior hypogastric plexus, superior mesenteric ganglion, superior mesenteric plexus, suprarenal plexus

Important networks of intersecting nerves in the abdominal sympathetic trunk include the abdominal aortic plexus, Auerbach's (myenteric) plexus, the celiac (solar) plexus, the gastric plexus, the hepatic plexus, the inferior hypogastric plexus, the inferior mesenteric plexus, Meissner's (submucous) plexus, the pancreatic plexus, the renal plexus, the splenic plexus, the superior hypogastric plexus, the superior mesenteric plexus, and the suprarenal plexus. The pelvic splanchnic nerve provides parasympathetic innervation to the hindgut. Additional nerve fiber bundles along the abdominal sympathetic trunk include the celiac ganglion, the inferior mesenteric ganglion, and the superior mesenteric ganglion.

Character Value — N, Lumbar Sympathetic Nerve

Associated Terms: Lumbar ganglion, lumbar splanchnic nerve

Lumbar ganglia along the lumbar sympathetic trunk give rise to the lumbar splanchnic nerves. These nerves innervate the glands and smooth muscle of the pelvic region.

Character Value — P, Sacral Sympathetic Nerve

Associated Terms: Ganglion impar (ganglion of Walther), pelvic splanchnic nerve, sacral ganglion, sacral splanchnic nerve

Sacral splanchnic nerves originate from the sacral ganglia along the sympathetic trunk, and their role is to provide innervation to the autonomic functions of the pelvic organs and muscles. Pelvic splanchnic nerves branch from the spinal nerves S2, S3, and S4, and their role is similar, providing innervation to the parasympathetic functions in the pelvis and genital organs. The ganglion impar is a small ganglion on the front of the coccyx.

Character Value — Q, Sacral Plexus

Associated Terms: Inferior gluteal nerve, posterior femoral cutaneous nerve, pudendal nerve

This group includes a large network of intersecting nerves from the fourth and fifth lumbar vertebrae and the first, second, and third sacral vertebrae. Nerves that originate in the sacral plexus include the inferior gluteal nerve, the posterior femoral cutaneous nerve, and the pudendal nerve.

Qualifier — Character 7

Like the central nervous system, the peripheral nervous system provides values for the 7th character for nerve transfer procedures. The body part found in the qualifier character represents the destination of the nerve grafting services. Nerve transfer characters are provided for nerves such as cervical, phrenic, ulnar, median, lumbar, femoral, tibial, etc. It is important for coders to understand the location of these nerves and how they relate to their corresponding body part values in character 4.

Representative ICD-10-PCS Code Examples

1. **Endoscopic transfer, median to ulnar nerve**

   01X54Z4   Transfer median nerve to ulnar nerve, percutaneous endoscopic approach

   Note: This PCS code is very specific, detailing the transfer procedure, with the nerve being transferred from represented by the 4th character body part and the nerve being transferred to represented by the 7th character qualifier. The specific approach is indicated as well, further differentiating the procedure.

2. **Open carpal tunnel release**

   01N50ZZ   Release median nerve, open approach

   Note: In order to assign the code for this procedure appropriately in ICD-10-PCS, the coder must know that a carpal tunnel release involves the median nerve.

3. **Suture repair of left posterior interosseous nerve laceration**

   01Q60ZZ   Repair of radial nerve, open approach

   Note: The Body Part Key provides instruction to use radial nerve for posterior interosseous nerve. The approach value is open, even though the surgical exposure may have been created by the wound itself.

4. **Open removal of lumbar sympathetic neurostimulator lead**

   01PY0MZ   Removal of neurostimulator lead device from peripheral nerve, open approach

   Note: The root operation removal can only be used for devices, not body parts. The only body part choice available in the removal table in the peripheral nervous system is ***peripheral nerve***. The sixth character M indicates that the neurostimulator lead is the type of device.

DEFINITIONS

peripheral nerves. Cord-like structures that contain nerve fibers that carry information from peripheral regions of the body to the spinal cord and back.

CODING AXIOM

ICD-10-PCS Official Coding Guideline—Root Operation B3.13: In the root operation release, the body part value coded is the body part being freed and not the tissue being manipulated or cut to free the body part.

Heart and Great Vessels (2)

Procedures included in the heart and great vessels body system section include coronary artery bypass surgery and pacemaker and automated implantable cardioverter-defibrillator implantations. It is important to note exactly where in the heart or vessels the procedure is performed, as there are several different body part characters, and even different body system characters depending on the anatomy. A compiled table for body system character 2 Heart and great vessels, provides all of the valid characters for that system in ICD-10-PCS.

> **DEFINITIONS**
>
> **papillary muscle.** One of the rounded muscles attached to the chordae tendinae that help to open and close the valves of the heart.

Operation–Character 3	Body Part–Character 4	Approach–Character 5	Device–Character 6	Qualifier–Character 7
1 Bypass	0 Coronary Artery, One Site	0 Open	0 Monitoring Device, Pressure Sensor	0 Allogeneic
5 Destruction	1 Coronary Artery, Two Sites	3 Percutaneous	2 Monitoring Device	1 Syngeneic
7 Dilation	2 Coronary Artery, Three Sites	4 Percutaneous Endoscopic	3 Infusion Device	2 Zooplastic
8 Division	3 Coronary Artery, Four or More Sites	X External	4 Intraluminal Device, Drug-eluting	3 Coronary Artery
B Excision	4 Coronary Vein		7 Autologous Tissue Substitute	4 Coronary Vein
C Extirpation	5 Atrial Septum		8 Zooplastic Tissue	5 Coronary Circulation
F Fragmentation	6 Atrium, Right		9 Autologous Venous Tissue	6 Bifurcation
H Insertion	7 Atrium, Left		A Autologous Arterial Tissue	7 Atrium, Left
J Inspection	8 Conduction Mechanism		C Extraluminal Device	8 Internal Mammary, Right
K Map	9 Chordae Tendineae		D Intraluminal Device	9 Internal Mammary, Left
L Occlusion	A Heart		J Synthetic Substitute OR Cardiac Lead, Pacemaker (for root operation INSERTION only)	B Subclavian
N Release	B Heart, Right		K Nonautologous Tissue Substitute OR Cardiac Lead, Defibrillator (for root operation INSERTION only)	C Thoracic Artery
P Removal	C Heart, Left		M Cardiac Lead	D Carotid
Q Repair	D *Papillary Muscle*		Q Implantable Heart Assist System	F Abdominal Artery
R Replacement	F Aortic Valve		R External Heart Assist System	H Transapical
S Reposition	G Mitral Valve		T Intraluminal Device, Radioactive	K Left Atrial Appendage
T Resection	H Pulmonary Valve		Z No Device	P Pulmonary Trunk
U Supplement	J Tricuspid Valve			Q Pulmonary Artery, Right
V Restriction	K Ventricle, Right			R Pulmonary Artery, Left
W Revision	L Ventricle, Left			S Biventricular
Y Transplantation	M Ventricular Septum			T Ductus Arteriosus
	N Pericardium			W Aorta
	P Pulmonary Trunk			X Diagnostic
	Q Pulmonary Artery, Right			Z No Qualifier
	R Pulmonary Artery, Left			
	S Pulmonary Vein, Right			
	T Pulmonary Vein, Left			
	V Superior Vena Cava			
	W Thoracic Aorta			
	Y Great Vessel			

© 2015 Optum360, LLC

Comprehensive Anatomy and Physiology for ICD-10-CM and ICD-10-PCS Coding

📖 **DEFINITIONS**

great vessel. Any of the large vessels entering and leaving the heart, such as the aorta, the superior or inferior vena cava, or the pulmonary arteries or veins.

Body Part — Character 4

The body part character in the heart and great vessels section details the various structures in the heart, as well as provides a listing for many of the **great vessels**. Each character is not reviewed in detail, as some are self-explanatory or have great detail provided in the ICD-10-CM anatomy and physiology section. See chapter 7 for additional information on the anatomy of the heart and great vessels.

Figure 15.8: Coronary Arteries

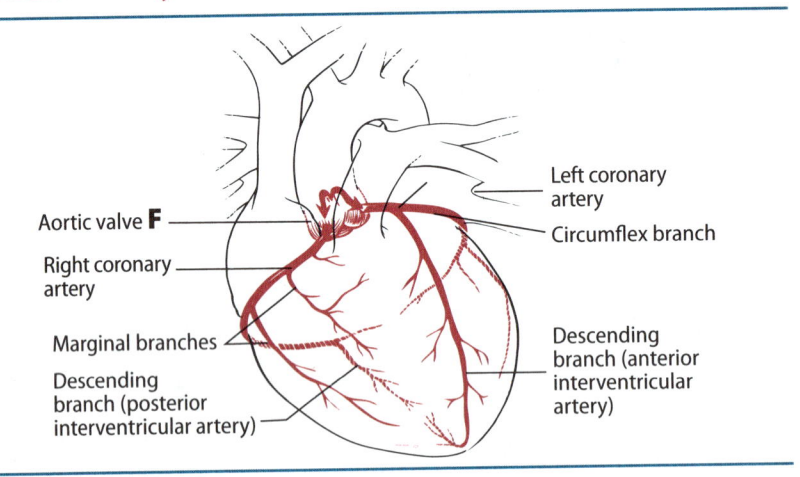

Labels: Aortic valve **F**, Right coronary artery, Marginal branches, Descending branch (posterior interventricular artery), Left coronary artery, Circumflex branch, Descending branch (anterior interventricular artery)

Character Value — 0, Coronary Artery, One Site

Character Value — 1, Coronary Artery, Two Sites

Character Value — 2, Coronary Artery, Three Sites

Character Value — 3, Coronary Artery, Four or More Sites

These body part characters are typically used in conjunction with coronary artery bypass procedures to describe the number of sites being grafted, as well as other procedures performed on the coronary arteries. Be aware there are specific coding guidelines in ICD-10-PCS regarding the use of these characters.

🕯 **CODING AXIOM**

ICD-10-PCS Official Coding Guideline—Root Operation B3.6b: Coronary arteries are classified by number of distinct sites treated, rather than number of coronary arteries or anatomic name of a coronary artery (e.g., left anterior descending). Coronary artery bypass procedures are coded differently than other bypass procedures (see Guideline B3.6a). Rather than identifying the body part bypassed from, the body part identifies the number of coronary artery sites bypassed to, and the qualifier specifies the vessel bypassed from.

Example: Aortocoronary artery bypass of one site on the left anterior descending coronary artery and one site on the obtuse marginal coronary artery is classified in the body part axis of classification as two coronary artery sites and the qualifier specifies the aorta as the body part bypassed from.

Figure 15.9: Heart Anatomy

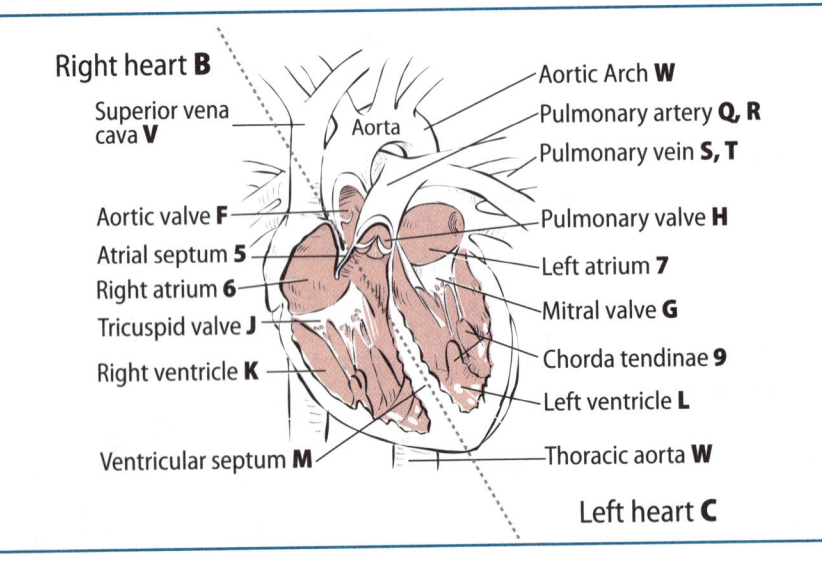

Labels: Right heart **B**, Superior vena cava **V**, Aorta, Aortic valve **F**, Atrial septum **5**, Right atrium **6**, Tricuspid valve **J**, Right ventricle **K**, Ventricular septum **M**, Aortic Arch **W**, Pulmonary artery **Q, R**, Pulmonary vein **S, T**, Pulmonary valve **H**, Left atrium **7**, Mitral valve **G**, Chorda tendinae **9**, Left ventricle **L**, Thoracic aorta **W**, Left heart **C**

Character Value — 5, Atrial Septum

Associated Terms: Interatrial septum

The atrial septum, also known as the interatrial septum, is the partition of tissue between the left and the right atria of the heart.

Character Value — 6, Atrium, Right

Associated Terms: Atrium dextrum cordis, right auricular appendix, sinus venosus

Deoxygenated blood is transported by the vessels to the right atrium of the heart, also known as the atrium dextrum cordis. The sinus venosus is part of the embryonic heart that becomes part of the right atrium as the embryo develops. The right auricular appendix is a small pouch of muscle attached to the right atrium of the heart.

Character Value — 7, Atrium, Left

Associated Terms: Atrium pulmonale, left auricular appendix

Oxygenated blood is received by the left atrium, also known as atrium pulmonale, from the pulmonary veins. The left auricular appendix is a small pouch of muscle attached to the left atrium of the heart.

Character Value — 8, Conduction Mechanism

Associated Terms: Atrioventricular node, bundle of HIS, bundle of Kent, sinoatrial node

Electrical conduction of the heart begins in the sinoatrial (SA) node in the right atrium. The SA node is known as the "pacemaker" of the conduction mechanism. The electrical impulse travels through the atria to the atrioventricular (AV) node. From there, it travels to the bundle of HIS, and then along to the remainder of the conduction pathway. The bundle of Kent is an abnormal conduction pathway seen in patients with Wolff-Parkinson-White syndrome.

Character Value—9, Chordae Tendineae

The chordae tendineae are tendinous chords attached to the cusps of the mitral and tricuspid valves of the heart that attach the valves to the papillary muscles of the ventricles.

Character Value — B, Heart, Right

Associated Terms: Right coronary sulcus

The right heart consists of the anatomy on the right side of the heart, including the right atrium and ventricle. The right coronary sulcus is the surface groove that separates the right atrium from the right ventricle.

Character Value — C, Heart, Left

Associated Terms: Left coronary sulcus, obtuse margin

The left heart includes the anatomy on the left side of the heart, such as the left atrium and ventricle, as well as the left coronary sulcus. The obtuse margin, or the left margin of the heart, is formed by the **left ventricle** and atrium, and is shorter than the right border of the heart.

Character Value — F, Aortic Valve

Associated Terms: Aortic annulus

Blood flows between the left ventricle and the aorta through the aortic valve. The aortic annulus attaches the aortic root to the left ventricle. The annulus is a ring-shaped portion of fibrous tissue.

DEFINITIONS

left ventricle. Responsible for pumping blood back through the aorta and therefore through the body.

Comprehensive Anatomy and Physiology for ICD-10-CM and ICD-10-PCS Coding

Character Value — G, Mitral Valve

Associated Terms: Bicuspid valve, left atrioventricular valve, mitral annulus

The mitral valve, also known as the left atrioventricular valve, is a bicuspid valve through which blood flows from the left atrium to the left ventricle. The mitral annulus is a fibrous ring that is attached to the mitral valve cusps to assist in complete closure of the valve.

Character Value — H, Pulmonary Valve

Associated Terms: Pulmonary annulus, pulmonic valve

Blood flows from the right ventricle into the pulmonary artery through the pulmonary valve, also known as the pulmonic valve. This blood then goes to the lungs to be re-oxygenated. The pulmonary annuli are ring-shaped fibrous tissue structures around the pulmonary valve.

Character Value — J, Tricuspid Valve

Associated Terms: Right atrioventricular valve, tricuspid annulus

Blood flows from the right atrium to the right ventricle through the tricuspid valve, also known as the right atrioventricular valve. The tricuspid annulus is a ring-shaped fibrous tissue structure around the tricuspid valve.

Character Value — K, Ventricle, Right

Associated Terms: Conus arteriosus

Deoxygenated blood travels from the right atrium to the right ventricle via the tricuspid valve. The conus arteriosus is a pouch in the upper left of the right ventricle of the embryonic heart from which the **pulmonary trunk** is formed.

Character Value — M, Ventricular septum

Associated Terms: Interventricular septum

A ventricular septum, also known as an interventricular septum, is the partition of tissue between the left and right ventricles of the heart.

Character Value — Q, Pulmonary Artery, Right

Character Value — R, Pulmonary Artery, Left

Associated Terms: Arterial canal (duct), Botallo's duct, pulmoaortic canal

The right pulmonary artery supplies the right lung, and the left pulmonary artery supplies the left lung with oxygenated blood to function properly. In a developing fetus, there are several vessels that develop into various portions of the pulmonary arterial system. The arterial canal (duct), Botallo's duct, and the pulmoaortic canal are all terms associated with embryonic vessel development.

Character Value — S, Pulmonary Vein, Right

Character Value — T, Pulmonary Vein, Left

Associated Terms: Left inferior pulmonary vein, left superior pulmonary vein, right inferior pulmonary vein, right superior pulmonary vein

The right pulmonary vein carries oxygenated blood from the right side of the lung back to the heart. It branches into both the right inferior pulmonary vein and the right superior pulmonary vein. The left pulmonary vein carries oxygenated blood from the left side of the lung back to the heart. It branches into both the left inferior pulmonary vein and the left superior pulmonary vein.

DEFINITIONS

pulmonary trunk. Short wide vessel that moves deoxygenated blood from the heart directly to the lungs.

Character Value — V, Superior Vena Cava

Associated Terms: Precava

Returning deoxygenated blood from the entire upper half of the body to the right atrium, the superior vena cava is the second largest vein in the body. It is also known as the precava or SVC.

Character Value — W, Thoracic Aorta

Associated Terms: Aortic arch, aortic intercostal artery, ascending aorta, bronchial artery, esophageal artery, subcostal artery

Supplying blood to many parts of the body, the thoracic aorta has many sections as well as branches. The ascending aorta comes out of the left ventricle, and then the aortic arch continues further down with the remainder of the thoracic aorta. Branches from the thoracic aorta include the aortic intercostal artery, the bronchial artery, the esophageal artery, and the subcostal artery.

Device — Character 6

The heart and great vessels section of PCS contains many values for device character 6, including those related to cardiac pacemakers, defibrillators and associated leads, monitoring devices, intraluminal stents, as well as various types of tissue used to assist in the performance of these procedures. Coders should be familiar with the different types of cardiac devices on the market today and also aware of the PCS definitions related to the devices and tissues represented by this character.

Qualifier — Character 7

The 7th character represents the destination of bypass procedures for the heart and great vessels body system, and it is important to note the difference between this and the 4th character root operation. For the root operation bypass, the 4th character body part provides values for the number of sites within the coronary arteries that are bypassed, including one site, two sites, three sites, and four or more sites. For those body part values, the corresponding 7th character represents the vessel bypassed from, for example, aorta, internal mammary artery, and abdominal artery. Other significant 7th character values include left atrial appendage for destruction, excision, and occlusion procedures. The 7th character also differentiates the sources used for heart transplant procedures, such as allogeneic (tissue from the same species), syngeneic (tissue with identical genes), or zooplastic (from another species).

Representative ICD-10-PCS Code Examples

1. **Coronary artery bypass graft X 2 (with saphenous vein graft), one aorta to LAD, one left internal mammary artery bypass, open approach**

   021009W Bypass coronary artery, one site from aorta with autologous venous tissue, open approach

   0210099 Bypass coronary artery, one site from left internal mammary with autologous venous tissue, open approach

   Note: Code separately excision of saphenous vein graft.

2. **Heart transplant, utilizing porcine heart**

   02YA0Z2 Transplantation of heart, zooplastic, open approach

3. **PTCA of the LAD and RCA both with drug-eluting stents**

   027134Z Dilation of coronary artery, two sites, with drug-eluting intraluminal device, percutaneous approach

4. **Heart catheterization with cardiac mapping**

   02K83ZZ Map Conduction Mechanism, percutaneous approach

   Note: The table for the root operation map only has one choice for body part: Conduction mechanism.

> **CODING AXIOM**
>
> **ICD-10-PCS Official Coding Guideline—Body Part B4.4:** The coronary arteries are classified as a single body part that is further specified by number of sites treated and not by name or number of arteries. Separate body part values are used to specify the number of sites treated when the same procedure is performed on multiple sites in the coronary arteries.
>
> *Example:* Angioplasty of two distinct sites in the left anterior descending coronary artery with placement of two stents is coded as dilation of coronary arteries, two sites, with intraluminal device.
>
> Angioplasty of two distinct sites in the left anterior descending coronary artery, one with stent placed and one without, is coded separately as dilation of coronary artery, one site with intraluminal device, and dilation of coronary artery, one site with no device.

5. **Percutaneous placement of PICC (peripherally inserted central catheter) into the cephalic vein and threaded to the superior vena cava**

    02HV33Z Insertion of infusion device into superior vena cava, percutaneous approach

    Note: The correct body part character for coding central venous catheters is determined by where the tip of the device ultimately resides, not the insertion point.

Upper Arteries (3)

Procedures involving the upper arteries, such as a carotid endarterectomy, bypasses of various upper arteries, and thrombectomies, are commonly seen throughout this body system section. When making character value assignments, pay close attention to the laterality, as it is used in more than one character section of the code. A compiled table for body system character 3 Upper arteries, shows all of the valid characters for that system in ICD-10-PCS.

> **DEFINITIONS**
>
> **common carotid artery.** Artery that supplies the head and neck with oxygenated blood; it divides in the neck to form the external and internal carotid arteries.

Operation–Character 3	Body Part–Character 4	Approach–Character 5	Device–Character 6	Qualifier–Character 7
1 Bypass	0 Internal Mammary Artery, Right	0 Open	0 Drainage Device	0 Upper Arm Artery, Right
5 Destruction	1 Internal Mammary Artery, Left	3 Percutaneous	2 Monitoring Device	1 Upper Arm Artery, Left
7 Dilation	2 Innominate Artery	4 Percutaneous Endoscopic	3 Infusion Device	2 Upper Arm Artery, Bilateral
9 Drainage	3 Subclavian Artery, Right	X External	4 Intraluminal Device, Drug-eluting	3 Lower Arm Artery, Right
B Excision	4 Subclavian Artery, Left		7 Autologous Tissue Substitute	4 Lower Arm Artery, Left
C Extirpation	5 Axillary Artery, Right		9 Autologous Venous Tissue	5 Lower Arm Artery, Bilateral
H Insertion	6 Axillary Artery, Left		A Autologous Arterial Tissue	6 Upper Leg Artery, Right
J Inspection	7 Brachial Artery, Right		B Intraluminal Device, Bioactive	7 Upper Leg Artery, Left
L Occlusion	8 Brachial Artery, Left		C Extraluminal Device	8 Upper Leg Artery, Bilateral
N Release	9 Ulnar Artery, Right		D Intraluminal Device	9 Lower Leg Artery, Right
P Removal	A Ulnar Artery, Left		J Synthetic Substitute	B Lower Leg Artery, Left
Q Repair	B Radial Artery, Right		K Nonautologous Tissue Substitute	C Lower Leg Artery, Bilateral
R Replacement	C Radial Artery, Left		M Stimulator Lead	D Upper Arm Vein
S Reposition	D Hand Artery, Right		Z No Device	F Lower Arm Vein
U Supplement	F Hand Artery, Left			G Intracranial Artery
V Restriction	G Intracranial Artery			J Extracranial Artery, Right
W Revision	H **Common Carotid Artery**, Right			K Extracranial Artery, Left
	J Common Carotid Artery, Left			M Pulmonary Artery, Right
	K Internal Carotid Artery, Right			N Pulmonary Artery, Left
	L Internal Carotid Artery, Left			X Diagnostic
	M External Carotid Artery, Right			Z No Qualifier
	N External Carotid Artery, Left			
	P Vertebral Artery, Right			
	Q Vertebral Artery, Left			
	R Face Artery			
	S Temporal Artery, Right			
	T Temporal Artery, Left			
	U Thyroid Artery, Right			
	V Thyroid Artery, Left			
	Y Upper Artery			

Body Part — Character 4

The body part characters in the upper arteries detail the various arteries in the upper body (above the diaphragm), stemming from the aorta.

Figure 15.10: Map of Upper Arteries

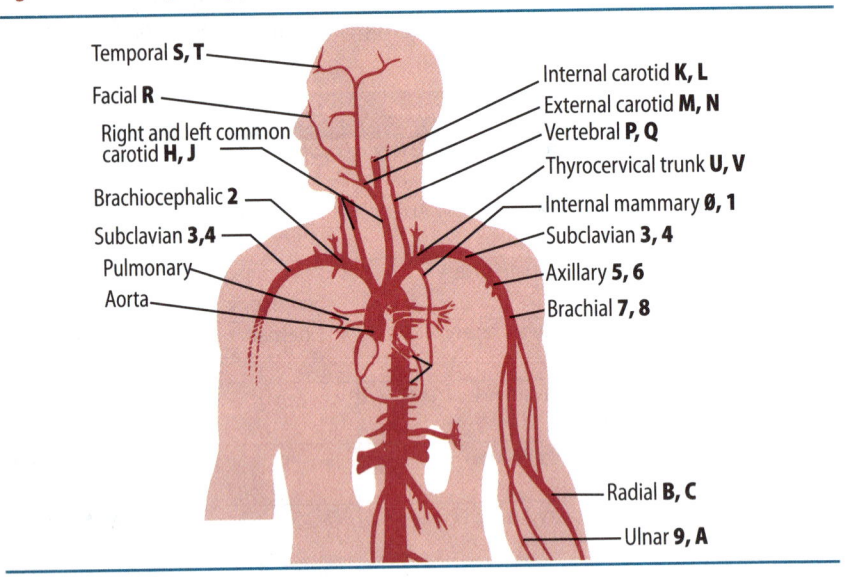

Temporal **S, T**
Facial **R**
Right and left common carotid **H, J**
Brachiocephalic **2**
Subclavian **3, 4**
Pulmonary
Aorta
Internal carotid **K, L**
External carotid **M, N**
Vertebral **P, Q**
Thyrocervical trunk **U, V**
Internal mammary **Ø, 1**
Subclavian **3, 4**
Axillary **5, 6**
Brachial **7, 8**
Radial **B, C**
Ulnar **9, A**

DEFINITIONS

pericardium. Thin and slippery case in which the heart lies that is lined with fluid so that the heart is free to pulse and move as it beats.

Character Value — Ø, 1, Internal Mammary Artery, Left & Right

Associated Terms: Anterior intercostal artery, internal thoracic artery, musculophrenic artery, pericardiophrenic artery, superior epigastric artery

Also called the internal thoracic arteries, the internal mammary arteries supply blood to the pectoral muscles, the breasts, the **pericardium**, and the abdominal muscles. They break into several branches, some of which are the anterior intercostal artery, the musculophrenic artery, the pericardiophrenic artery, and the superior epigastric artery.

Character Value — 2, Innominate Artery

Associated Terms: Brachiocephalic artery, brachiocephalic trunk

The innominate artery, also known as the brachiocephalic artery or the brachiocephalic trunk, branches directly off the arch of the aorta and supplies blood to the head and neck, as well as the right arm.

Character Value — 3, 4, Subclavian Artery, Left & Right

Associated Terms: Costocervical trunk, dorsal scapular artery, internal thoracic artery

Although they stem from different locations, the left and right subclavian arteries both branch into six similar vessels whose purpose is to supply blood to the ear, the vertebral column, the spinal cord, and the brain. Some of the branches include the costocervical trunk and the dorsal scapular artery.

Character Value — 5, 6, Axillary Artery, Left & Right

Associated Terms: Anterior circumflex humeral artery, lateral thoracic artery, posterior circumflex humeral artery, subscapular artery, superior thoracic artery, thoracoacromial artery

Continuations of the subclavian arteries, the left and right axillary arteries become the brachial artery after passing through the axillary area. Prior to becoming the brachial artery, several branches separate, including the anterior circumflex humeral artery, the lateral thoracic artery, the posterior circumflex humeral artery, the subscapular artery, the superior thoracic artery, and the thoracoacromial artery.

Character Value — 7, 8, Brachial Artery, Left & Right

Associated Terms: Inferior ulnar collateral artery, profunda brachii, superior ulnar collateral artery

After continuing on from the axillary arteries, the left and right brachial arteries continue down the upper arm, branching into the inferior ulnar collateral artery, the profunda brachii, and the superior ulnar collateral artery. Finally, the brachial artery ends at a bifurcation into the radial and ulnar arteries.

Character Value — 9, A, Ulnar Artery, Left & Right

Associated Terms: Anterior ulnar recurrent artery, common interosseous artery, posterior ulnar recurrent artery

A terminal branch from the brachial artery, the left and right ulnar arteries supply blood to the muscles in the forearm, wrist, and hand. They have several branches, including the anterior ulnar recurrent artery, the common interosseous artery, and the posterior ulnar recurrent artery.

Character Value — B, C, Radial Artery, Left & Right

Associated Terms: Radial recurrent artery

Also a terminal branch from the brachial artery, the left and right radial arteries supply blood to the forearm, wrist, and hand. There are many branches to the radial arteries, including the radial recurrent artery, which supplies blood to the arm and elbow.

Character Value — D, F, Hand Artery, Left & Right

Associated Terms: Deep palmar arch, princeps pollicis artery, radialis indicis, superficial palmar arch

The radial and ulnar arteries run into the hand and combine to make the deep palmar arch and the superficial palmar arch. The princeps pollicis artery and the radialis indicis branch off the radial artery in the hand.

Figure 15.11: Cerebrovascular Arteries

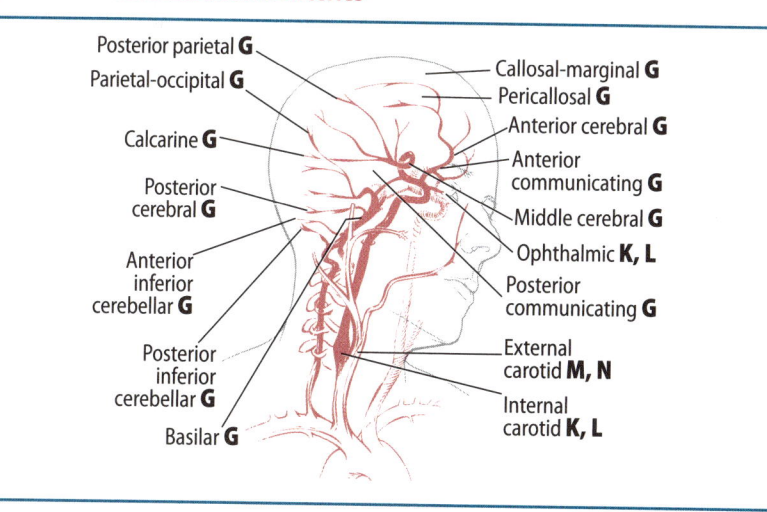

Figure 15.12: Circle of Willis

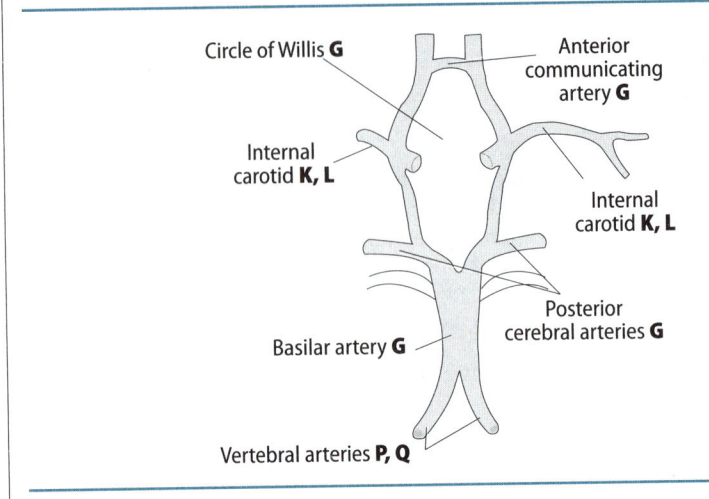

- Circle of Willis **G**
- Anterior communicating artery **G**
- Internal carotid **K, L**
- Internal carotid **K, L**
- Basilar artery **G**
- Posterior cerebral arteries **G**
- Vertebral arteries **P, Q**

Character Value — G, Intracranial Artery

Associated Terms: Anterior cerebral artery, anterior choroidal artery, anterior communicating artery, basilar artery, Circle of Willis, middle cerebral artery, posterior cerebral artery, posterior communicating artery, posterior inferior cerebellar artery (PICA)

Several arteries are considered intracranial arteries, and it is important for coders to be aware of the terminology used to describe these vessels. Terms such as anterior cerebral artery, anterior choroidal artery, anterior communicating artery, basilar artery, middle cerebral artery, posterior cerebral artery, posterior communicating artery, and posterior inferior cerebellar artery (PICA) may all be used to describe the arteries in the intracranial character set. The term Circle of Willis may be used, but be aware that not all elements of the Circle of Willis are contained in the intracranial artery set. Examine the documentation closely to determine which vessels the procedure involves.

Character Value — K, L, Internal Carotid Artery, Left & Right

Associated Terms: Caroticotympanic artery, carotid sinus, ophthalmic artery

On each side of the head and neck, the internal carotid arteries supply the brain with blood. They have several branches, some of which are the caroticotympanic artery, the carotid sinus, and the ophthalmic artery.

Figure 15.13: External Carotid

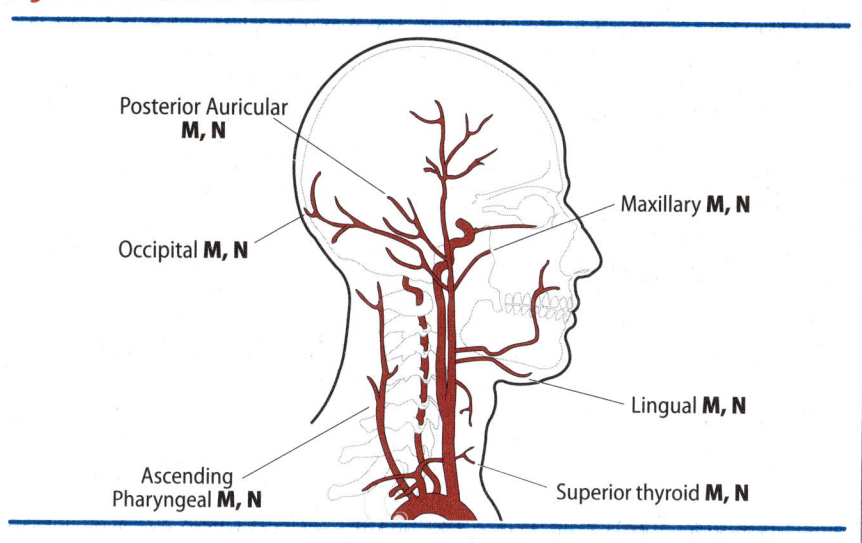

Posterior Auricular **M, N**
Occipital **M, N**
Ascending Pharyngeal **M, N**
Maxillary **M, N**
Lingual **M, N**
Superior thyroid **M, N**

Character Value — M, N, External Carotid Artery, Left & Right

Associated Terms: Ascending pharyngeal artery, internal maxillary artery, lingual artery, maxillary artery, occipital artery, posterior auricular artery, superior thyroid artery

The external carotid artery travels up the side of the head and neck and branches into several different smaller order vessels, including the ascending pharyngeal artery, the internal maxillary artery, the lingual artery, the maxillary artery, the occipital artery, the posterior auricular artery, and the superior thyroid artery.

Character Value — P, Q, Vertebral Artery, Left & Right

Associated Terms: Anterior spinal artery, posterior spinal artery

Branching from the subclavian arteries, the left and right vertebral arteries supply blood to the deep neck muscles, the spinal cord and membranes, and the cerebellum. They branch and eventually form the anterior spinal artery and the posterior spinal artery.

Character Value — R, Face Artery

Associated Terms: Angular artery, ascending palatine artery, external maxillary artery, facial artery, inferior labial artery, submental artery, superior labial artery

The facial artery, also known as the external maxillary artery, stems from the external carotid artery and supplies blood to many tissues and structures in the head. It has many branches, some of which include the angular artery, the ascending palatine artery, the inferior labial artery, the submental artery, and the superior labial artery.

Character Value — S, T, Temporal Artery, Left & Right

Associated Terms: Middle temporal artery, superficial temporal artery, transverse facial artery

Temporal arteries, such as the superficial temporal artery and the middle temporal artery, branch off from the external carotid artery and continue on to be one of the major arteries of the head. Branches of the temporal artery include the transverse facial artery.

Character Value — U, V, Thyroid Artery

Associated Terms: Cricothyroid artery, hyoid artery, sternocleidomastoid artery, superior laryngeal artery, superior thyroid artery, thyrocervical trunk

There are two sections of thyroid arteries: those arising from the external carotid and those arising from the subclavian artery. The superior thyroid artery stems from the external carotid artery, and from that vessel branches the cricothyroid artery, the hyoid artery, the sternocleidomastoid artery, and the superior laryngeal artery. The thyrocervical trunk is a branch of the subclavian artery, and divides into the inferior thyroid artery.

Qualifier — Character 7

In the upper arteries body system there are values for the 7th character for arterial bypass procedures. The body part found in the qualifier character represents the destination of the bypass procedure. The 7th character values for the bypass procedures include such sites as upper arm artery, lower leg artery, and extracranial artery, along with designations for laterality (right, left, and bilateral). It is important for coders to understand the location of these body sites and how they relate to their corresponding body part values in character 4.

Representative ICD-10-PCS Code Examples

1. **Percutaneous thrombectomy of arterial portion of dialysis AV graft, right lower arm**

   03CY3ZZ   Extirpation of matter from upper artery, percutaneous approach

   Note: The thrombus material was removed from the artery, meeting the definition of root operation extirpation (e.g., removal of solid matter from a tubular body part).

2. **Endovascular repair of right vertebral artery aneurysm with bioactive embolization coils**

   03VP3BZ   Restriction of right vertebral artery with bioactive intraluminal device, percutaneous approach

   Note: The bioactive coils are threaded through a catheter and coiled up inside the aneurysm cavity, where thrombin and clot formation on the coils prevent rupture of the aneurysmal sac. Since the procedure is performed on the inside of the vessel, the device (6th character) value assigned is B Bioactive Intraluminal Device.

3. **Percutaneous dilation with stenting of middle cerebral artery**

   037G3DZ   Dilation of intracranial artery with intraluminal device, percutaneous approach

   Note: According to the body part key, the middle cerebral artery is an intracranial artery. The root operation dilation is used with the device character—intraluminal device for the stent.

4. **Open, right common carotid endarterectomy**

   03CH0ZZ   Extirpation of matter from right common carotid artery, open approach

Chapter 15. ICD-10-PCS: Nervous and Circulatory Systems

Lower Arteries (4)

The lower arteries body system section includes many of the same types of procedures as the upper arteries section. These vessels originate from the abdominal aorta, and reside in the lower half of the body. A compiled table for body system character 4 Lower arteries, provides all of the valid characters for that system in ICD-10-PCS.

Operation–Character 3	Body Part–Character 4	Approach–Character 5	Device–Character 6	Qualifier–Character 7
1 Bypass	0 Abdominal Aorta	0 Open	0 Drainage Device	0 Abdominal Aorta
5 Destruction	1 Celiac Artery	3 Percutaneous	1 Radioactive Element	1 Celiac Artery
7 Dilation	2 Gastric Artery	4 Percutaneous Endoscopic	2 Monitoring Device	2 Mesenteric Artery
9 Drainage	3 Hepatic Artery	X External	3 Infusion Device	3 Renal Artery, Right
B Excision	4 Splenic Artery		4 Intraluminal Device, Drug-eluting	4 Renal Artery, Left
C Extirpation	5 Superior Mesenteric Artery		7 Autologous Tissue Substitute	5 Renal Artery, Bilateral
H Insertion	6 Colic Artery, Right		9 Autologous Venous Tissue	6 Common Iliac Artery, Right
J Inspection	7 Colic Artery, Left		A Autologous Arterial Tissue	7 Common Iliac Artery, Left
L Occlusion	8 Colic Artery, Middle		C Extraluminal Device	8 Common Iliac Arteries, Bilateral
N Release	9 Renal Artery, Right		D Intraluminal Device	9 Internal Iliac Artery, Right
P Removal	A Renal Artery, Left		J Synthetic Substitute	B Internal Iliac Artery, Left
Q Repair	B Inferior Mesenteric Artery		K Nonautologous Tissue Substitute	C Internal Iliac Arteries, Bilateral
R Replacement	C Common Iliac Artery, Right		Z No Device	D External Iliac Artery, Right
S Reposition	D Common Iliac Artery, Left			F External Iliac Artery, Left
U Supplement	E Internal Iliac Artery, Right			G External Iliac Arteries, Bilateral
V Restriction	F Internal Iliac Artery, Left			H Femoral Artery, Right
W Revision	H External Iliac Artery, Right			J Femoral Artery, Left OR Temporary (for Root Operation RESTRICTION Only)
	J External Iliac Artery, Left			K Femoral Arteries, Bilateral
	K Femoral Artery, Right			L Popliteal Artery
	L Femoral Artery, Left			M Peroneal Artery
	M Popliteal Artery, Right			N Posterior Tibial Artery
	N Popliteal Artery, Left			P Foot Artery
	P Anterior Tibial Artery, Right			Q Lower Extremity Artery
	Q Anterior Tibial Artery, Left			R Lower Artery
	R Posterior Tibial Artery, Right			S Lower Extremity Vein

(Continued on next page)

© 2015 Optum360, LLC

Comprehensive Anatomy and Physiology for ICD-10-CM and ICD-10-PCS Coding

Operation–Character 3	Body Part–Character 4	Approach–Character 5	Device–Character 6	Qualifier–Character 7
(Continued)	S Posterior Tibial Artery, Left			T Uterine Artery, Right
	T Peroneal Artery, Right			U Uterine Artery, Left
	U Peroneal Artery, Left			X Diagnostic
	V Foot Artery, Right			Z No Qualifier
	W Foot Artery, Left			
	Y Lower Artery			

Body Part — Character 4

The body part characters that fall within the lower arteries detail the various arteries in the lower body, stemming from the abdominal aorta as mentioned previously.

Figure 15.14: Lower Arteries

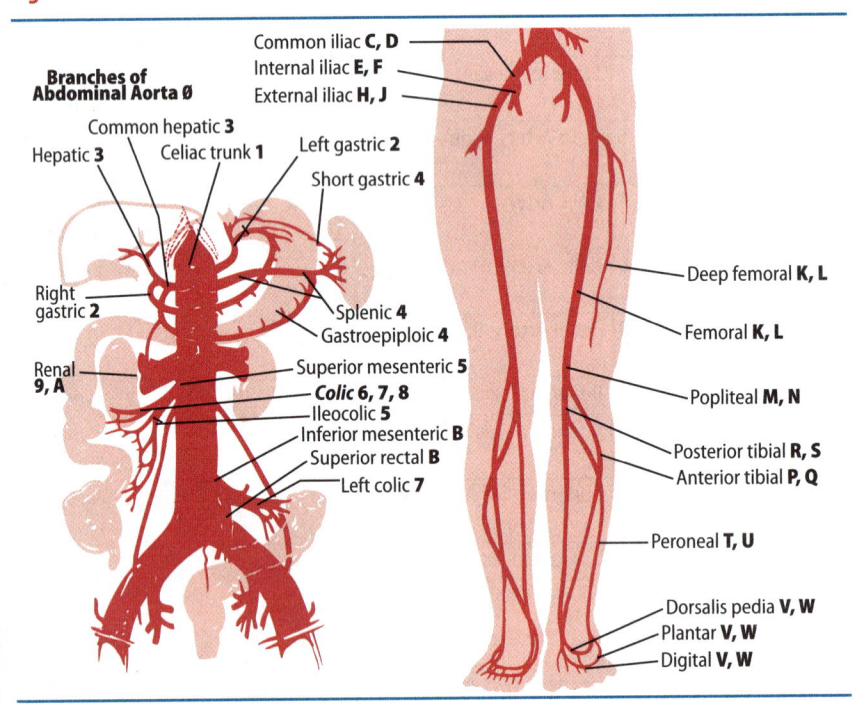

> **DEFINITIONS**
>
> **colic arteries.** Vessels that are branches of the mesenteric artery and feed oxygenated blood to different portions of the colon.

Branches of Abdominal Aorta 0
Common hepatic 3
Hepatic 3
Celiac trunk 1
Left gastric 2
Short gastric 4
Right gastric 2
Splenic 4
Gastroepiploic 4
Renal 9, A
Superior mesenteric 5
Colic 6, 7, 8
Ileocolic 5
Inferior mesenteric B
Superior rectal B
Left colic 7
Common iliac C, D
Internal iliac E, F
External iliac H, J
Deep femoral K, L
Femoral K, L
Popliteal M, N
Posterior tibial R, S
Anterior tibial P, Q
Peroneal T, U
Dorsalis pedia V, W
Plantar V, W
Digital V, W

Character Value — Ø, Abdominal Aorta

Associated Terms: Inferior phrenic artery, lumbar artery, median sacral artery, middle suprarenal artery, ovarian artery, testicular artery

The abdominal aorta is the lower portion of the descending aorta, prior to its division into the *common iliac arteries*. It has several branches, some of which are the inferior phrenic artery, the lumbar artery, the median sacral artery, the middle suprarenal artery, and the gonadal artery (the ovarian artery in females and the testicular artery in males).

Character Value — 1, Celiac Artery

Associated Terms: Celiac trunk

As one of the branches of the abdominal aorta, the celiac artery supplies blood to many of the abdominal organs. It is also known as the celiac trunk.

> **DEFINITIONS**
>
> **common iliac arteries.** Two large arteries that arise directly from the aorta and bifurcate into the external and internal iliac arteries.

Character Value — 2, Gastric Artery

Associated Terms: Left gastric artery, right gastric artery

As they branch from the celiac trunk, the gastric arteries create a blood supply to the stomach and the lower esophagus. The left gastric artery is a direct branch of the celiac trunk, whereas the right gastric artery branches from the proper hepatic artery, which is a further branch from the celiac trunk.

Character Value — 3, Hepatic Artery

Associated Terms: Common hepatic artery, gastroduodenal artery, hepatic artery proper

The common hepatic artery branches from the celiac trunk. This vessel then branches into several components, including the gastroduodenal artery and the hepatic artery proper. These vessels supply many of the abdominal organs with their blood supply.

Character Value — 4, Splenic Artery

Associated Terms: Left gastroepiploic artery, pancreatic artery, short gastric artery

A branch of the celiac trunk, the splenic artery runs along the top of the pancreas on its way to the spleen. It branches in several locations, creating additional vessels such as the left gastroepiploic artery, the pancreatic artery, and the short gastric artery.

Character Value — 5, Superior Mesenteric Artery

Associated Terms: Ileal artery, ileocolic artery, inferior pancreaticoduodenal artery, jejunal artery

As a branch of the abdominal aorta, the superior mesenteric artery supplies blood to a large portion of the intestinal tract. This artery has several branches itself, including the ileal artery, the ileocolic artery, the inferior pancreaticoduodenal artery, and the jejunal artery.

Character Value — 9, A, Renal Artery, Left & Right

Associated Terms: Inferior suprarenal artery, renal segmental artery

Responsible for supplying the kidneys and ureters with blood, as well as some other surrounding structures, the left and right renal arteries stem directly from the abdominal aorta. They also branch into other vessels, such as the inferior suprarenal artery and the renal segmental artery.

Character Value — B, Inferior Mesenteric Artery

Associated Terms: Sigmoid artery, superior rectal artery

Like its counterpart the superior mesenteric artery, the inferior mesenteric artery also branches from the abdominal aorta and feeds a portion of the intestinal tract. This vessel provides blood to a lower portion of the intestinal tract, whereas the superior mesenteric artery provides blood to an upper portion of the intestinal tract. Branches of the inferior mesenteric artery include the sigmoid artery and the superior rectal artery.

Character Value — E, F, Internal Iliac Artery, Left & Right

Associated Terms: Deferential artery, hypogastric artery, iliolumbar artery, inferior gluteal artery, inferior vesical artery, internal pudendal artery, lateral sacral artery, middle rectal artery, obturator artery, superior gluteal artery, umbilical artery, uterine artery, vaginal artery

A division of the common iliac arteries, the right and left internal iliac arteries, also sometimes known as the hypogastric arteries, provide a blood supply to the pelvic area, the reproductive organs, the buttocks, and a portion of the upper thigh. Branches of the iliac arteries include the deferential artery, the iliolumbar artery, the inferior gluteal artery, the inferior vesical artery, the internal pudendal artery, the lateral sacral artery, the middle rectal artery, the obturator artery, the superior gluteal artery, the umbilical artery, the uterine artery, and the vaginal artery.

Character Value — H, J, External Iliac Artery, Left & Right

Associated Terms: Deep circumflex iliac artery, inferior epigastric artery

Another division of the common iliac arteries, the left and right external iliac arteries supply blood to the lower extremities. These arteries branch into vessels such as the deep circumflex iliac artery and the inferior epigastric artery.

Character Value — K, L, Femoral Artery, Left & Right

Associated Terms: Circumflex iliac artery, deep femoral artery, descending genicular artery, external pudendal artery, superficial epigastric artery

Branching from the external iliac arteries, the femoral arteries supply blood to many areas in the thigh and groin area. Branches of the femoral arteries include the circumflex iliac artery, the deep femoral artery, the descending genicular artery, the external pudendal artery, and the superficial epigastric artery.

Character Value — M, N, Popliteal Artery, Left & Right

Associated Terms: Inferior genicular artery, middle genicular artery, superior genicular artery, sural artery

Distally from the femoral arteries, the popliteal arteries supply blood to the thigh, knee, and calf. These arteries branch into vessels such as the inferior genicular artery, the middle genicular artery, the superior genicular artery, and the sural artery.

Character Value — P, Q, Anterior Tibial Artery, Left & Right

Associated Terms: Anterior lateral malleolar artery, anterior medial malleolar artery, anterior tibial recurrent artery, dorsalis pedis artery, ***posterior tibial*** recurrent artery

As one of the divisions of the popliteal artery, the left and right anterior tibial arteries supply blood to the anterior portion of the lower leg and foot. Branches of the anterior tibial arteries include the anterior lateral malleolar artery, the anterior medial malleolar artery, the anterior tibial recurrent artery, the dorsalis pedis artery, and the posterior tibial recurrent artery.

Character Value — T, U, Peroneal Artery, Left & Right

Associated Terms: Fibular artery

The peroneal artery, also known as the fibular artery, is typically a branch of the *posterior tibial artery,* but may also come from the popliteal artery in some people. This vessel supplies blood to the lower portion of the leg.

Character Value — V, W, Foot Artery, Left & Right

Associated Terms: Arcuate artery, dorsal metatarsal artery, lateral plantar artery, lateral tarsal artery, medial plantar artery

There are several arteries that bring oxygenated blood to the foot. The dorsalis pedis artery, a continuation of the anterior tibial artery, brings blood to the dorsal surface of the foot. Several other vessels bring blood to other various portions of the foot, such as the arcuate artery, the dorsal metatarsal artery, the lateral plantar artery, the lateral tarsal artery, and the medial plantar artery.

DEFINITIONS

posterior tibial artery. Found in the lower limb, this vessel carries blood to the posterior portion of the leg and plantar surface of the foot from the popliteal artery.

Qualifier — Character 7

In the lower arteries body system, the majority of the values for the 7th character are for arterial bypass procedures. The body part found in the qualifier character represents the destination of the bypass procedure. The 7th character values for the bypass procedures include such sites as upper arm artery, lower leg artery, and extracranial artery, along with designations for laterality (right, left, and bilateral). The other qualifier value of interest is found in the root operation table for occlusion procedures and designates the uterine artery as the site of the procedure, representing uterine artery embolization procedures. It is important for coders to understand the location of these body sites and how they relate to corresponding body part values in character 4.

Representative ICD-10-PCS Code Examples

1. **Endovascular uterine artery embolization using Embosphere, bilateral**

    04LE3DT Occlusion of right uterine artery with intraluminal device, percutaneous approach

    04LF3DU Occlusion of left uterine artery with intraluminal device, percutaneous approach

    Note: The ICD-10-PCS codes utilize the 4th character values of E and F Internal iliac artery, right and left, respectively. These values are derived from the body part key. When "uterine artery" is referenced, the valid PCS 4th character value routes the coder to the internal iliac artery. To fully represent the fact that the procedure was performed on the uterine arteries, those specific values in the 7th character are assigned.

2. **Open left femoral-popliteal bypass, using Gore-Tex graft**

    041L0JL Bypass left femoral artery to popliteal artery with synthetic substitute, open approach

    Note: The fourth character, body part, specifies the body part bypassed "from," and the seventh character, qualifier, specifies the body part bypassed "to."

3. **Open excision of abdominal aorta with Gore-Tex graft replacement**

    04R00JZ Replacement of abdominal aorta with synthetic substitute, open approach

    Note: The root operation replacement includes the excision of the body part.

Upper Veins (5)

The venous system is responsible for transporting deoxygenated blood back to the heart and thereby the lungs for reoxygenation. Procedures in the upper vein section involve many types of repairs, bypasses, dilations, extractions, and services that take place on the veins in the upper body. A compiled table for body system character 5 Upper veins, provides all of the valid characters for that system in ICD-10-PCS.

Operation–Character 3	Body Part–Character 4	Approach–Character 5	Device–Character 6	Qualifier–Character 7
1 Bypass	0 Azygos Vein	0 Open	0 Drainage Device	X Diagnostic
5 Destruction	1 Hemiazygos Vein	3 Percutaneous	2 Monitoring Device	Y Upper Vein
7 Dilation	3 Innominate Vein, Right	4 Percutaneous Endoscopic	3 Infusion Device	Z No Qualifier
9 Drainage	4 Innominate Vein, Left	X External	7 Autologous Tissue Substitute	
B Excision	5 Subclavian Vein, Right		9 Autologous Venous Tissue	
C Extirpation	6 Subclavian Vein, Left		A Autologous Arterial Tissue	
D Extraction	7 Axillary Vein, Right		C Extraluminal Device	
H Insertion	8 Axillary Vein, Left		D Intraluminal Device	
J Inspection	9 Brachial Vein, Right		J Synthetic Substitute	
L Occlusion	A Brachial Vein, Left		K Nonautologous Tissue Substitute	
N Release	B Basilic Vein, Right		Z No Device	
P Removal	C Basilic Vein, Left			
Q Repair	D Cephalic Vein, Right			
R Replacement	F Cephalic Vein, Left			
S Reposition	G Hand Vein, Right			
U Supplement	H Hand Vein, Left			
V Restriction	L Intracranial Vein			
W Revision	M Internal Jugular Vein, Right			
	N Internal Jugular Vein, Left			
	P External Jugular Vein, Right			
	Q External Jugular Vein, Left			
	R Vertebral Vein, Right			
	S Vertebral Vein, Left			
	T Face Vein, Right			
	V Face Vein, Left			
	Y Upper Vein			

Body Part — Character 4

The body part characters in the upper veins system detail the various veins in the upper body.

Figure 15.15: Map of Upper Veins

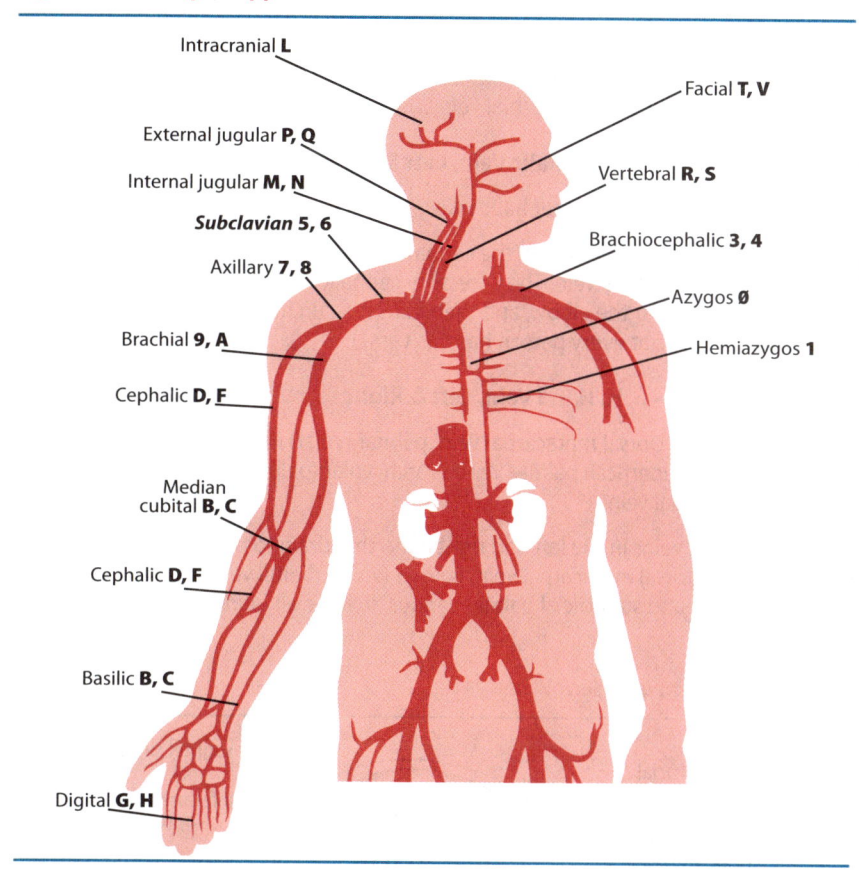

Intracranial **L**
Facial **T, V**
External jugular **P, Q**
Vertebral **R, S**
Internal jugular **M, N**
Subclavian **5, 6**
Brachiocephalic **3, 4**
Axillary **7, 8**
Azygos **Ø**
Brachial **9, A**
Hemiazygos **1**
Cephalic **D, F**
Median cubital **B, C**
Cephalic **D, F**
Basilic **B, C**
Digital **G, H**

> **DEFINITIONS**
>
> **subclavian vein.** Continuation of the axillary vein in the upper body, receiving deoxygenated blood from the external jugular vein and meeting up with the internal jugular vein to create the brachiocephalic vein.

Character Value — Ø, Azygos Vein

Associated Terms: Right ascending lumbar vein, right subcostal vein

Running up one side of the vertebral column, the azygos vein moves blood from the thorax and abdomen into the superior vena cava. The azygos vein is formed by the right ascending lumbar vein and the right subcostal vein.

Character Value — 1, Hemiazygos vein

Associated Terms: Left ascending lumbar vein, left subcostal vein

The hemiazygos vein begins in the left ascending lumbar vein, and receives blood from several of the intercostal veins on the left side of the body. One of the vessels that joins the hemiazygos vein is the left subcostal vein.

Character Value — 3, 4, Innominate Vein, Left & Right

Associated Terms: Brachiocephalic vein, inferior thyroid vein

Innominate veins are found on the left and right side of the neck, and they drain blood from the head, neck, and upper extremities. Also called the brachiocephalic veins, the inferior thyroid vein drains into the innominate veins, among other vessels.

Character Value — 9, A, Brachial Vein, Left & Right

Associated Terms: Radial vein, ulnar vein

Brachial veins travel alongside the brachial artery in the arm to drain the blood of the arm. The radial and ulnar veins empty into the brachial vein from the forearm, and the brachial vein empties into the axillary vein.

Character Value — B, C, Basilic Vein, Left & Right

Associated Terms: Median antebrachial vein, median cubital vein

The basilic veins run along the posterior surface of the arm, making it a popular choice for venipuncture. Several smaller veins in the arm and hand drain to the basilic vein, such as the median antebrachial vein and the median cubital vein.

Character Value — D, F, Cephalic Vein, Left & Right

Associated Terms: Accessory cephalic vein

Receiving blood from the forearm, the cephalic veins run through the upper limb, emptying into the axillary vein. The accessory cephalic vein is a vessel that branches from the cephalic near the elbow, and then joins it again higher up. It is a variable vein, meaning that not every person has this vessel.

Character Value — G, H, Hand Vein, Left & Right

Associated Terms: Dorsal metacarpal vein, palmar (volar) digital vein, palmar (volar) metacarpal vein, superficial palmar venous arch, volar (palmar) digital vein, volar (palmar) metacarpal vein

There are several veins in the left and right hand that drain to the various larger veins of the arm. The dorsal metacarpal vein, palmar (volar) digital vein, palmar (volar) metacarpal vein, and superficial palmar venous arch are all found in the hand.

Figure 15.16: Head and Neck Veins

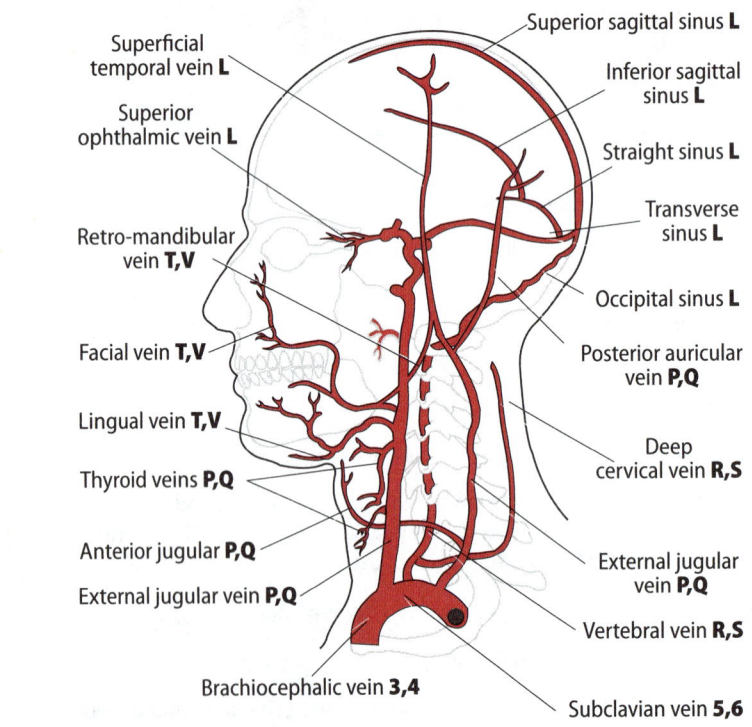

Character Value — L, Intracranial Vein

Associated Terms: Anterior cerebral vein, basal (internal) cerebral vein, dural venous sinus, great cerebral vein, inferior cerebellar vein, inferior cerebral vein, internal (basal) cerebral vein, middle cerebral vein, ophthalmic vein, superior cerebellar vein, superior cerebral vein

Various veins that are considered intracranial include the anterior cerebral vein, the basal (internal) cerebral vein, the dural venous sinus, the great cerebral vein, the inferior cerebellar vein, the inferior cerebral vein, the middle cerebral vein, the ophthalmic vein, the superior cerebellar vein, or the superior cerebral vein. This is not necessarily an all-inclusive list, however, so coders should refer to the body part key when assessing whether a vessel is considered an intracranial vein for purposes of this character value assignment.

Character Value — P, Q, External Jugular Vein, Left & Right

Associated Terms: Posterior auricular vein

Traversing up each side of the neck, the external jugular veins carry blood back to the heart from the exterior of the head and the facial tissues. The posterior auricular vein adjoins it near the ear.

Character Value — R, S, Vertebral Vein, Left & Right

Associated Terms: Deep cervical vein, suboccipital venous plexus

From the deep cervical vein, a network of four veins is created (including the vertebral vein) called the suboccipital venous plexus, which drains the deoxygenated blood from the back of the head. These veins drain into the brachiocephalic vein to lead back to the heart.

Character Value — T, V, Face Vein, Left & Right

Associated Terms: Angular vein, anterior facial vein, common facial vein, deep facial vein, frontal vein, posterior facial (retromandibular) vein, supraorbital vein

There are several veins in the face that drain blood, typically to the ***internal jugular vein***. The common facial and anterior facial veins are the largest veins in the face. Some of the smaller facial veins are the angular vein, the deep facial vein, the frontal vein, the posterior facial (retromandibular) vein, and the supraorbital vein.

> **DEFINITIONS**
>
> **internal jugular vein.** Vessel that unites with the subclavian vein to create the brachiocephalic vein.

Representative ICD-10-PCS Code Examples

1. **Percutaneous placement of central venous catheter (CVC) into left internal jugular vein**

   Ø5HN33Z Insertion of infusion device into left internal jugular vein, percutaneous approach

   Note: A central venous catheter is considered an infusion device, which is represented by character value 3 Infusion Device, in the 6th character position.

2. **Percutaneous right axillary vein thrombectomy**

   Ø5C73ZZ Extirpation of matter from right axillary vein, percutaneous approach

3. **Phlebotomy of the left median cubital vein for polycythemia vera**

   Ø59A3ZZ Drainage of left brachial vein, percutaneous approach

   Note: The median cubital vein is a branch of the brachial vein and is therefore coded to the brachial vein. See Body Part Key for reference.

> **CODING AXIOM**
>
> According to the guideline for the root operation "bypass," body part, character four, indicates the body part bypassed "from" and qualifier, character seven, represents the body part bypassed "to." When an arterial-venous anastomosis is created for the purpose of hemodialysis, it is helpful for the coder to know that blood generally flows "from" the artery "to" the vein (high pressure to low pressure).
>
> *Coding Clinic,* 1Q, 13, 27

4. **Anastomosis for hemodialysis of the left deep cephalic vein and the left radial artery (AV fistula), open approach**

   031C0ZF Bypass left radial artery to left lower arm vein, open approach

   Note: This example is coded to the upper artery body system with radial artery as the body part and uses the qualifier to indicate the lower arm vein. Note that there is no seventh character value for deep cephalic vein so the more general lower arm vein must be used. See the *Coding Clinic* reference in the coding axiom.

Lower Veins (6)

The lower venous system, like the upper venous system, returns deoxygenated blood to the heart. For the lower veins, the blood comes mainly from the lower extremities and the lower half of the abdomen. A compiled table for body system character 6 Lower veins, provides all of the valid characters for that system in ICD-10-PCS.

> **DEFINITIONS**
>
> **esophageal vein.** Vessel that carries deoxygenated blood away from the esophagus to the azygos vein to eventually return to the heart.

Operation–Character 3	Body Part–Character 4	Approach–Character 5	Device–Character 6	Qualifier–Character 7
1 Bypass	0 Inferior Vena Cava	0 Open	0 Drainage Device	5 Superior Mesenteric Vein
5 Destruction	1 Splenic Vein	3 Percutaneous	2 Monitoring Device	6 Inferior Mesenteric Vein
7 Dilation	2 Gastric Vein	4 Percutaneous Endoscopic	3 Infusion Device	9 Renal Vein, Right
9 Drainage	3 **Esophageal Vein**	X External	7 Autologous Tissue Substitute	B Renal Vein, Left
B Excision	4 Hepatic Vein		9 Autologous Venous Tissue	C Hemorrhoidal Plexus
C Extirpation	5 Superior Mesenteric Vein		A Autologous Arterial Tissue	T Via Umbilical Vein
D Extraction	6 Inferior Mesenteric Vein		C Extraluminal Device	X Diagnostic
H Insertion	7 Colic Vein		D Intraluminal Device	Y Lower Vein
J Inspection	8 Portal Vein		J Synthetic Substitute	Z No Qualifier
L Occlusion	9 Renal Vein, Right		K Nonautologous Tissue Substitute	
N Release	B Renal Vein, Left		Z No Device	
P Removal	C Common Iliac Vein, Right			
Q Repair	D Common Iliac Vein, Left			
R Replacement	F External Iliac Vein, Right			
S Reposition	G External Iliac Vein, Left			
U Supplement	H Hypogastric Vein, Right			
V Restriction	J Hypogastric Vein, Left			
W Revision	M Femoral Vein, Right			
	N Femoral Vein, Left			
	P Greater Saphenous Vein, Right			
	Q Greater Saphenous Vein, Left			
	R Lesser Saphenous Vein, Right			
	S Lesser Saphenous Vein, Left			
	T Foot Vein, Right			
	V Foot Vein, Left			
	Y Lower Vein			

© 2015 Optum360, LLC

Comprehensive Anatomy and Physiology for ICD-10-CM and ICD-10-PCS Coding

Body Part — Character 4

The body part characters detail the various veins in the lower body.

Figure 15.17: Map of Lower Veins

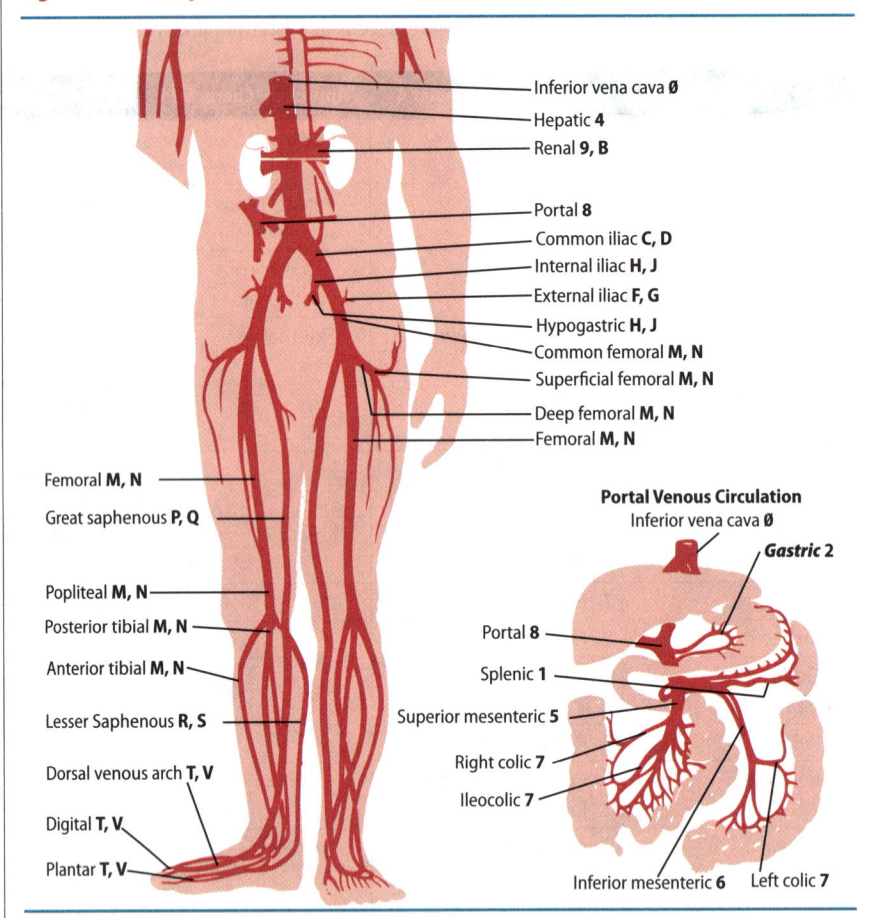

- Inferior vena cava **Ø**
- Hepatic **4**
- Renal **9, B**
- Portal **8**
- Common iliac **C, D**
- Internal iliac **H, J**
- External iliac **F, G**
- Hypogastric **H, J**
- Common femoral **M, N**
- Superficial femoral **M, N**
- Deep femoral **M, N**
- Femoral **M, N**
- Femoral **M, N**
- Great saphenous **P, Q**
- Popliteal **M, N**
- Posterior tibial **M, N**
- Anterior tibial **M, N**
- Lesser Saphenous **R, S**
- Dorsal venous arch **T, V**
- Digital **T, V**
- Plantar **T, V**

Portal Venous Circulation
- Inferior vena cava **Ø**
- *Gastric* **2**
- Portal **8**
- Splenic **1**
- Superior mesenteric **5**
- Right colic **7**
- Ileocolic **7**
- Inferior mesenteric **6**
- Left colic **7**

> **DEFINITIONS**
>
> **gastric vein.** Left and right gastric veins carry deoxygenated blood away from the stomach. The left gastric vein is more commonly known as the coronary vein, and the right gastric vein is more commonly known as the pyloric vein.

Character Value — Ø, Inferior Vena Cava

Associated Terms: Postcava, right inferior phrenic vein, right ovarian vein, right second lumbar vein, right suprarenal vein, right testicular vein

Responsible for returning blood into the heart from the lower half of the body, the inferior vena cava (postcava) is formed by the junction of the two common iliac veins. There are many other veins that join the inferior vena cava as well, such as the right inferior phrenic vein, the right ovarian vein, the right second lumbar vein, the right suprarenal vein, and the right testicular vein.

Character Value — 1, Splenic Vein

Associated Terms: Left gastroepiploic vein, pancreatic vein

The splenic vein is responsible for draining blood from the spleen, emptying into the **hepatic** portal vein. The left gastroepiploic vein and pancreatic vein are both smaller veins that drain into the splenic vein.

Character Value — 5, Superior Mesenteric Vein

Associated Terms: Right gastroepiploic vein

Draining the blood from much of the small intestine, the superior mesenteric vein has many tributaries, including the right gastroepiploic vein.

Character Value — 6, Inferior Mesenteric Vein

Associated Terms: Sigmoid vein, superior rectal vein

Responsible for draining blood from the lower intestines, the inferior mesenteric vein empties into the splenic vein. Smaller veins such as the sigmoid vein and the superior rectal vein empty into the inferior mesenteric vein.

Character Value — 7, Colic Vein

Associated Terms: Ileocolic vein, left colic vein, middle colic vein, right colic vein

Draining deoxygenated blood from the colon and surrounding area, the colic veins are tributaries of two different veins. The ileocolic, middle colic, and right colic veins all drain into the superior mesenteric vein. The left colic vein drains into the inferior mesenteric vein.

Character Value — 8, Portal Vein

Associated Terms: Hepatic portal vein

Different than most veins, the portal vein (or hepatic portal vein) feeds blood into the liver. The blood is then sent to the heart through the **hepatic veins**.

Character Value — 9, B, Renal Vein, Right & Left

Associated Terms: Left inferior phrenic vein, left ovarian vein, left second lumbar vein, left suprarenal vein, left testicular vein

There is not symmetry between the right and left sides of the body with regard to the **renal veins.** The inferior vena cava is found on the right side of the body, so the left renal vein is the longer of the two renal veins. The left inferior phrenic vein, left ovarian vein, left second lumbar vein, left suprarenal vein, and left testicular vein all drain into the left renal vein. The right renal vein is able to drain directly into the inferior cava, as are the counterparts of those other vessels.

Character Value — H, J, Hypogastric Vein, Right & Left

Associated Terms: Gluteal vein, internal iliac vein, internal pudendal vein, lateral sacral vein, middle hemorrhoidal vein, obturator vein, uterine vein, vaginal vein, vesical vein

Also known as the internal iliac veins, the hypogastric veins (right and left) join the external iliac veins to create the common iliac veins. Their tributaries include the gluteal vein, internal pudendal vein, lateral sacral vein, middle hemorrhoidal vein, obturator vein, uterine vein, vaginal vein, and vesical vein.

Character Value — M, N, Femoral Vein, Right & Left

Associated Terms: Deep femoral (profunda femoris) vein, popliteal vein, profunda femoris (deep femoral) vein

A continuation of the popliteal vein, the femoral vein runs along the thigh to drain the lower extremity of blood. The deep femoral vein joins with it, as well as other vessels, to eventually drain to the external iliac vein.

Character Value — P, Q, Greater Saphenous Vein, Right & Left

Associated Terms: External pudendal vein, great saphenous vein, superficial circumflex iliac vein, superficial epigastric vein

One of the longest veins in the body, the greater (or great) saphenous vein runs through the leg and thigh. The saphenous vein is often used in vessel grafting procedures because of its long-term patency. Some of the veins that drain into the saphenous vein are the external pudendal vein, the superficial circumflex iliac vein, and the superficial epigastric vein.

DEFINITIONS

hepatic vein. Vessels that drain the deoxygenated blood from the liver into the inferior vena cava.

renal vein. Vessels that remove deoxygenated blood from the kidneys and carry it to the inferior vena cava for return to the heart.

KEY POINT

A portion of the greater saphenous vein is often harvested from the thigh for use in vessel grafting, such as coronary artery bypass procedures. It is a preferred choice as graft material because of its long term patency. At times, the lesser saphenous vein may also be used as graft material. The coder can recognize which of the veins were obtained by the location of the graft harvest. If the vein was obtained in the thigh, the greater saphenous vein was used. The lesser saphenous vein would be harvested from the posterior lower leg since it terminates near the knee.

Character Value — R, S, Lesser Saphenous Vein, Right & Left

Associated Terms: Small saphenous vein

The lesser or small saphenous veins of the lower extremities run along the back of the leg just under the skin and drain into the popliteal vein near the knee.

Character Value — T, V, Foot Vein, Right & Left

Associated Terms: Common digital vein, dorsal metatarsal vein, dorsal venous arch, plantar digital vein, plantar metatarsal vein, plantar venous arch

There are several veins in the feet, serving to drain the deoxygenated blood from the various portions of the foot. Some of these veins include the common digital vein, the dorsal metatarsal vein, the dorsal venous arch, the plantar digital vein, the plantar metatarsal vein, and the plantar venous arch.

Representative ICD-10-PCS Code Examples

1. **Transjugular intrahepatic portosystemic shunt (TIPS)**
   06183DY Bypass portal vein to lower vein with intraluminal device, percutaneous approach

   Note: TIPS is a shunt (tube) placed between the portal vein, which carries blood from the intestines and intraabdominal organs to the liver, and the hepatic vein, which carries blood from the liver back to the vena cava and the heart. It results in a percutaneously created connection within the liver between the portal and systemic circulations. Because the route of passage of a tubular body part (the vein) is being changed, the root operation bypass is assigned. The bypass procedure begins with the portal vein so 4th character body part value 8 Portal Vein, is assigned. An expandable metal stent is used in these procedures, which is considered an intraluminal device in PCS; assign value D Intraluminal device, for the 6th character. The 7th character qualifier represents the site at the end of the bypass procedure, which is the hepatic vein. Note that there is no 7th character value for hepatic vein; the more general value of Y Lower Vein, must be assigned.

2. **Percutaneous right leg greater and lesser saphenous vein stripping**
   06DP3ZZ Extraction of right greater saphenous vein, percutaneous approach
   06DR3ZZ Extraction of right lesser saphenous vein, percutaneous approach

   Note: The ligation and stripping procedure commonly performed for varicose veins translates to an extraction root operation in ICD-10-PCS. Two codes must be assigned, one for the greater saphenous vein and the other for the lesser saphenous vein.

3. **Endoscopic banding of esophageal varices for esophageal bleeding**
   06L34CZ Occlusion of esophageal vein with extraluminal device, percutaneous endoscopic approach

   Note: The occlusion is of the vein of the esophagus, not the esophagus itself. The bands are considered extraluminal devices. There currently is no choice within the cardiovascular tables for the approach "via natural or artificial opening" so the approach of percutaneous endoscopic should be used according to the advice in *Coding Clinic,* 4Q, 13, 112.

4. **Endoscopic harvest of the right saphenous vein in thigh for graft**
   06BP4ZZ Excision of right greater saphenous vein, percutaneous endoscopic approach

   Note: The greater saphenous vein would be the appropriate choice since the lesser saphenous vein does not extend into the thigh.

Summary

The seven body systems outlined in this chapter and their associated tables in the ICD-10-PCS coding system cover the majority of procedures performed on the nervous and circulatory systems. Knowing how anatomy correlates to key coding components, such as the body part character or the qualifier character, is vital to accurate coding. Becoming educated on the terms found in the ICD-10-PCS manual itself, as well as the associated terms defined throughout this chapter, will assist in training for future success in ICD-10-PCS coding.

Knowledge Assessment Questions

1. If a patient has a procedure performed on the third cranial nerve, which body part character in the central nervous system is reported?
   a. H Oculomotor nerve
   b. L Abducens nerve
   c. J Trochlear nerve
   d. M Facial nerve

2. Which of the following terms is NOT included in the foot artery body part in the lower arteries body system?
   a. Arcuate artery
   b. Lateral tarsal artery
   c. Medial plantar artery
   d. Fibular artery

3. If a procedure is performed on the tentorium cerebelli, it would likely be assigned to body part character value 2 in the central nervous system section.
   a. True
   b. False

4. A procedure performed on the pelvic splanchnic nerve would be assigned to which body part character in which section of ICD-10-PCS?
   a. Character K under the peripheral nervous system
   b. Character M under the peripheral nervous system
   c. Character Q under the central nervous system
   d. Character R under the central nervous system

5. In the qualifier section (character 7) for the central and peripheral nervous system, the nerves listed detail the site the graft was transferred from.
   a. True
   b. False

6. Which procedure is defined as "expanding an orifice or the lumen of a tubular body part"?
   a. Bypass
   b. Insertion
   c. Division
   d. Dilation

7. In the heart and great vessels section, a procedure performed on the right ventricle uses the same body part character as a procedure performed on the left ventricle.
   a. True
   b. False

8. A procedure performed on the posterior communicating artery would likely be assigned to which body part character in the upper arteries body system?
   a. R Face artery
   b. G Intracranial artery
   c. K Internal carotid artery
   d. M External carotid artery

9. What root operation is defined as "putting in a nonbiological appliance that monitors, assists, performs, or prevents a physiological function but does not physically take the place of a body part"?

    a. Insertion
    b. Restriction
    c. Occlusion
    d. Destruction

10. A procedure performed on the Scarpa's ganglion would be assigned to body part character N in the central nervous system.

    a. True
    b. False

Chapter 16. ICD-10-PCS: Lymphatic, Sense Organ, and Respiratory Systems

Lymphatic and Hemic Systems (7)*

Procedures performed in the lymphatic and hemic systems include excisions of lymph nodes, bone marrow biopsies, or splenectomy. It is important to be familiar with terms that are used to describe procedures in the lymphatic and hemic systems section for accuracy in coding in conjunction with procedures in other sections. For example, a radical neck dissection may be coded in conjunction with an excision of a malignant neoplasm. A compiled table for body system character 7 Lymphatic and hemic systems, provides all of the valid characters for that system in ICD-10-PCS.

Operation–Character 3	Body Part–Character 4	Approach–Character 5	Device–Character 6	Qualifier–Character 7
2 Change	0 Lymphatic, Head	0 Open	0 Drainage Device	0 Allogeneic
5 Destruction	1 Lymphatic, Right Neck	3 Percutaneous	3 Infusion Device	1 Syngeneic
9 Drainage	2 Lymphatic, Left Neck	4 Percutaneous Endoscopic	7 Autologous Tissue Substitute	2 Zooplastic
B Excision	3 Lymphatic, Right Upper Extremity	X External	C Extraluminal Device	X Diagnostic
C Extirpation	4 Lymphatic, Left Upper Extremity		D Intraluminal Device	Z No Qualifier
D Extraction	5 Lymphatic, Right Axillary		J Synthetic Substitute	
H Insertion	6 Lymphatic, Left Axillary		K Nonautologous Tissue Substitute	
J Inspection	7 Lymphatic, Thorax		Y Other Device	
L Occlusion	8 Lymphatic, Internal Mammary, Right		Z No Device	
N Release	9 Lymphatic, Internal Mammary, Left			
P Removal	B Lymphatic, Mesenteric			
Q Repair	C Lymphatic, Pelvis			
S Reposition	D Lymphatic, Aortic			
T Resection	F Lymphatic, Right Lower Extremity			
U Supplement	G Lymphatic, Left Lower Extremity			
V Restriction	H Lymphatic, Right Inguinal			
W Revision	J Lymphatic, Left Inguinal			
Y Transplantation	K Thoracic Duct			

(Continued on next page)

---

* Includes lymph vessels and lymph nodes.

Operation–Character 3	Body Part–Character 4	Approach–Character 5	Device–Character 6	Qualifier–Character 7
(Continued)	L Cisterna Chyli			
	M Thymus			
	N Lymphatic			
	P Spleen			
	Q **Bone Marrow**, Sternum			
	R Bone Marrow, Iliac			
	S Bone Marrow, Vertebral			
	T Bone Marrow			

Body Part — Character 4

The body part characters specified in the lymphatic and hemic system table detail the various portions of the lymphatic and hemic systems of the body.

Character Value — 0, Lymphatic, Head

Associated Terms: Buccinator lymph node, infraauricular lymph node, infraparotid lymph node, parotid lymph node, preauricular lymph node, submandibular lymph node, submaxillary lymph node, submental lymph node, subparotid lymph node, suprahyoid lymph node

The lymph nodes mainly associated with the head are the buccinator lymph node, the infraauricular lymph node, the intraparotid lymph node, the parotid lymph node, the preauricular lymph node, the submandibular lymph node, the submaxillary lymph node, the submental lymph node, the subparotid lymph node, and the suprahyoid lymph node.

Figure 16.1: Lymphatic System

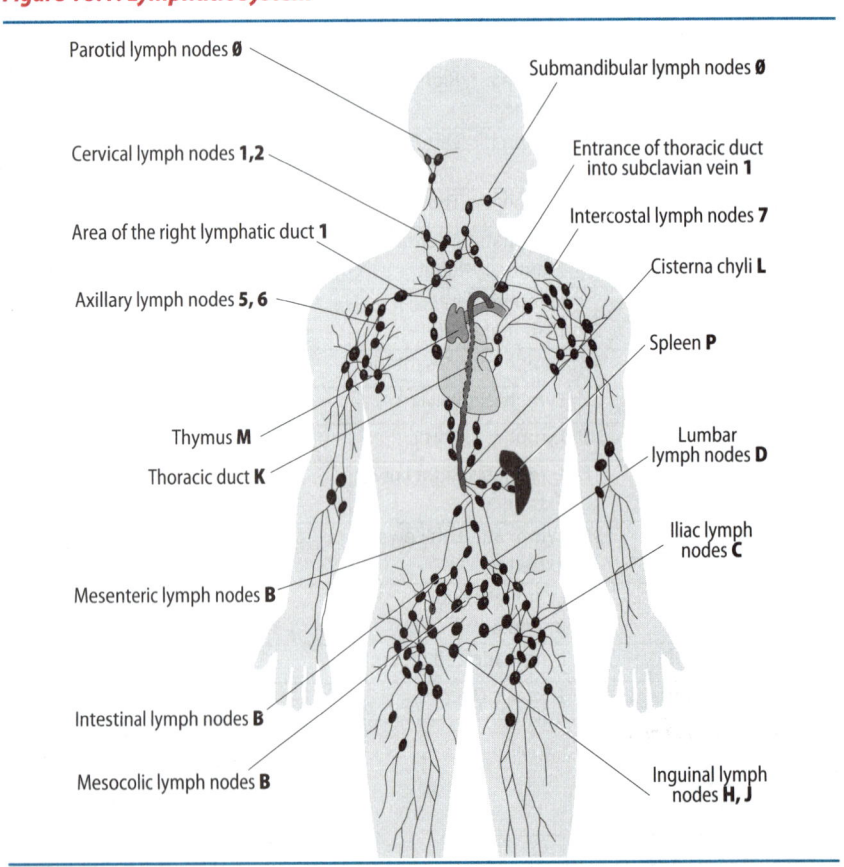

Parotid lymph nodes 0
Submandibular lymph nodes 0
Cervical lymph nodes 1,2
Entrance of thoracic duct into subclavian vein 1
Area of the right lymphatic duct 1
Intercostal lymph nodes 7
Cisterna chyli L
Axillary lymph nodes 5, 6
Spleen P
Thymus M
Lumbar lymph nodes D
Thoracic duct K
Iliac lymph nodes C
Mesenteric lymph nodes B
Intestinal lymph nodes B
Mesocolic lymph nodes B
Inguinal lymph nodes H, J

DEFINITIONS

bone marrow. Soft tissue found filling the cavities of bones, consisting of two types: yellow and red. Red bone marrow is a hematopoietic tissue that manufactures various cellular components of blood, such as platelets and red and white blood cells. Yellow marrow consists mostly of fat cells and is found in the medullary cavities of large bones. Bone marrow is a network of connective tissue of branching fibers forming a frame-like structure, filled with marrow cells. Bone marrow is harvested and transplanted for its progenitor or stem cells in cases of leukemia and other diseases. Marrow is used in spinal fusion to provide osteoprogenitor cells to mix with the allograft and form strong bone fusion. Bone marrow is biopsied to help diagnose many diseases of the blood, based on the distribution and formation of various blood cells.

Chapter 16. ICD-10-PCS: Lymphatic, Sense Organ, and Respiratory Systems

Character Value — 1, Lymphatic, Right Neck

Associated Terms: Cervical lymph node, jugular lymph node, mastoid (postauricular) lymph node, occipital lymph node, postauricular (mastoid) lymph node, retropharyngeal lymph node, right jugular trunk, right lymphatic duct, right subclavian trunk, supraclavicular (Virchow's) lymph node, Virchow's (supraclavicular) lymph node

Typically found on the right side of the neck are the following lymph nodes: cervical lymph node, jugular lymph node, mastoid (postauricular) lymph node, occipital lymph node, retropharyngeal lymph node, right jugular trunk, right lymphatic duct, right subclavian trunk, and the supraclavicular (Virchow's) lymph node.

Character Value — 2, Lymphatic, Left Neck

Associated Terms: Cervical lymph node, jugular lymph node, mastoid (postauricular) lymph node, occipital lymph node, postauricular (mastoid) lymph node, retropharyngeal lymph node, supraclavicular (Virchow's) lymph node, Virchow's (supraclavicular) lymph node

Found on the left side of the neck are the following lymph nodes: cervical lymph node, jugular lymph node, mastoid (postauricular) lymph node, occipital lymph node, retropharyngeal lymph node, and Virchow's (supraclavicular) lymph node.

Character Value — 3, 4, Lymphatic, Right & Left Upper Extremity

Associated Terms: Cubital lymph node, deltopectoral (infraclavicular) lymph node, epitrochlear lymph node, infraclavicular (deltopectoral) lymph node, supratrochlear lymph node

Lymph nodes associated with the right and left upper extremities are the cubital lymph node, the deltopectoral (infraclavicular) lymph node, the epitrochlear lymph node, and the supratrochlear lymph node.

Character Value — 5, 6, Lymphatic, Left & Right Axillary

Associated Terms: Anterior (pectoral) lymph node, apical (subclavicular) lymph node, brachial (lateral) lymph node, central axillary lymph node, lateral (brachial) lymph node, pectoral (anterior) lymph node, posterior (subscapular) lymph node, subclavicular (apical) lymph node, subscapular (posterior) lymph node

Associated lymph nodes in the axillary region are the anterior (pectoral) lymph node, the apical (subclavicular) lymph node, the brachial (lateral) lymph node, the central axillary lymph node, and the posterior (subscapular) lymph node.

Character Value — 7, Lymphatic, Thorax

Associated Terms: Intercostal lymph node, mediastinal lymph node, parasternal lymph node, paratracheal lymph node, tracheobronchial lymph node

The following lymph nodes are found in the thorax: intercostal lymph node, mediastinal lymph node, parasternal lymph node, paratracheal lymph node, tracheobronchial lymph node

Character Value — B, Lymphatic, Mesenteric

Associated Terms: Inferior mesenteric lymph node, pararectal lymph node, superior mesenteric lymph node

Lymph nodes associated with the lower abdomen and mesentery include the inferior mesenteric lymph node, pararectal lymph node, and superior mesenteric lymph node.

Character Value — C, Lymphatic, Pelvis

Associated Terms: Common iliac (subaortic) lymph node, gluteal lymph node, iliac lymph node, inferior epigastric lymph node, obturator lymph node, sacral lymph node, subaortic (common iliac) lymph node, suprainguinal lymph node

The pelvic lymph nodes include the following: common iliac (subaortic) lymph node, gluteal lymph node, iliac lymph node, inferior epigastric lymph node, obturator lymph node, sacral lymph node, and suprainguinal lymph node.

Character Value — D, Lymphatic, Aortic

Associated Terms: Celiac lymph node, gastric lymph node, hepatic lymph node, lumbar lymph node, pancreaticosplenic lymph node, paraaortic lymph node, retroperitoneal lymph node

Lymph nodes that are found in relation to the aorta are the celiac lymph node, the gastric lymph node, the hepatic lymph node, the lumbar lymph node, the pancreaticosplenic lymph node, the paraaortic lymph node, and the retroperitoneal lymph node.

Character Value — F, G, Lymphatic, Left & Right Lower Extremity

Associated Terms: Femoral lymph node, popliteal lymph node

The following lymph nodes are associated with the lower extremities: femoral lymph node and popliteal lymph node.

Character Value — K, Thoracic Duct

Associated Terms: Left jugular trunk, left subclavian trunk

The thoracic duct is the largest lymphatic vessel in the body. This vessel meets with other groups of smaller lymphatic vessels, such as the left jugular trunk or the left subclavian trunk, and eventually drains into the blood circulation system.

Character Value — L, Cisterna Chyli

Associated Terms: Intestinal lymphatic trunk, lumbar lymphatic trunk

Lymph from the lymphatic system flows through the lymphatic system, into the thoracic duct, and into the cisterna chyli, which is a dilated sac. Specifically, the lymphatic trunks, such as the intestinal lymphatic trunk and the lumbar lymphatic trunk, feed lymph into this sac, where the lymph is acted upon by chyle that is transported by the intestines. This functions as part of the digestion process.

Character Value — M, Thymus

Associated Terms: Thymus gland

The thymus gland is the primary gland of the lymphatic system, and works as an important part of the body's immune system. It is found in the chest, just above the heart.

Character Value — P, Spleen

Associated Terms: Accessory spleen

Located in the left upper quadrant of the abdomen, the spleen is an organ that is considered to be part of the hemic system. It has roles related to red blood cell recycling, destruction, and storage, as well as some related to the immune system. An accessory spleen occurs in some patients, where a small portion of splenic tissue has grown elsewhere in the body.

Representative ICD-10-PCS Code Examples

1. **Radical dissection right inguinal groin lymphatics, open**
   07TH0ZZ   Resection of right inguinal lymphatic, open approach
   Note: A radical dissection of lymphatics involves the removal of the entire lymph chain, which translates to the PCS definition of root operation resection.

2. **Fine needle aspiration biopsy, left axillary region**
   07963ZX   Drainage of left axillary lymphatic, percutaneous approach, diagnostic
   Note: Root operation drainage is defined in PCS as taking or letting out fluids and/or gases from a body part. An aspirational fine needle biopsy meets this definition. Assign character value 9 Drainage; the qualifier 7th character value of X Diagnostic, is assigned to represent the biopsy procedure.

3. **Open right axillary sentinel lymph node biopsy**
   07B50ZX   Excision right axillary lymph node, open, diagnostic

4. **Percutaneous drainage of left mastoid lymph node**
   07923ZZ   Drainage of left neck lymph node, percutaneous approach
   Note: Left mastoid lymph node is listed in the body part key as being part of the left neck lymph node.

Eye (8)

Procedures involving the eye can include the eye itself, such as with repair of a retinal detachment or a cataract extraction; the eyelids, such as with a blepharoptosis repair; or the extraocular muscles, such as in the case of strabismus surgery. A compiled table for body system character 8 Eye, provides all of the valid characters for that system in ICD-10-PCS.

Operation–Character 3	Body Part–Character 4	Approach–Character 5	Device–Character 6	Qualifier–Character 7
0 Alteration	0 Eye, Right	0 Open	0 Drainage Device OR Synthetic Substitute, Intraocular Telescope (for root operation REPLACEMENT only)	3 Nasal Cavity
1 Bypass	1 Eye, Left	3 Percutaneous	1 Radioactive Element	4 Sclera
2 Change	2 Anterior Chamber, Right	7 Via Natural or Artificial Opening	3 Infusion Device	X Diagnostic
5 Destruction	3 Anterior Chamber, Left	8 Via Natural or Artificial Opening Endoscopic	5 Epiretinal Visual Prosthesis	Z No Qualifier
7 Dilation	4 Vitreous, Right	X External	7 Autologous Tissue Substitute	
9 Drainage	5 Vitreous, Left		C Extraluminal Device	
B Excision	6 Sclera, Right		D Intraluminal Device	
C Extirpation	7 Sclera, Left		J Synthetic Substitute	
D Extraction	8 Cornea, Right		K Nonautologous Tissue Substitute	
F Fragmentation	9 Cornea, Left		Y Other Device	
H Insertion	A Choroid, Right		Z No Device	
J Inspection	B Choroid, Left			
L Occlusion	C Iris, Right			
M Reattachment	D Iris, Left			
N Release	E Retina, Right			
P Removal	F Retina, Left			
Q Repair	G Retinal Vessel, Right			
R Replacement	H Retinal Vessel, Left			
S Reposition	J Lens, Right			
T Resection	K Lens, Left			
U Supplement	L Extraocular Muscle, Right			
V Restriction	M Extraocular Muscle, Left			
W Revision	N Upper Eyelid, Right			
X Transfer	P Upper Eyelid, Left			
	Q Lower Eyelid, Right			
	R Lower Eyelid, Left			
	S Conjunctiva, Right			
	T Conjunctiva, Left			
	V Lacrimal Gland, Right			
	W Lacrimal Gland, Left			
	X Lacrimal Duct, Right			
	Y Lacrimal Duct, Left			

Body Part — Character 4

The body part characters specified in the eye table detail the eye and surrounding structures.

Figure 16.2: Eye

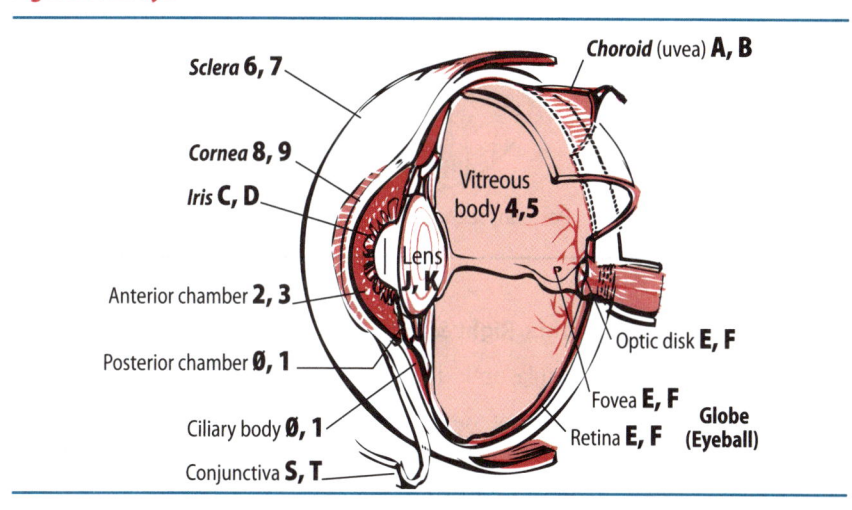

Sclera **6, 7**
Cornea **8, 9**
Iris **C, D**
Anterior chamber **2, 3**
Posterior chamber **0, 1**
Ciliary body **0, 1**
Conjunctiva **S, T**
Choroid (uvea) **A, B**
Vitreous body **4, 5**
Lens **J, K**
Optic disk **E, F**
Fovea **E, F**
Retina **E, F**
Globe (Eyeball)

Character Value — 0, 1, Eye, Right & Left

Associated Terms: Ciliary body, posterior chamber

Eyes are made up of multiple components, many of which have their own characters in ICD-10-PCS. However, two of the components that do not have their own character and may fall within the more "generic" listing of eye are the ciliary body and posterior chamber. These terms may be used in an operative note, but would likely be classified to this general PCS character.

Character Value — 2, 3, Anterior Chamber, Right & Left

Associated Terms: Aqueous humour

Part of the anterior cavity of the eye, the anterior chamber is the portion of the eye that holds the aqueous humor, a clear, watery fluid that moves throughout the anterior and posterior chambers of the eye.

Character Value — 4, 5, Vitreous, Right & Left

Associated Terms: Vitreous body

The vitreous, also referred to as the vitreous body or vitreous humor, is a semigelatinous substance that fills the cavity between the lens of the eye and the retina.

DEFINITIONS

choroid. Thin, nourishing vascular layer of the eye that supplies blood to the retina, arteries, and nerves to structures in the anterior part of the eye.

cornea. Five-layered, transparent structure that forms the anterior or front part of the *sclera* of the eye.

iris. Pigmented membrane behind the cornea and in front of the lens that contracts and expands to enlarge or shrink the size of the pupil to regulate the light entering the eye.

sclera. White, fibrous, outer coating of the eye continuous with the cornea anteriorly and the optic nerve sheath posteriorly that is covered with conjunctival tissue.

Comprehensive Anatomy and Physiology for ICD-10-CM and ICD-10-PCS Coding

📖 **DEFINITIONS**
retinal vessel. The retina has its own blood supply, provided by the ophthalmic artery. There are various vessels within the retina that could be affected by illness or injury.

Figure 16.3: Retina (E, F)

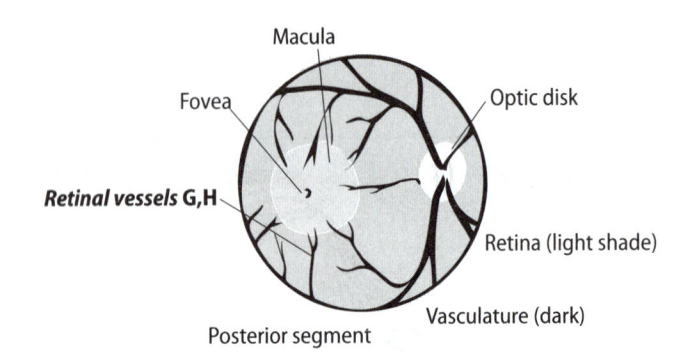

Labels: Macula, Fovea, Optic disk, Retinal vessels G,H, Retina (light shade), Vasculature (dark), Posterior segment

Character Value — E, F, Retina, Right & Left

Associated Terms: Fovea, macula, optic disc

The retina is a portion of the back of the eye that is a network of nervous tissue. It receives images of external objects and transmits them through the optic nerve to the brain. There are several components to the retina, such as the fovea, the macula, and the optic disc, among others.

Character Value — J, K, Lens, Right & Left

Associated Terms: Zonule of Zinn

The lens lies immediately behind the pupil and refracts light rays onto the retina. By changing shape, the lens helps the eye focus on objects at various distances. The Zonule of Zinn is a ring of fibrous strands that serves as a ligament to help anchor the lens in place to the ciliary body.

Figure 16.4: Eye Musculature

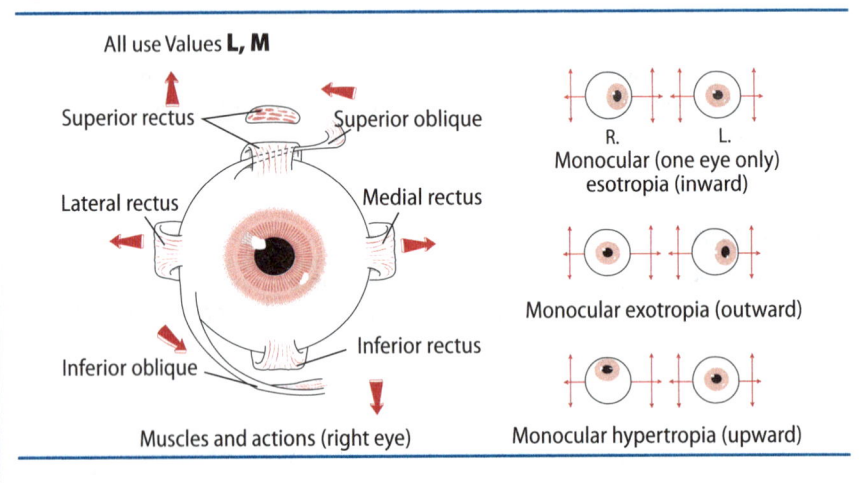

*Labels: All use Values **L, M**; Superior rectus, Superior oblique, Lateral rectus, Medial rectus, Inferior oblique, Inferior rectus, Muscles and actions (right eye)*

R. L. Monocular (one eye only) esotropia (inward)
Monocular exotropia (outward)
Monocular hypertropia (upward)

Character Value — L, M, Extraocular Muscle, Right & Left

Associated Terms: Inferior oblique muscle, inferior rectus muscle, lateral rectus muscle, medial rectus muscle, superior oblique muscle, superior rectus muscle

Extraocular muscles work to control the movements of the eyes. There are six muscles, including the inferior oblique muscle, the inferior rectus muscle, the lateral rectus muscle, the medial rectus muscle, the superior oblique muscle, and the superior rectus muscle.

Character Value — N, P, Upper Eyelid, Right & Left

Associated Terms: Lateral canthus, levator palpebrae superioris muscle, orbicularis oculi muscle, superior tarsal plate

The upper eyelid is made of very thin tissue. The superior tarsal plate is a piece of dense connective tissue that forms and supports the eyelid. The lateral canthus is the outermost point of the upper eyelid, where it meets the lower lid. The levator palpebrae superioris muscle and the orbicularis oculi muscle are two of the muscles that control the upper lid function.

Character Value — Q, R, Lower Eyelid, Right & Left

Associated Terms: Inferior tarsal plate, medial canthus

The lower eyelid is supported by the connective tissue of the inferior tarsal plate. The medial canthus is the innermost point of the eyelids, where the upper and lower eyelids meet near the nose.

Character Value — S, T, Conjunctiva, Right & Left

Associated Terms: Plica semilunaris

The conjunctiva is a mucous membrane that lines the inner surface of the eyelids, as well as a portion of the sclera, and creates mucous to help the ***lacrimal glands*** keep the eyes moist and keep dust and debris out. The plica semilunaris is a small portion of separate conjunctiva found on the eye, a vestigial remnant of a previous type of membrane.

> **DEFINITIONS**
>
> **lacrimal gland.** Tear-producing gland that provides lubrication and flushing of the eyes and nasal cavities.

Figure 16.5: Lacrimal System

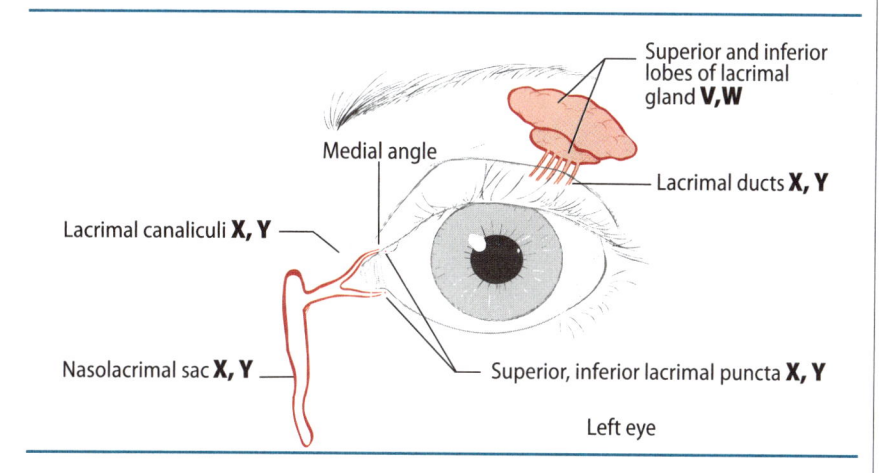

*Labels: Superior and inferior lobes of lacrimal gland **V, W**; Medial angle; Lacrimal ducts **X, Y**; Lacrimal canaliculi **X, Y**; Nasolacrimal sac **X, Y**; Superior, inferior lacrimal puncta **X, Y**; Left eye*

Character Value — X, Y, Lacrimal Duct, Right & Left

Associated Terms: Lacrimal canaliculus, lacrimal punctum, lacrimal sac, nasolacrimal duct

Responsible for draining tears from the lacrimal gland into the eyes, the lacrimal ducts play an important role in keeping the conjunctiva moist and clean. The lacrimal puncta are the "exit" on the other end of the lacrimal ducts, where the tears are able to drain from the eye into the lacrimal canaliculi and then into the lacrimal sac. They then make their way into the nasolacrimal duct and into the nasal tract.

Representative ICD-10-PCS Code Examples

1. **Right eye extracapsular cataract extraction with synchronous intraocular lens placement**

    Ø8RJ3JZ   Replacement of right lens with synthetic substitute, percutaneous approach

    Note: In ICD-9-CM, cataract extraction with synchronous lens placement requires two codes. In ICD-10-PCS, when the cataract extraction is followed by a lens implant, the procedure should be coded to replacement only. ICD-10-PCS defines the root operation replacement as putting in or on biological or synthetic material that physically takes the place and/or function of all or a portion of a body part. Extraction would not be reported in a replacement procedure, as the intent of the root operation extraction is to pull out or off some or all of a body part without replacement. A right eye extracapsular cataract extraction without a synchronous intraocular lens implant would be reported with code Ø8DJ3ZZ Extraction of right lens, percutaneous approach.

2. **Left eye laser photocoagulation iridotomy, for glaucoma**

    Ø85D3ZZ   Destruction of left iris, percutaneous approach

3. **Transnasal stent placement with dilation of right lacrimal duct**

    Ø87X7DZ   Dilation of lacrimal duct, right, with insertion of intraluminal device, via natural or artificial opening

4. **Removal of foreign body from right cornea**

    Ø8C8XZZ   Extirpation of foreign body from right cornea, external approach

Ear, Nose, and Sinus (9)*

Procedures on the ear, nose, and sinus include items such as a myringotomy, turbinectomy, or frontal sinusotomy. As with any section involving potential bilateral procedures, it is important to pay close attention to documentation to verify any laterality issues for each procedure. A compiled table for body system character 9 Ear, nose and sinus, provides all of the valid characters for those systems in ICD-10-PCS.

Operation–Character 3	Body Part–Character 4	Approach–Character 5	Device–Character 6	Qualifier–Character 7
0 Alteration	0 External Ear, Right	0 Open	0 Drainage Device	0 Endolymphatic
1 Bypass	1 External Ear, Left	3 Percutaneous	4 Hearing Device, Bone Conduction	X Diagnostic
2 Change	2 External Ear, Bilateral	4 Percutaneous Endoscopic	5 Hearing Device, Single Channel Cochlear Prosthesis	Z No Qualifier
5 Destruction	3 External Auditory Canal, Right	7 Via Natural or Artificial Opening	6 Hearing Device, Multiple Channel Cochlear Prosthesis	
7 Dilation	4 External Auditory Canal, Left	8 Via Natural or Artificial Opening Endoscopic	7 Autologous Tissue Substitute	
8 Division	5 Middle Ear, Right	X External	B Intraluminal Device, Airway	
9 Drainage	6 Middle Ear, Left		D Intraluminal Device	
B Excision	7 Tympanic Membrane, Right		J Synthetic Substitute	
C Extirpation	8 Tympanic Membrane, Left		K Nonautologous Tissue Substitute	
D Extraction	9 Auditory Ossicle, Right		S Hearing Device	
H Insertion	A Auditory Ossicle, Left		Y Other Device	
J Inspection	B Mastoid Sinus, Right		Z No Device	
M Reattachment	C Mastoid Sinus, Left			
N Release	D Inner Ear, Right			
P Removal	E Inner Ear, Left			
Q Repair	F Eustachian Tube, Right			
R Replacement	G Eustachian Tube, Left			
S Reposition	H Ear, Right			
T Resection	J Ear, Left			
U Supplement	K Nose			
W Revision	L Nasal Turbinate			
	M Nasal Septum			
	N Nasopharynx			
	P Accessory Sinus			
	Q Maxillary Sinus, Right			
	R Maxillary Sinus, Left			
	S Frontal Sinus, Right			
	T Frontal Sinus, Left			
	U Ethmoid Sinus, Right			
	V Ethmoid Sinus, Left			
	W Sphenoid Sinus, Right			
	X Sphenoid Sinus, Left			
	Y Sinus			

* Includes sinus ducts.

Body Part — Character 4

The body part characters specified in the ear, nose, and sinus systems table detail the various components of the ears, nose, and sinuses.

Figure 16.6: Ear Anatomy

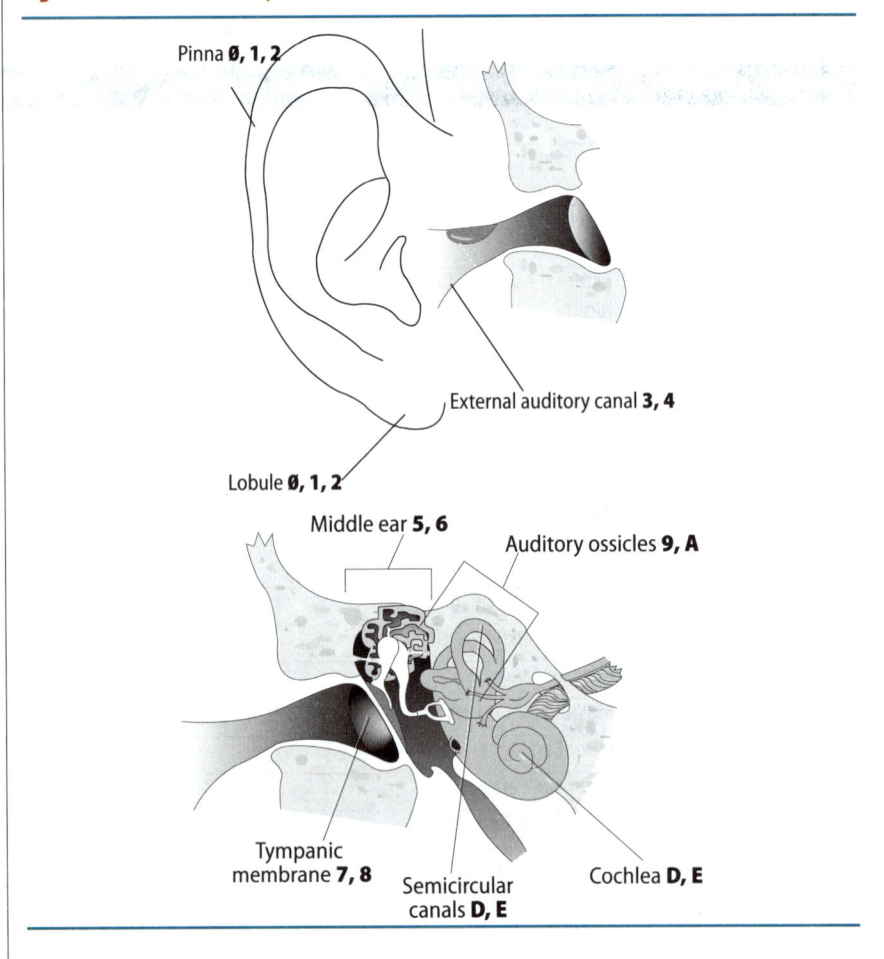

- Pinna Ø, 1, 2
- External auditory canal 3, 4
- Lobule Ø, 1, 2
- Middle ear 5, 6
- Auditory ossicles 9, A
- Tympanic membrane 7, 8
- Semicircular canals D, E
- Cochlea D, E

Character Value — Ø, 1, 2, External Ear, Right, Left, Bilateral

Associated Terms: Antihelix, antitragus, auricle, earlobe, helix, pinna, tragus

The external portion of the ear is made up of many components, including the antihelix, the antitragus, the auricle, the earlobe, the helix, the pinna, and the tragus.

Character Value — 3, 4, External Auditory Canal, Right & Left

Associated Terms: External auditory meatus

Running from the external ear to the middle ear, the external auditory canal is a tube that varies in size and shape by individual. It is also known as the external auditory meatus.

Character Value — 5, 6, Middle Ear, Right & Left

Associated Terms: Oval window, tympanic cavity

An air-filled cavity between the tympanic membrane and the inner ear, the middle ear includes many components. In conjunction with the ossicles, the middle ear equalizes air pressure and transfers sound from air to fluid. Components such as the oval window and the tympanic cavity are also classified to the middle ear PCS character value.

Character Value — 7, 8, Tympanic Membrane, Right & Left

Associated Terms: Pars flaccida

Responsible for transmitting sound vibrations to the inner ear, the tympanic membrane is a vital component of the sense of hearing. The pars flaccida is one small triangular piece of the tympanic membrane, found above the malleolar folds.

Figure 16.7: Middle and Inner Ear

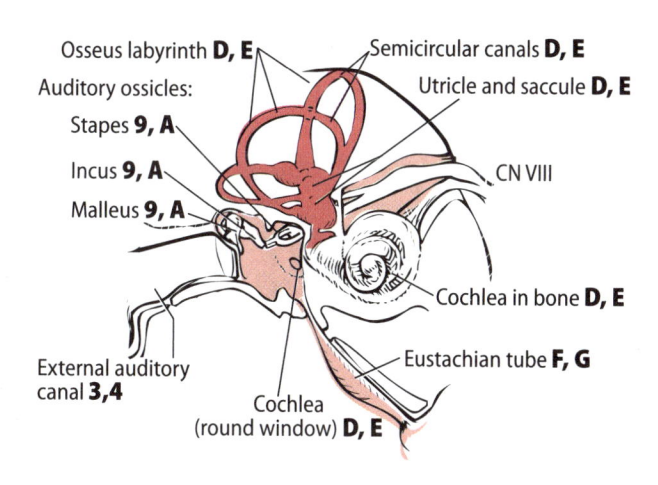

Character Value — 9, A, Auditory Ossicle, Right & Left

Associated Terms: Incus, malleus, ossicular chain, stapes

A series of three small bones in the middle ear, the ossicular chain components articulate with one another to transmit the sound waves received from the tympanic membrane onto the cochlea. The three bones are called the incus, the malleus, and the stapes.\

Character Value — B, C, Mastoid Sinus, Right & Left

Associated Terms: Mastoid air cells

The mastoid sinuses, also called mastoid air cells, are air pockets in the temporal bone, behind the ear. They aren't like "traditional" sinuses, but hollow pockets in the temporal bone that connect to the inner ear and the Eustachian tube.

Character Value — D, E, Inner Ear, Right & Left

Associated Terms: Bony labyrinth, bony vestibule, cochlea, round window, semicircular canal

The inner ear is the innermost part of the ear consisting of the cochlea and the vestibular system and encased in the temporal bone. It includes the vestibule, the cochlea, and the semicircular canal. The function of the inner ear is twofold: hearing and balance. Other terms associated with the inner ear include the bony labyrinth (the vestibule, semicircular canals, and the cochlea combined), the bony vestibule, and the round window.

Character Value — F, G, Eustachian Tube, Right & Left

Associated Terms: Auditory tube, pharyngotympanic tube

Joining the nasopharynx and the middle ear, the Eustachian tube is typically closed but opens when a person yawns, chews, or swallows so that air pressure can equalize. It is also called the auditory tube or the pharyngotympanic tube.

Character Value — K, Nose

Associated Terms: Columella, external naris, greater alar cartilage, internal naris, lateral nasal cartilage, lesser alar cartilage, nasal cavity, nostril

There are several elements to the nose, from the external portions, such as the columella, the external naris, and the nostrils, to the more internal portions, such as the nasal cavity itself. Other important structures include the greater alar cartilage, the lateral cartilage, and the lesser alar cartilage.

Figure 16.8: Nasal Turbinates

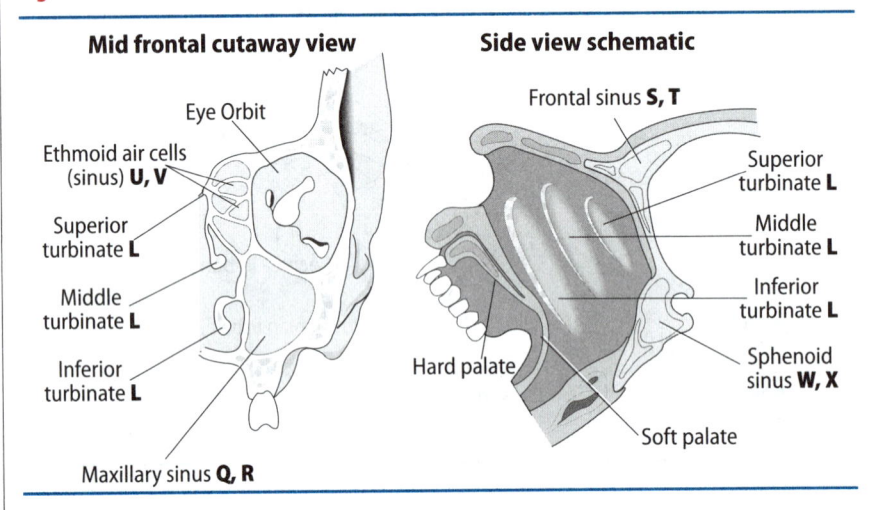

Mid frontal cutaway view

- Eye Orbit
- Ethmoid air cells (sinus) **U, V**
- Superior turbinate **L**
- Middle turbinate **L**
- Inferior turbinate **L**
- Maxillary sinus **Q, R**

Side view schematic

- Frontal sinus **S, T**
- Superior turbinate **L**
- Middle turbinate **L**
- Inferior turbinate **L**
- Sphenoid sinus **W, X**
- Hard palate
- Soft palate

Character Value — L, Nasal Turbinate

Associated Terms: Inferior turbinate, middle turbinate, nasal concha, superior turbinate

Turbinates are bone shelves in the nasal passages that direct air flow into the sinuses. Also known as nasal concha, turbinates are divided into the inferior turbinate, the middle turbinate, and the superior turbinate.

Character Value — M, Nasal Septum

Associated Terms: Quadrangular cartilage, septal cartilage, vomer bone

The nasal septum is a membrane made of cartilage, bone, and mucosa that partitions the two nostrils, or nasal cavities, down the middle. The septal or quadrangular cartilage and the vomer bone are parts of the nasal septum.

Character Value — N, Nasopharynx

Associated Terms: Choana, fossa of Rosenmüller, pharyngeal recess, rhinopharynx

A membranous passage above the level of the soft palate, the nasopharynx (sometimes called the rhinopharynx) is the uppermost region of the throat. Some of the other key components of this area are the choana, as well as the fossa of Rosenmüller (pharyngeal recess).

Character Value — P, Accessory Sinus

Associated Terms: Paranasal sinus

Accessory sinus is the general term used to describe the group of paired, air-filled cavities found surrounding the nasal cavity. The maxillary sinus, frontal sinus, ethmoid sinus, and sphenoid sinus are all found through the various bones within the facial structure.

Figure 16.9: Paranasal/Accessory sinuses

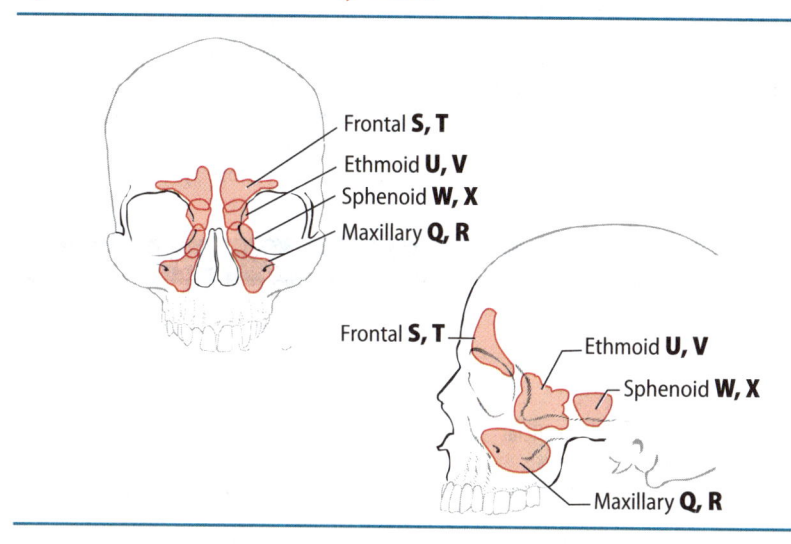

Frontal **S, T**
Ethmoid **U, V**
Sphenoid **W, X**
Maxillary **Q, R**

Frontal **S, T**
Ethmoid **U, V**
Sphenoid **W, X**
Maxillary **Q, R**

Character Value — Q, R, Maxillary Sinus, Right & Left

Associated Terms: Antrum of Highmore

Large sinus cavities in the body of the maxilla, the maxillary sinuses are typically the lowest on the face and extend through the zygomatic arch region. They are sometimes referred to as the antrum of Highmore.

Character Value — S, T, Frontal Sinus, Right & Left

The frontal sinuses are the air-filled cavities between the lamina of the frontal bone of the face, slightly above and between the eyes. They drain into the nose, via the ethmoid sinuses.

Character Value — U, V, Ethmoid Sinus, Right & Left

Associated Terms: Ethmoidal air cell

The ethmoid sinuses, also known as ethmoidal air cells, lie between the upper part of the nasal cavities and the orbits on both the right and left sides of the face.

Character Value — W, X, Sphenoid Sinus, Right & Left

The **sphenoid sinuses** are found deep within the skull, behind the ethmoid sinuses. Critical structures, such as the optic nerve and intracranial blood vessels, lie in close proximity to the sphenoid sinuses, making surgery in this area high risk.

Representative ICD-10-PCS Code Examples

1. **Right side epistaxis cautery**
   Ø95KXZZ   Destruction of nose, external approach

2. **Endoscopic bilateral total frontal sinusectomy**
   Ø9TS4ZZ   Resection of right frontal sinus, percutaneous endoscopic approach
   Ø9TT4ZZ   Resection of left frontal sinus, percutaneous endoscopic approach

---

DEFINITIONS

sphenoid sinuses. One of a pair of sinus cavities in the head, lined with mucous membrane, found in the sphenoid bone of the skull.

Respiratory System (B)

As the nose itself is included in a separate body system chapter, the respiratory system begins with the trachea and proceeds through the remainder of the organs of respiration. Procedures involving the respiratory system include tracheostomies, bronchial biopsies, and lung transplants. A compiled table for body system character B Respiratory system, provides all of the valid characters for those systems in ICD-10-PCS.

Operation–Character 3	Body Part–Character 4	Approach–Character 5	Device–Character 6	Qualifier–Character 7
1 Bypass	0 Tracheobronchial Tree	0 Open	0 Drainage Device	0 Allogeneic
2 Change	1 Trachea	3 Percutaneous	1 Radioactive Element	1 Syngeneic
5 Destruction	2 Carina	4 Percutaneous Endoscopic	2 Monitoring Device	2 Zooplastic
7 Dilation	3 Main Bronchus, Right	7 Via Natural or Artificial Opening	3 Infusion Device	4 Cutaneous
9 Drainage	4 Upper Lobe Bronchus, Right	8 Via Natural or Artificial Opening Endoscopic	7 Autologous Tissue Substitute	6 Esophagus
B Excision	5 Middle Lobe Bronchus, Right	X External	C Extraluminal Device	X Diagnostic
C Extirpation	6 Lower Lobe Bronchus, Right		D Intraluminal Device	Z No Qualifier
D Extraction	7 Main Bronchus, Left		E Intraluminal Device, Endotracheal Airway	
F Fragmentation	8 Upper Lobe Bronchus, Left		F Tracheostomy Device	
H Insertion	9 Lingula Bronchus		G Intraluminal Device, Endobronchial Valve	
J Inspection	B Lower Lobe Bronchus, Left		J Synthetic Substitute	
L Occlusion	C Upper Lung Lobe, Right		K Nonautologous Tissue Substitute	
M Reattachment	D Middle Lung Lobe, Right		M Diaphragmatic Pacemaker Lead	
N Release	F Lower Lung Lobe, Right		Y Other Device	
P Removal	G Upper Lung Lobe, Left		Z No Device	
Q Repair	H Lung Lingula			
S Reposition	J Lower Lung Lobe, Left			
T Resection	K Lung, Right			
U Supplement	L Lung, Left			
V Restriction	M Lungs, Bilateral			
W Revision	N Pleura, Right			
Y Transplantation	P Pleura, Left			
	Q Pleura			
	R Diaphragm, Right			
	S Diaphragm, Left			
	T Diaphragm			

Body Part — Character 4

The body part characters specified in the respiratory system table detail the various components of the respiratory system.

Character Value — 1, Trachea

Associated Terms: Cricoid cartilage

The **trachea** connects the larynx to the lungs and creates a pathway for air exchange. It is made up of many cartilaginous rings, which help it to maintain a more rigid structure.

Character Value — 2, Carina

Associated Terms: Annular ligaments, tracheal rings

The carina is the ridge at the junction of the trachea and the bronchi formed by a projection of the lowest tracheal cartilage separating the openings of the two bronchi. Other structures in the area include the tracheal rings and the annular ligaments.

Figure 16.10: Bronchi

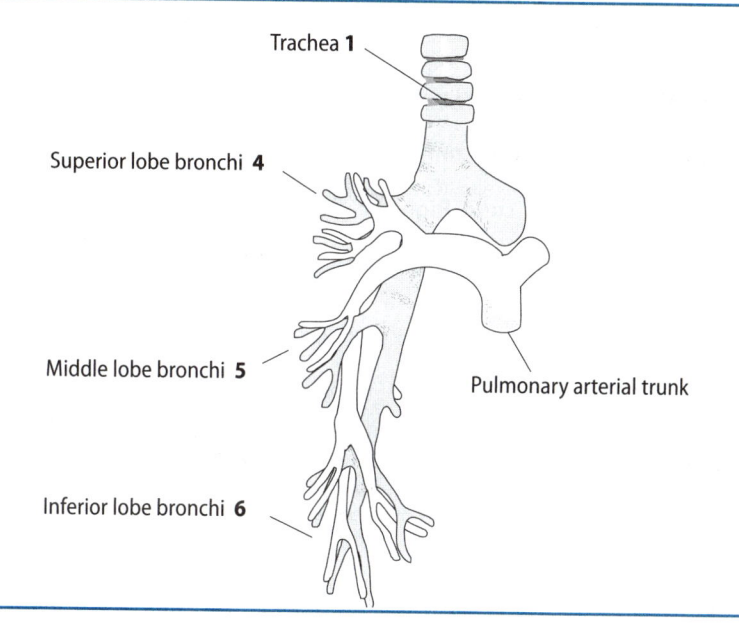

Character Value — 4, 5, 6, Right Bronchus, Upper, Middle, Lower Lobe

Associated Terms: Bronchi

Plural for bronchus, the bronchi of the upper, middle, and lower lobes are tubes that are found in the various lobes of the right lung and provide appropriate air exchange. It is important to note that there are three levels of bronchi on the right side, but only two on the left side.

Character Value — 8, 9, B, Upper Lobe Bronchus, Left; Lingula Bronchus; Lower Lobe Bronchus, Left

Associated Terms: Hyaline cartilage

On the left side, there are only two bronchial lobes. The bronchi only need to split into those two lobular areas. However, there is a small section of the left lobe of the lung known as the lingua, and there are bronchi that reach that area as well. Also,

---

> **KEY POINT**
>
> Except for Trachea, CMS has not provided any "official" definitions for any of the body parts in the respiratory section. Optum360 has provided some common terms associated with the body parts in this section but be aware: most of the terms in this section under "Associated Terms" will not be found in the Body Part Key or the Body Part Definitions table.

> **DEFINITIONS**
>
> **trachea.** Tube descending from the larynx and branching into the right and left main bronchi.

hyaline cartilage is present in the bronchi and may be mentioned in the procedural documentation.

Figure 16.11: Lungs

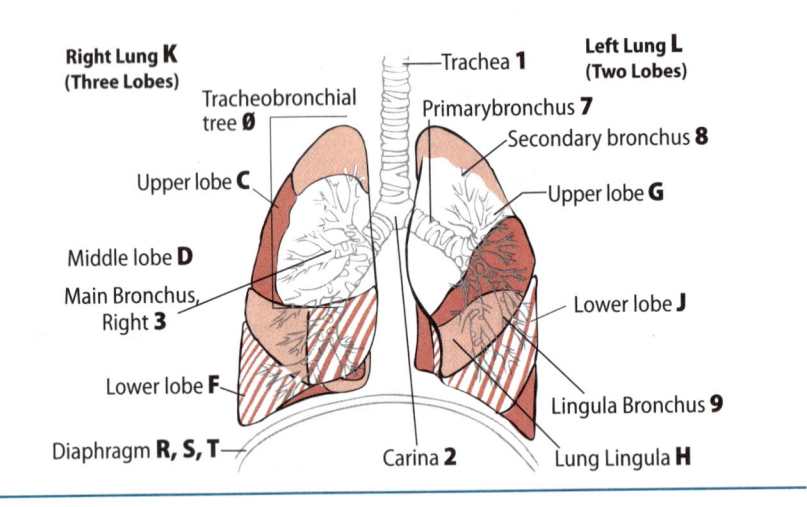

Right Lung K (Three Lobes)
- Tracheobronchial tree Ø
- Upper lobe C
- Middle lobe D
- Main Bronchus, Right 3
- Lower lobe F
- Diaphragm R, S, T

- Trachea 1
- Carina 2

Left Lung L (Two Lobes)
- Primarybronchus 7
- Secondary bronchus 8
- Upper lobe G
- Lower lobe J
- Lingula Bronchus 9
- Lung Lingula H

Character Value — C, D, F, Right Lung, Upper, Middle, Lower Lobe

Character Value — G, H, J, Left Lung, Upper, Lower Lobe, Lung Lingula

Character Value — K, L, M, Lung, Right, Left, Bilateral

The lungs are a pair of air filled sacs in the chest that enclose the bronchi, and like the bronchi, are composed of two lobes on the left and three lobes on the right.

Character Value — N, P, Q, Pleura, Right; Pleura, Left; Pleura

Associated Terms: Parietal pleura, pleural cavity, pleural fluid, visceral pleura

A thin membrane covering the lungs and lining the inside of the chest wall, the pleura is composed of two layers. The inner layer is known as the visceral pleura and the outer layer is known as the parietal pleura. The space between these two layers, known as the pleural cavity, contains a small amount of a viscous fluid, called pleural fluid.

Character Value — R, S, T, Diaphragm, Right & Left; Diaphragm

Associated Terms: Inferior thoracic aperture

Aiding in respiration by moving up and down, the diaphragm is the muscular wall separating the thorax and its structures from the abdomen. The opening closed by the diaphragm is known as the inferior thoracic aperture.

Representative ICD-10-PCS Code Examples

1. **Tracheoscopy with intraluminal dilation of tracheal stenosis**

   0B718ZZ   Dilation of trachea, via natural or artificial opening endoscopic

2. **Diagnostic bronchoscopy**

   0BJ08ZZ   Inspection of tracheobronchial tree, via natural or artificial opening endoscopic

3. **Right lung transplant using organ donor match**

   0BYK0Z0   Transplant of lung, open approach with allogeneic donor

   Note: Allogeneic is from one individual to another of the same species. Syngeneic is genetically identical individuals (e.g., identical twins). Zooplastic is from an animal of another species.

4. **Formation of tracheostomy with tracheostomy tube placement, percutaneous**

   0B113F4   Bypass from trachea, with tracheostomy device, to cutaneous, percutaneous approach

5. **Insertion of brachytherapy seeds, via bronchoscopy into right main bronchus**

   0BH081Z   Insertion into tracheobronchial tree, of radioactive element, via endoscopic artificial or natural opening

   Note: Even though right main bronchus is a choice in this table, it is not a valid code since the only device value listed in this row is endobronchial valve. Since the appropriate device is radioactive element, the code must be selected from the row with the more general body part of tracheobronchial tree. All of the values needed to construct a valid code must be chosen from the same set of cells in the same row.

Summary

This chapter reviews the root operations, body parts, and approach characters associated with the lymphatic, sense organ, and respiratory systems, and details the characters from an anatomy and physiology perspective. Understanding the anatomy and physiology associated with these body areas is essential to precise coding. Additional information regarding ICD-10-PCS coding can be found in Optum360's *Detailed Instruction for Appropriate ICD-10-PCS Coding*.

Knowledge Assessment Questions

1. Which approach is defined as "entry of instrumentation through a natural or artificial external opening to reach the site of the procedure"?

    a. Open

    b. Percutaneous

    c. Via natural or artificial opening

    d. External

2. Which root operation is defined as "taking or letting out fluid and/or gases from a body part"?

    a. Extirpation

    b. Release

    c. Change

    d. Drainage

3. What body part character would be assigned for a procedure performed in the lymphatic and hemic systems on the bone marrow of the sternum?

    a. T Bone marrow

    b. Q Bone marrow, sternum

    c. 7 Lymphatic, thorax

    d. S Bone marrow, vertebral

4. Which procedure is defined as "putting back in or on all or a portion of a separated body part to its normal location or other suitable location"?

    a. Reattachment

    b. Alteration

    c. Revision

    d. Transfer

5. A procedure is performed on the antrum of Highmore and is assigned to body part character Q or R in the ear, nose, and sinus body system.

    a. True

    b. False

6. A patient has a procedure performed on the left side of the diaphragm. Which of the following body part characters would be the most appropriate choice from the respiratory body system?

    a. T Diaphragm

    b. 2 Carina

    c. S Diaphragm, left

    d. L Lung, left

7. The lung pleura is the ridge at the junction of the trachea and the bronchi formed by a projection of the lowest tracheal cartilage separating the openings of the two bronchi.

    a. True

    b. False

8. Which procedure involves modifying the anatomic structure of a body part without affecting function?
   a. Bypass
   b. Alteration
   c. Map
   d. Reposition

9. If a procedure is performed on the zonule of Zinn on the right side, which body part character from the eye body system would likely be assigned?
   a. J Lens, right
   b. E Retina, right
   c. K Lens, left
   d. L Extraocular muscle, right

10. A procedure performed on the optic disc would be assigned to one of the lens body part characters in the eye body system.
    a. True
    b. False

Chapter 17. ICD-10-PCS: Digestive and Endocrine Systems

Mouth and Throat (C)

Procedures on the mouth and throat include services such as cleft palate repair, tonsillectomy with adenoidectomy, or a labial frenectomy. A compiled table for body system character C Mouth and throat, provides all of the valid characters for those systems in ICD-10-PCS.

Operation–Character 3	Body Part–Character 4	Approach–Character 5	Device–Character 6	Qualifier–Character 7
0 Alteration	0 Upper Lip	0 Open	0 Drainage Device	0 Single
2 Change	1 Lower Lip	3 Percutaneous	1 Radioactive Element	1 Multiple
5 Destruction	2 Hard Palate	4 Percutaneous Endoscopic	5 External Fixation Device	2 All
7 Dilation	3 Soft Palate	7 Via Natural or Artificial Opening	7 Autologous Tissue Substitute	X Diagnostic
9 Drainage	4 Buccal Mucosa	8 Via Natural or Artificial Opening Endoscopic	B Intraluminal Device, Airway	Z No Qualifier
B Excision	5 Upper Gingiva	X External	C Extraluminal Device	
C Extirpation	6 Lower Gingiva		D Intraluminal Device	
D Extraction	7 Tongue		J Synthetic Substitute	
F Fragmentation	8 Parotid Gland, Right		K Nonautologous Tissue Substitute	
H Insertion	9 Parotid Gland, Left		Y Other Device	
J Inspection	A Salivary Gland		Z No Device	
L Occlusion	B Parotid Duct, Right			
M Reattachment	C Parotid Duct, Left			
N Release	D Sublingual Gland, Right			
P Removal	F Sublingual Gland, Left			
Q Repair	G Submaxillary Gland, Right			
R Replacement	H Submaxillary Gland, Left			
S Reposition	J Minor Salivary Gland			
T Resection	M Pharynx			
U Supplement	N Uvula			
V Restriction	P Tonsils			
W Revision	Q Adenoids			
X Transfer	R Epiglottis			
	S Larynx			
	T Vocal Cord, Right			
	V Vocal Cord, Left			
	W Upper Tooth			
	X Lower Tooth			
	Y Mouth and Throat			

Comprehensive Anatomy and Physiology for ICD-10-CM and ICD-10-PCS Coding

Body Part — Character 4

The body part characters specified in the mouth and throat table detail the various subcomponents of the mouth and throat.

Figure 17.1: Mouth Frontal View (Upper)

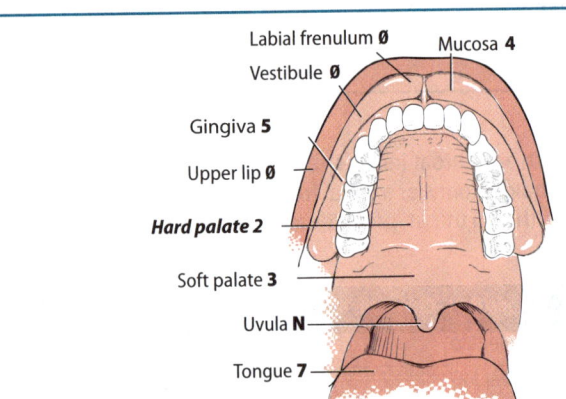

Figure 17.2: Mouth Frontal View (Lower)

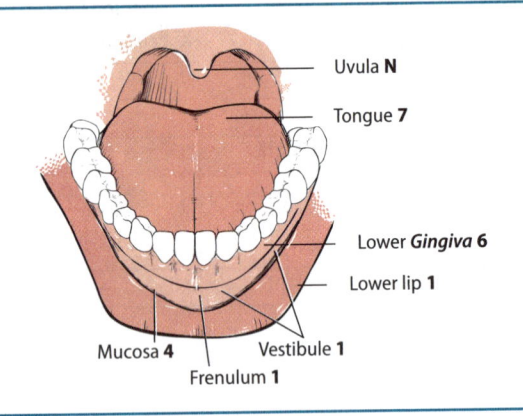

DEFINITIONS

gingiva. Soft tissues surrounding the crowns of unerupted teeth and necks of erupted teeth.

hard palate. Bony portion of the roof of the mouth.

Character Value — 0, 1, Upper Lip, Lower Lip

Associated Terms: Frenulum labii inferioris (lower), frenulum labii superioris (upper), labial gland, vermilion border

The lips are the fleshy areas at the opening of the mouth, delimited by the vermillion border. The labial glands are found around the mouth. The frenulum labii superioris is a small fold of tissue that restricts the movement of the upper lip away from the inside of the mouth. The frenulum labii inferioris is the same type of tissue restricting movement of the lower lip.

Character Value — 2, Hard Palate

Character Value — 3, Soft Palate

Associated Terms: Velum

The palate is the roof of the mouth. The front portion is known as the hard palate, due to the bony plate beneath. The back portion is known as the soft palate, as it is made up of muscle fiber and mucous membrane.

452 © 2015 Optum360, LLC

Character Value — 4, Buccal Mucosa

Associated Terms: Buccal gland, molar gland, palatine gland

Tissue from the mucous membranes on the inside of the cheek, the buccal mucosa are supplied with their secretions by several different glands, including the buccal gland, the molar gland, and the palatine gland.

Figure 17.3: Oral Anatomy

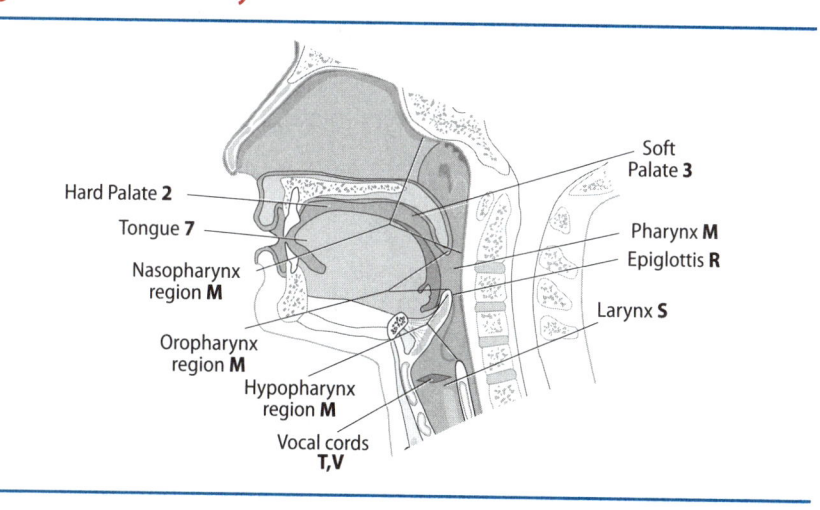

Hard Palate **2**
Tongue **7**
Nasopharynx region **M**
Oropharynx region **M**
Hypopharynx region **M**
Vocal cords **T, V**
Soft Palate **3**
Pharynx **M**
Epiglottis **R**
Larynx **S**

Character Value — 7, Tongue

Associated Terms: Frenulum linguae, lingual tonsil

Used to manipulate food for purposes of eating, as well as to serve several other purposes, the tongue is quite important to daily life. The lingual tonsils are found at the back of the tongue and are masses of lymphatic tissue. The frenulum linguae is a small fold of tissue that restricts the movement of tongue from the bottom of the mouth.

Figure 17.4: Mandibular Glands

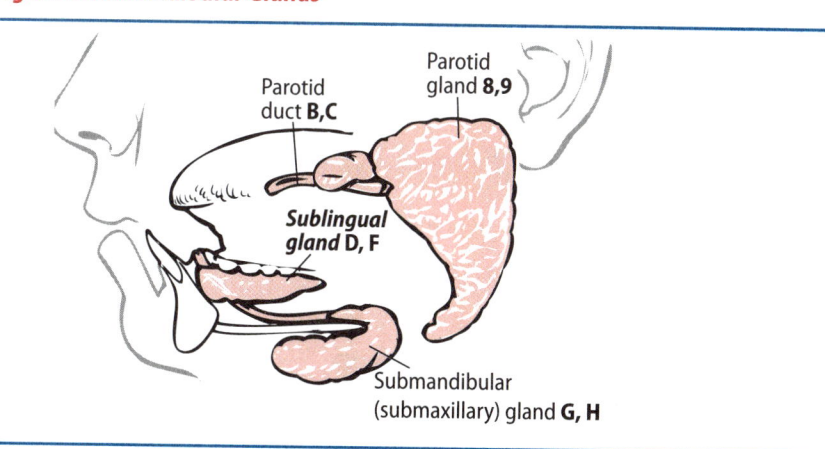

Parotid duct **B, C**
Parotid gland **8, 9**
Sublingual gland **D, F**
Submandibular (submaxillary) gland **G, H**

> **DEFINITIONS**
>
> **parotid gland.** Salivary gland located near the ear.
>
> **sublingual gland.** Small salivary gland found under the tongue.

Character Value — B, C, Parotid Duct, Left & Right

Associated Terms: Stensen's duct

The parotid ducts, also known as Stensen's ducts, route saliva from the ***parotid gland*** to the mouth.

Comprehensive Anatomy and Physiology for ICD-10-CM and ICD-10-PCS Coding

DEFINITIONS

soft palate. Fleshy portion of the roof of the mouth extending from the back of the hard palate and from which the uvula is suspended at the posterior edge.

Character Value — G, H, Submaxillary Gland, Left & Right

Associated Terms: Submandibular gland

Located beneath the floor of the mouth, the submaxillary glands provide saliva. They are also known as the submandibular glands.

Figure 17.5: Pharynx

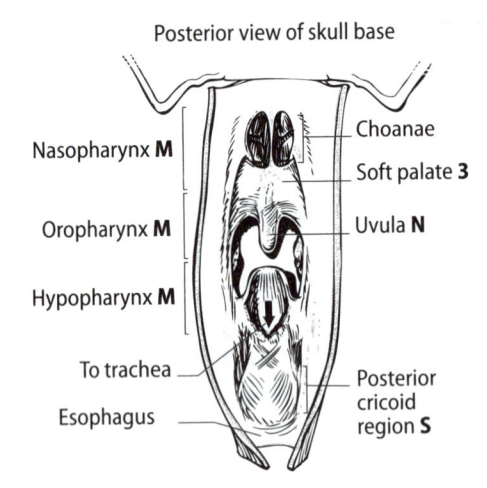

Posterior view of skull base

- Nasopharynx **M**
- Oropharynx **M**
- Hypopharynx **M**
- To trachea
- Esophagus
- Choanae
- Soft palate **3**
- Uvula **N**
- Posterior cricoid region **S**

Character Value — J, Minor Salivary Gland

Associated Terms: Anterior lingual gland.

Character Value — M, Pharynx

Associated Terms: Hypopharynx, laryngopharynx, oropharynx, piriform recess (sinus)

The musculomembranous passage of the throat consists of three regions: the nasopharynx is the passage at the back of the nostrils, as discussed in the ear, nose, and sinus system; the oropharynx is the region between the **soft palate** and the edge of the epiglottis; and the hypopharynx or laryngopharynx is the region of the epiglottis at the juncture of the larynx and esophagus. The piriform recess is found on either side of the larynx.

Character Value — N, Uvula

Associated Terms: Palatine uvula

The uvula is a pendulous fleshy mass at the back of the throat, also referred to as the palatine uvula.

Character Value — P, Tonsils

Associated Terms: Palatine tonsils

Tonsils are small masses of lymphoid tissue that are found in the oropharynx. They are also commonly called palatine tonsils, although there are other types of tonsils found in the throat as well.

Character Value — Q, Adenoids

Associated Terms: Pharyngeal tonsils

Adenoids are masses of lymphoid tissue situated on the back wall and roof of the nasopharynx, also commonly known as pharyngeal tonsils.

Character Value — R, Epiglottis

Associated Terms: Glossoepiglottic fold

A lid-like cartilaginous tissue that covers the entrance to the larynx, the epiglottis blocks food from entering the trachea. It is covered with mucous membrane that is partly attached to the wall of the pharynx through the glossoepiglottic fold.

Character Value — S, Larynx

Associated Terms: Aryepiglottic fold, arytenoid cartilage, corniculate cartilage, cuneiform cartilage, false vocal cord, glottis, rima glottidis, thyroid cartilage, ventricular fold

The larynx is a musculocartilaginous structure between the trachea and the pharynx that functions as the valve preventing food and other particles from entering the respiratory tract, as well as the voice mechanism. It is composed of three single cartilages: cricoid, epiglottis, and thyroid; and three paired cartilages: arytenoid, corniculate, and cuneiform. Other structures in and around the larynx include the ventricular fold or false vocal cord, the aryepiglottic fold, the glottis, and the rima glottidis.

Character Value — T, V, Vocal Cord, Left & Right

Associated Terms: Vocal fold

Vocal cords, also known as vocal folds, are foldings of mucous membrane stretched horizontally across the larynx that vibrate causing phonation.

Representative ICD-10-PCS Code Examples

1. **Tonsillectomy and adenoidectomy**

   ØCTPXZZ Resection of tonsils, external approach
   ØCTQXZZ Resection of adenoids, external approach

   Note: There is no 4th character body part value that combines tonsils and adenoids; the two procedures must be coded separately. Since it is possible to visualize and perform the procedure without the aid of any instrumentation, the appropriate approach 5th character value is X External.

2. **Percutaneous marsupialization of right submaxillary gland cyst**

   ØC9G3ZZ Drainage of right submaxillary gland, percutaneous approach

   Note: When marsupializing a cyst, it is opened by a puncture or small incision, thus draining its contents. This translates to the root operation drainage in ICD-10-PCS.

Comprehensive Anatomy and Physiology for ICD-10-CM and ICD-10-PCS Coding

Gastrointestinal System (D)

The gastrointestinal system table begins with the esophagus and makes its way through the gastrointestinal tract all the way to the anus. Procedures that may be found in this section include gastrotomy, repair of esophageal strictures, colonoscopies, and appendectomies. A compiled table for body system character D Gastrointestinal system, shows all of the valid characters for those systems under ICD-10-PCS.

Operation–Character 3	Body Part–Character 4	Approach–Character 5	Device–Character 6	Qualifier–Character 7
1 Bypass	0 Upper Intestinal Tract	0 Open	0 Drainage Device	0 Allogeneic
2 Change	1 Esophagus, Upper	3 Percutaneous	1 Radioactive Element	1 Syngeneic
5 Destruction	2 Esophagus, Middle	4 Percutaneous Endoscopic	2 Monitoring Device	2 Zooplastic
7 Dilation	3 Esophagus, Lower	7 Via Natural or Artificial Opening	3 Infusion Device	3 Vertical
8 Division	4 Esophagogastric Junction	8 Via Natural or Artificial Opening Endoscopic	7 Autologous Tissue Substitute	4 Cutaneous
9 Drainage	5 Esophagus	X External	B Intraluminal Device, Airway	5 Esophagus
B Excision	6 Stomach		C Extraluminal Device	6 Stomach
C Extirpation	7 Stomach, Pylorus		D Intraluminal Device	9 Duodenum
F Fragmentation	8 Small Intestine		J Synthetic Substitute	A Jejunum
H Insertion	9 Duodenum		K Nonautologous Tissue Substitute	B Ileum
J Inspection	A Jejunum		L Artificial Sphincter	H Cecum
L Occlusion	B Ileum		M Stimulator Lead	K Ascending Colon
M Reattachment	C *Ileocecal Valve*		U Feeding Device	L Transverse Colon
N Release	D Lower Intestinal Tract		Y Other Device	M Descending Colon
P Removal	E Large Intestine		Z No Device	N Sigmoid Colon
Q Repair	F Large Intestine, Right			P Rectum
R Replacement	G Large Intestine, Left			Q Anus
S Reposition	H Cecum			X Diagnostic
T Resection	J Appendix			Z No Qualifier
U Supplement	K Ascending Colon			
V Restriction	L Transverse Colon			
W Revision	M Descending Colon			
X Transfer	N Sigmoid Colon			
Y Transplantation	P Rectum			
	Q Anus			
	R Anal Sphincter			
	S Greater Omentum			
	T Lesser Omentum			
	U Omentum			
	V Mesentery			
	W Peritoneum			

Definitions

ileocecal valve. Sphincter between the ileum of the small intestine and the cecum of the large intestine.

© 2015 Optum360, LLC

Body Part — Character 4

The body part characters specified in the gastrointestinal system table detail the various components of the GI system.

Figure 17.6: Gastrointestinal System: Upper Intestinal Tract, Lower Intestinal Tract

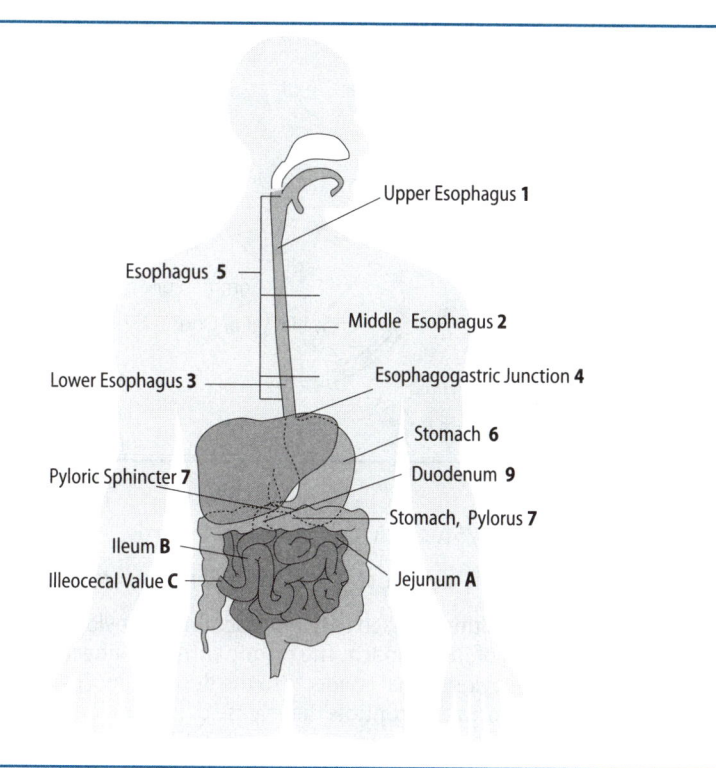

> **KEY POINT**
>
> For the root operations of change, inspection, removal, and revision, the upper and lower intestinal tract are provided as body part values. In PCS, the upper intestinal tract includes the area from the esophagus down to and including the duodenum. The lower intestinal tract includes the area from the jejunum down to and including the rectum and anus.

- Upper Esophagus **1**
- Esophagus **5**
- Middle Esophagus **2**
- Lower Esophagus **3**
- Esophagogastric Junction **4**
- Stomach **6**
- Pyloric Sphincter **7**
- Duodenum **9**
- Stomach, Pylorus **7**
- Ileum **B**
- Illeocecal Value **C**
- Jejunum **A**

Character Value — 1, 2, 3, 5, Esophagus, Upper, Middle, Lower; Esophagus

Associated Terms: Abdominal esophagus (lower), cervical esophagus (upper), thoracic esophagus (middle)

The esophagus is a muscular tube that carries swallowed liquids and foods from the pharynx to the stomach, and is divided into three separate components: upper, middle, and lower. The upper esophagus is also known as the cervical esophagus, the middle esophagus is also known as the thoracic esophagus, and the lower esophagus is also known as the abdominal esophagus.

Character Value — 4, Esophagogastric Junction

Associated Terms: Cardia, cardioesophageal junction, gastroesophageal (GE) junction

The esophagogastric junction is located between the esophagus and the stomach (also known as the cardia), and it functions somewhat like a valve. The esophagogastric junction is also known as the cardioesophageal junction or the GE junction.

Figure 17.7: Stomach and Pylorus

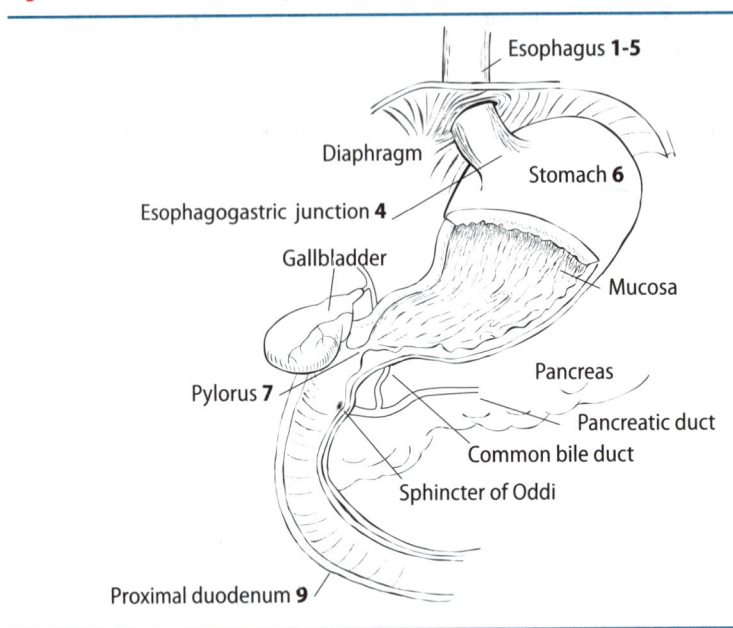

Diagram labels: Esophagus 1-5, Diaphragm, Stomach 6, Esophagogastric junction 4, Gallbladder, Mucosa, Pylorus 7, Pancreas, Pancreatic duct, Common bile duct, Sphincter of Oddi, Proximal duodenum 9

Character Value — 6, 7, Stomach, and Stomach, Pylorus

Associated Terms: Pyloric antrum, pyloric canal, pyloric sphincter

Connecting the body of the stomach to the duodenum, the pylorus is a narrow, nearly tubular portion of the stomach. The pyloric antrum connects to the body of the stomach, and the pyloric canal connects to the duodenum. The pyloric sphincter is at the end of the pylorus and controls the release of food products into the duodenum.

Character Value — 9, Duodenum

Associated Terms: Duodenal bulb

The duodenum is a short (approximately 10 inch) portion of the small intestine that connects the stomach to the rest of the intestinal tract. It is shaped like a "C" and connects with the jejunum. The duodenum is important to the digestive process as bile and pancreatic juices are introduced to the system at this point.

Figure 17.8: Lower GI

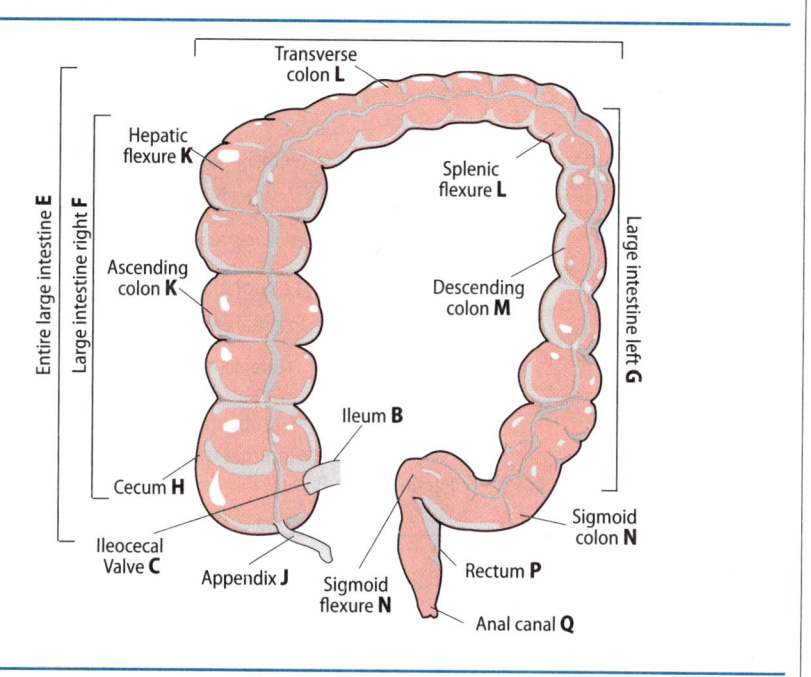

Diagram of the lower GI tract with labeled parts: Transverse colon L, Hepatic flexure K, Splenic flexure L, Ascending colon K, Descending colon M, Entire large intestine E, Large intestine right F, Large intestine left G, Ileum B, Cecum H, Ileocecal Valve C, Appendix J, Sigmoid flexure N, Sigmoid colon N, Rectum P, Anal canal Q.

Character Value — A, Jejunum

Associated Terms: Duodenojejunal flexure

The jejunum is a highly vascular, intermediate section of the small intestine, and extends from the duodenum to the ileum. The duodenum and jejunum meet at the duodenojejunal flexure. The junction of the duodenum and jejunum is also often referred to as the ligament of Treitz.

Character Value — J, Appendix

Associated Terms: Vermiform appendix

An appendage of the cecum, the appendix is a pouch-like structure that doesn't serve any significant purpose in the GI system. It is also referred to as the vermiform appendix.

Character Value — E, F, G, H, Large Intestine; Large Intestine, Right; Large Intestine, Left; Cecum

Character Value — K, Ascending Colon

Associated Terms: Hepatic flexure

Character Value — L, Transverse Colon

Associated Terms: Splenic flexure

Character Value — M, Descending Colon

Character Value — N, Sigmoid Colon

Associated Terms: Rectosigmoid junction, sigmoid flexure

The colon is a portion of the large intestine that extends from the cecum to the rectum, and consists of four components: ascending colon, transverse colon, descending colon, and sigmoid colon. The points at which the colon changes direction are known as various flexures, such as the hepatic flexure, the splenic flexure, and the sigmoid flexure. The rectosigmoid junction is the point where the rectum and the sigmoid colon join together.

Comprehensive Anatomy and Physiology for ICD-10-CM and ICD-10-PCS Coding

Figure 17.9: Rectum and Anus

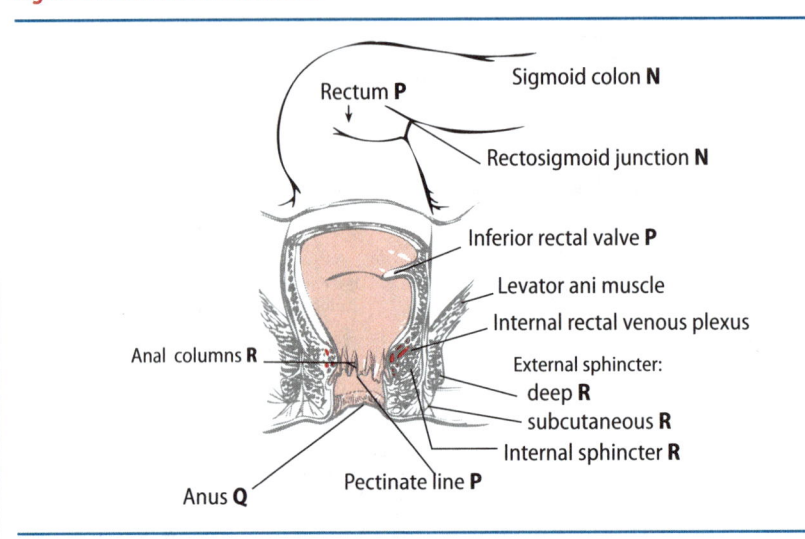

Character Value — P, Rectum

Associated Terms: Anorectal junction

The rectum is the end portion of the large intestine from the rectosigmoid junction to the anus. The junction between the rectum and the anus is known as the anorectal junction.

Character Value — Q, Anus

Associated Terms: Anal orifice

The anus or anal orifice is the opening at the end of the anal canal that serves as the external opening to the gastrointestinal system through which one is able to expel waste products from the body.

Character Value — R, Anal Sphincter

Associated Terms: External anal sphincter, internal anal sphincter

The anal sphincters have their own individual functions. The external anal sphincter is mainly tasked with keeping the anal canal and orifice closed. The internal anal sphincter moves feces along the canal to expel it through the anus, as well as helps keep the canal and orifice closed.

Character Value — S, Greater Omentum

Associated Terms: Gastrocolic ligament, gastrocolic omentum, gastrophrenic ligament, gastrosplenic ligament

A fold of peritoneal membrane, the greater omentum covers the outside of the greater curvature of the stomach all the way to the transverse colon. Also known as the gastrocolic omentum, the greater omentum helps seal off infections or hernias. The gastrocolic ligament, gastrophrenic ligament, and gastrosplenic ligament are also parts of the greater omentum.

Character Value — T, Lesser Omentum

Associated Terms: Gastrohepatic omentum, hepatogastric ligament

Also a fold of peritoneal membrane, the lesser omentum (gastrohepatic omentum) covers the area from the liver to the lesser curvature of the stomach and the duodenum. The hepatogastric ligament is part of the lesser omentum.

> ✓ **QUICK TIP**
>
> An important fact to know, especially when coding lysis of adhesions, is that the greater omentum is below the stomach and the lesser omentum is above the stomach.

Character Value — V, Mesentery

Associated Terms: Mesoappendix, mesocolon

The mesentery consists of two layers of peritoneum that fold to attach organs to the abdominal wall. The mesentery may be known by additional terms based on nearby organs. Mesoappendix and mesocolon are portions of the mesentery.

Character Value — W, Peritoneum

Associated Terms: Epiploic foramen

The peritoneum is a strong, continuous membrane that forms the lining of the abdominal and pelvic cavity. The parietal peritoneum, or outer layer, is attached to the abdominopelvic walls, and the visceral peritoneum, or inner layer, surrounds the organs inside the abdominal cavity. The peritoneum has two sacs: the general greater sac and the lesser omental sac. These two regions of peritoneum are connected by the epiploic foramen.

Representative ICD-10-PCS Code Examples

1. **Open colocutaneous colostomy formation, using transverse colon**

   0D1L0Z4   Bypass transverse colon to cutaneous, open approach

   Note: A colocutaneous colostomy formation connects the colon to the outside surface of the skin. Body part value L Transverse colon, is the body site bypassed from, and qualifier value Cutaneous, should be assigned for the body site bypassed to.

2. **Laparoscopic vertical sleeve gastrectomy**

   0DB64Z3   Excision of stomach, percutaneous endoscopic approach, vertical

   Note: Qualifier character value 3 Vertical, differentiates this procedure from other types of gastrectomies.

3. **Laparoscopic lysis of adhesions up to the ligament of Treitz to free the small bowel**

   0DNA4ZZ   Release of jejunum, percutaneous endoscopic approach

   Note: The appropriate body part is jejunum because the small bowel is being freed "up to" the ligament of Treitz. The coder needs to know that the ligament of Treitz is the junction between the jejunum and duodenum. The duodenojejunal flexure, also where the duodenum and jejunum meet, is associated with "jejunum" in the body part key.

4. **Total resection of anorectal junction**

   0DTP0ZZ   Resection of Rectum, open approach

   Note: Per the body part key, anorectal junction is coded to the body part value P Rectum.

Hepatobiliary System and Pancreas (F)

Procedures on the hepatobiliary system and pancreas include services such as a cholecystectomy, hepatectomy, or a pancreatic transplant. A compiled table for body system character F Hepatobiliary system and pancreas, provides all of the valid characters for those systems in ICD-10-PCS.

> **DEFINITIONS**
>
> **hepatobiliary duct.** Commonly known as the hepatic duct or the common hepatic duct, the hepatobiliary duct combines with the cystic duct to form the common bile duct. It carries bile from the liver.

Operation–Character 3	Body Part–Character 4	Approach–Character 5	Device–Character 6	Qualifier–Character 7
1 Bypass	0 Liver	0 Open	0 Drainage Device	0 Allogeneic
2 Change	1 Liver, Right Lobe	3 Percutaneous	1 Radioactive Element	1 Syngeneic
5 Destruction	2 Liver, Left Lobe	4 Percutaneous Endoscopic	2 Monitoring Device	2 Zooplastic
7 Dilation	4 Gallbladder	7 Via Natural or Artificial Opening	3 Infusion Device	3 Duodenum
8 Division	5 Hepatic Duct, Right	8 Via Natural or Artificial Opening Endoscopic	7 Autologous Tissue Substitute	4 Stomach
9 Drainage	6 Hepatic Duct, Left	X External	C Extraluminal Device	5 Hepatic Duct, Right
B Excision	8 Cystic Duct		D Intraluminal Device	6 Hepatic Duct, Left
C Extirpation	9 Common Bile Duct		J Synthetic Substitute	7 Hepatic Duct, Caudate
F Fragmentation	B *Hepatobiliary Duct*		K Nonautologous Tissue Substitute	8 Cystic Duct
H Insertion	C Ampulla of Vater		Y Other Device	9 Common Bile Duct
J Inspection	D Pancreatic Duct		Z No Device	B Small Intestine
L Occlusion	F Pancreatic Duct, Accessory			C Large Intestine
M Reattachment	G Pancreas			X Diagnostic
N Release				Z No Qualifier
P Removal				
Q Repair				
R Replacement				
S Reposition				
T Resection				
U Supplement				
V Restriction				
W Revision				
Y Transplantation				

Body Part — Character 4

The body part characters specified in the hepatobiliary system and pancreas table detail the specific components of the liver, biliary, and pancreatic systems.

Figure 17.10: Liver

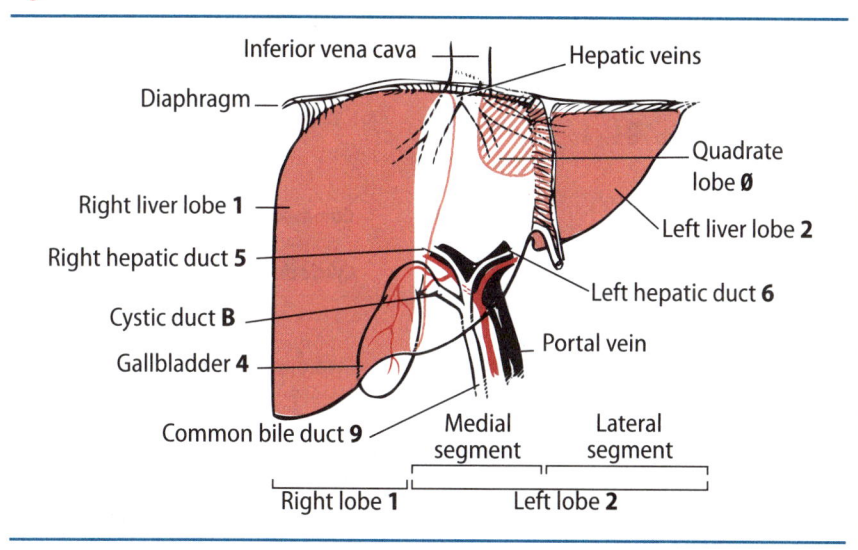

Character Value — 0, 1, 2, Liver; Liver, Right Lobe; Liver, Left Lobe

Associated Terms: Caudate lobe, quadrate lobe

The liver is responsible for many different functions, including detoxification and synthesis of proteins, and is most commonly divided into right and left lobes. There are also quadrate and caudate lobes, which function somewhat differently and have separate blood supplies.

Character Value — 4, Gallbladder

The gallbladder is a pouch found just under the liver. It is a reservoir for bile, produced by the liver, to be stored until it is needed by the digestive tract.

Figure 17.11: Gallbladder and Ducts

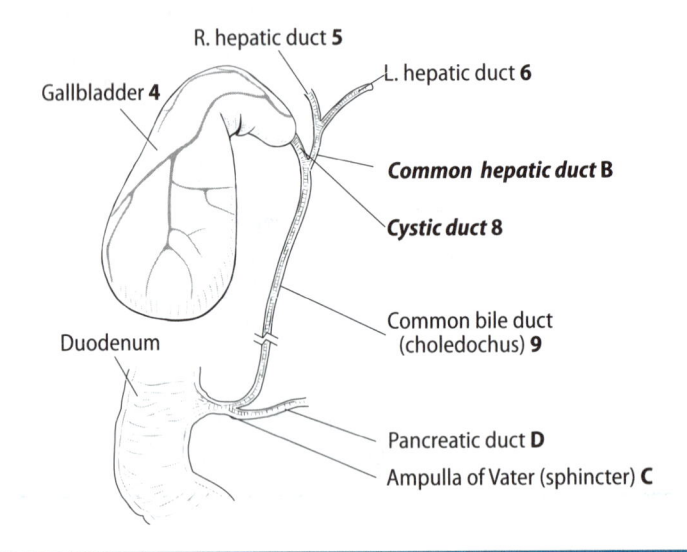

Character Value — C, Ampulla of Vater

Associated Terms: Duodenal ampulla, hepatopancreatic ampulla

The ampulla of Vater, also known as the duodenal ampulla or the hepatopancreatic ampulla, is a tubular structure with flask-like dilation where the common bile and pancreatic ducts join before emptying into the duodenum.

Figure 17.12: Pancreas

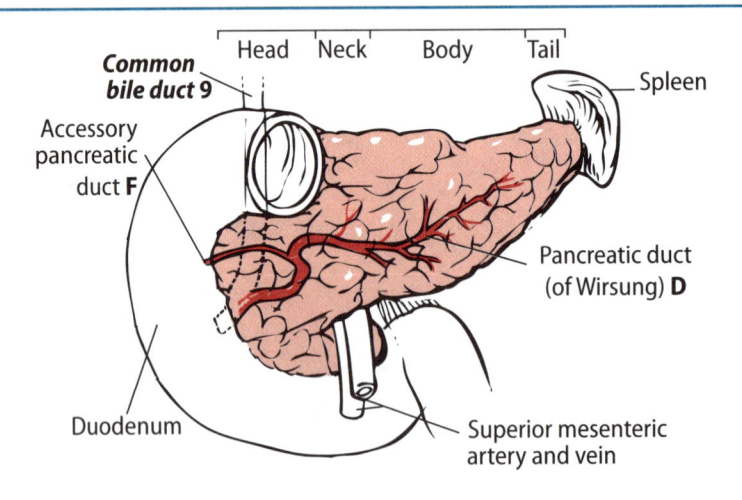

DEFINITIONS

common bile duct. Formed from the union of the cystic and hepatic ducts, this common bile duct's main function is to carry bile to the duodenum.

cystic duct. Joins the gallbladder to the common bile duct; bile can flow in both directions in this duct.

hepatic duct. Duct that carries bile from the liver into the common bile duct, and conveys it to the duodenum.

Character Value — D, Pancreatic Duct

Associated Terms: Duct of Wirsung

Joining the pancreas to the common bile duct, the pancreatic duct supplies pancreatic enzymes for the purpose of digestion. It is also called the duct of Wirsung.

Character Value — F, Pancreatic Duct, Accessory

Associated Terms: Duct of Santorini

In some patients, an accessory pancreatic duct exists, connecting the pancreas directly to the duodenum. The functioning of this second duct varies by patient. It is also called the duct of Santorini.

Representative ICD-10-PCS Code Examples

1. **Percutaneous needle core biopsy of the left lobe of the liver**

    0FB23ZX   Excision of left lobe liver, percutaneous approach, diagnostic

    Note: There is another body part value for liver, if the specific lobe is not identified. Coders should assign the most specific character value available, if possible. For biopsy procedures, the 7th character qualifier value X Diagnostic, is assigned.

2. **Total cholecystectomy, laparoscopic converted to open**

    0FT40ZZ   Resection of gallbladder, open approach

    0FJ44ZZ   Inspection of gallbladder, percutaneous endoscopic approach

    Note: Refer to coding guideline B3.2.d: When an intended root operation is attempted using one approach, but is converted to a different approach, assign separate codes, one with the root operation inspection with the initial approach value coded.

3. **ERCP with lithotripsy of Duct of Wirsung stone**

    0FFD8ZZ   Fragmentation of Pancreatic Duct stone, via natural or artificial opening, endoscopic approach

    Note: Per the body part key, duct of Wirsung refers to the pancreatic duct.

Definitions

aortic body. One of several small structures along the aortic arch that is sensitive to the chemical composition of the arterial blood due to the makeup of its neural tissue.

para-aortic body. Small mass of chromaffin tissue found near the sympathetic ganglia along the abdominal aorta.

paraganglion. Collection of chromaffin cells derived from neural ectoderm, occurring outside the adrenal medulla, usually somewhere near the sympathetic ganglia.

Endocrine System (G)

The endocrine system is responsible for secreting hormones to fulfill a variety of functions throughout the body. Procedures performed in the endocrine system may include thyroidectomy, biopsy of the pineal gland, or repair of the adrenal gland. A compiled table for body system character G Endocrine system, provides all of the valid characters for those systems in ICD-10-PCS.

Operation–Character 3	Body Part–Character 4	Approach–Character 5	Device–Character 6	Qualifier–Character 7
2 Change	0 Pituitary Gland	0 Open	0 Drainage Device	X Diagnostic
5 Destruction	1 Pineal Body	3 Percutaneous	2 Monitoring Device	Z No Qualifier
8 Division	2 Adrenal Gland, Left	4 Percutaneous Endoscopic	3 Infusion Device	
9 Drainage	3 Adrenal Gland, Right	X External	Y Other Device	
B Excision	4 Adrenal Glands, Bilateral		Z No Device	
C Extirpation	5 Adrenal Gland			
H Insertion	6 Carotid Body, Left			
J Inspection	7 Carotid Body, Right			
M Reattachment	8 Carotid Bodies, Bilateral			
N Release	9 *Para-aortic Body*			
P Removal	B Coccygeal Glomus			
Q Repair	C Glomus Jugulare			
S Reposition	D *Aortic Body*			
T Resection	F *Paraganglion* Extremity			
W Revision	G Thyroid Gland Lobe, Left			
	H Thyroid Gland Lobe, Right			
	J Thyroid Gland Isthmus			
	K Thyroid Gland			
	L Superior Parathyroid Gland, Right			
	M Superior Parathyroid Gland, Left			
	N Inferior Parathyroid Gland, Right			
	P Inferior Parathyroid Gland, Left			
	Q Parathyroid Glands, Multiple			
	R Parathyroid Gland			
	S Endocrine Gland			

Body Part — Character 4

The body part characters specified in the endocrine system table detail the various glands and structures within the endocrine system.

Figure 17.13: Endocrine System

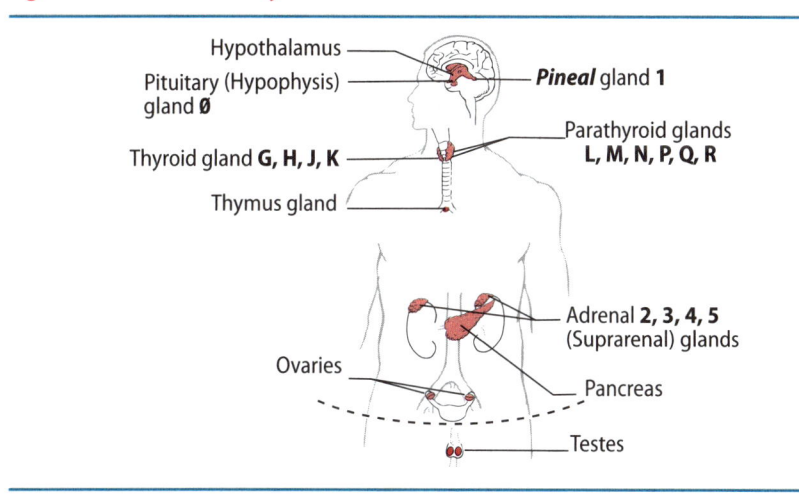

Character Value — 0, Pituitary Gland

Associated Terms: Adenohypophysis, hypophysis, neurohypophysis

The pituitary gland, or hypophysis, is a hormone-controlling epithelial body located within the sella turcica at the base of the brain. It secretes most of the body's hormones and regulates neurohormones received from the hypothalamus. The pituitary gland is divided into two components: the anterior pituitary or adenohypophysis and the posterior pituitary or neurohypophysis.

Figure 17.14: Adrenal Glands

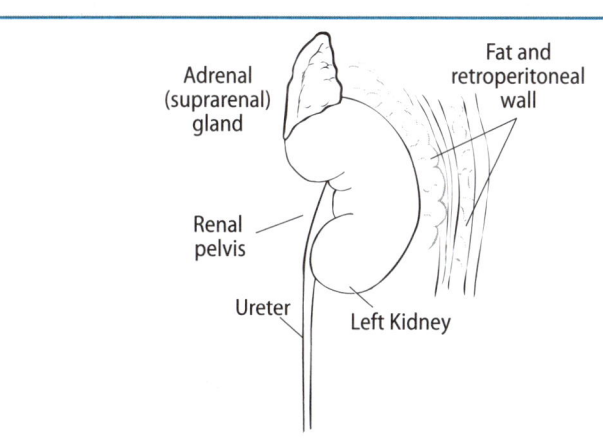

Character Value — 2, 3, 4, 5, Adrenal Gland, Left, Right, Bilateral

Associated Terms: Suprarenal gland

The adrenal glands, also known as suprarenal glands, are a specialized group of secretory cells located above the kidneys that produce hormones to regulate metabolism, maintain fluid balance, and control blood pressure. They also produce slight amounts of androgens, estrogens, and progesterone.

> ✓ **QUICK TIP**
>
> Many of the body part values in the endocrine system, such as the para-aortic body, glomus jugulare, and paraganglion, may be unfamiliar terms. Using the Character Meaning Table is very useful in determining whether these body part values are contained in this body system.

> 📖 **DEFINITIONS**
>
> **pineal body.** Cone-shaped gland in the brain responsible for synthesizing and secreting melatonin.

Character Value — 6, 7, 8, Carotid Body, Left, Right, Bilateral

Associated Terms: Carotid glomus

The carotid body is a small neurovascular structure located at the fork of the carotid arteries. Its primary function is to monitor the oxygen content of the blood, which helps to regulate respiration, blood pressure, and heart rate in response to changes in hydrogen and carbon dioxide levels. The carotid body is also called the carotid glomus.

Character Value — B, Coccygeal Glomus

Associated Terms: Coccygeal body

The coccygeal glomus is a grouping of cells near the tip of the coccyx, also referred to as the coccygeal body.

Character Value — C, Glomus Jugulare

Associated Terms: Jugular body

The glomus jugulare is a grouping of cells located in and around the jugular foramen of the temporal bone.

> **DEFINITIONS**
>
> **parathyroid gland.** Small glands, typically four, attached to the dorsal surfaces of the lateral lobes of the thyroid glands.

Figure 17.15: Thyroid and Parathyroid Glands

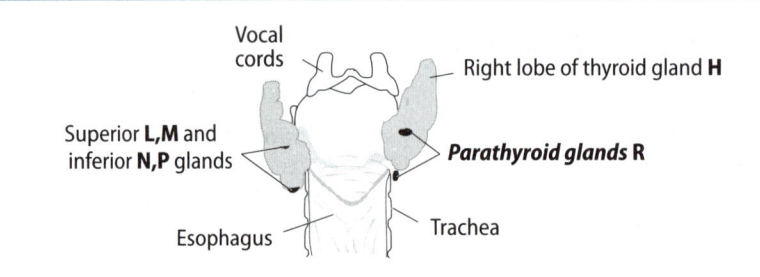

Posterior view of parathyroid glands
- Vocal cords
- Right lobe of thyroid gland **H**
- Superior **L,M** and inferior **N,P** glands
- **Parathyroid glands R**
- Esophagus
- Trachea

Figure 17.16: Thyroid (Frontal)

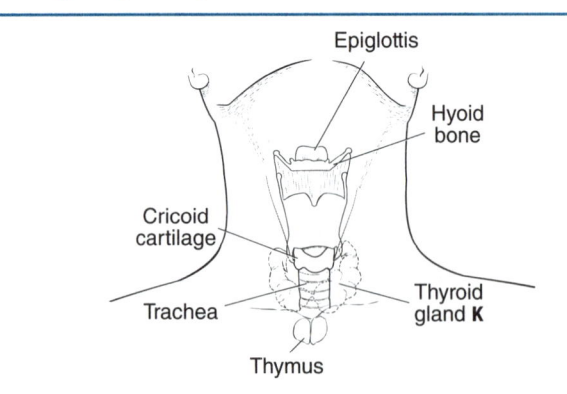

- Epiglottis
- Hyoid bone
- Cricoid cartilage
- Trachea
- Thyroid gland **K**
- Thymus

Representative ICD-10-PCS Code Examples

1. **Open transsphenoidal total excision of pituitary gland**

   0GT00ZZ Resection of pituitary gland, open approach

   Note: Because the entire pituitary gland was removed, the most appropriate root operation is resection, regardless of whether it is documented as such. Both transfrontal and transsphenoidal approaches are classified to the 0 Open, character value in ICD-10-PCS.

2. **Partial parathyroidectomy, right superior gland, open approach**

   0GBL0ZZ Excision of right superior parathyroid gland, open approach

Summary

This chapter provides an overview of the mouth and throat, gastrointestinal system, hepatobiliary system and pancreas, and endocrine system. Understanding the various anatomical structures within these body areas and organ systems can aid coders in a successful transition to the ICD-10-PCS code set, providing an excellent base from which to learn more about the methods of ICD-10-PCS coding. It also alerts providers about potential issues or confusion with documentation in the future.

Knowledge Assessment Questions

1. What root operation is defined as "freeing a body part from an abnormal physical constraint by cutting or by use of force"?
   a. Release
   b. Division
   c. Removal
   d. Revision

2. How many codes are necessary to code EGD biopsies of the stomach, including the antrum, cardia, and fundus? _____

3. The vermillion border is the area around the _____?
   a. Teeth
   b. Lips
   c. Tonsils
   d. Larynx

4. Which procedure involves putting in or on all or a portion of a living body part taken from another individual or animal to physically take the place and/or function of all or a portion of a similar body part?
   a. Transplantation
   b. Transfer
   c. Reposition
   d. Reattachment

5. A procedure performed on the duct of Wirsung would likely be assigned to body part character D in the hepatobiliary system and pancreas body system.
   a. True
   b. False

6. Inspection of the suprarenal glands bilaterally is assigned to which body part character in the endocrine system table?
   a. S Endocrine gland
   b. 5 Adrenal gland
   c. 4 Adrenal glands, bilateral
   d. 8 Carotid bodies, bilateral

7. A resection involves cutting out or off, without replacement, a portion of a body part.
   a. True
   b. False

8. Documentation provides information on a procedure performed on the epiploic foramen. Where is this found in the gastrointestinal system?
   a. Ascending colon
   b. Esophagogastric junction
   c. Rectum
   d. Abdominal cavity, connecting the two layers of peritoneum

9. Which procedure involves putting in or on biological or synthetic material that physically takes the place and/or function of all or a portion of a body part?

    a. Change
    b. Replacement
    c. Insertion
    d. Transfer

10. A procedure performed on the anorectal junction would likely be assigned to body part character R in the gastrointestinal body system.

    a. True
    b. False

Chapter 18. ICD-10-PCS: Skin, Subcutaneous Tissue, and Musculoskeletal Systems

Skin and Breast (H) *

The skin is the largest organ system of the body, covering the entire external structure. Procedures on the skin and breast include services such as repairs, grafts and flaps, breast reconstructions, and mastectomies. A compiled table for body system character H Skin and breast, provides all of the valid characters for those systems in ICD-10-PCS.

Operation–Character 3	Body Part–Character 4	Approach–Character 5	Device–Character 6	Qualifier–Character 7
0 Alteration	0 Skin, Scalp	0 Open	0 Drainage Device	3 Full Thickness
2 Change	1 Skin, Face	3 Percutaneous	1 Radioactive Element	4 Partial Thickness
5 Destruction	2 Skin, Right Ear	7 Via Natural or Artificial Opening	7 Autologous Tissue Substitute	5 Latissimus Dorsi Myocutaneous Flap
8 Division	3 Skin, Left Ear	8 Via Natural or Artificial Opening Endoscopic	J Synthetic Substitute	6 Transverse Rectus Abdominis Myocutaneous Flap
9 Drainage	4 Skin, Neck	X External	K Nonautologous Tissue Substitute	7 Deep Inferior Epigastric Artery Perforator Flap
B Excision	5 Skin, Chest		N Tissue Expander	8 Superficial Inferior Epigastric Artery Flap
C Extirpation	6 Skin, Back		Y Other Device	9 Gluteal Artery Perforator Flap
D Extraction	7 Skin, Abdomen		Z No Device	D Multiple
H Insertion	8 Skin, Buttock			X Diagnostic
J Inspection	9 Skin, Perineum			Z No Qualifier
M Reattachment	A Skin, Genitalia			
N Release	B Skin, Right Upper Arm			
P Removal	C Skin, Left Upper Arm			
Q Repair	D Skin, Right Lower Arm			
R Replacement	E Skin, Left Lower Arm			
S Reposition	F Skin, Right Hand			
T Resection	G Skin, Left Hand			
U Supplement	H Skin, Right Upper Leg			
W Revision	J Skin, Left Upper Leg			
X Transfer	K Skin, Right Lower Leg			
	L Skin, Left Lower Leg			
	M Skin, Right Foot			

(Continued on next page)

---

* Includes skin and breast glands and ducts.

Comprehensive Anatomy and Physiology for ICD-10-CM and ICD-10-PCS Coding

Operation–Character 3	Body Part–Character 4	Approach–Character 5	Device–Character 6	Qualifier–Character 7
(Continued)	N Skin, Left Foot			
	P Skin			
	Q Finger Nail			
	R Toe Nail			
	S *Hair*			
	T Breast, Right			
	U Breast, Left			
	V Breast, Bilateral			
	W Nipple, Right			
	X Nipple, Left			
	Y *Supernumerary Breast*			

Definitions

hair. Strand of keratin developed from a specialized follicle in the skin.

supernumerary breast. Having an additional or extra breast, sometimes referred to as an accessory breast or polymastia.

Body Part — Character 4

The body part characters specified in the skin and breast table detail the various elements and locations of the skin and breast.

Figure 18.1: Integumentary Anatomy (Ø-9, A-P)

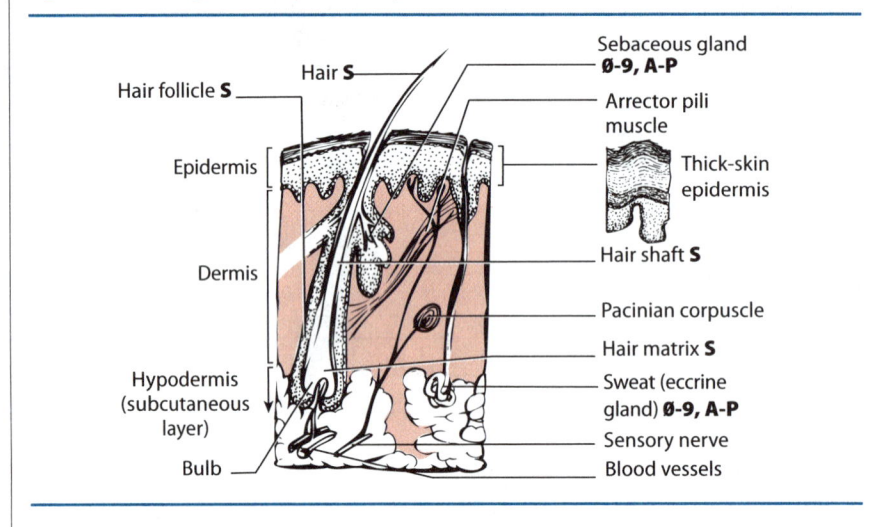

Character Value — Ø-9, A-P, Skin, Various Regions

Associated Terms: Dermis, epidermis, sebaceous gland, sweat gland

These various character values cover skin in many different sites across the body. The two main layers of the skin are the epidermis and the dermis, with the subcutaneous tissue located underneath. Procedures that extend to the subcutaneous tissue should be coded from the next table: J Subcutaneous tissue and fascia. Sebaceous glands and sweat glands are found within the structure of the skin as well.

Figure 18.2: Nail Anatomy (Q, R)

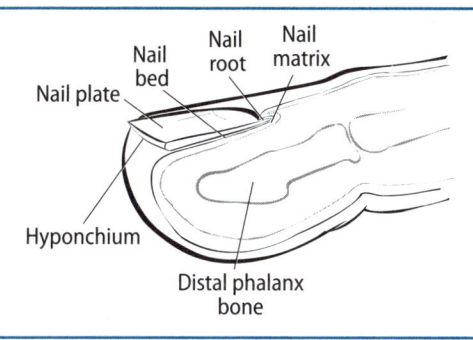

Character Value — Q, R, Finger Nail, Toe Nail

Associated Terms: Nail bed, nail plate

Nails are thin, horny plates on the dorsal side of the **phalanx** of the distal toes (toenails) and fingers (fingernails). The nail root is the proximal end under the cuticle or skin fold. The nail bed is the area of dermal layer beneath the nail, and the nail plate is the body of the nail itself.

> **DEFINITIONS**
>
> **phalanx.** Bones of the digits (fingers or toes).

Figure 18.3: Breast (T-X)

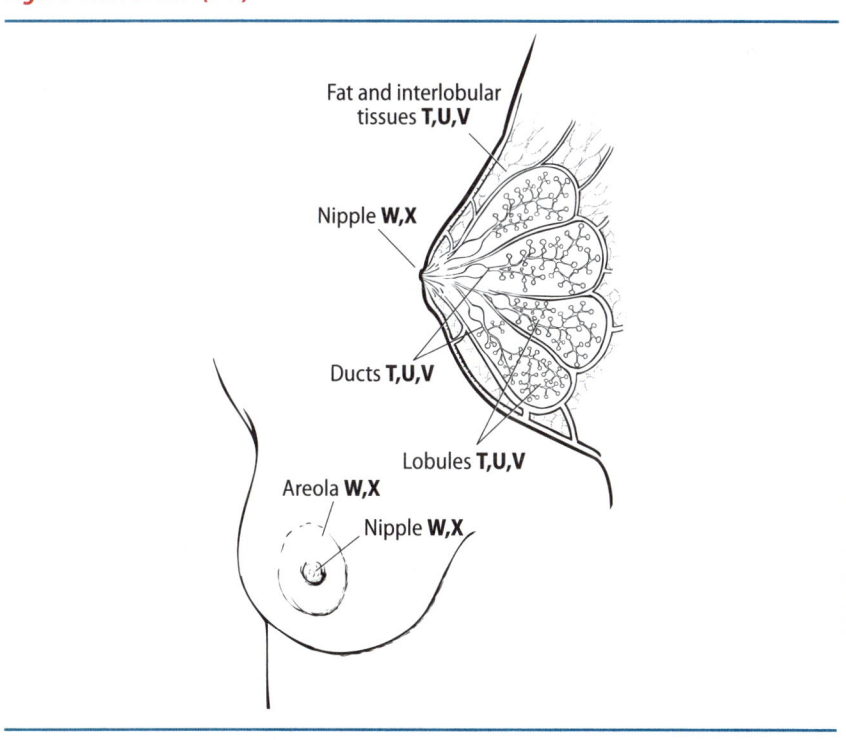

Character Value — T, U, V, Breast, Left, Right, Bilateral

Associated Terms: Mammary duct, mammary gland

The breasts are found on the anterior aspect of the chest surface. In females, they also contain the mammary glands and ducts.

Character Value — W, X, Nipple, Right, Left

Associated Terms: Areola

Opening to the lactiferous ducts below (in females), the nipple is a small, pigmented cylindrical structure near the center of each breast. It is surrounded by another pigmented round area called the areola.

Qualifier — Character 7

In the skin and breast body system section, the qualifier character is used for various types of grafting procedures. The information provided in the qualifier character details the thickness of the graft or the site and type of graft in some flap grafts. The grafts in the skin and breast section are typically assigned to root operation characters R Replacement, U Supplement, and X Transfer. For allogenic and autogenic tissue grafts, as well as synthetic grafts of the skin, qualifiers 3 and 4 are used to indicate full-thickness and partial-thickness grafts. For breast procedures, the following qualifiers are used:

- 5 Latissimus dorsi myocutaneous flap: This includes skin, fat, vessels, and muscle located in the back, behind the arm pit, and below the shoulder, which is tunneled under the skin to the chest.
- 6 Transverse rectus abdominis myocutaneous flap (TRAM): This includes skin, fat, vessels, and either all or a portion of the rectus muscle from the lower abdomen.
- 7 Deep inferior epigastric artery perforator flap (DIEP): This includes taking fat, skin, and deep blood vessels, but no muscle, from the lower abdominal wall.
- 8 Superficial inferior epigastric artery flap (SIEA or SIEP): This is the same as DIEP, except that it uses vessels that are not as deep, making it less invasive. However, because the more superficial vessels are not as large as the deep vessels, they are not always adequate for this procedure.
- 9 Gluteal artery perforator flap: This free flap procedure includes skin, fat, and vessels from the buttocks.

It is important for coders to understand the location of these various qualifier characters and how they relate to the corresponding body part values in character 4.

Representative ICD-10-PCS Code Examples

1. **Left total mastectomy with free TRAM flap reconstruction**

   0HRU076 Replacement of left breast using TRAM flap, open approach

   Note: As the entire breast was removed and the reconstructed breast takes the place of the removed breast, the root operation replacement is assigned. The TRAM is a free flap from the same patient and is considered an autologous tissue substitute. The replacement procedure also includes taking out the original body part, so the mastectomy is not coded separately.

2. **Excision of malignant melanoma from skin of right ear**

   0HB2XZZ Excision of right ear skin, external approach

3. **Right scalp advancement flap to right temple**

   0HX0XZZ Transfer of skin of scalp, external approach

4. **Incision of scar contracture, right elbow**

   0HNDXZZ Release of skin of lower arm, external approach

   Note: The skin of the elbow region is coded to lower arm (see guideline B4.6).

Subcutaneous Tissue and Fascia (J)

The subcutaneous tissue is the innermost layer of the integumentary system, and the fascia lie between the subcutaneous tissue and the muscle. Procedures performed on the subcutaneous tissue and fascia are similar to those performed on the skin, such as repairs, flaps, and grafts. A compiled table for body system character J Subcutaneous tissue and fascia, provides all of the valid characters for those systems in ICD-10-PCS.

Operation–Character 3	Body Part–Character 4	Approach–Character 5	Device–Character 6	Qualifier–Character 7
0 Alteration	0 Subcutaneous Tissue and Fascia, Scalp	0 Open	0 Drainage Device OR Monitoring Device, Hemodynamic (for root operation INSERTION only)	B Skin and Subcutaneous Tissue
2 Change	1 Subcutaneous Tissue and Fascia, Face	3 Percutaneous	1 Radioactive Element	C Skin, Subcutaneous Tissue and Fascia
5 Destruction	4 Subcutaneous Tissue and Fascia, Anterior Neck	X External	2 Monitoring Device	X Diagnostic
8 Division	5 Subcutaneous Tissue and Fascia, Posterior Neck		3 Infusion Device	Z No Qualifier
9 Drainage	6 Subcutaneous Tissue and Fascia, Chest		4 Pacemaker, Single Chamber	
B Excision	7 Subcutaneous Tissue and Fascia, Back		5 Pacemaker, Single Chamber Rate Responsive	
C Extirpation	8 Subcutaneous Tissue and Fascia, Abdomen		6 Pacemaker, Dual Chamber	
D Extraction	9 Subcutaneous Tissue and Fascia, Buttock		7 Autologous Tissue Substitute OR Cardiac Resynchronization Pacemaker Pulse Generator (for root operation INSERTION only)	
H Insertion	B Subcutaneous Tissue and Fascia, Perineum		8 Defibrillator Generator	
J Inspection	C Subcutaneous Tissue and Fascia, Pelvic Region		9 Cardiac Resynchronization Defibrillator Pulse Generator	
N Release	D Subcutaneous Tissue and Fascia, Right Upper Arm		A Contractility Modulation Device	
P Removal	F Subcutaneous Tissue and Fascia, Left Upper Arm		B Stimulator Generator, Single Array	
Q Repair	G Subcutaneous Tissue and Fascia, Right Lower Arm		C Stimulator Generator, Single Array Rechargeable	
R Replacement	H Subcutaneous Tissue and Fascia, Left Lower Arm		D Stimulator Generator, Multiple Array	
W Revision	J Subcutaneous Tissue and Fascia, Right Hand		E Stimulator Generator, Multiple Array Rechargeable	
X Transfer	K Subcutaneous Tissue and Fascia, Left Hand		H Contraceptive Device	
	L Subcutaneous Tissue and Fascia, Right Upper Leg		J Synthetic Substitute	
	M Subcutaneous Tissue and Fascia, Left Upper Leg		K Nonautologous Tissue Substitute	

(Continued on next page)

Operation–Character 3	Body Part–Character 4	Approach–Character 5	Device–Character 6	Qualifier–Character 7
(Continued)	N Subcutaneous Tissue and Fascia, Right Lower Leg		M Stimulator Generator	
	P Subcutaneous Tissue and Fascia, Left Lower Leg		N Tissue Expander	
	Q Subcutaneous Tissue and Fascia, Right Foot		P Cardiac Rhythm Related Device	
	R Subcutaneous Tissue and Fascia, Left Foot		V Infusion Device, Pump	
	S Subcutaneous Tissue and Fascia, Head and Neck		W Vascular Access Device, Reservoir	
	T Subcutaneous Tissue and Fascia, Trunk		X Vascular Access Device	
	V Subcutaneous Tissue and Fascia, Upper Extremity		Y Other Device	
	W Subcutaneous Tissue and Fascia, Lower Extremity		Z No Device	

Body Part — Character 4

The body part characters specified in the subcutaneous tissue and fascia table detail the various locations of subcutaneous tissue and fascia.

Character Value — 0, Subcutaneous Tissue and Fascia, Scalp

Associated Terms: Galea aponeurotica

A fibrous membrane that covers the upper part of the cranium, the galea aponeurotica is one of the specific terms that may appear in physician documentation for these procedures. It may also be called epicranial aponeurosis.

Character Value — 1, Subcutaneous Tissue and Fascia, Face

Associated Terms: Masseteric fascia, orbital fascia

The masseteric fascia, located on the side of the face, and the orbital fascia, located around the orbit, are two important tissue areas in the facial region.

Character Value — 4, Subcutaneous Tissue and Fascia, Anterior Neck

Associated Terms: Deep cervical fascia, pretracheal fascia

The deep cervical fascia is found on the side of the anterior neck while the pretracheal fascia is located along the front of the neck, in front of the trachea.

Character Value — 5, Subcutaneous Tissue and Fascia, Posterior Neck

Associated Terms: Prevertebral fascia

The prevertebral fascia is found in the back of the neck, and passes in front of the prevertebral muscles.

Character Value — 6, Subcutaneous Tissue and Fascia, Chest

Associated Terms: Pectoral fascia

Covering the pectoral muscles and other portions of the chest, the pectoral fascia covers a large area and varies in thickness based on the area it is covering.

Character Value — D, F, Subcutaneous Tissue and Fascia, Right & Left Upper Arm

Associated Terms: Axillary fascia, deltoid fascia, infraspinatus fascia, subscapular aponeurosis, supraspinatus fascia

The axillary fascia is found in the axilla or armpit region. The deltoid, infraspinatus, and supraspinatus fascia are found covering those specified muscle groups in the upper body. On the concave portion of the inside of the scapula there is a membrane known as the subscapular aponeurosis.

Character Value — G, H, Subcutaneous Tissue and Fascia, Right & Left Lower Arm

Associated Terms: Antebrachial fascia, bicipital aponeurosis

A general term for the *fascia* in the forearm, the antebrachial fascia is a general sheath for the muscles in this area. The bicipital aponeurosis is a structure in the elbow that protects the brachial artery and median nerve underneath.

Character Value — J, K, Subcutaneous Tissue and Fascia, Right & Left Hand

Associated Terms: Palmar fascia (aponeurosis)

The palmar fascia, also known as the palmar aponeurosis, is a sheet of fascia that is found under the skin of the palm and also surrounds the muscles.

Character Value — L, M, Subcutaneous Tissue and Fascia, Right & Left Upper Leg

Associated Terms: Crural fascia, fascia lata, iliac fascia, iliotibial tract (band)

The crural fascia is the deep fascia of the leg found between the knee and ankle, and is continuous with the fascia lata, which is the deep fascia of the thigh. The iliac fascia is found in the pelvic area. The iliotibial band or tract is a fibrous band of connective tissue that runs along the outside of the thigh from the knee to the iliac crest.

Character Value — Q, R, Subcutaneous Tissue and Fascia, Right & Left Foot

Associated Terms: Plantar fascia (aponeurosis)

Plantar fascia, also called plantar aponeurosis, is tough fascia that surrounds the muscles on the soles of the feet.

Character Value — T, Subcutaneous Tissue and Fascia, Trunk

Associated Terms: External oblique aponeurosis, transversalis fascia

There are several different fascias in the trunk region, including the external oblique aponeurosis and the transversalis fascia.

> **DEFINITIONS**
>
> **fascia.** Fibrous sheet or band of tissue that envelops organs, muscles, and groupings of muscles.

Representative ICD-10-PCS Code Examples

1. **Open placement of dual chamber pacemaker generator in chest wall**

   0JH606Z Insertion of pacemaker, dual chamber into chest subcutaneous tissue and fascia, open approach

   Note: Although the reason for the placement of a pacemaker isn't related to the subcutaneous tissue or fascia, the device placement itself is related to these body areas. The device character (6) is also important in this area of coding, as this tells which type of device was implanted in the patient.

2. **Percutaneous fascia transfer to fill defect, anterior neck**

   0JX43ZZ Transfer anterior neck subcutaneous tissue and fascia, percutaneous approach

Comprehensive Anatomy and Physiology for ICD-10-CM and ICD-10-PCS Coding

📖 DEFINITIONS

autologous. Tissue or structure derived from the same individual.

nonautologous. Derived from a source other than the same individual or recipient (e.g., cells, tissue, blood vessels, and other organs donated from another human).

Muscles (K)

Muscles serve several different functions within the body, depending on the type of muscle and the location. Procedures that are performed on muscles include myotomies, reattachments, and repairs. A compiled table for body system character K Muscles, provides all of the valid characters for those systems in ICD-10-PCS.

Operation–Character 3	Body Part–Character 4	Approach–Character 5	Device–Character 6	Qualifier–Character 7
2 Change	0 Head Muscle	0 Open	0 Drainage Device	0 Skin
5 Destruction	1 Facial Muscle	3 Percutaneous	7 **Autologous** Tissue Substitute	1 Subcutaneous Tissue
8 Division	2 Neck Muscle, Right	4 Percutaneous Endoscopic	J Synthetic Substitute	2 Skin and Subcutaneous Tissue
9 Drainage	3 Neck Muscle, Left	X External	K **Nonautologous** Tissue Substitute	6 Transverse Rectus Abdominis Myocutaneous Flap
B Excision	4 Tongue, Palate, Pharynx Muscle		M Stimulator Lead	X Diagnostic
C Extirpation	5 Shoulder Muscle, Right		Y Other Device	Z No Qualifier
H Insertion	6 Shoulder Muscle, Left		Z No Device	
J Inspection	7 Upper Arm Muscle, Right			
M Reattachment	8 Upper Arm Muscle, Left			
N Release	9 Lower Arm and Wrist Muscle, Right			
P Removal	B Lower Arm and Wrist Muscle, Left			
Q Repair	C Hand Muscle, Right			
S Reposition	D Hand Muscle, Left			
T Resection	F Trunk Muscle, Right			
U Supplement	G Trunk Muscle, Left			
W Revision	H Thorax Muscle, Right			
X Transfer	J Thorax Muscle, Left			
	K Abdomen Muscle, Right			
	L Abdomen Muscle, Left			
	M Perineum Muscle			
	N Hip Muscle, Right			
	P Hip Muscle, Left			
	Q Upper Leg Muscle, Right			
	R Upper Leg Muscle, Left			
	S Lower Leg Muscle, Right			
	T Lower Leg Muscle, Left			
	V Foot Muscle, Right			
	W Foot Muscle, Left			
	X Upper Muscle			
	Y Lower Muscle			

Body Part — Character 4

The body part characters specified in the muscle table detail the various locations of muscles throughout the body.

Figure 18.4: Muscles

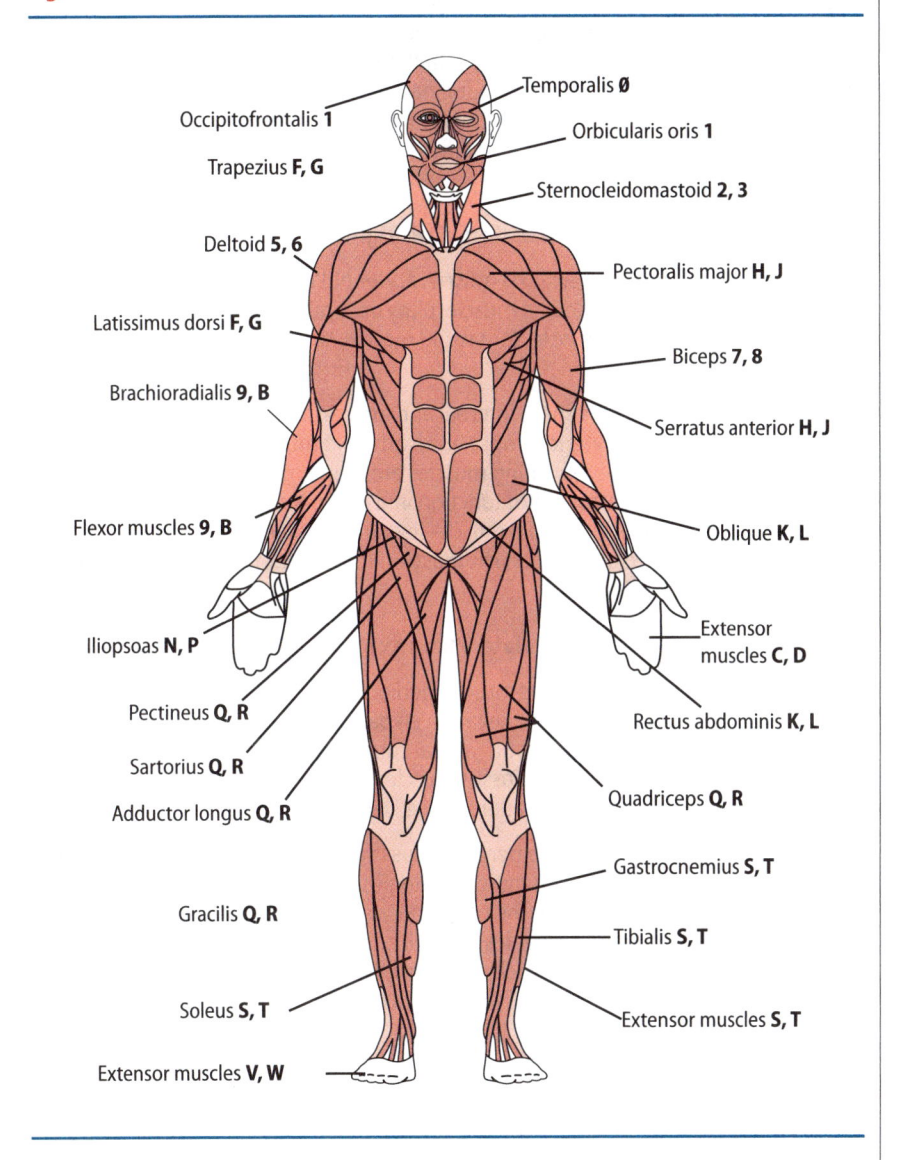

- Temporalis 0
- Occipitofrontalis 1
- Orbicularis oris 1
- Trapezius F, G
- Sternocleidomastoid 2, 3
- Deltoid 5, 6
- Pectoralis major H, J
- Latissimus dorsi F, G
- Biceps 7, 8
- Brachioradialis 9, B
- Serratus anterior H, J
- Flexor muscles 9, B
- Oblique K, L
- Extensor muscles C, D
- Iliopsoas N, P
- Pectineus Q, R
- Rectus abdominis K, L
- Sartorius Q, R
- Adductor longus Q, R
- Quadriceps Q, R
- Gastrocnemius S, T
- Gracilis Q, R
- Tibialis S, T
- Soleus S, T
- Extensor muscles S, T
- Extensor muscles V, W

Character Value — 0, Head Muscle

Associated Terms: Auricularis muscle, masseter muscle, pterygoid muscle, splenius capitis muscle, temporalis muscle, temporoparietalis muscle

There are several different sets of muscles in the head. The masseter, temporalis, and medial and lateral pterygoid muscles assist in closing the jaw. The auricularis muscles surround the ear, and the temporoparietalis muscle runs directly above it. The splenius capitis muscle runs across the back of the neck.

Character Value — 1, Facial Muscle

Associated Terms: Buccinator muscle, corrugator supercilii muscle, depressor anguli oris muscle, depressor labii inferioris muscle, depressor septi nasi muscle, depressor supercilii muscle, levator anguli oris muscle, levator labii superioris alaeque nasi muscle, levator labii superioris muscle, mentalis muscle, nasalis muscle, occipitofrontalis muscle, orbicularis oris muscle, procerus muscle, risorius muscle, zygomaticus muscle

Muscles in the facial region are numerous. In and around the mouth are the buccinator muscle, depressor anguli oris muscle, depressor labii inferioris muscle, levator anguli oris muscle, orbicularis oris muscle, risorius muscle, and zygomaticus muscle. In and around the eye are the corrugator supercilii muscle, depressor supercilii muscle, and the procerus muscle. In the nasal region are the depressor septi nasi muscle, levator labii superioris alaeque nasi muscle, and the nasalis muscle. In the remainder of the facial regions are the levator labii superioris muscle and the mentalis muscle in the area of the cheek and the occipitofrontalis muscle in and around the forehead.

Character Value — 2, 3, Neck Muscle, Left & Right

Associated Terms: Anterior vertebral muscle, arytenoid muscle, cricothyroid muscle, infrahyoid muscle, levator scapulae muscle, platysma muscle, scalene muscle, splenius cervicis muscle, sternocleidomastoid muscle, suprahyoid muscle, thyroarytenoid muscle

Some muscles in the neck are more internal and are part of the larynx and the throat structures, including the arytenoid muscle, cricothyroid muscle, and the thyroarytenoid muscle. The remaining muscles are found mainly along the external portion of the neck, to control motor function in these areas. These muscles are the anterior vertebral muscle, infrahyoid muscle, levator scapulae muscle, platysma muscle, scalene muscle, splenius cervicis muscle, sternocleidomastoid muscle, and suprahyoid muscle.

Character Value — 4, Tongue, Palate, Pharynx Muscle

Associated Terms: Chondroglossus muscle, genioglossus muscle, hyoglossus muscle, inferior longitudinal muscle, levator veli palatini muscle, palatoglossal muscle, palatopharyngeal muscle, pharyngeal constrictor muscle, salpingopharyngeus muscle, styloglossus muscle, stylopharyngeus muscle, superior longitudinal muscle, tensor veli palatini muscle, verticalis linguae

The tongue itself is made up of the genioglossus muscle, hyoglossus muscle, inferior longitudinal muscle, palatoglossal muscle, styloglossus muscle, superior longitudinal muscle, and the verticalis linguae. The other muscles of the palate and pharynx include the chondroglossus muscle, levator veli palatini muscle, palatopharyngeal muscle, pharyngeal constrictor muscle, salpingopharyngeus muscle, stylopharyngeus muscle, and sensor veli palatini muscle.

Character Value — 5, 6, Shoulder Muscle, Left & Right

Associated Terms: Deltoid muscle, infraspinatus muscle, subscapularis muscle, supraspinatus muscle, teres major muscle, teres minor muscle

There are several important muscles in the shoulder that are commonly referenced in operative reports. The four muscles that make up the rotator cuff are the infraspinatus muscle, the subscapularis muscle, the supraspinatus muscle, and the teres minor muscle. The deltoid muscle comes across the top of the shoulder, making the rounded surface. The teres major muscle comes up through the axilla to the bottom of the shoulder, creating the axillary surface.

Character Value — 7, 8, Upper Arm Muscle, Left & Right

Associated Terms: Biceps brachii muscle, brachialis muscle, coracobrachialis muscle, triceps brachii muscle

Character Value — 9, B, Lower Arm Muscle, Left & Right

Associated Terms: Anatomical snuffbox, brachioradialis muscle, extensor carpi radialis muscle, extensor carpi ulnaris muscle, flexor carpi radialis muscle, flexor carpi ulnaris muscle, flexor pollicis longus muscle, palmaris longus, pronator quadratus muscle, pronator teres muscle

The anatomical snuffbox is a depression found on the hand when the thumb is abducted and extended. This is caused by the tendons in the hand. The palmaris longus is one of the most variable muscles in the body, and its function is to flex the hand at the wrist. Muscles that are found in the forearm include the brachioradialis muscle, extensor carpi radialis muscle, extensor carpi ulnaris muscle, flexor carpi radialis muscle, flexor carpi ulnaris muscle, flexor pollicis longus muscle, pronator quadratus muscle, and pronator teres muscle.

Character Value — C, D, Hand Muscle, Left & Right

Associated Terms: Hypothenar muscle, palmar interosseous muscle, thenar muscle

Character Value — F, G, Trunk Muscle, Left & Right

Associated Terms: Coccygeus muscle, erector spinae muscle, interspinalis muscle, intertransversarius muscle, latissimus dorsi muscle, levator ani muscle, quadratus lumborum muscle, rhomboid major muscle, rhomboid minor muscle, serratus posterior muscle, transversospinalis muscle, trapezius muscle

Muscles in the pelvic area of the trunk include the coccygeus muscle and the levator ani muscle. Muscles in the back include the erector spinae muscle, interspinalis muscle, intertransversarius muscle, latissimus dorsi muscle, quadratus lumborum muscle, rhomboid major and minor muscles, serratus posterior muscle, transversospinalis muscle, and trapezius muscle.

Character Value — H, J, Thorax Muscle, Left & Right

Associated Terms: Intercostal muscle, levatores costarum muscle, pectoralis major muscle, pectoralis minor muscle, serratus anterior muscle, subclavius muscle, subcostal muscle, transverse thoracis muscle

Character Value — K, L, Abdomen Muscle, Left & Right

Associated Terms: External oblique muscle, internal oblique muscle, pyramidalis muscle, rectus abdominis muscle, transversus abdominis muscle

The rectus abdominis muscle is a body part included in the abdomen muscle group and is also a qualifier when used for a TRAM flap (root operation—transfer).

Character Value — M, Perineum Muscle

Associated Terms: Bulbospongiosus muscle, cremaster muscle, deep transverse perineal muscle, ischiocavernosus muscle, superficial transverse perineal muscle

Character Value — N, P, Hip Muscle, Left & Right

Associated Terms: Gemellus muscle, gluteus maximus muscle, gluteus medius muscle, gluteus minimus muscle, iliacus muscle, obturator muscle, piriformis muscle, psoas muscle, quadratus femoris muscle, tensor fasciae latae muscle

The muscles of the hip help with motor functions of the legs and trunk.

Character Value — Q, R, Upper Leg Muscle, Left & Right

Associated Terms: Adductor brevis muscle, adductor longus muscle, adductor magnus muscle, biceps femoris muscle, gracilis muscle, pectineus muscle, quadriceps (femoris) rectus femoris muscle, sartorius muscle, semimembranosus muscle, semitendinosus muscle, vastus intermedius muscle, vastus lateralis muscle, vastus medialis muscle

Character Value — S, T, Lower Leg Muscle, Left & Right

Associated Terms: Extensor digitorum longus muscle, extensor hallucis longus muscle, fibularis brevis muscle, fibularis longus muscle, flexor digitorum longus muscle, flexor hallucis longus muscle, gastrocnemius muscle, peroneus brevis muscle, peroneus longus muscle, popliteus muscle, soleus muscle, tibialis anterior muscle, tibialis posterior muscle

Character Value — V, W, Foot Muscle, Left & Right

Associated Terms: Abductor hallucis muscle, adductor hallucis muscle, extensor digitorum brevis muscle, extensor hallucis brevis muscle, flexor digitorum brevis muscle, flexor hallucis brevis muscle, quadratus plantae muscle

Representative ICD-10-PCS Code Examples

1. **Percutaneous biopsy of right gastrocnemius muscle**

   0KBS3ZX   Excision of right lower leg muscle, percutaneous approach, diagnostic

   Note: In this instance, the ICD-10-PCS code is much more detailed than that in ICD-9-CM. It provides information not only related to the specific procedure performed, but also the site, the approach, and even laterality. The coder may need to reference the body part key to determine that the gastrocnemius muscle is classified as a lower leg muscle in ICD-10-PCS.

2. **Open bilateral TRAM pedicle flap reconstruction (muscle only), status post mastectomy**

   0KXK0Z6   Transfer right abdomen muscle, TRAM flap, open approach
   0KXL0Z6   Transfer left abdomen muscle, TRAM flap, open approach

   Note: A bilateral TRAM flap uses both the left and right abdominal muscles and requires two separate PCS codes. Since the mastectomy was performed at an earlier surgical episode, this procedure is not coded with the root operation replacement. Instead, it is classified as a transfer procedure; the muscle flap remains attached to its vascular and nervous supply.

Tendons (L) *

Tendons are bands of dense fibrous tissue that connect muscle to bone. Procedures performed on tendons include tenotomies, reattachments of tendons, or tendon releases. A compiled table for body system character L Tendons, provides all of the valid characters for those systems in ICD-10-PCS.

Operation–Character 3	Body Part–Character 4	Approach–Character 5	Device–Character 6	Qualifier–Character 7
2 Change	0 Head and Neck Tendon	0 Open	0 Drainage Device	X Diagnostic
5 Destruction	1 Shoulder Tendon, Right	3 Percutaneous	7 Autologous Tissue Substitute	Z No Qualifier
8 Division	2 Shoulder Tendon, Left	4 Percutaneous Endoscopic	J Synthetic Substitute	
9 Drainage	3 Upper Arm Tendon, Right	X External	K Nonautologous Tissue Substitute	
B Excision	4 Upper Arm Tendon, Left		Y Other Device	
C Extirpation	5 Lower Arm and Wrist Tendon, Right		Z No Device	
J Inspection	6 Lower Arm and Wrist Tendon, Left			
M Reattachment	7 Hand Tendon, Right			
N Release	8 Hand Tendon, Left			
P Removal	9 Trunk Tendon, Right			
Q Repair	B Trunk Tendon, Left			
R Replacement	C Thorax Tendon, Right			
S Reposition	D Thorax Tendon, Left			
T Resection	F Abdomen Tendon, Right			
U Supplement	G Abdomen Tendon, Left			
W Revision	H Perineum Tendon			
X Transfer	J Hip Tendon, Right			
	K Hip Tendon, Left			
	L Upper Leg Tendon, Right			
	M Upper Leg Tendon, Left			
	N Lower Leg Tendon, Right			
	P Lower Leg Tendon, Left			
	Q Knee Tendon, Right			
	R Knee Tendon, Left			
	S Ankle Tendon, Right			
	T Ankle Tendon, Left			
	V Foot Tendon, Right			
	W Foot Tendon, Left			
	X Upper Tendon			
	Y Lower Tendon			

* Includes synovial membrane.

Body Part — Character 4

The body part characters specified in the tendons table detail the various locations of tendons throughout the body. The most appropriate way for coders to determine the accurate body part characters within the tendon table is to use the body part key for muscles. This can assist in finding the most appropriate general grouping and a corresponding PCS character value for tendons. A full body part key is found in appendix B.

Details on the various character values in the muscles table can be found in the muscles section as well. The following illustrations can provide some insight into the location of tendons throughout various sites in the body.

Figure 18.5: Wrist and Forearm Cross-section

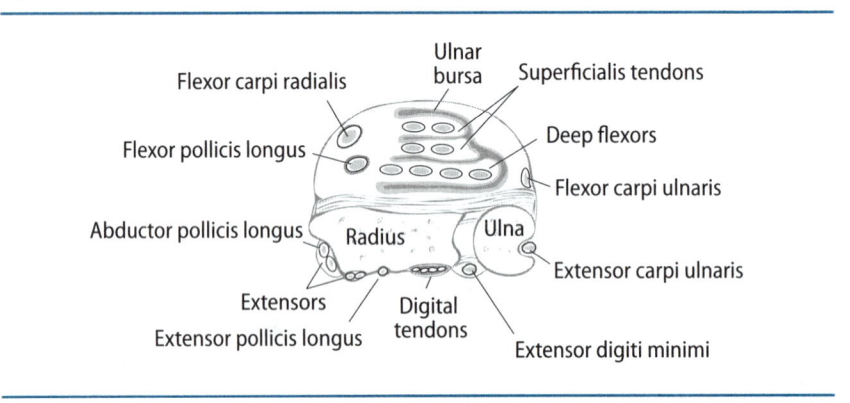

Figure 18.6: Tendons of the Wrist and Hand

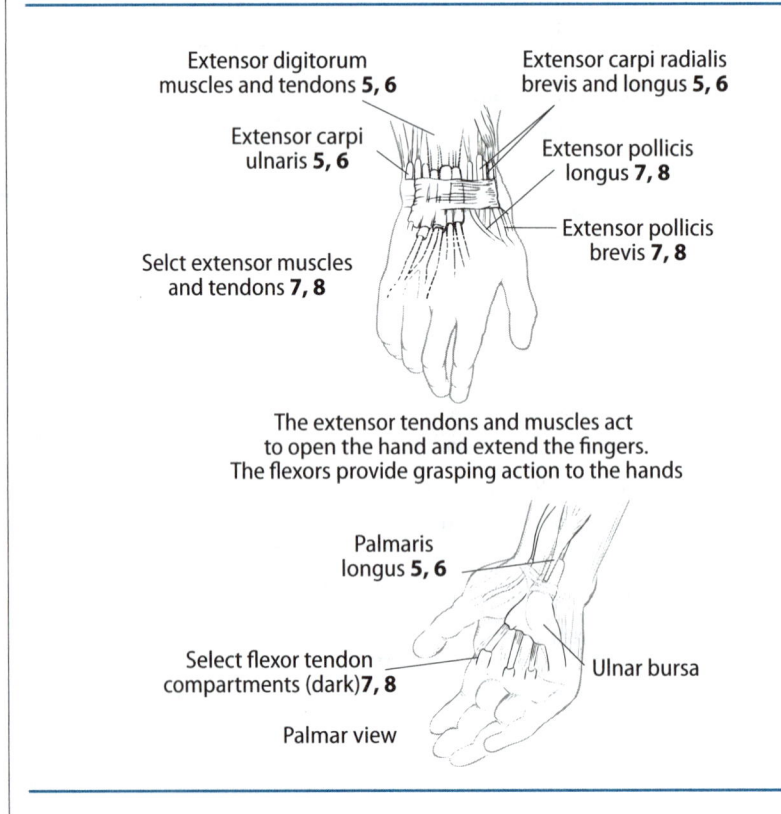

Figure 18.7: Shoulder Tendons

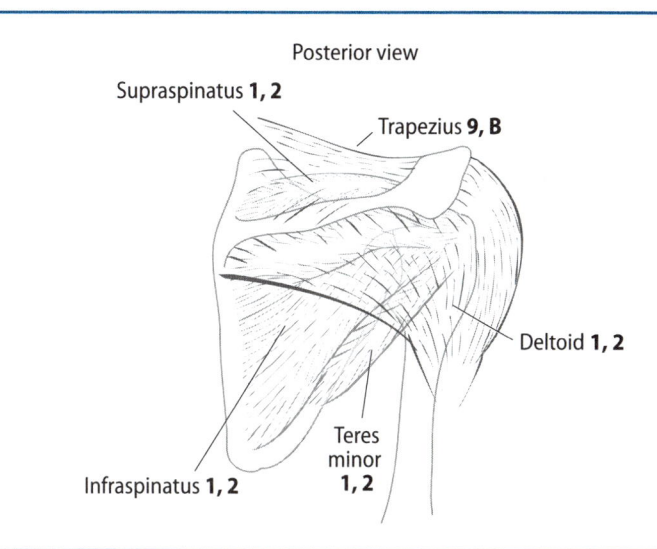

Posterior view

- Supraspinatus **1, 2**
- Trapezius **9, B**
- Deltoid **1, 2**
- Teres minor **1, 2**
- Infraspinatus **1, 2**

Figure 18.8: Leg Muscles and Tendons

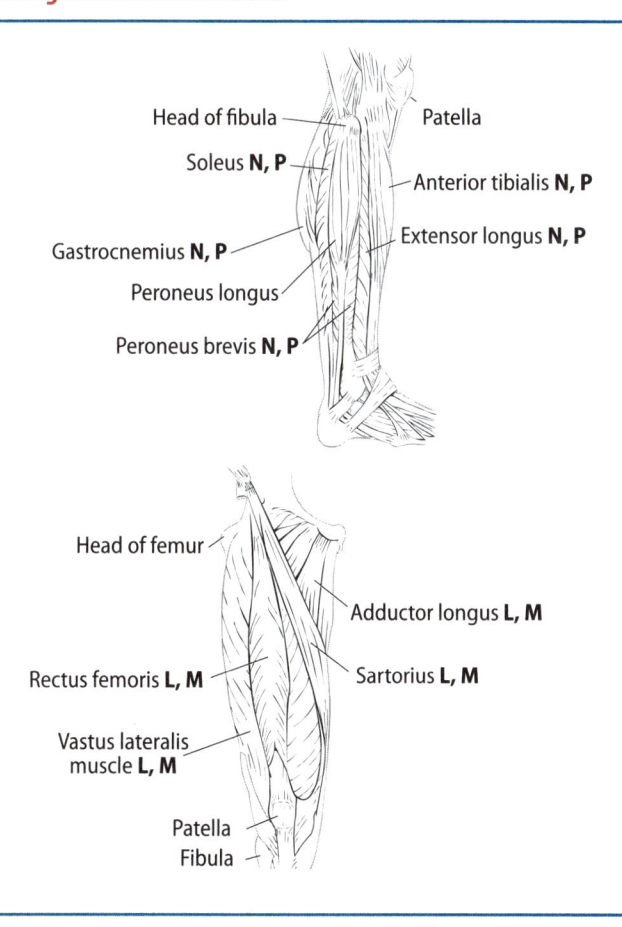

- Head of fibula
- Patella
- Soleus **N, P**
- Anterior tibialis **N, P**
- Gastrocnemius **N, P**
- Extensor longus **N, P**
- Peroneus longus
- Peroneus brevis **N, P**

- Head of femur
- Adductor longus **L, M**
- Rectus femoris **L, M**
- Sartorius **L, M**
- Vastus lateralis muscle **L, M**
- Patella
- Fibula

Figure 18.9: Lower Leg Tendons

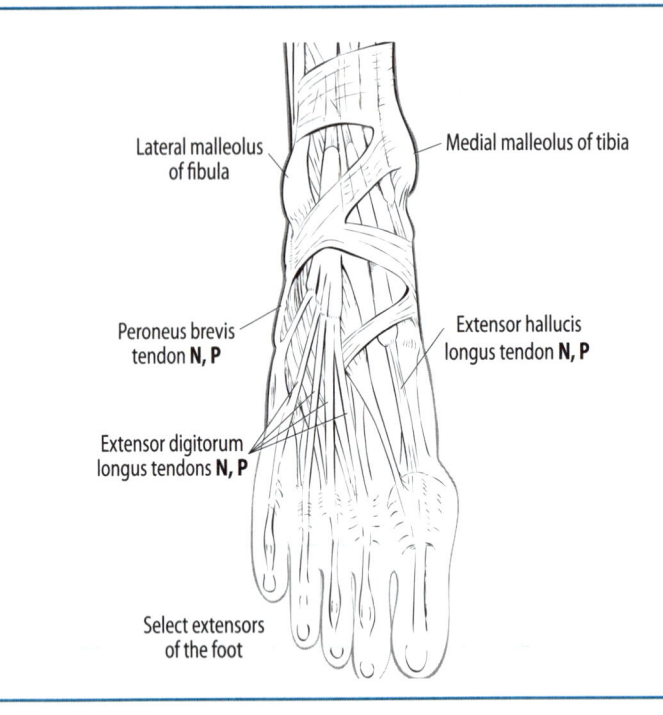

Lateral malleolus of fibula
Medial malleolus of tibia
Peroneus brevis tendon **N, P**
Extensor hallucis longus tendon **N, P**
Extensor digitorum longus tendons **N, P**
Select extensors of the foot

Representative ICD-10-PCS Code Examples

1. **Right wrist open palmaris longus tendon transfer**

   0LX50ZZ Transfer right lower arm and wrist tendon, open approach

   Note: The palmaris longus is a tendon found in the wrist, as seen in the illustration "Tendons of the Wrist and Hand." These tendons help to give the hand motion.

2. **Percutaneous left Achilles tendon release**

   0LNP3ZZ Release left lower leg tendon, percutaneous approach

Bursae and Ligaments (M)*

Ligaments are fibrous tissue that bind joints together and connect articular bones and cartilages. A bursa is a sac between a tendon and the bone beneath it that can act as a cushion. Procedures performed on bursae and ligaments may include bursectomy and bursotomy, repair and reconstruction, and suturing. A compiled table for body system character M Bursae and ligaments, provides all of the valid characters for those systems in ICD-10-PCS.

> **DEFINITIONS**
>
> **transverse ligament of perineum.** Thickened front border of the urogenital diaphragm, formed by the fusion of its two fascial layers.

Operation–Character 3	Body Part–Character 4	Approach–Character 5	Device–Character 6	Qualifier–Character 7
2 Change	0 Head and Neck Bursa and Ligament	0 Open	0 Drainage Device	X Diagnostic
5 Destruction	1 Shoulder Bursa and Ligament, Right	3 Percutaneous	7 Autologous Tissue Substitute	Z No Qualifier
8 Division	2 Shoulder Bursa and Ligament, Left	4 Percutaneous Endoscopic	J Synthetic Substitute	
9 Drainage	3 Elbow Bursa and Ligament, Right	X External	K Nonautologous Tissue Substitute	
B Excision	4 Elbow Bursa and Ligament, Left		Y Other Device	
C Extirpation	5 Wrist Bursa and Ligament, Right		Z No Device	
D Extraction	6 Wrist Bursa and Ligament, Left			
J Inspection	7 Hand Bursa and Ligament, Right			
M Reattachment	8 Hand Bursa and Ligament, Left			
N Release	9 Upper Extremity Bursa and Ligament, Right			
P Removal	B Upper Extremity Bursa and Ligament, Left			
Q Repair	C Trunk Bursa and Ligament, Right			
S Reposition	D Trunk Bursa and Ligament, Left			
T Resection	F Thorax Bursa and Ligament, Right			
U Supplement	G Thorax Bursa and Ligament, Left			
W Revision	H Abdomen Bursa and Ligament, Right			
X Transfer	J Abdomen Bursa and Ligament, Left			
	K *Perineum Bursa and Ligament*			
	L Hip Bursa and Ligament, Right			
	M Hip Bursa and Ligament, Left			
	N Knee Bursa and Ligament, Right			
	P Knee Bursa and Ligament, Left			
	Q Ankle Bursa and Ligament, Right			

(Continued on next page)

---

* Includes synovial membrane

Comprehensive Anatomy and Physiology for ICD-10-CM and ICD-10-PCS Coding

Operation–Character 3	Body Part–Character 4	Approach–Character 5	Device–Character 6	Qualifier–Character 7
(Continued)	R Ankle Bursa and Ligament, Left			
	S Foot Bursa and Ligament, Right			
	T Foot Bursa and Ligament, Left			
	V Lower Extremity Bursa and Ligament, Right			
	W Lower Extremity Bursa and Ligament, Left			
	X Upper Bursa and Ligament			
	Y Lower Bursa and Ligament			

Body Part — Character 4

The body part characters specified in the bursae and ligament table detail the various locations of these structures throughout the body.

Character Value — 0, Head and Neck Bursa and Ligament

Associated Terms: Alar ligament of axis, cervical interspinous ligament, cervical intertransverse ligament, cervical ligamentum flavum, interspinous ligament, lateral temporomandibular ligament, sphenomandibular ligament, stylomandibular ligament, transverse ligament of atlas

Ligaments found in the neck are the alar ligament of axis, cervical interspinous ligament, cervical intertransverse ligament, cervical ligamentum flavum, and the transverse ligament of atlas. Ligaments found in the jaw area are the lateral temporomandibular ligament, sphenomandibular ligament, and stylomandibular ligament.

Figure 18.10: Shoulder Anatomy

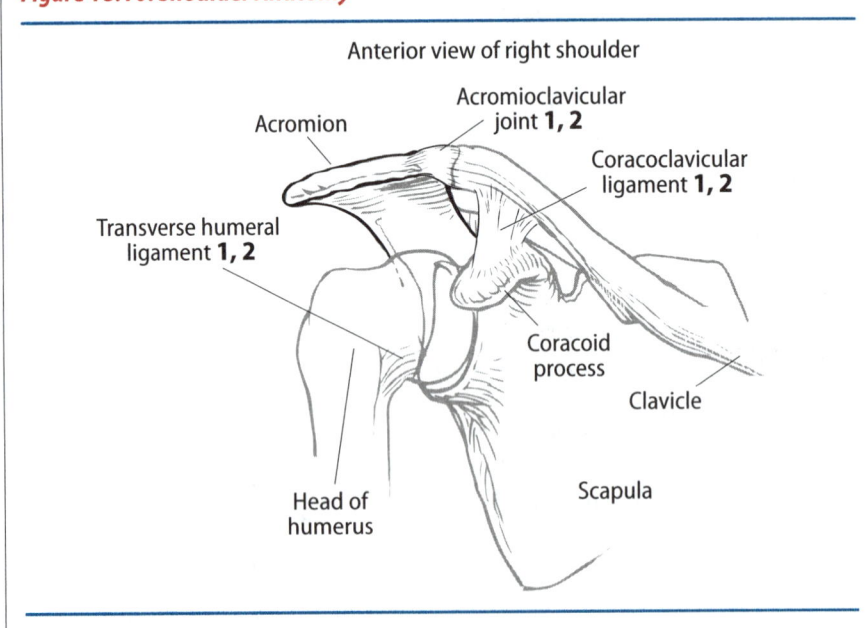

Character Value — 1, 2, Shoulder Bursa and Ligament, Right & Left

Associated Terms: Acromioclavicular ligament, coracoacromial ligament, coracoclavicular ligament, coracohumeral ligament, costoclavicular ligament, glenohumeral ligament, interclavicular ligament, sternoclavicular ligament, subacromial bursa, transverse humeral ligament, transverse scapular ligament

The subacromial bursa is found in the shoulder area. Ligaments in the shoulder region include the acromioclavicular ligament, coracoacromial ligament, coracoclavicular ligament, coracohumeral ligament, costoclavicular ligament, glenohumeral ligament, glenoid ligament (labrum), interclavicular ligament, sternoclavicular ligament, transverse humeral ligament, and transverse scapular ligament.

Character Value — 3, 4, Elbow Bursa and Ligament, Right & Left

Associated Terms: Annular ligament, olecranon bursa, radial collateral ligament, ulnar collateral ligament

Ligaments in the elbow region include the annular ligament, the radial collateral ligament, and the ulnar collateral ligament. The bursa in the elbow is the olecranon bursa.

Character Value — 5, 6, Wrist Bursa and Ligament, Right & Left

Associated Terms: Palmar ulnocarpal ligament, radial collateral carpal ligament, radiocarpal ligament, radioulnar ligament, ulnar collateral carpal ligament

Figure 18.11: Wrist Ligaments

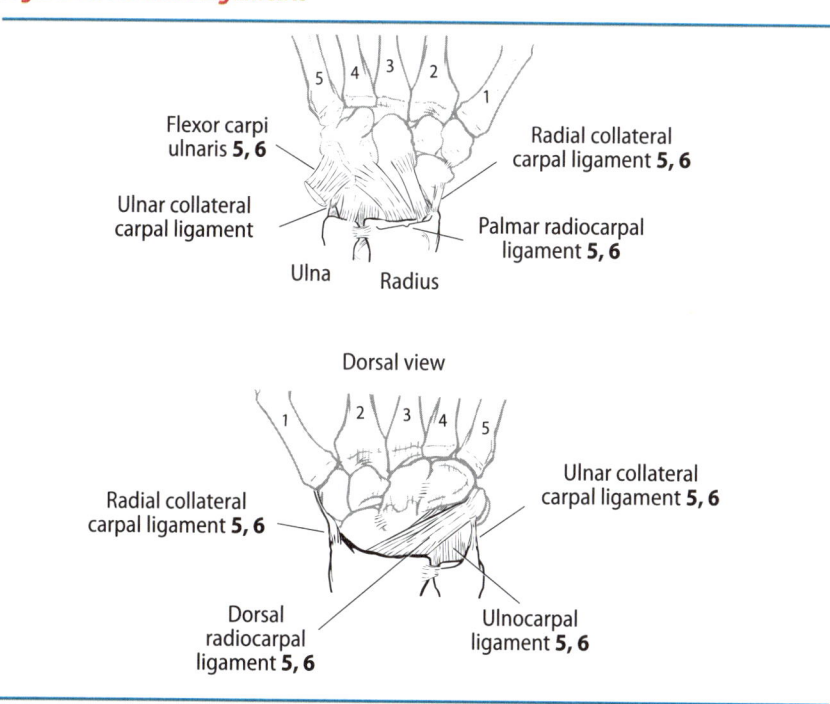

Character Value — 7, 8, Hand Bursa and Ligament, Right & Left

Associated Terms: Carpometacarpal ligament, intercarpal ligament, interphalangeal ligament, lunotriquetral ligament, **metacarpal** ligament, metacarpophalangeal ligament, pisohamate ligament, pisometacarpal ligament, scapholunate ligament, scaphotrapezium ligament

DEFINITIONS

metacarpal. Five long bones of the hand that join with the carpal bones and with the proximal phalanges of the fingers.

Character Value — C, D, Trunk Bursa and Ligament, Right & Left

Associated Terms: Iliolumbar ligament, interspinous ligament, intertransverse ligament, ligamentum flavum, pubic ligament, sacrococcygeal ligament, sacroiliac ligament, sacrospinous ligament, sacrotuberous ligament, supraspinous ligament

Character Value — F, G, Thorax Bursa and Ligament, Right & Left

Associated Terms: Costotransverse ligament, costoxiphoid ligament, sternocostal ligament

Character Value — L, M, Hip Bursa and Ligament, Right & Left

Associated Terms: Iliofemoral ligament, ischiofemoral ligament, pubofemoral ligament, transverse acetabular ligament, trochanteric bursa

The bursa in the hip is the trochanteric bursa. Ligaments in the hip include the iliofemoral ligament, the ischiofemoral ligament, the pubofemoral ligament, and the transverse acetabular ligament.

Figure 18.12: Knee Bursae

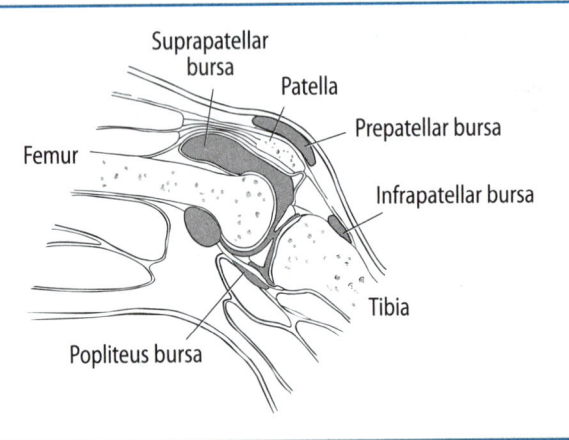

Character Value — N, P, Knee Bursa and Ligament, Right & Left

Associated Terms: Anterior cruciate ligament (ACL), lateral collateral ligament (LCL), ligament of head of fibula, medial collateral ligament (MCL), patellar ligament, popliteal ligament, posterior cruciate ligament (PCL), prepatellar bursa

The prepatellar bursa is one of the bursae of the knee. Ligaments of the knee include the ACL, the LCL, the ligament of head of fibula, the MCL, the patellar ligament, the popliteal ligament, and the PCL.

Figure 18.13: Knee Ligaments

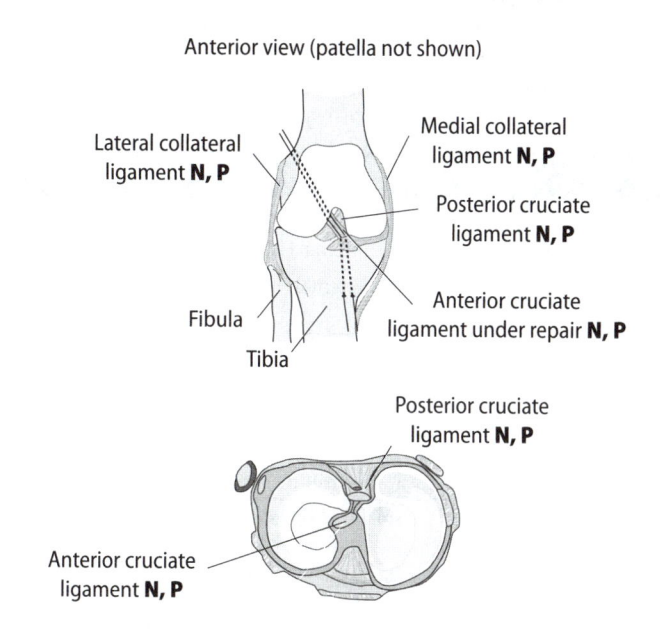

Anterior view (patella not shown)

- Lateral collateral ligament **N, P**
- Medial collateral ligament **N, P**
- Posterior cruciate ligament **N, P**
- Anterior cruciate ligament under repair **N, P**
- Fibula
- Tibia
- Posterior cruciate ligament **N, P**
- Anterior cruciate ligament **N, P**

Character Value — Q, R, Ankle Bursa and Ligament, Right & Left

Associated Terms: Calcaneofibular ligament, deltoid ligament, ligament of the lateral malleolus, talofibular ligament

Character Value — S, T, Foot Bursa and Ligament, Right & Left

Associated Terms: Calcaneocuboid ligament, cuneonavicular ligament, intercuneiform ligament, interphalangeal ligament, metatarsal ligament, metatarsophalangeal ligament, subtalar ligament, talocalcaneal ligament, talocalcaneonavicular ligament, tarsometatarsal ligament

Representative ICD-10-PCS Code Examples

1. **Right shoulder arthroscopy with coracoacromial ligament release**

    ØMN14ZZ Release right shoulder bursa and ligament, percutaneous endoscopic approach

    Note: When the body part key is referenced, the coracoacromial ligament is classified in ICD-10-PCS to the character values for shoulder bursa and ligament.

2. **Left knee arthroscopy with reposition of anterior cruciate ligament**

    ØMSP4ZZ Reposition left knee bursa and ligament, percutaneous endoscopic approach

    Note: The percutaneous endoscopic (arthroscopic) approaches are popular for the bursae and ligaments, as well as for the joint procedures. Pay careful attention in the documentation to the approach used, and report it with approach character 5.

Head and Facial Bones (N)

Procedures that could be performed on the head and facial bones include a mandibulectomy, treatment of orbital fracture, or various types of bone grafting to facial bones. A compiled table for body system character N Head and facial bones, provides all of the valid characters for those systems in ICD-10-PCS.

Operation–Character 3	Body Part–Character 4	Approach–Character 5	Device–Character 6	Qualifier–Character 7
2 Change	0 Skull	0 Open	0 Drainage Device	X Diagnostic
5 Destruction	1 Frontal Bone, Right	3 Percutaneous	4 Internal Fixation Device	Z No Qualifier
8 Division	2 Frontal Bone, Left	4 Percutaneous Endoscopic	5 External Fixation Device	
9 Drainage	3 **Parietal Bone**, Right	X External	7 Autologous Tissue Substitute	
B Excision	4 Parietal Bone, Left		J Synthetic Substitute	
C Extirpation	5 Temporal Bone, Right		K Nonautologous Tissue Substitute	
H Insertion	6 Temporal Bone, Left		M Bone Growth Stimulator	
J Inspection	7 Occipital Bone, Right		N Neurostimulator Generator	
N Release	8 Occipital Bone, Left		S Hearing Device	
P Removal	B Nasal Bone		Y Other Device	
Q Repair	C Sphenoid Bone, Right		Z No Device	
R Replacement	D Sphenoid Bone, Left			
S Reposition	F Ethmoid Bone, Right			
T Resection	G Ethmoid Bone, Left			
U Supplement	H Lacrimal Bone, Right			
W Revision	J Lacrimal Bone, Left			
	K Palatine Bone, Right			
	L Palatine Bone, Left			
	M Zygomatic Bone, Right			
	N Zygomatic Bone, Left			
	P Orbit, Right			
	Q Orbit, Left			
	R Maxilla, Right			
	S Maxilla, Left			
	T Mandible, Right			
	V Mandible, Left			
	W Facial Bone			
	X **Hyoid Bone**			

Definitions

hyoid bone. Single, u-shaped bone palpable in the neck above the larynx and below the mandible (lower jaw) with various muscles attached but not articulating with any other bone.

parietal bones. Pair of bones that form the sides of the cranium.

Chapter 18. ICD-10-PCS: Skin, Subcutaneous Tissue, and Musculoskeletal Systems

Body Part — Character 4

The body part characters specified in the head and facial bones table detail the various bone structures in the head and face.

Figure 18.14: Head and Facial Bones

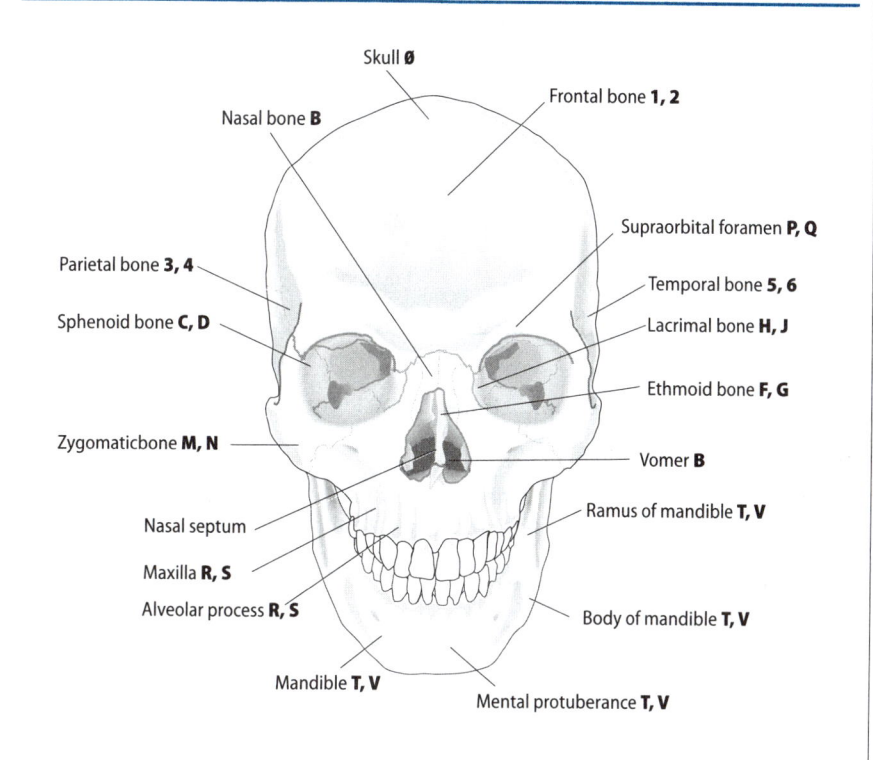

Skull **0**
Frontal bone **1, 2**
Nasal bone **B**
Supraorbital foramen **P, Q**
Parietal bone **3, 4**
Temporal bone **5, 6**
Sphenoid bone **C, D**
Lacrimal bone **H, J**
Ethmoid bone **F, G**
Zygomatic bone **M, N**
Vomer **B**
Nasal septum
Ramus of mandible **T, V**
Maxilla **R, S**
Alveolar process **R, S**
Body of mandible **T, V**
Mandible **T, V**
Mental protuberance **T, V**

Character Value — 1, 2, Frontal Bone, Left & Right

Associated Terms: Zygomatic process of frontal bone

Covering the majority of the space above the eyes to the top of the head, the frontal bone forms the front of the skull. The zygomatic process of the frontal bone is where the frontal bone and the ***zygomatic bone*** meet, near the temple.

Character Value — 5, 6, Temporal Bone, Left & Right

Associated Terms: Mastoid process, petrous part of temporal bone, tympanic part of temporal bone, zygomatic process of temporal bone

The temporal bones are a pair of large bones forming the lower sides and base of the cranium, and contain various cavities and recesses associated with the ear. Terms associated with the temporal bone include the mastoid process, the petrous part of temporal bone, and the tympanic part of temporal bone. The zygomatic process of temporal bone is where the temporal bone meets the zygomatic bone.

DEFINITIONS

zygomatic bones. Zygomatic process of the temporal bone that creates the cheekbone.

© 2015 Optum360, LLC

Figure 18.15: Skull Bones

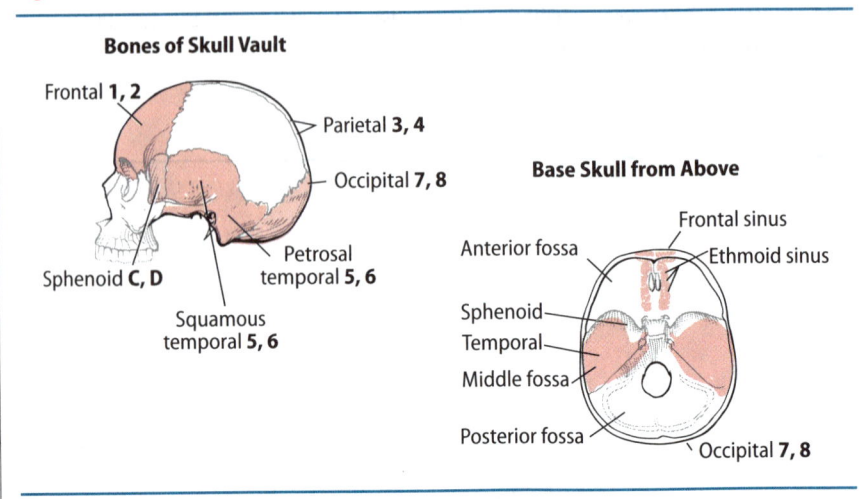

Bones of Skull Vault

Frontal **1, 2**
Parietal **3, 4**
Occipital **7, 8**
Petrosal temporal **5, 6**
Sphenoid **C, D**
Squamous temporal **5, 6**

Base Skull from Above

Frontal sinus
Ethmoid sinus
Anterior fossa
Sphenoid
Temporal
Middle fossa
Posterior fossa
Occipital **7, 8**

Character Value — 7, 8, Occipital Bone, Left & Right

Associated Terms: Foramen magnum

The occipital bones are located at the base of the skull that contains the foramen magnum, the oval opening in the bone that allows the spinal cord to join the brain.

Character Value — B, Nasal Bone

Associated Terms: Vomer of nasal septum

Nasal bones are small oblong bones that form the bridge of the nose. The vomer of the nasal septum is the flat bone that forms the lower, posterior portion of the nasal septum.

Character Value — C, D, Sphenoid Bone, Left & Right

Associated Terms: Greater wing, lesser wing, optic foramen, pterygoid process, sella turcica

The sphenoid bone is an irregular, wedge-shaped bone in the skull base that has several components, including the greater wing, lesser wing, optic foramen, pterygoid process, and sella turcica.

Character Value — F, G, Ethmoid Bone, Left & Right

Associated Terms: Cribriform plate

A cube-shaped bone located between the orbits, the ethmoid bone forms the roof and some of the walls of the nasal cavity. The cribriform plate is a portion of the ethmoid bone.

Character Value — P, Q, Orbit, Left & Right

Associated Terms: Bony orbit, orbital portion of ethmoid bone, orbital portion of frontal bone, orbital portion of **lacrimal bone**, orbital portion of maxilla, orbital portion of **palatine bone**, orbital portion of sphenoid bone, orbital portion of zygomatic bone

The orbit is a bony cavity that contains the eyeball, formed by seven bones of the skull: frontal, sphenoid, maxilla, zygomatic, palatine, lacrimal, and ethmoid.

DEFINITIONS

lacrimal bone. Located at the back of the orbit, it is the smallest and most fragile bone of the face.

palatine bones. Irregularly shaped bones that form the posterior part of the hard palate and contribute to the formation of the nasal cavity and floors of the orbits.

Character Value — R, S, Maxilla, Left & Right

Associated Terms: Alveolar process of maxilla

The maxilla is a pyramidally shaped bone forming the upper jaw, part of the eye orbit, nasal cavity, and palate, and also lodges the upper teeth. The alveolar process of the maxilla is the ridge of bone in the maxilla that contains the tooth sockets.

Character Value — T, V, Mandible, Left & Right

Associated Terms: Alveolar process of mandible, condyloid process, mandibular notch, mental foramen

The mandible is the lower jawbone, which gives structure to the floor of the oral cavity. The alveolar process of the mandible is the ridge of bone containing the tooth sockets for the lower teeth. Other portions of the mandible include the condyloid process, the mandibular notch, and the mental foramen.

Representative ICD-10-PCS Code Examples

1. **Percutaneous biopsy of the left side of the mandible**
   ØNBV3ZX   Excision of left mandible, percutaneous approach, diagnostic
   Note: Root operation excision appropriately reflects the partial excision of tissue for the diagnostic testing purpose indicated in this example.

2. **External closed reduction of a nasal fracture**
   ØNSBXZZ   Reposition nasal bone, external approach
   Note: In ICD-10-PCS, all closed reduction procedures for displaced fractures are coded with root operation reposition, which is defined as "Moving to its normal location or other suitable location all or a portion of a body part."

Upper Bones (P)

Procedures that might be performed on the bones of the upper body include osteotomy of the hand, placement of an external fixation device for an ulnar fracture, or insertion of a bone growth stimulator. A compiled table for body system character P Upper bones, provides all of the valid characters for those systems in ICD-10-PCS.

Operation–Character 3	Body Part–Character 4	Approach–Character 5	Device–Character 6	Qualifier–Character 7
2 Change	0 Sternum	0 Open	0 Drainage Device OR Internal Fixation Device, Rigid Plate (for root operation INSERTION or REPOSITION only)	X Diagnostic
5 Destruction	1 Rib, Right	3 Percutaneous	4 Internal Fixation Device	Z No Qualifier
8 Division	2 Rib, Left	4 Percutaneous Endoscopic	5 External Fixation Device	
9 Drainage	3 Cervical Vertebra	X External	6 Internal Fixation Device, Intramedullary	
B Excision	4 Thoracic Vertebra		7 Autologous Tissue Substitute	
C Extirpation	5 Scapula, Right		8 External Fixation Device, Limb Lengthening	
H Insertion	6 Scapula, Left		B External Fixation Device, Monoplanar	
J Inspection	7 Glenoid Cavity, Right		C External Fixation Device, Ring	
N Release	8 Glenoid Cavity, Left		D External Fixation Device, Hybrid	
P Removal	9 Clavicle, Right		J Synthetic Substitute	
Q Repair	B Clavicle, Left		K Nonautologous Tissue Substitute	
R Replacement	C Humeral Head, Right		M Bone Growth Stimulator	
S Reposition	D Humeral Head, Left		Y Other Device	
T Resection	F Humeral Shaft, Right		Z No Device	
U Supplement	G Humeral Shaft, Left			
W Revision	H Radius, Right			
	J Radius, Left			
	K Ulna, Right			
	L Ulna, Left			
	M Carpal, Right			
	N Carpal, Left			
	P Metacarpal, Right			
	Q Metacarpal, Left			
	R Thumb Phalanx, Right			
	S Thumb Phalanx, Left			
	T Finger Phalanx, Right			
	V Finger Phalanx, Left			
	Y Upper Bone			

Chapter 18. ICD-10-PCS: Skin, Subcutaneous Tissue, and Musculoskeletal Systems

Body Part — Character 4

The body part characters specified in the upper bones table detail the various bone structures in the upper portion of the body (above the diaphragm).

Character Value — 0, Sternum

Associated Terms: Manubrium, suprasternal notch, xiphoid process

The sternum is a flat, long bone in the middle of the thorax that is connected to the *rib* bones via cartilage. The manubrium is the top portion of the sternal bone, with the suprasternal notch at the very top. The xiphoid process is at the bottom end of the sternal bone.

Character Value — 3, 4, Cervical, Thoracic Vertebrae

Associated Terms: Spinous process, vertebral arch, vertebral foramen, vertebral lamina, vertebral pedicle

Vertebrae are divided into various sections, based on their location along the spinal column. The seven cervical vertebrae and 12 thoracic vertebrae are included in the upper bone system. The bony structure of each vertebra includes components such as the spinous process, the vertebral arch, the vertebral foramen, the vertebral lamina, and the vertebral pedicle.

> **DEFINITIONS**
>
> **rib.** Series of long curved bones of the chest that are attached to the vertebrae and occur in pairs.

Figure 18.16: Humerus and Scapula

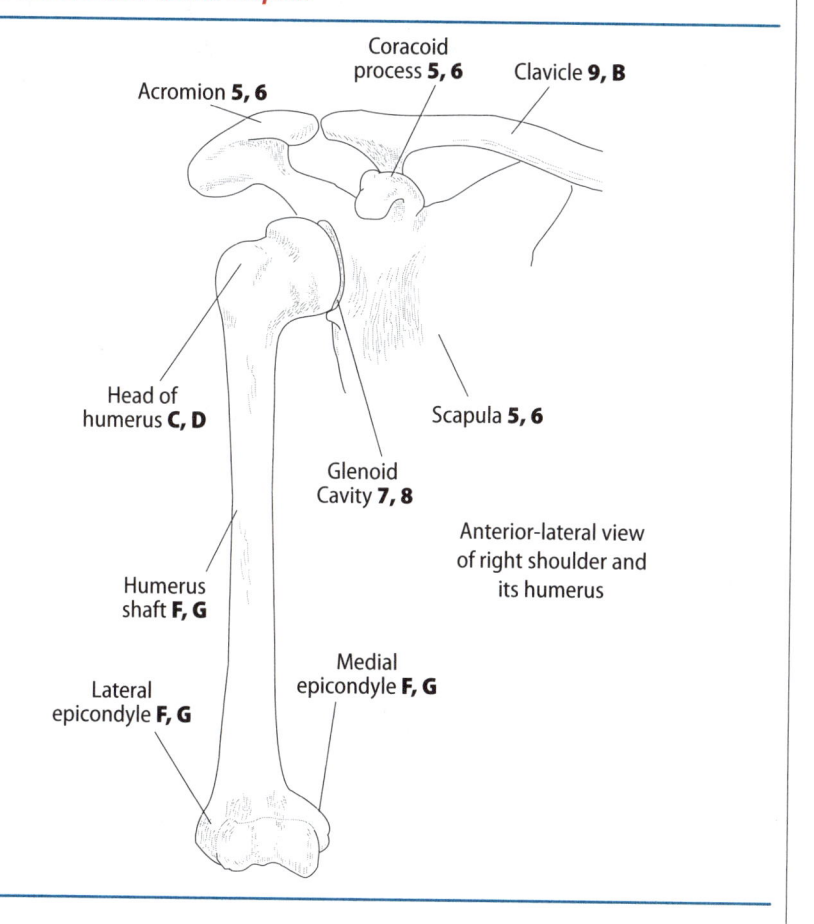

Acromion **5, 6**
Coracoid process **5, 6**
Clavicle **9, B**
Head of humerus **C, D**
Scapula **5, 6**
Glenoid Cavity **7, 8**
Humerus shaft **F, G**
Lateral epicondyle **F, G**
Medial epicondyle **F, G**

Anterior-lateral view of right shoulder and its humerus

Comprehensive Anatomy and Physiology for ICD-10-CM and ICD-10-PCS Coding

> **DEFINITIONS**
>
> **clavicle.** Long curved horizontal bone located directly above the first rib. It articulates with the sternum and the scapula.

Character Value — 5, 6, Scapula, Right & Left

Associated Terms: Acromion (process), coracoid process

A triangular bone commonly referred to as the shoulder blade, the scapula connects the humerus and the **clavicle.** Other portions of the scapular area include the acromion (process) and the coracoid process.

Character Value — 7, 8, Glenoid Cavity, Right & Left

Associated Terms: Glenoid fossa (of scapula)

The glenoid cavity, also known as the glenoid fossa of the scapula, is a shallow depressed area on the lateral edge of the scapula that forms the junction with the head of the humerus.

Character Value — C, D, Humeral Head, Right & Left

Associated Terms: Greater tuberosity, lesser tuberosity, neck of humerus (anatomical)(surgical)

The upper rounded portion of the humerus is known as the humeral head. The greater and lesser tuberosities are around the sides of the humeral head, and the neck of the humerus is just below the head portion.

Character Value — F, G, Humeral Shaft, Right & Left

Associated Terms: Lateral epicondyle of humerus, medial epicondyle of humerus

As the long straight portion of the humerus, the humeral shaft makes up the majority of the bone. The lateral and medial epicondyles of the humerus are at the end of the bone, at the elbow joint.

Figure 18.17: Radius and Ulna

> **CODING AXIOM**
>
> Since ICD-10-CM and PCS require specificity of body part values, laterality, and types of fractures, it is important to remember that it is appropriate to use the x-ray report to obtain additional specificity, provided that the physician has already diagnosed the condition (e.g., physician documents fracture of humerus and x-ray report confirms a displaced fracture of the right humeral head).
>
> *Coding Clinic,* 1Q, 13, 28

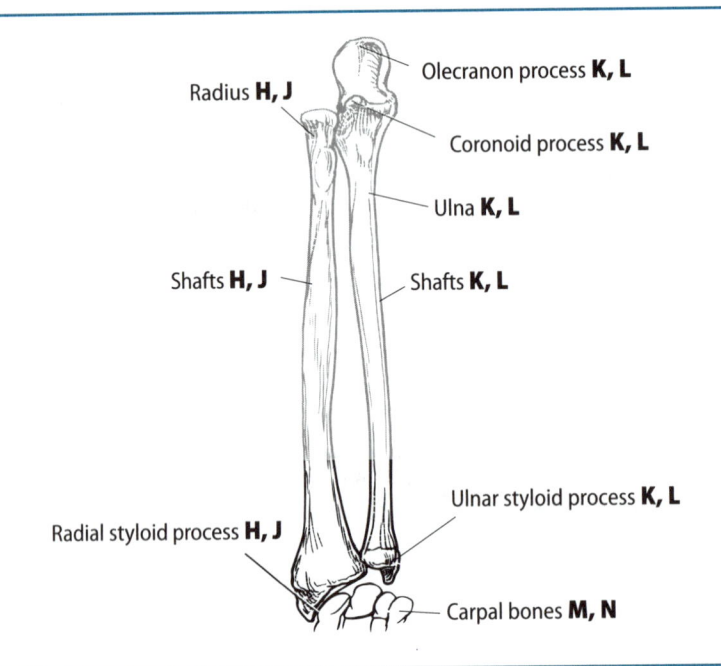

Labels on figure:
- Radius **H, J**
- Olecranon process **K, L**
- Coronoid process **K, L**
- Ulna **K, L**
- Shafts **H, J**
- Shafts **K, L**
- Ulnar styloid process **K, L**
- Radial styloid process **H, J**
- Carpal bones **M, N**

Character Value — H, J, Radius, Right & Left

Associated Terms: Ulnar notch

The radius is the shorter of the two bones in the forearm. The point where it articulates with the ulna is called the ulnar notch.

Character Value — K, L, Ulna, Right & Left

Associated Terms: Olecranon process, radial notch

The ulna is the longer of the two bones in the forearm, and lies parallel to the radius. The end of the ulna that projects beyond the humerus and forms the tip of the elbow is the olecranon process. The radial notch is the point along the ulna where the radius and ulna articulate.

Figure 18.18: Hand Bones

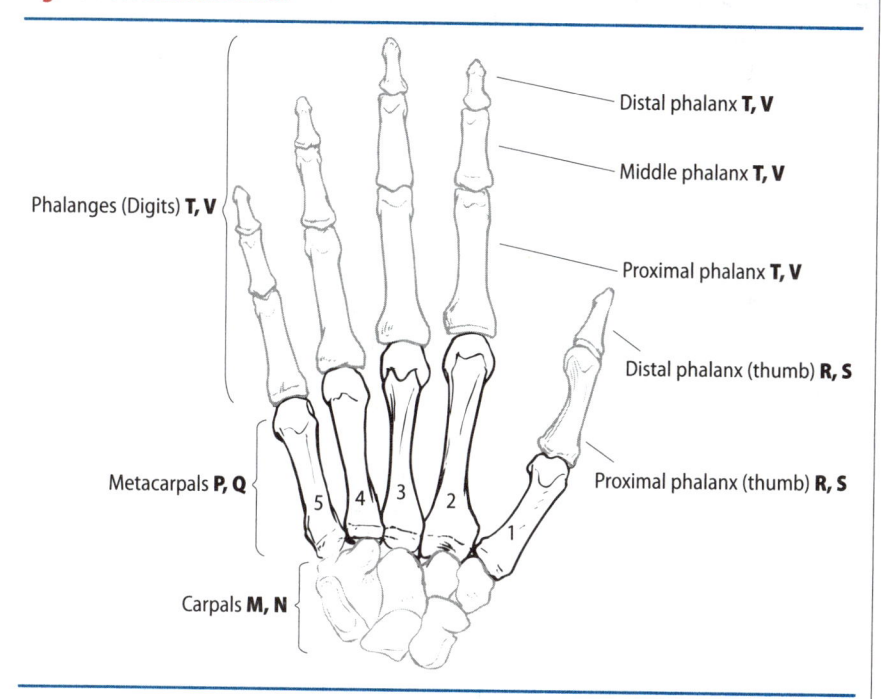

Character Value — M, N, Carpal, Right & Left

Associated Terms: Capitate bone, hamate bone, lunate bone, pisiform bone, scaphoid bone, trapezium bone, trapezoid bone, triquetral bone

The wrist area has many small bones called the carpals. Although there are many bones, including the accessory carpal bones, the eight main carpals are the capitate bone, the hamate bone, the lunate bone, the pisiform bone, the scaphoid bone, the trapezium bone, the trapezoid bone, and the triquetral bone.

Representative ICD-10-PCS Code Examples

1. **Open fracture reduction, right radius and ulna**
   0PSH0ZZ   Reposition right radius, open approach
   0PSK0ZZ   Reposition right ulna, open approach

   Note: Unlike ICD-9-CM, procedures performed on the radius and ulna bones must be coded separately in ICD-10-PCS, since they are identified by separate body part values.

2. **Open osteotomy of the trapezoid bone, left hand**
   0P8N0ZZ   Division of left carpal, open approach

Lower Bones (Q)

Procedures that may be performed on the bones of the lower body include open fracture reduction for a right femur fracture, removal of previously placed internal fixation of the left medial malleolus, or an osteotomy of distal phalanx of the foot. A compiled table for body system character Q Lower bones, provides all of the valid characters for those systems in ICD-10-PCS.

Operation–Character 3	Body Part–Character 4	Approach–Character 5	Device–Character 6	Qualifier–Character 7
2 Change	0 Lumbar Vertebra	0 Open	0 Drainage Device	X Diagnostic
5 Destruction	1 Sacrum	3 Percutaneous	4 Internal Fixation Device	Z No Qualifier
8 Division	2 Pelvic Bone, Right	4 Percutaneous Endoscopic	5 External Fixation Device	
9 Drainage	3 Pelvic Bone, Left	X External	6 Internal Fixation Device, Intramedullary	
B Excision	4 Acetabulum, Right		7 Autologous Tissue Substitute	
C Extirpation	5 Acetabulum, Left		8 External Fixation Device, Limb Lengthening	
H Insertion	6 Upper Femur, Right		B External Fixation Device, Monoplanar	
J Inspection	7 Upper Femur, Left		C External Fixation Device, Ring	
N Release	8 Femoral Shaft, Right		D External Fixation Device, Hybrid	
P Removal	9 Femoral Shaft, Left		J Synthetic Substitute	
Q Repair	B Lower Femur, Right		K Nonautologous Tissue Substitute	
R Replacement	C Lower Femur, Left		M Bone Growth Stimulator	
S Reposition	D Patella, Right		Y Other Device	
T Resection	F Patella, Left		Z No Device	
U Supplement	G Tibia, Right			
W Revision	H Tibia, Left			
	J Fibula, Right			
	K Fibula, Left			
	L Tarsal, Right			
	M Tarsal, Left			
	N Metatarsal, Right			
	P Metatarsal, Left			
	Q Toe Phalanx, Right			
	R Toe Phalanx, Left			
	S Coccyx			
	Y Lower Bone			

Body Part — Character 4

The body part characters specified in the lower bones table detail the various bone structures in the lower portion of the body (below the diaphragm).

Character Value — 0, Lumbar Vertebra

Associated Terms: Spinous process, vertebral arch, vertebral foramen, vertebral lamina, vertebral pedicle

There are five lumbar vertebrae in the lower portion of the vertebral column. Each vertebra is made up of several components, such as the spinous process, the vertebral arch, the vertebral foramen, the vertebral lamina, and the vertebral pedicle.

Figure 18.19: Hip Bone Anatomy

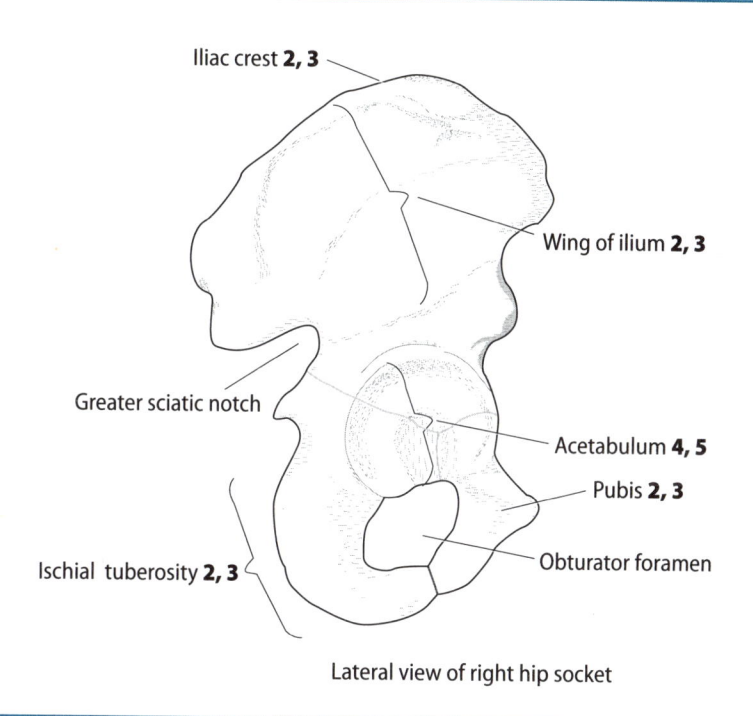

Lateral view of right hip socket

- Iliac crest **2, 3**
- Wing of ilium **2, 3**
- Greater sciatic notch
- Acetabulum **4, 5**
- Pubis **2, 3**
- Obturator foramen
- Ischial tuberosity **2, 3**

Character Value — 2, 3, Pelvic Bone, Left & Right

Associated Terms: Iliac crest, ilium, ischium, pubis

A combination of three different bones, the pelvis is made up of the ilium, the ischium, and the pubis. The iliac crest is the edge of the "wing" of the ilium.

Comprehensive Anatomy and Physiology for ICD-10-CM and ICD-10-PCS Coding

> **DEFINITIONS**
>
> **acetabulum.** Cup-shaped socket in the hipbone into which the head of the femur fits, forming a ball-and-socket joint.
>
> **sacrum.** Lower portion of the spine composed of five fused vertebrae designated as S1-S5.

Figure 18.20: Pelvic and Lower Bones

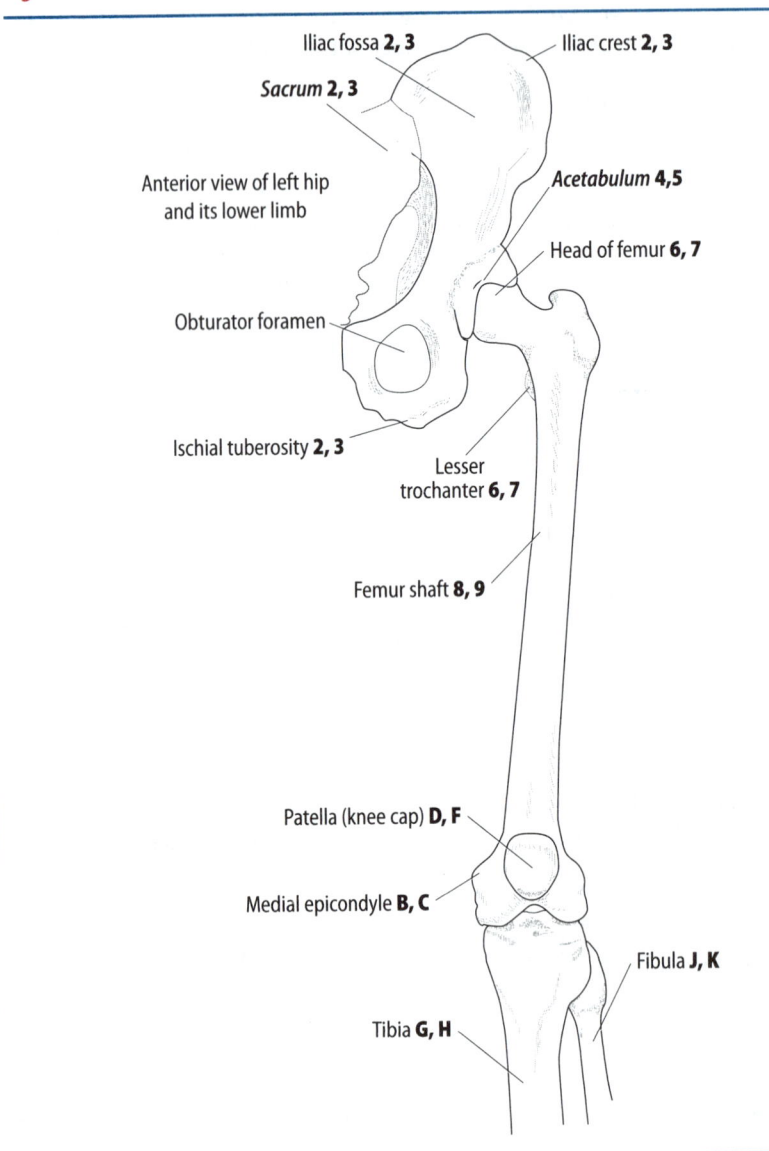

Iliac fossa **2, 3**
Iliac crest **2, 3**
Sacrum **2, 3**
Anterior view of left hip and its lower limb
Acetabulum **4, 5**
Head of femur **6, 7**
Obturator foramen
Ischial tuberosity **2, 3**
Lesser trochanter **6, 7**
Femur shaft **8, 9**
Patella (knee cap) **D, F**
Medial epicondyle **B, C**
Fibula **J, K**
Tibia **G, H**

Character Value — 6, 7, Upper Femur, Left & Right

Associated Terms: Femoral head, greater trochanter, lesser trochanter, neck of femur

As the longest bone in the body, the femur has been divided into six different body part characters. The upper femur includes the femoral head and neck, as well as the greater and lesser trochanters.

Character Value — 8, 9, Femoral Shaft, Left & Right

Associated Terms: Body of femur

The main body of the femur, also known as the shaft of the femur, is the lengthy, narrow portion in the middle of the bone.

Character Value — B, C, Lower Femur, Left & Right

Associated Terms: Lateral condyle of femur, lateral epicondyle of femur, medial condyle of femur, medial epicondyle of femur

The point of articulation with the lower leg is found in the lower portion of the femur, specifically the condyles, which are projections of the lower end of the femur that interact with the ligaments and bursae in the knee. These condyles are called the lateral condyle of femur, the lateral epicondyle of femur, the medial condyle of femur, and the medial epicondyle of femur.

Character Value — G, H, Tibia, Left & Right

Associated Terms: Lateral condyle of tibia, medial condyle of tibia, medial malleolus

The tibia is the larger of the two bones in the lower leg and runs parallel to the fibula. The lateral and medial condyles are points of the bone where they articulate with the fibula. The medial malleolus is the rounded portion of the bottom of the tibia that makes up the bony prominence of the inside of the ankle.

Character Value — J, K, Fibula, Left & Right

Associated Terms: Body of fibula, head of fibula, lateral malleolus

Thinner than the tibia, the fibula is somewhat triangular in shape. The head of the fibula is on the upper end, just below the knee, and the body of the fibula makes up the long portion of the bone. The lateral malleolus is at the bottom of the fibula and is the bony prominence on the outside of the ankle.

Figure 18.21: Foot Bones

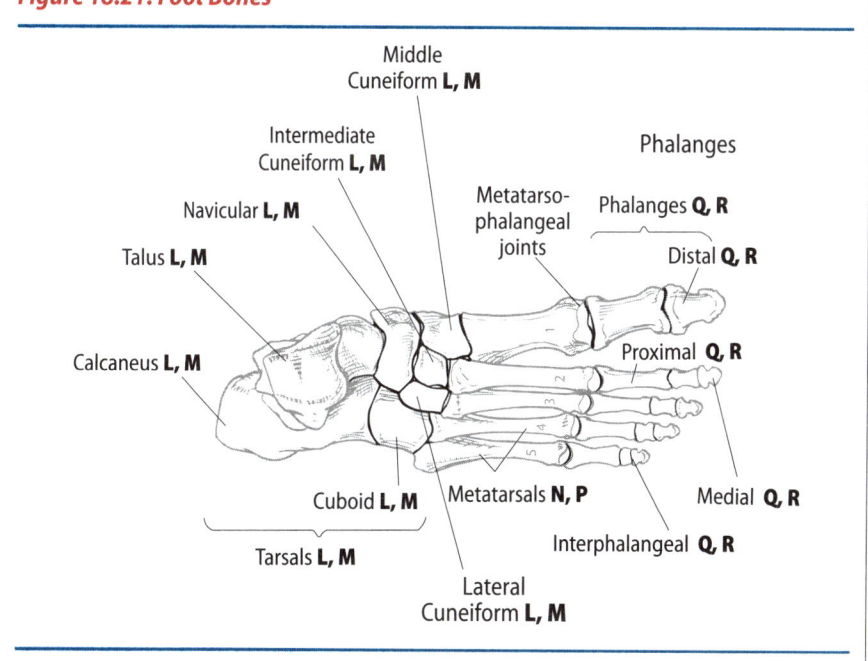

Character Value — L, M, Tarsal, Left & Right

Associated Terms: Calcaneus, cuboid bone, intermediate cuneiform bone, lateral cuneiform bone, medial cuneiform bone, navicular bone, talus bone

The tarsals consist of seven bones that make up the ankle and heel: the posterior talus, the calcaneus, the anterior cuboid, navicular, and three cuneiform (medial, intermediate, and lateral) bones.

Representative ICD-10-PCS Code Examples

1. **Open reduction of the right femoral shaft with placement of a plate and four bone screws**

    0QS804Z   Reposition right femoral shaft with internal fixation device, open approach

2. **Incision with removal of K-wire fixation, right first metatarsal**

    0QPN04Z   Removal of internal fixation device from right metatarsal, open approach

    Note: The notation that this removal was done via an incision tells the coder that this is an open procedure. Paying close attention to this level of detail is vital to accurate coding in ICD-10-PCS.

3. **ORIF of bimalleolar right ankle fracture**

    0QSG04Z   Reposition with internal fixation of right tibia, open approach
    0QSJ04Z   Reposition with internal fixation of right fibula, open approach

    Note: A bimalleolar fracture involves the tibia and fibula. Since they each have a separate body part value in ICD-10-PCS, it is necessary to use two separate codes.

Upper Joints (R)*

Joints, or the articulations between bones, occur throughout the body. This body system includes joints in the upper portion of the body (above the diaphragm). Procedures on joints in the upper body include anterior interbody arthrodesis on the cervical vertebrae or arthroscopy of the shoulder. A compiled table for body system character R Upper joints, provides all of the valid characters for those systems under ICD-10-PCS.

Operation–Character 3	Body Part–Character 4	Approach–Character 5	Device–Character 6	Qualifier–Character 7
2 Change	0 *Occipital-cervical Joint*	0 Open	0 Drainage Device OR Synthetic Substitute, Reverse Ball and Socket (for root operation REPLACEMENT only)	0 Anterior Approach, Anterior Column
5 Destruction	1 Cervical Vertebral Joint	3 Percutaneous	3 Infusion Device	1 Posterior Approach, Posterior Column
9 Drainage	2 Cervical Vertebral Joint, 2 or more	4 Percutaneous Endoscopic	4 Internal Fixation Device	6 Humeral Surface
B Excision	3 Cervical Vertebral Disc	X External	5 External Fixation Device	7 Glenoid Surface
C Extirpation	4 Cervicothoracic Vertebral Joint		7 Autologous Tissue Substitute	J Posterior Approach, Anterior Column
G Fusion	5 Cervicothoracic Vertebral Disc		8 Spacer	X Diagnostic
H Insertion	6 Thoracic Vertebral Joint		A Interbody Fusion Device	Z No Qualifier
J Inspection	7 Thoracic Vertebral Joint, 2 to 7		B Spinal Stabilization Device, Interspinous Process	
N Release	8 Thoracic Vertebral Joint, 8 or more		C Spinal Stabilization Device, Pedicle-Based	
P Removal	9 Thoracic Vertebral Disc		D Spinal Stabilization Device, Facet Replacement	
Q Repair	A Thoracolumbar Vertebral Joint		J Synthetic Substitute	
R Replacement	B Thoracolumbar Vertebral Disc		K Nonautologous Tissue Substitute	
S Reposition	C *Temporomandibular Joint*, Right		Y Other Device	
T Resection	D Temporomandibular Joint, Left		Z No Device	
U Supplement	E *Sternoclavicular Joint*, Right			
W Revision	F Sternoclavicular Joint, Left			
	G *Acromioclavicular Joint*, Right			
	H Acromioclavicular Joint, Left			
	J Shoulder Joint, Right			
	K Shoulder Joint, Left			
	L Elbow Joint, Right			
	M Elbow Joint, Left			
	N Wrist Joint, Right			
	P Wrist Joint, Left			

(Continued on next page)

---

* Includes synovial membrane.

Operation–Character 3	Body Part–Character 4	Approach–Character 5	Device–Character 6	Qualifier–Character 7
(Continued)	Q Carpal Joint, Right			
	R Carpal Joint, Left			
	S Metacarpocarpal Joint, Right			
	T Metacarpocarpal Joint, Left			
	U *Metacarpophalangeal Joint*, Right			
	V Metacarpophalangeal Joint, Left			
	W Finger Phalangeal Joint, Right			
	X Finger Phalangeal Joint, Left			
	Y Upper Joint			

DEFINITIONS

acromioclavicular joint. Junction between the clavicle and the scapula. The acromion is the projection from the back of the scapula that forms the highest point of the shoulder and connects with the clavicle. Trauma or injury to the acromioclavicular joint is often referred to as a dislocation of the shoulder. This is not correct, however, as a dislocation of the shoulder is a disruption of the glenohumeral joint.

metacarpophalangeal joint. Joint at the base of each finger.

occipital-cervical joint. Articulation between the occiput at the base of the skull and the first cervical vertebrae.

sternoclavicular joint. Articulation between the sternum and the clavicle. This joint allows movement in three planes: anteroposterior, vertical, and some limited rotation.

temporomandibular joint. Joint or hinge formed by the connection of the lower jaw to the temporal bone of the cranium, located in front of the ear on both sides of the face.

Body Part — Character 4

The body part characters specified in the upper joints table detail the various articulations in the upper portion of the body (above the diaphragm).

Character Value — 1, 2, Cervical Vertebral Joint; 2 or more

Associated Terms: Atlantoaxial joint, cervical facet joint

The atlantoaxial joint is located between the atlas (C1) and the axis (C2), the first two cervical vertebrae. The facet joints are smooth surface areas where the transverse and articular processes of the cervical vertebrae articulate with the next vertebra. Each vertebra has two sets of facet joints: one on the left and one on the right.

Character Value — 4, Cervicothoracic Vertebral Joint

Associated Terms: Cervicothoracic facet joint

The cervicothoracic vertebral joint is located between C7 and T1 in the vertebral column. The cervicothoracic facet joints are located at this articulation.

Figure 18.22: Vertebral Joint

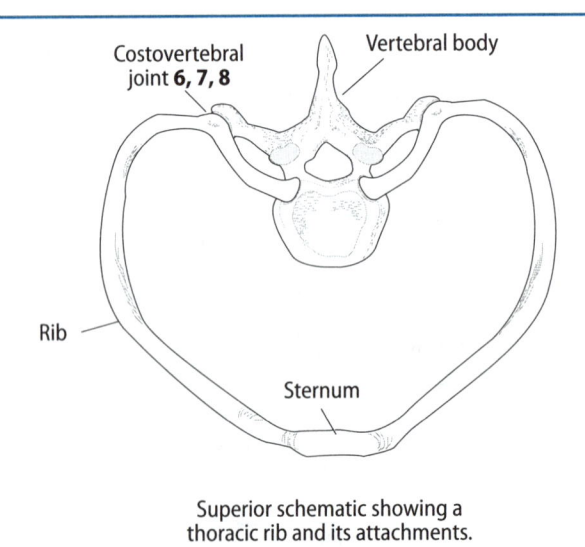

Superior schematic showing a thoracic rib and its attachments.

Character Value — 6, 7, 8, Thoracic Vertebral Joint; 2 to 7; 8 or more

Associated Terms: Costotransverse joint, costovertebral joint, thoracic facet joint

There are 12 vertebrae in the thoracic portion of the spinal column, along with corresponding joint articulations. The thoracic portion of the spinal column is where the rib cage interacts with the vertebrae; articulations known as costotransverse and costovertebral joints are where these bones intersect. The facet joints in the thoracic vertebrae are known as thoracic facet joints.

Character Value — A, Thoracolumbar Vertebral Joint

Associated Terms: Thoracolumbar facet joint

The thoracolumbar vertebral joint is located at the point where T12 articulates with L1. The facet joints at this location are referred to as the thoracolumbar facet joints.

Figure 18.23: Shoulder Joint

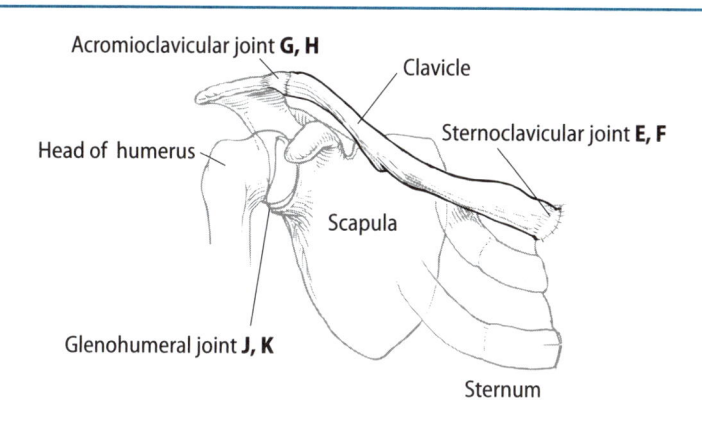

Character Value — J, K, Shoulder Joint, Left & Right

Associated Terms: Glenohumeral joint, glenoid ligament (labrum)

The shoulder joint is a ball and socket joint where the head of the humerus meets the scapula, also known as the glenohumeral joint.

Character Value — L, M, Elbow Joint, Left & Right

Associated Terms: Humeroradial joint, humeroulnar joint, proximal radioulnar joint

The elbow joint is made up of three different articulations, and involves the humerus of the upper arm and the radius and ulna of the forearm. The three joints of the elbow are the humeroradial joint (humerus/radius), the humeroulnar joint (humerus/ulna), and the proximal radioulnar joint (radius/ulna).

Character Value — N, P, Wrist Joint, Left & Right

Associated Terms: Distal radioulnar joint, radiocarpal joint

The wrist joint, or radiocarpal joint, is the articulation formed by the radius and the carpal bones. The distal radioulnar joint is an articulation in the area of the wrist between the radius and the ulna.

Figure 18.24: Hand Joints

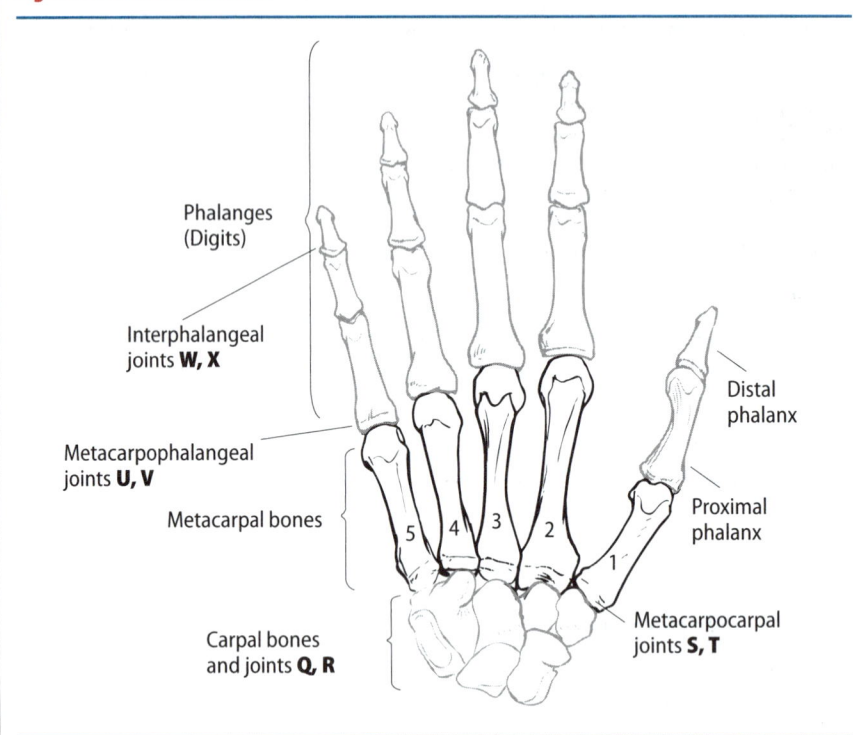

- Phalanges (Digits)
- Interphalangeal joints **W, X**
- Metacarpophalangeal joints **U, V**
- Metacarpal bones
- Carpal bones and joints **Q, R**
- Distal phalanx
- Proximal phalanx
- Metacarpocarpal joints **S, T**

Character Value — Q, R, Carpal Joint, Left & Right

Associated Terms: Intercarpal joint, midcarpal joint

Creating one of the most complex articulations in the body, the carpals operate in various manners based on which section of the wrist they are in. Some of them slide over one another, while others are locked together by ligaments and move more in unison. There are two main carpal joints: the intercarpal joint and the midcarpal joint.

Character Value — S, T, Metacarpocarpal Joint, Left & Right

Associated Terms: Carpometacarpal (CMC) joint

The metacarpocarpal joint, also known as the carpometacarpal joint, forms the articulations between the distal row of the carpal bones and the base of the metacarpals.

Character Value — W, X, Finger Phalangeal Joint, Left & Right

Associated Terms: Interphalangeal (IP) joint

Hinge type articulations, the phalangeal joints are located between the phalanges of the fingers. They are also known as interphalangeal joints.

Qualifier — Character 7

In the joints sections (upper and lower), qualifier values are available in the 7th character field to indicate the approach and column for spinal fusion (root operation character G). Qualifier 0 indicates anterior approach, anterior column; 1 indicates posterior approach, posterior column; and J indicates posterior approach, anterior column. Fusion procedures are only performed on joints, so there are a limited number of procedures that use this root operation. When coding spinal fusion procedures, pay special attention to the sixth- and seventh-character device and qualifier values. When multiple vertebral joints are fused but use different device or qualifier values, they should be coded separately, so it is vital to understand the anatomy and physiology surrounding these joints. Provider arthrodesis documentation should provide the detail required to appropriately code these qualifier values.

Representative ICD-10-PCS Code Examples

1. **Anterior column cervical fusion of C3 through C5 with bone bank grafting and open anterior approach**

    0RG20K0 Fusion of 2 or more cervical vertebral joints with nonautologous tissue substitute, anterior approach, anterior column, open approach

    Note: This scenario is an example of when to use 7th character qualifier 0 Anterior approach and anterior column.

2. **Diagnostic arthroscopy of right shoulder**

    0RJJ4ZZ Inspection of right shoulder joint, percutaneous endoscopic approach

Comprehensive Anatomy and Physiology for ICD-10-CM and ICD-10-PCS Coding

Lower Joints (S)*

The articulations in the lower body are detailed in this section. Procedures performed on the lower joints may include a sacrococcygeal fusion with bone graft, an exploratory arthroscopy of the left knee, and an open revision of a right hip replacement with readjustment of the prosthesis. A compiled table for body system character S Lower joints, provides all of the valid characters for those systems in ICD-10-PCS.

Operation–Character 3	Body Part–Character 4	Approach–Character 5	Device–Character 6	Qualifier–Character 7
2 Change	0 Lumbar Vertebral Joint	0 Open	0 Drainage Device OR Synthetic Substitute, Polyethylene (for root operation REPLACEMENT only)	0 Anterior Approach, Anterior Column
5 Destruction	1 Lumbar Vertebral Joint, 2 or more	3 Percutaneous	1 Synthetic Substitute, Metal	1 Posterior Approach, Posterior Column
9 Drainage	2 Lumbar Vertebral Disc	4 Percutaneous Endoscopic	2 Synthetic Substitute, Metal on Polyethylene	9 Cemented
B Excision	3 Lumbosacral Joint	X External	3 Infusion Device OR Synthetic Substitute, Ceramic (for root operation REPLACEMENT only)	A Uncemented
C Extirpation	4 Lumbosacral Disc		4 Internal Fixation Device OR Synthetic Substitute, Ceramic on Polyethylene (for root operation REPLACEMENT only)	C Patellar Surface
G Fusion	5 Sacrococcygeal Joint		5 External Fixation Device	J Posterior Approach, Anterior Column
H Insertion	6 Coccygeal Joint		7 Autologous Tissue Substitute	X Diagnostic
J Inspection	7 Sacroiliac Joint, Right		8 Spacer	Z No Qualifier
N Release	8 Sacroiliac Joint, Left		9 Liner	
P Removal	9 Hip Joint, Right		A Interbody Fusion Device	
	A Hip Joint, Acetabular Surface, Right		B Resurfacing Device OR Spinal Stabilization Device, Interspinous Process (for root operation INSERTION only)	
Q Repair	B Hip Joint, Left		C Spinal Stabilization Device, Pedicle-Based	
R Replacement	C Knee Joint, Right		D Spinal Stabilization Device, Facet Replacement	
S Reposition	D Knee Joint, Left		J Synthetic Substitute	
	E Hip Joint, Acetabular Surface, Left		K Nonautologous Tissue Substitute	
T Resection	F Ankle Joint, Right		Y Other Device	
U Supplement	G Ankle Joint, Left		Z No Device	
W Revision	H Tarsal Joint, Right			
	J Tarsal Joint, Left			
	K Metatarsal-Tarsal Joint, Right			
	L Metatarsal-Tarsal Joint, Left			
	M Metatarsal-Phalangeal Joint, Right			

(Continued on next page)

* Includes synovial membrane.

Operation–Character 3	Body Part–Character 4	Approach–Character 5	Device–Character 6	Qualifier–Character 7
(Continued)	N Metatarsal-Phalangeal Joint, Left			
	P Toe Phalangeal Joint, Right			
	Q Toe Phalangeal Joint, Left			
	R Hip Joint, Femoral Surface, Right			
	S Hip Joint, Femoral Surface, Left			
	T Knee Joint, Femoral Surface, Right			
	U Knee Joint, Femoral Surface, Left			
	V Knee Joint, Tibial Surface, Right			
	W Knee Joint, Tibial Surface, Left			
	Y Lower Joint			

Body Part — Character 4

The body part characters specified in the lower joints table detail the various articulations in the lower portion of the body (below the diaphragm).

Character Value — 0, 1, Lumbar Vertebral Joint; 2 or more

Associated Terms: Lumbar facet joint

The facet joints are smooth surface areas where the transverse and articular processes of the vertebrae articulate with other vertebrae. Each vertebra has two sets of facet joints, one on the left and one on the right. The facet joints in the lumbar spine are referred to as lumbar facet joints.

Character Value — 3, Lumbosacral Joint

Associated Terms: Lumbosacral facet joint

Located between the final lumbar vertebra and the first sacral vertebra, the lumbosacral joint is the articulation between L5 and S1. The facet joints between these vertebrae are referred to as the lumbosacral facet joints.

Character Value — 5, Sacrococcygeal Joint

Associated Terms: Sacrococcygeal symphysis

The sacrococcygeal joint, also referred to as the sacrococcygeal symphysis, is an articulation between the apex of the sacrum and the base of the *coccyx*.

> **DEFINITIONS**
>
> **coccyx.** Small triangular bone at the base of the spinal column, formed by the fusion of the remnants of vestigial vertebrae.
>
> **sacroiliac joint.** Joint formed by the sacrum and the ilium where they meet on either side of the lower back.

Figure 18.25: Hip Joint

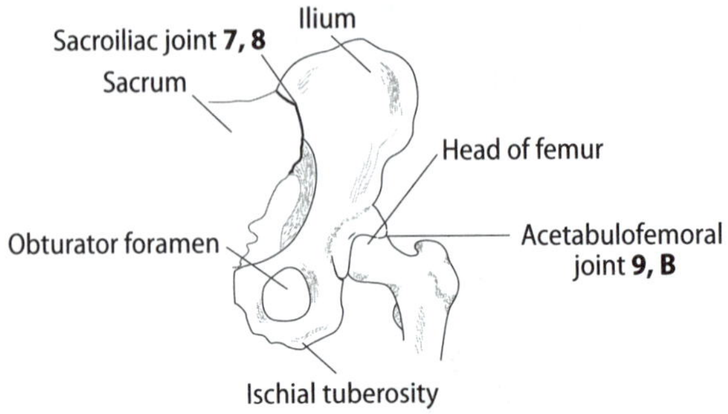
Ilium
Sacroiliac joint 7, 8
Sacrum
Head of femur
Obturator foramen
Acetabulofemoral joint 9, B
Ischial tuberosity

Character Value — 9, B, Hip Joint, Left & Right

Associated Terms: Acetabulofemoral joint

Character Value — A, E Hip Joint, Acetabular Surface, Right & Left

Character Value — R, S Hip Joint, Femoral Surface, Right & Left

A ball and socket type of articulation, the hip joint is formed by the head of the femur and the acetabulum of the pelvis. It is also referred to as the acetabulofemoral joint.

Figure 18.26: Knee Joint (C, D)

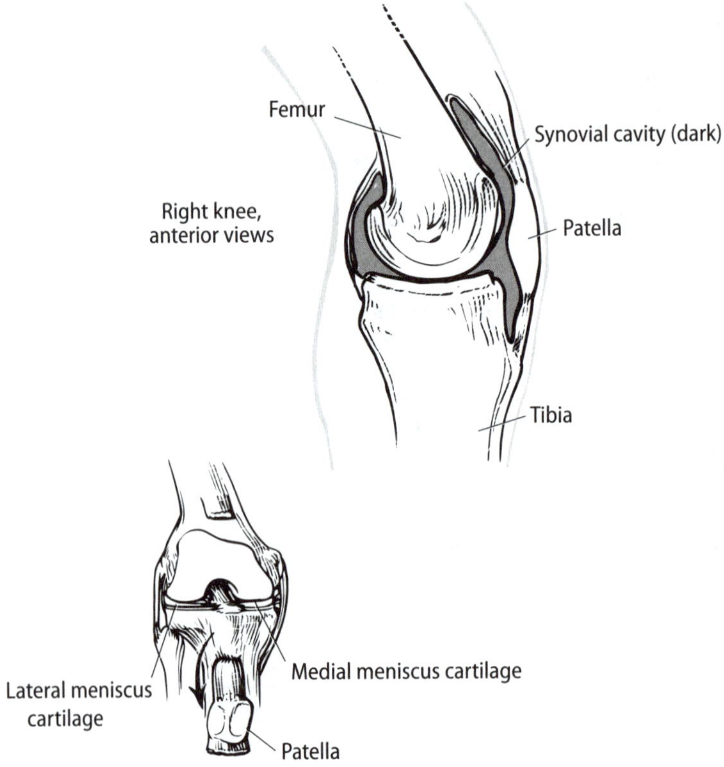
Femur
Synovial cavity (dark)
Right knee, anterior views
Patella
Tibia
Lateral meniscus cartilage
Medial meniscus cartilage
Patella

Figure 18.27: Lateral View, Knee (C, D)

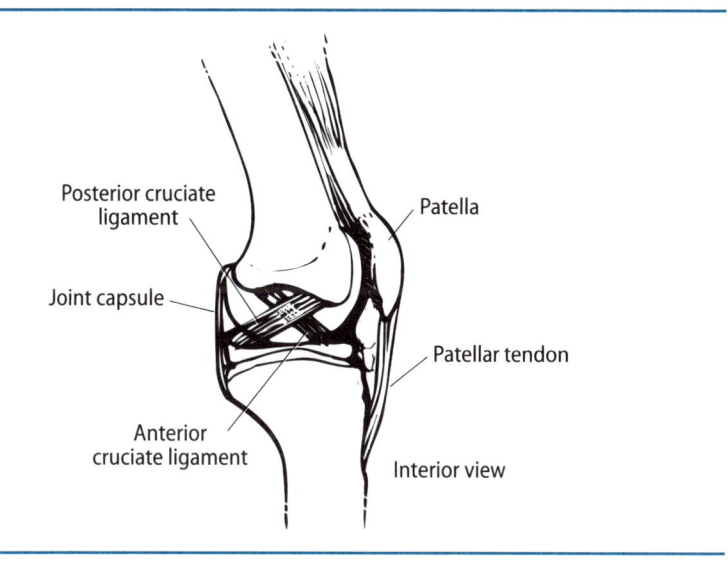

- Posterior cruciate ligament
- Patella
- Joint capsule
- Patellar tendon
- Anterior cruciate ligament
- Interior view

Character Value — C, D, Knee Joint, Left & Right

Character Value — T, U Knee Joint, Femoral Surface, Right & Left

Character Value — V, W Knee Joint, Tibial Surface, Right & Left

Associated Terms: Femoropatellar joint, femorotibial joint, lateral meniscus, medial meniscus, patellofemoral joint, tibiofemoral joint

A complicated articulation, the knee joint is made up of many components. The femoropatellar joint articulates the *patella* and the femur. The femorotibial joint articulates the femur and the tibia. The lateral and medial menisci are discs of fibrous cartilage that exist in the knee compartment to protect the ends of the bones from rubbing on one another.

Character Value — F, G, Ankle Joint, Left & Right

Associated Terms: Inferior tibiofibular joint, talocrural joint

The ankle joint, also known as the talocrural joint, is a hinge type of joint that connects the tibia and fibula with the bones of the foot. The inferior tibiofibular joint is an articulation where the tibia and fibula join together in the ankle region.

DEFINITIONS

patella. Large flat bone at the front of the knee joint.

Comprehensive Anatomy and Physiology for ICD-10-CM and ICD-10-PCS Coding

Figure 18.28: Foot

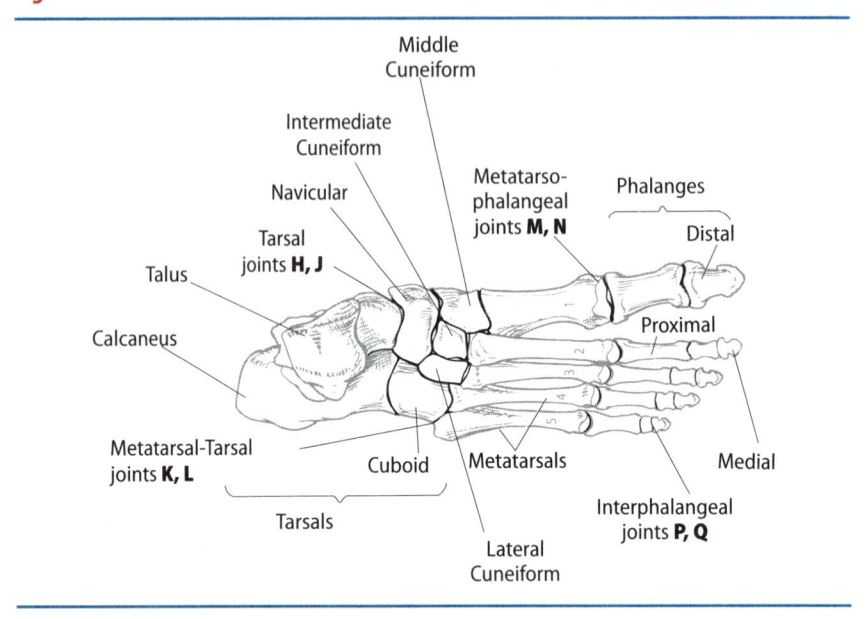

(Anatomical diagram of the foot showing: Talus, Calcaneus, Navicular, Tarsal joints H, J, Intermediate Cuneiform, Middle Cuneiform, Lateral Cuneiform, Cuboid, Metatarsal-Tarsal joints K, L, Tarsals, Metatarsals, Metatarsophalangeal joints M, N, Phalanges (Distal, Proximal, Medial), Interphalangeal joints P, Q)

Character Value — H, J, Tarsal Joint, Left & Right

Associated Terms: Calcaneocuboid joint, cuboideonavicular joint, cuneonavicular joint, intercuneiform joint, subtalar (talocalcaneal) joint, talocalcaneal (subtalar) joint, talocalcaneonavicular joint

There are several joints in the tarsal bones in the foot that allow for its complex motion, including the calcaneocuboid joint, the cuboideonavicular joint, the cuneonavicular joint, the intercuneiform joint, the subtalar (talocalcaneal) joint, and the talocalcaneonavicular joint.

Character Value — K, L, Metatarsal - Tarsal Joint, Left & Right

Associated Terms: Tarsometatarsal joint

The articulation between the cuboid or one of the cuneiform bones and the *metatarsals* is referred to as the metatarsal-tarsal joint or the tarsometatarsal joint.

Character Value — M, N, Metatarsal - Phalangeal Joint, Left & Right

Associated Terms: Metatarsophalangeal (MTP) joint

The articulations between the metatarsals and the phalanges are known as the metatarsal-phalangeal joints or the metatarsophalangeal (MTP) joints.

Character Value — P, Q, Toe Phalangeal Joint, Left & Right

Associated Terms: Interphalangeal (IP) joint

The phalangeal joints, also known as the interphalangeal joints, are hinge type articulations between the phalanges of the toes.

DEFINITIONS

metatarsals. Five long bones in the foot between the ankle bones and the phalanges, or toes.

Representative ICD-10-PCS Code Examples

1. **Total left knee arthroplasty with insertion of total knee prosthesis**

   0SRD0JZ Replacement of left knee joint with synthetic substitute, open approach

   Note: In this example, device character value 6 is used to indicate the synthetic knee prosthetic.

2. **Open revision of right hip replacement, with readjustment of prosthesis**

   0SW90JZ Revision of synthetic substitute in right hip joint, open approach

Summary

The skin, subcutaneous tissue, and musculoskeletal systems have been divided into 10 body system sections, and the majority of ICD-10-PCS procedures performed on these body areas are coded using these characters. An understanding of the anatomical sites outlined in these body systems is vital to accurate coding, as small nuances in the anatomy can mean a variance in the body part character. Laterality is also important to musculoskeletal system character selection. Additional information regarding ICD-10-PCS coding can be found in Optum360's *Detailed Instruction for Appropriate ICD-10-PCS Coding*.

Knowledge Assessment Questions

1. A patient has a procedure performed on the right platysma muscle. Which body part character in the muscle system table (K) would be utilized?
   a. C Hand muscle, right
   b. 2 Neck muscle, right
   c. F Trunk muscle, right
   d. V Foot muscle, right

2. Qualifiers (character 7) in the skin and breast body system are used, when appropriate, to describe grafting procedures, such as specific thickness of the graft or site and type of graft.
   a. True
   b. False

3. A procedure performed on the galea aponeurotica would be assigned to which body part character in the subcutaneous tissue and fascia body system?
   a. T Subcutaneous tissue and fascia, trunk
   b. 6 Subcutaneous tissue and fascia, chest
   c. 0 Subcutaneous tissue and fascia, scalp
   d. 1 Subcutaneous tissue and fascia, face

4. Which procedure involves restoring, to the extent possible, a body part to its normal anatomic structure and function?
   a. Repair
   b. Reposition
   c. Revision
   d. Supplement

5. The quadratus lumborum muscle is found in what part of the body?
   a. Calf
   b. Arm
   c. Thigh
   d. Back

6. The scalene muscle is assigned to body part character 1 under the muscle body system.
   a. True
   b. False

7. A repair procedure is performed on the extensor digitorum longus tendon on the left leg. What is the appropriate body part character assignment from the tendons body system table?
   a. W Foot tendon, left
   b. T Ankle tendon, left
   c. P Lower leg tendon, left
   d. Y Lower tendon

8. Which procedure involves joining together portions of an articular body part rendering the articular body part immobile?
   a. Fragmentation
   b. Extirpation
   c. Destruction
   d. Fusion

9. The olecranon process is part of the elbow, but is classified in ICD-10-PCS to the body part character for ulna.
   a. True
   b. False

10. A procedure performed at the calcaneocuboid joint on the left side is assigned to which body part character from the lower joints body system?
    a. C Knee joint, left
    b. J Tarsal joint, left
    c. L Metatarsal-tarsal joint, left
    d. Y Lower joint

Chapter 19. ICD-10-PCS: Genitourinary Systems

Urinary System (T)

The role of the urinary system is to create, store, and transport urine out of the body. Procedures performed on the urinary system include a percutaneous needle core biopsy of the left kidney, a transurethral cystoscopy with fragmentation of bladder calculus, or a cystoscopy with retrieval of left ureteral stent. A compiled table for body system character T Urinary system, provides all of the valid characters for that system in ICD-10-PCS.

Operation–Character 3	Body Part–Character 4	Approach–Character 5	Device–Character 6	Qualifier–Character 7
1 Bypass	0 Kidney, Right	0 Open	0 Drainage Device	0 Allogeneic
2 Change	1 Kidney, Left	3 Percutaneous	2 Monitoring Device	1 Syngeneic
5 Destruction	2 Kidneys, Bilateral	4 Percutaneous Endoscopic	3 Infusion Device	2 Zooplastic
7 Dilation	3 Kidney Pelvis, Right	7 Via Natural or Artificial Opening	7 Autologous Tissue Substitute	3 Kidney Pelvis, Right
8 Division	4 Kidney Pelvis, Left	8 Via Natural or Artificial Opening Endoscopic	C Extraluminal Device	4 Kidney Pelvis, Left
9 Drainage	5 Kidney	X External	D Intraluminal Device	6 Ureter, Right
B Excision	6 Ureter, Right		J Synthetic Substitute	7 Ureter, Left
C Extirpation	7 Ureter, Left		K Nonautologous Tissue Substitute	8 Colon
D Extraction	8 Ureters, Bilateral		L Artificial Sphincter	9 Colocutaneous
F Fragmentation	9 Ureter		M Stimulator Lead	A Ileum
H Insertion	B Bladder		Y Other Device	B Bladder
J Inspection	C Bladder Neck		Z No Device	C Ileocutaneous
L Occlusion	D Urethra			D Cutaneous
M Reattachment				X Diagnostic
N Release				Z No Qualifier
P Removal				
Q Repair				
R Replacement				
S Reposition				
T Resection				
U Supplement				
V Restriction				
W Revision				
Y Transplantation				

Body Part — Character 4

The body part characters specified in the urinary system table detail the various components and structures of the urinary system.

Figure 19.1: Genitourinary System

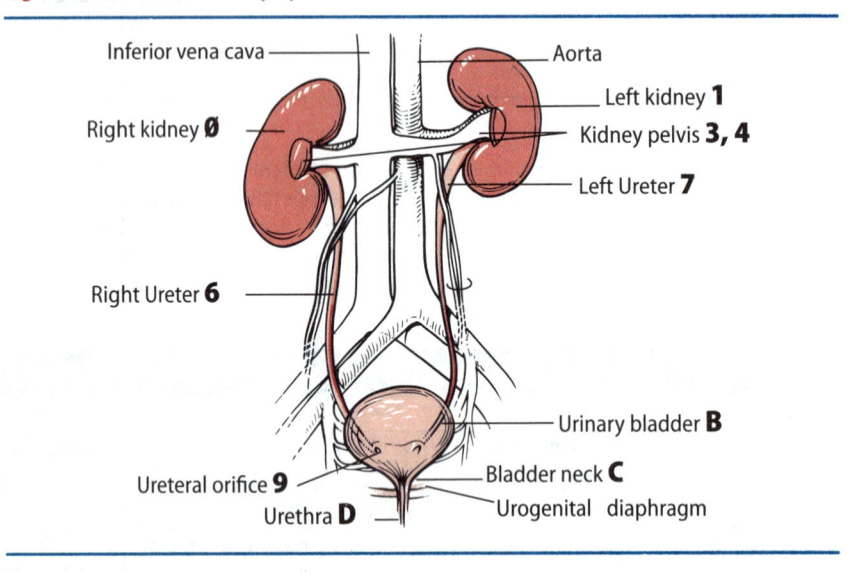

Character Value — 0, 1, 2, 5, Kidney; Right, Left, Bilateral

Associated Terms: Renal calyx, renal capsule, renal cortex, renal segment

Located in the dorsal part of the abdomen, the main function of the kidneys is to filter the blood and help eliminate wastes. There are several components to the kidneys, such as the renal calyx, the renal capsule, the renal cortex, and the renal segment.

Figure 19.2: Kidney

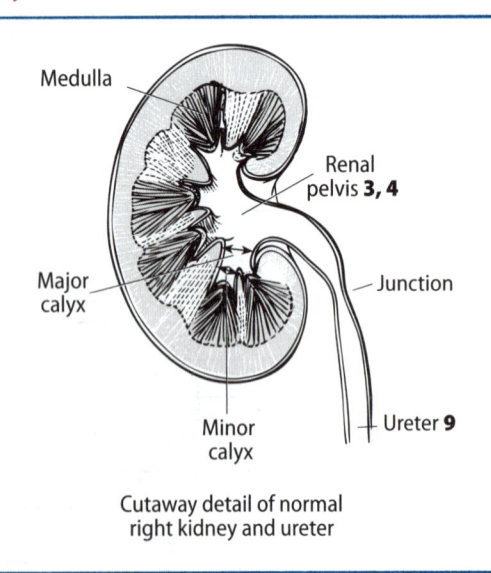

Cutaway detail of normal right kidney and ureter

Character Value — 3, 4, Kidney Pelvis, Left & Right

Associated Terms: Ureteropelvic junction (UPJ)

The kidney or renal pelvis is a funnel-like tube that leads from the kidney to the ureter and funnels urine from the kidney to the bladder. The ureteropelvic junction is the junction between the renal pelvis and the ureter.

Figure 19.3: Bladder

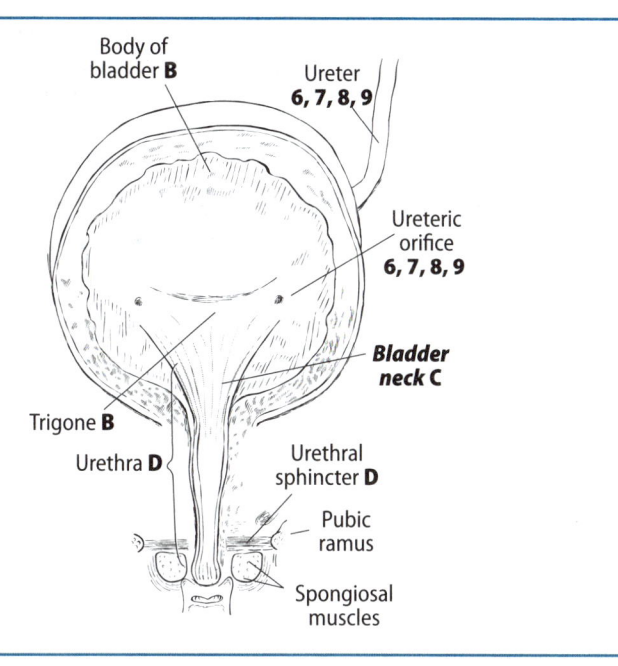

> **DEFINITIONS**
>
> **bladder neck.** Area of the bladder where it begins to narrow and the bladder and urethra connect.

Character Value — 6, 7, 8, 9, Ureter; Right, Left, Bilateral

Associated Terms: Ureteral orifice, ureterovesical orifice

Each ureter, a tube leading from the kidney to the urinary bladder, is made up of three layers of tissue, and enters the bladder through a narrow valve-like orifice that prevents the backflow of urine to the kidney. This orifice is known as the ureteral orifice or the ureterovesical orifice.

Character Value — B, Bladder

Associated Terms: Trigone of bladder

The bladder is a muscular sac that resides in the pelvis and stores urine for discharge through the urethra. The trigone of the urinary bladder is a triangular portion of the internal bladder that is bounded by the openings to the ureters and the internal urethral orifice.

Character Value — D, Urethra

Associated Terms: Bulbourethral (Cowper's) gland, Cowper's (bulbourethral) gland, external urethral sphincter, internal urethral sphincter, membranous urethra, penile urethra, prostatic urethra

The urethra is a small tube lined with mucous membrane that leads from the bladder to the exterior of the body. In the male, it is approximately 20 cm long and passes through the prostate gland just below the bladder, where it joins the ejaculatory ducts. Urine is prevented from mixing with semen during ejaculation by the reflex closure of the sphincter muscles guarding the opening into the bladder. In the female, the urethra lies directly behind the symphysis pubis and in front of the vagina, and is only about 3 cm long. The membranous urethra, penile urethra, and prostatic urethra are all different segments of the urethra, and are found in males only. The bulbourethral (Cowper's) gland is found in the area of the urethra of males as well. The external urethral sphincter and internal urethral sphincter are found in males and females, which function to control the flow of urine.

Representative ICD-10-PCS Code Examples

1. **Percutaneous needle core biopsy of right kidney**

    ØTBØ3ZX   Excision of right kidney, percutaneous approach, diagnostic

    Note: The root operation excision simply means "cutting out or off, without replacement, a portion of a body part." It may seem somewhat extreme for a biopsy, but this is the appropriate root operation for an excisional biopsy in ICD-10-PCS, along with 7th character qualifier value X Diagnostic.

2. **Transurethral cystoscopy with removal of bladder stone**

    ØTCB8ZZ   Extirpation of matter from bladder, via natural or artificial opening endoscopic

Female Reproductive System (U)

The female reproductive system includes internal and external structures, represented in the body part characters. Procedures that may be performed on the female reproductive system include laparoscopy with excision of an endometrial implant from the left ovary, a diagnostic hysteroscopy with D&C, or placement of a transvaginal intraluminal cervical cerclage. A compiled table for body system character U Female reproductive system, provides all of the valid characters for that system in ICD-10-PCS.

> **DEFINITIONS**
>
> **cul-de-sac.** Blind pouch or sac formed by the caudal portion of the parietal peritoneum.

Operation–Character 3	Body Part–Character 4	Approach–Character 5	Device–Character 6	Qualifier–Character 7
1 Bypass	0 Ovary, Right	0 Open	0 Drainage Device	0 Allogeneic
2 Change	1 Ovary, Left	3 Percutaneous	1 Radioactive Element	1 Syngeneic
5 Destruction	2 Ovaries, Bilateral	4 Percutaneous Endoscopic	3 Infusion Device	2 Zooplastic
7 Dilation	3 Ovary	7 Via Natural or Artificial Opening	7 Autologous Tissue Substitute	5 Fallopian Tube, Right
8 Division	4 Uterine Supporting Structure	8 Via Natural or Artificial Opening Endoscopic	C Extraluminal Device	6 Fallopian Tube, Left
9 Drainage	5 Fallopian Tube, Right	F Via Natural or Artificial Opening With Percutaneous Endoscopic Assistance	D Intraluminal Device	9 Uterus
B Excision	6 Fallopian Tube, Left	X External	G Intraluminal Device, Pessary	X Diagnostic
C Extirpation	7 Fallopian Tubes, Bilateral		H Contraceptive Device	Z No Qualifier
D Extraction	8 Fallopian Tube		J Synthetic Substitute	
F Fragmentation	9 Uterus		K Nonautologous Tissue Substitute	
H Insertion	B Endometrium		Y Other Device	
J Inspection	C Cervix		Z No Device	
L Occlusion	D Uterus and Cervix			
M Reattachment	F *Cul-de-sac*			
N Release	G Vagina			
P Removal	H Vagina and Cul-de-sac			
Q Repair	J Clitoris			
S Reposition	K Hymen			
T Resection	L Vestibular Gland			
U Supplement	M Vulva			
V Restriction	N Ova			
W Revision				
Y Transplantation				

Body Part — Character 4

The body part characters specified in the female reproductive system table detail the various components and structures of the female reproductive system.

Figure 19.4: Female Reproductive System

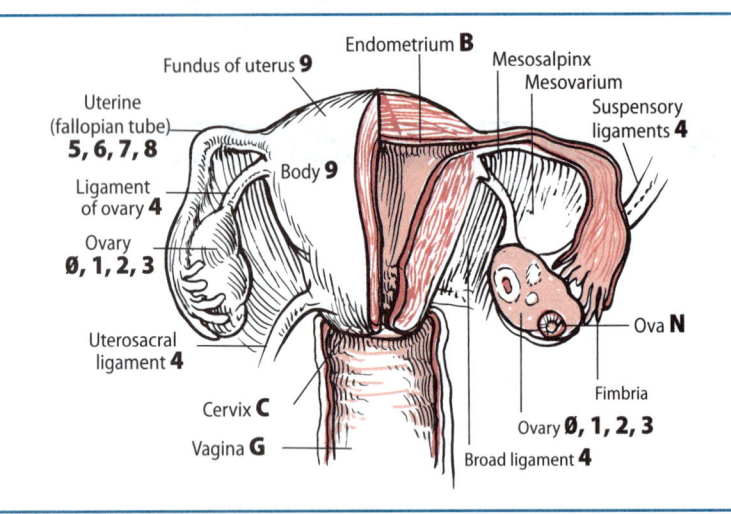

Character Value — 4, Uterine Supporting Structure

Associated Terms: Broad ligament, infundibulopelvic ligament, ovarian ligament, round ligament of uterus

The broad ligament is a fold of peritoneum extending from the side of the uterus to the wall of the pelvis. The infundibulopelvic ligament, ovarian ligament, and round ligament of uterus are all found within this broad ligament, and all act to support the uterus in the abdominal cavity.

Character Value — 5, 6, 7, 8, Fallopian Tube; Right, Left, Bilateral

Associated Terms: Oviduct, salpinx, uterine tube

The fallopian tubes, also referred to as oviducts, salpinx, or uterine tubes, are bilateral, paired tubes that extend from the uterus to the ovaries, through which an ovum released from the follicle travels to the uterus during ovulation.

Character Value — 9, Uterus

Associated Terms: Fundus uteri, myometrium, perimetrium, uterine cornu

The uterus is a pear shaped, hollow organ made up of three layers: the **endometrium**, the myometrium, and the perimetrium. The fundus uteri is the top portion of the uterus, furthest away from the cervix. The uterine cornua are the points where the uterus and the fallopian tubes meet.

Character Value — L, Vestibular Gland

Associated Terms: Bartholin's (greater vestibular) gland, greater vestibular (Bartholin's) gland, paraurethral (Skene's) gland, Skene's (paraurethral) gland

Located on either side of the vaginal orifice, the vestibular glands are found in pairs, including the greater vestibular (Bartholin's) glands and the paraurethral (Skene's) glands.

DEFINITIONS

endometrium. Lining of the uterus that thickens in preparation for fertilization. A fertilized ovum embeds into the thickened endometrium. When no fertilization takes place, the endometrial lining sheds during the process of menstruation.

Figure 19.5: Female External Structures

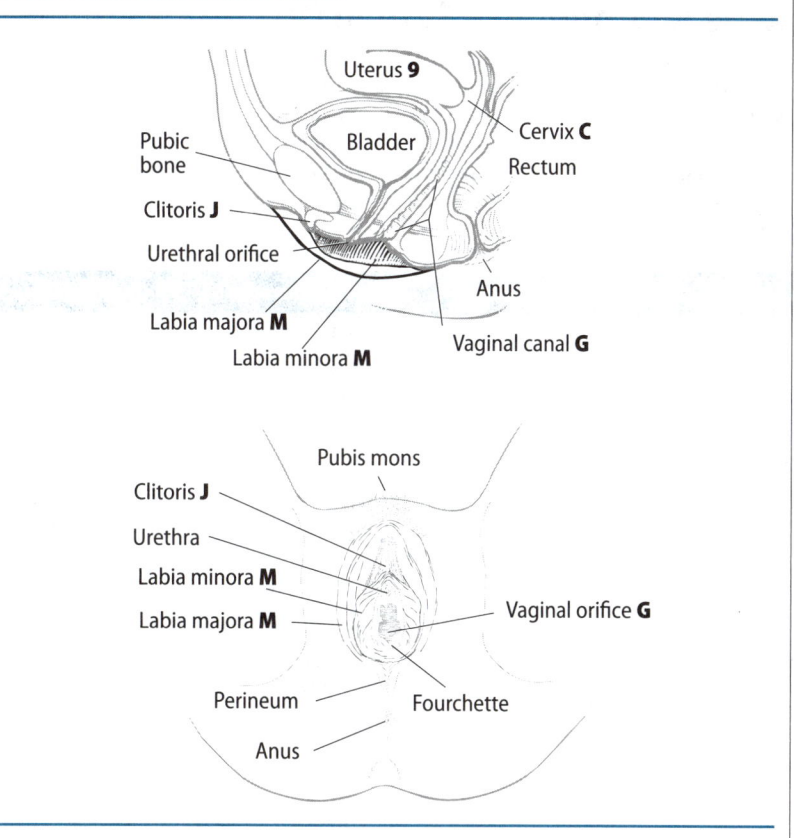

Character Value — M, Vulva

Associated Terms: Labia majora, labia minora

The vulva is the external genitalia of a female and is composed of many elements, two of which are the labia majora and minora. The labia majora and minora are folds of skin appearing on the outside of the vaginal orifice.

Representative ICD-10-PCS Code Examples

1. **Hysteroscopy with balloon dilation of bilateral fallopian tubes**

    0U778ZZ Dilation of bilateral fallopian tubes, via natural or artificial opening endoscopic

    Note: Laterality, as well as approach and mechanism of surgery, are all included in this code, as well as the procedure itself.

2. **Laparoscopic-assisted total vaginal hysterectomy**

    0UT9FZZ Resection of uterus, via natural or artificial opening with percutaneous endoscopic assistance

    0UTCFZZ Resection of cervix, via natural or artificial opening with percutaneous endoscopic assistance

> **CODING AXIOM**
>
> If only "total hysterectomy" is documented on the operative report, it is appropriate to code the resection of the uterus and cervix as removal of both organs is included in a total hysterectomy. Two codes are needed as the uterus and cervix each have a unique body part value.
>
> *Coding Clinic,* 3Q, 13, 28

Male Reproductive System (V)

Like the female reproductive system, the male reproductive system includes internal and external structures, represented in the body part characters. Procedures on the male reproductive system may include services such as a transurethral endoscopic laser ablation of the prostate, cystoscopy with placement of brachytherapy seeds in the prostate gland, or a vasectomy. A compiled table for body system character V Male reproductive system, provides all of the valid characters for that system in ICD-10-PCS.

Operation–Character 3	Body Part–Character 4	Approach–Character 5	Device–Character 6	Qualifier–Character 7
1 Bypass	0 Prostate	0 Open	0 Drainage Device	J Epididymis, Right
2 Change	1 Seminal Vesicle, Right	3 Percutaneous	1 Radioactive Element	K Epididymis, Left
5 Destruction	2 Seminal Vesicle, Left	4 Percutaneous Endoscopic	3 Infusion Device	N Vas Deferens, Right
7 Dilation	3 Seminal Vesicles, Bilateral	7 Via Natural or Artificial Opening	7 Autologous Tissue Substitute	P Vas Deferens, Left
9 Drainage	4 Prostate and Seminal Vesicles	8 Via Natural or Artificial Opening Endoscopic	C Extraluminal Device	X Diagnostic
B Excision	5 Scrotum	X External	D Intraluminal Device	Z No Qualifier
C Extirpation	6 Tunica Vaginalis, Right		J Synthetic Substitute	
H Insertion	7 Tunica Vaginalis, Left		K Nonautologous Tissue Substitute	
J Inspection	8 Scrotum and Tunica Vaginalis		Y Other Device	
L Occlusion	9 Testis, Right		Z No Device	
M Reattachment	B Testis, Left			
N Release	C Testes, Bilateral			
P Removal	D Testis			
Q Repair	F Spermatic Cord, Right			
R Replacement	G Spermatic Cord, Left			
S Reposition	H Spermatic Cords, Bilateral			
T Resection	J Epididymis, Right			
U Supplement	K Epididymis, Left			
W Revision	L Epididymis, Bilateral			
	M Epididymis and Spermatic Cord			
	N Vas Deferens, Right			
	P Vas Deferens, Left			
	Q Vas Deferens, Bilateral			
	R Vas Deferens			
	S Penis			
	T Prepuce			

Body Part — Character 4

The body part characters specified in the male reproductive system table detail the various components and structures of the male reproductive system.

Figure 19.6: Male Reproductive System

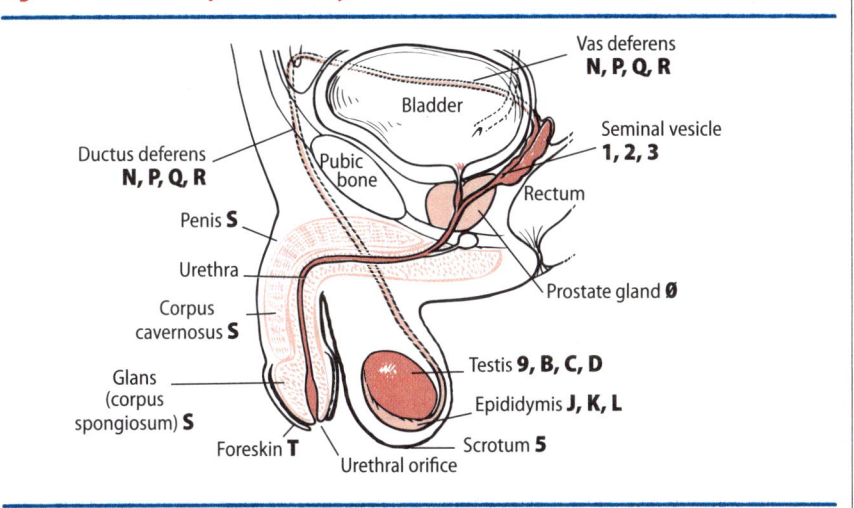

Character Value — F, G, H, Spermatic Cord, Right, Left, Bilateral

Associated Terms: Pampiniform plexus

Traversing from the abdomen to the testicles, the spermatic cord contains several important structures, including the testicular, differential, and cremasteric arteries, as well as the cremaster and testicular nerves, the vas deferens, the pampiniform plexus, lymphatic vessels, and the ***tunica vaginalis***.

Character Value — N, P, Q, R, Vas Deferens, Right, Left, Bilateral

Associated Terms: Ductus deferens, ejaculatory duct

The vas deferens, also referred to as the ductus deferens, is a duct that arises in the tail of the ***epididymis***, whose main function is to store and carry sperm from the epididymis to the urethra. The ejaculatory duct is formed where the vas deferens meets the ***seminal vesicle***.

Character Value — S, Penis

Associated Terms: Corpus cavernosum, corpus spongiosum

The penis is a male reproductive and urinary excretion organ that is composed of three structures enclosed by fascia and skin: two parallel cylindrical bodies (the corpora cavernosa) and the corpus spongiosum lying underneath them, through which the urethra passes.

DEFINITIONS

epididymis. Coiled tube on the back of the testis that is the site of sperm maturation and storage and where spermatozoa are propelled into the vas deferens toward the ejaculatory duct by contraction of smooth muscle.

seminal vesicles. Paired glands located at the base of the bladder in males that release the majority of fluid into semen through ducts that join with the vas deferens forming the ejaculatory duct.

tunica vaginalis. Serous membrane that partially covers the testes formed by an outpocketing of the peritoneum when the testes descend.

Figure 19.7: Penis

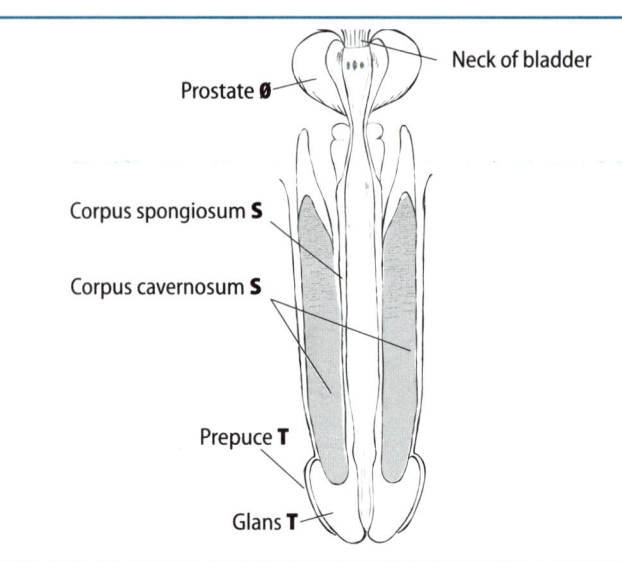

- Neck of bladder
- Prostate 0
- Corpus spongiosum S
- Corpus cavernosum S
- Prepuce T
- Glans T

Character Value — T, Prepuce

Associated Terms: Foreskin, glans penis

The prepuce, also known as the foreskin, is a fold of penile skin covering the glans penis. The glans penis is the distal end or head of the penis.

Representative ICD-10-PCS Code Examples

1. **Transurethral endoscopic laser ablation of the prostate gland**

   0V508ZZ   Destruction of prostate, via natural or artificial opening endoscopic

   Note: The ICD-10-PCS code indicates a destruction root operation versus an excision or resection, meaning that a direct use of energy was applied to eradicate the tissue.

2. **Cystoscopy with placement of brachytherapy seeds in prostate gland**

   0VH081Z   Insertion of radioactive element into prostate, via natural or artificial opening endoscopic

   Note: The coder must understand the purpose of the device being inserted; in this case, the brachytherapy seeds are considered a radioactive element reported in the 6th character value.

Summary

In this chapter, the urinary system, the female reproductive system, and the male reproductive system have been reviewed. The majority of procedures performed on these systems are coded in ICD-10-PCS using the characters in this chapter. Each section provides a review of the root operation, body part, and approach characters, and details the anatomy and physiology involved in character selection. Having a clear understanding of the different characters and the terminology associated with each character provides a great base from which to learn more about the methods for ICD-10-PCS coding.

Knowledge Assessment Questions

1. What root operation is defined as "completely closing an orifice or lumen of a tubular body part"?
   a. Insertion
   b. Restriction
   c. Occlusion
   d. Destruction

2. What body part character is reported for a procedure performed on the left oviduct in the female reproductive system?
   a. D Uterus and cervix
   b. 6 Fallopian tube, left
   c. 1 Ovary, left
   d. G Vagina

3. What body part character is reported when a procedure is performed on the renal capsule on the left side?
   a. 1 Kidney, left
   b. 2 Kidneys, bilateral
   c. 5 Kidney
   d. 4 Kidney pelvis, left

4. A procedure performed on the Cowper's gland is assigned to body part character 9 in the urinary system.
   a. True
   b. False

5. A procedure performed on the salpinx bilaterally is assigned to which body part character in the female reproductive system?
   a. 3 Ovary
   b. F Cul-de-sac
   c. 2 Ovaries, bilateral
   d. 7 Fallopian tubes, bilateral

6. Which procedure is defined as "cutting into a body part without draining fluids and/or gases from the body part in order to separate or transect a body part"?
   a. Detachment
   b. Division
   c. Occlusion
   d. Resection

7. A procedure performed on the Bartholin's gland is assigned to which body part character in the female reproductive system?
   a. L Vestibular gland
   b. F Cul-de-sac
   c. B Endometrium
   d. V Ova

8. A procedure performed on the renal pelvis is assigned to the body part character for kidney.
   a. True
   b. False

9. Which root operation could be described as "breaking solid matter in a body part into pieces"?
   a. Extirpation
   b. Resection
   c. Fragmentation
   d. Removal

10. The cul-de-sac is a blind pouch or sac formed by the caudal portion of the parietal peritoneum in the lower abdomen.
    a. True
    b. False

Chapter 20. ICD-10-PCS: Anatomical Regions Systems

Anatomical Regions

In the remaining tables in ICD-10-PCS, the body systems contain generic anatomical regions only. These tables will not be reviewed in their entirety as the listings are self-explanatory.

Qualifier — Character 7

In the upper and lower extremities anatomical regions tables (body systems X & Y), there are options for 7th character qualifier assignment based on the location for each extremity. These qualifier values are specifically related to the root operation detachment, and indicate the exact location of the amputation. For example, a high detachment of the leg is defined as an amputation at the proximal portion of the shaft of the femur. The following table details the definitions of each of the detachment body parts found in the lower and upper extremities anatomical regions tables.

	Qualifier Definition	Arm	Leg
1	**High:** Amputation at the proximal portion of the shaft of the:	Humerus	Femur
2	**Mid:** Amputation at the middle portion of the shaft of the:	Humerus	Femur
3	**Low:** Amputation at the distal portion of the shaft of the:	Humerus	Femur
	Qualifier Definition	Hand	Foot
0	Complete 1st through 5th Rays Ray: digit of hand or foot with corresponding metacarpus or metatarsus	Through carpo-metacarpal joint, **Wrist**	Through tarso-metatarsal Joint, **Ankle**
4	Complete 1st Ray	Through carpo-metacarpal joint, **Thumb**	Through tarso-metatarsal joint, **Great Toe**
5	Complete 2nd Ray	Through carpo-metacarpal joint, **Index Finger**	Through tarso-metatarsal joint, **2nd Toe**
6	Complete 3rd Ray	Through carpo-metacarpal joint, **Middle Finger**	Through tarso-metatarsal joint, **3rd Toe**
7	Complete 4th Ray	Through carpo-metacarpal joint, **Ring Finger**	Through tarso-metatarsal joint, **4th Toe**
8	Complete 5th Ray	Through carpo-metacarpal joint, **Little Finger**	Through tarso-metatarsal joint, **Little Toe**
9	Partial 1st Ray	Anywhere along shaft or head of metacarpal bone, **Thumb**	Anywhere along shaft or head of metatarsal bone, **Great Toe**
B	Partial 2nd Ray	Anywhere along shaft or head of metacarpal bone, **Index Finger**	Anywhere along shaft or head of metatarsal bone, **2nd Toe**
C	Partial 3rd Ray	Anywhere along shaft or head of metacarpal bone, **Middle Finger**	Anywhere along shaft or head of metatarsal bone, **3rd Toe**
D	Partial 4th Ray	Anywhere along shaft or head of metacarpal bone, **Ring Finger**	Anywhere along shaft or head of metatarsal bone, **4th Toe**
F	Partial 5th Ray	Anywhere along shaft or head of metacarpal bone, **Little Finger**	Anywhere along shaft or head of metatarsal bone, **Little Toe**

DEFINITIONS

complete amputation of the toe. Detachment through the metatarsal-phalangeal joint.

partial amputation of the foot. Detachment anywhere through the shaft or head of the metatarsal bone of the foot.

KEY POINT

If the surgeon uses the word "toe" to describe an amputation, but the operative report says he extends the amputation to the midshaft of the fifth metatarsal, the appropriate body part value is the foot. The qualifier is then used to describe the partial fifth ray.

	Qualifier Definition	Finger or Thumb	Toe
0	**Complete:** Amputation at the metacarpophalangeal metatarsal-phalangeal joint	Finger or Thumb, any one 1st -5th	Toe, any one 1st -5th
1	**High:** Amputation anywhere along the proximal phalanx	Finger or Thumb, any one 1st -5th	Toe, any one 1st -5th
2	**Mid:** Amputation through the proximal intraphalangeal joint or anywhere along the middle phalanx	Finger or Thumb, any one 1st -5th	Toe, any one 1st -5th
3	**Low:** Amputation through the distal intraphalangeal joint or anywhere along the distal phalanx	Finger or Thumb, any one 1st -5th	Toe, any one 1st -5th

Representative ICD-10-PCS Code Examples

1. **Open repair of a previous mid-thigh amputation, right leg**

   ØYQCØZZ   Repair right upper leg, open approach

2. **Control of hemorrhage in the throat following a tonsillectomy/adenoidectomy**

   ØW33XZZ   Control bleeding in oral cavity and throat, external approach

   Note: The root operation control (of postprocedural hemorrhage) is only valid for the anatomical regions body systems in ICD-10-PCS; many postoperative hemorrhages involve body regions instead of specific body parts. The approach is external because the tonsillectomy area may be visualized through the mouth from an external standpoint without the use of instrumentation.

3. **Right leg and hip amputation through ischium**

   ØY62ØZZ   Detachment, right hindquarter, open approach

   Note: The hindquarter body part includes amputation along any part of the hip bone.

4. **Fifth ray carpometacarpal joint amputation, left hand**

   ØX6KØZ8   Detachment of complete 5th ray of left hand, open approach

   Note: A complete ray amputation is through the carpometacarpal joint.

Summary

This chapter touches on the section in ICD-10-PCS that covers the general anatomical regions. It does not focus on any particular portion of the anatomy, but simply more generic regions of the body. However, there are some important anatomical points to note in this chapter. Be sure to review the qualifier definitions associated with amputations, as it can often be the key to accurate coding. There are also specific types of root operations that are only found in these body systems, making an understanding of the root operations vital to successful coding.

Knowledge Assessment Questions

1. Which root operation is defined as "taking or cutting out solid matter from a body part"?

    a. Excision

    b. Extirpation

    c. Extraction

    d. Fragmentation

2. In the hand, detachment of the complete third ray is defined as an amputation of the middle finger through the carpometacarpal joint.

    a. True

    b. False

3. Which procedure is described as "stopping, or attempting to stop, post-procedural bleeding"?

    a. Insertion

    b. Repair

    c. Control

    d. Alteration

4. Which approach involves "entry, by puncture or minor incision, of instrumentation through the skin or mucous membrane and/or any other body layers necessary to reach and visualize the site of the procedure"?

    a. Percutaneous

    b. External

    c. Open

    d. Percutaneous endoscopic

Appendix A. Knowledge Assessment Answers

Chapter 1. Introduction to the Human Body

1. The following are all levels of structural organization *except*:
   a. Chemical
   b. Organ
   c. Organismal
   d. Anatomical

   Rationale: Chemical, organ, and organismal are all levels of structural organization of the human body, but anatomical is not.

2. The principal parts of a cell are the plasma membrane, cytoplasm, and the nucleus.

   Rationale: The principal parts of a cell are the plasma membrane, the cytoplasm, and the nucleus, where DNA is housed. These cells are the building blocks for all of our organs, muscles, blood, and more.

3. All of the following are basic types of tissue found in the body, *except*:
   a. DNA
   b. Connective
   c. Muscle
   d. Nervous

   Rationale: DNA is not a tissue found in the body. It is genetic material found in the nucleus of a cell. Connective, muscle, and nervous are all types of tissue.

4. Metabolism takes place in two parts: catabolism and anabolism.

   Rationale: Catabolism and anabolism are the two elements of metabolism. Catabolism is the process of breaking down a very complex chemical substance into a more simple one, such as breaking down protein in food into its component parts such as amino acids. Anabolism is the opposite—it takes those smaller component parts and creates complex chemical substances.

5. Growth refers only to adding additional cells to the body.
   a. True
   b. False

   Rationale: Growth can occur by adding additional cells, by having existing cells grow larger, or by having the material that surrounds the cells expand, such as in the case of bone growth.

6. A patient who is face down on the examining room table would be in the prone position.

   Rationale: Being face down in a reclining position is referred to as being in the prone position.

© 2015 Optum360, LLC

7. When the body is standing upright with palms forward, this is the anatomical position.

   Rationale: The anatomical position is when the patient is in the forward facing position, with the head level, and eyes facing forward. The patient's feet are flat on the floor and the palms are turned forward.

8. Write the correct term or terms that denote relationships, compare positions, or denote movement.

   a. Toward the back of the body Posterior, caudal, or dorsal
   b. Toward the front of the body Anterior or ventral
   c. Farther from the middle Lateral
   d. Toward the middle Medial
   e. Toward the top of the body Superior, cranial, or cephalic
   f. Toward the lower part of the body Inferior
   g. Farthest from the point of origin Distal
   h. Nearest to the point of origin Proximal
   i. Farthest from the center Exterior
   j. Nearest to the center Interior
   k. Closest to the surface Superficial
   l. Conveying toward the center Afferent
   m. Conveying away from the center Efferent
   n. The movement causing decreased angle of a joint Flexion
   o. The movement causing straightening of a joint Extension
   p. Movement away from the median plane Abduction
   q. Movement toward the median plane Adduction
   r. Movement of lower arm that rotates the palm and forearm anteriorly Supination
   s. Movement of the lower arm that rotates the palm and forearm posteriorly Pronation
   t. Movement of the foot at the ankle away from the medial plane Eversion
   u. Movement of the foot at the ankle toward the medial plane Inversion

9. The left arm and left leg would be ipsilateral to one another.

   a. True
   b. False

   Rationale: This statement is true, as ipsilateral means on the same side of the body as another structure.

10. Because we consciously control our own skeletal muscle tissues, this type of muscle is often referred to as voluntary muscle.

    Rationale: Skeletal muscle is commonly referred to as voluntary muscle because its activity, either contraction or relaxation, is under conscious control.

Chapter 2. ICD-10-CM: Integumentary System

1. A furuncle is also known as a boil and is typically found in a gland or a hair follicle.

   Rationale: Furuncles are localized skin infections that exist mainly in glands and hair follicles where a core of dead tissue is formed, which causes pain, redness, and swelling.

2. The following are all layers of the skin and subcutaneous tissue, except:
   a. Epidermis
   b. Dermis
   c. Muscle and fascia
   d. Hypodermis

   Rationale: The muscle and fascia are not layers of the skin and subcutaneous tissue. They are in layers underneath the subcutaneous tissue.

3. What is the key role of the sudoriferous glands in the body?
   a. Releasing oil onto the skins surface
   b. Releasing perspiration to cool the body
   c. Assisting in hair growth
   d. Serving as a sensory receptor

   Rationale: The sudoriferous glands are the sweat glands, whose main responsibility is to produce perspiration to cool the body.

4. Which type of response to solar radiation causes hives or wheals in response to UV radiation?
   a. Drug photoallergic response
   b. Photocontact dermatitis
   c. Drug phototoxic response
   d. Solar urticaria

   Rationale: Solar urticaria is a condition classified as hives or wheals caused specifically by exposure to the sun or UV radiation.

5. Lichenification is a thickening and hardening of the epidermis of the skin.

   Rationale: Lichenification is a symptom of many of the skin disorders examined in this chapter.

6. The most common form of psoriasis is:
   a. Psoriasis vulgaris
   b. Palmoplantar psoriasis
   c. Pustular psoriasis
   d. Guttate psoriasis

   Rationale: Psoriasis vulgaris is the most common form of psoriasis, affecting 80 to 90 percent of patients with a psoriasis diagnosis.

7. Acne vulgaris affects adolescents, not adult patients.
   a. True
   b. **False**

   Rationale: Many adult patients deal with this common form of acne, beginning in their adolescent years or as adults.

8. Treatment for all types of alopecia is cosmetic in nature.
   a. True
   b. **False**

   Rationale: Although treatment for androgenic alopecia is typically cosmetic in nature, treatment for other types of medical hair loss, such as alopecia areata or anagen effluvium, may not be considered cosmetic.

9. Which stage of pressure ulcer involves a full-thickness skin loss extending through the subcutaneous tissue but not to the muscle and bone?
   a. First stage
   b. Second stage
   c. **Third stage**
   d. Fourth stage

   Rationale: A pressure ulcer with a full-thickness skin loss extending through the subcutaneous tissue but not to the muscle and bone is a Stage 3 pressure ulcer.

10. What is another name for a "pins and needles" feeling in the skin?
    a. Anesthesia
    b. **Paraesthesia**
    c. Hyperesthesia
    d. Skin disturbance

    Rationale: Paraesthesia is a tingling or prickling feeling in the affected area, often referred to as pins and needles.

11. Where is the axillary tail found?
    a. Nail
    b. Anywhere on the skin
    c. With a neoplasm
    d. **Breast**

    Rationale: The axillary tail is a portion of the breast tissue that extends from the upper outer quadrant to the axilla or armpit.

Chapter 3. ICD-10-CM: Skeletal Systems and Articulations

1. The mandible is the only bone in the face that moves.
   a. **True**
   b. False

   Rationale: The face consists of 13 stationary bones and one that is mobile. The mandible (jawbone) is the only facial bone that moves, and it is also the largest and strongest bone of the face.

2. The bony spine is also called the **vertebral** column, named after the 24 individual bones that it comprises.

   Rationale: The vertebral column is the support for the head and trunk of the body, as well as protection for the spinal cord. It is composed of 26 individual bones. Of these bones, 24 are vertebrae that are separated by cartilage called intervertebral discs.

3. There are how many vertebrae in each section of spine?
   a. **7** cervical
   b. **12** thoracic
   c. **5** lumbar

   Rationale: The vertebrae can be divided into three groups: 7 cervical (C1-C7; C1 is also known as atlas, C2 as axis), 12 thoracic (T1-T12), 5 lumbar (L1-L5).

4. The **clavicle** and **scapula** form the shoulder girdle.

   Rationale: The shoulder girdle consists of two bones on each side, the clavicle, or collar bone, and the scapula, or shoulder blade. The clavicle is found on the anterior side of the shoulder and the scapula on the posterior.

5. What is the lowest portion of the coxal bones called? **ischium**

   Rationale: This area is identified in the illustration of the pelvis.

6. The acetabulum is where the head of the **femur** sits to form the **hip** joint.

   Rationale: Where the three parts of the pelvic bone fuse together is referred to as the acetabulum. It is a deep-seated pocket that accepts the rounded upper epiphysis of the thigh bone, or femoral head, to form the hip joint.

7. Both the thumb and big toe have more phalanges than the other toes.
   a. True
   b. **False**

   Rationale: There are three phalanges in all fingers, except thumbs, which have only two. Similar to the fingers, all of the toes have three phalanges— proximal, middle, and distal—with the exception of the great toe, or hallux.

8. The two sections of the skeleton are **axial** and **appendicular**.

   Rationale: The 206 bones that make up the adult skeleton can be divided into two classifications: the axial skeleton and appendicular skeleton.

9. A ligament attaches bone to muscle.
   a. True
   b. False

   Rationale: Ligament is fibrous tissue binding joints together that connects bone to bone or bone to cartilage.

10. The shoulder is a pivot joint.
    a. True
    b. False

    Rationale: The shoulder (humeral head and glenoid depression of the scapula) and hip joints (femoral head and acetabulum of a coxa bone) are ball-and-socket articulations. The articulation between the C1 and C2 vertebrae that allows the head to move back and forth is a pivot joint.

11. There are two types of etiology of fractures: traumatic and pathological.

    Rationale: A traumatic fracture is the result of an external cause, while a pathological fracture is the result of another disease process weakening the bone. Although an external cause or trauma may initiate a pathological fracture, it is the weakening of the bone due to the underlying disease process that makes the bone susceptible to breakage and not necessarily the trauma itself.

12. A malunion of a fracture is when it has healed or is healing in an incorrect position.

    Rationale: A malunion is a fractured bone that has healed or is healing in an incorrect position.

13. A nonunion of a fracture is when it has failed to heal.

    Rationale: A nonunion is a fractured bone that has failed to heal.

14. A type IIIA open fracture requires skin grafting.
    a. True
    b. False

    Rationale: In a type IIIA fracture there is enough local soft tissue to cover the wound and bone without the need for skin grafting.

15. A peripheral meniscus tear affects the outer third of the meniscus.

    Rationale: Peripheral tears are located in the peripheral or outer third of the meniscus. This area is very susceptible to healing as it has access to a rich blood supply.

16. When a joint becomes inflamed as a reaction to another disease, it is referred to as reactive arthropathy.

    Rationale: Occasionally the joint is impacted by an infection elsewhere. Inflammation of the joint as a reaction to another disease is referred to as reactive arthropathy.

17. When osteoarthritis is due to the aging process, it is considered secondary.
    a. True
    b. False

    Rationale: As the human body ages, the cartilage of the joints begins to degenerate and lose its elasticity from wear and tear and the natural aging process. This degeneration is referred to as primary osteoarthritis.

18. Spondylosis is degenerative osteoarthritis of the spine.

    Rationale: When degenerative osteoarthritis occurs in the spine, it is called spondylosis.

19. Spinal stenosis is a narrowing of the vertebral foramen, or space that the spinal nerves occupy.

    Rationale: Stenosis is the narrowing of a foramen of the spine, putting pressure on the nerves and causing pain, numbness, and weakness of limbs.

20. The three types of spinal curvature abnormalities are:
    a. Scoliosis
    b. Lordosis
    c. Kyphosis

    Rationale: Sometimes the normal curvatures in the spine become deformed. There are three types of these deformities: scoliosis, a lateral curvature of the spine; kyphosis, an abnormal posterior convex curvature of the spine; and lordosis, an exaggerated inward curvature of the lower back.

Chapter 4. ICD-10-CM: Muscular System

1. The three types of muscle are cardiac, smooth, and skeletal.

   Rationale: There are three types of muscle tissue: cardiac, smooth, and skeletal (or striated). Each type shares one or more of four functional characteristics.

2. Cardiac muscle is found only in the heart.

   Rationale: Cardiac muscle forms the heart walls and performs the contractions that push blood through the vessels of the body.

3. Smooth muscle is located lining the inside of hollow organs.

   Rationale: Smooth muscle is involuntary in its movements but is not striated, hence the name "smooth" muscle. This type of muscle lines the hollow organs of the body and contracts to force fluids and other bodily substances through the proper channels. It is found in organs such as the gastrointestinal tract, the uterus, urinary bladder, and blood vessels.

4. The basic components of muscle are:
   - Muscle tissue
   - Nerves
   - Blood vessels
   - Connective tissue

   Rationale: All skeletal muscles are composed of muscle tissue, nerves, blood vessels, and substantial amounts of connective tissue.

5. A tendon connects a muscle to bone.

   Rationale: In some cases, the fascia extends past the muscle it surrounds, forming a cordlike structure that attaches to the periosteum of a bone. This cord is referred to as a tendon.

6. An aponeurosis connects muscle to muscle.

   Rationale: In other cases, the fascia extends past its muscle to form broad, thick sheets of connective tissue that connect the muscle to an adjacent muscle, called aponeurosis.

7. Bursae are located where muscles and tendons make contact with the bone.

   Rationale: In certain instances, mainly where muscles and tendons make contact with bone, there are fluid-filled sacs called bursae, which reduce friction between the muscle or tendon and the bone it moves across.

8. The four distinctions that determine a muscle's movement are:
   - Origin
   - Insertion
   - Shape
   - Coordination with other muscles

   Rationale: Muscles provide various movements based not only their origins, insertions, and shape but also on coordination with other muscles.

9. Abduction is moving away from midline, and adduction is moving toward midline.

   Rationale: Abduction means moving away from midline (reaching out with the arm), whereas adduction means moving closer to midline (pulling the arm close to the body).

10. Skeletal muscles are usually named for one or more of the following characteristics:
    - Size
    - Shape
    - Action
    - Location
    - Attachments

    Rationale: It is important to point out that the names of skeletal muscles are based on their basic characteristics: size, shape, action, location, and/or attachments. Understanding the meaning of a muscle's name gives a clue to that muscle's specific attributes.

11. The muscles in the head are responsible only for facial expression.
    a. True
    b. False

    Rationale: The muscles in the head are responsible for three main functions: facial expression, mastication, and movement of the eyes.

12. The diaphragm is the dome-shaped muscle dividing the abdominal and thoracic cavities and aids in respiration.

    Rationale: The diaphragm is a dome-shaped divider between the thoracic and abdominal cavities. This muscle flattens when it contracts, making more space available to the lungs during inhalation.

13. The trapezius is found in both the neck and thoracic regions.

    Rationale: Most superior in the back of the neck and connecting to the tops of the shoulders, forming the "crook" of the neck, is the trapezius muscle. This muscle stabilizes and controls movements of the shoulder. Although its superior location is the neck, it extends into the posterior thorax musculature.

14. The intrinsic muscles of the hand move the fingers.

    Rationale: The muscles in the forearm tend to control the less delicate hand movements, but the intrinsic muscles in the hands perform the precise and fluid movements of the fingers.

15. A sprain is an injury to a ligament whereas a strain is an injury of muscle or tendon.

    Rationale: A sprain occurs when there is a stretch or tear of a ligament, the tissue that connects bone to bone. A strain is an injury to a muscle or tendon, usually due to overexertion, twisting, or pulling.

16. A rotator cuff tear usually involves the supraspinatus muscle.

    Rationale: A rotator cuff tear is a very common injury, sometimes classified as a sprain. It occurs in the shoulder region and usually involves the supraspinatus muscle but can occur in the other muscles or tendons in the shoulder.

17. Tendinitis and tenosynovitis are synonymous.
    a. True
    b. False

    Rationale: Tendinitis is slightly different from tenosynovitis, in that it affects only the tendon without swelling of the tendon sheath.

18. Calcification can occur without ossification.

    a. True
    b. False

    Rationale: The process of calcification occurs during the ossification process, but they are not synonymous. Calcification can occur without ossification being present.

19. A cramp is a more severe form of a spasm.

    Rationale: Both cramps and spasms are a contraction of a muscle; the difference is the duration and whether or not there is associated pain. A spasm is a brief contraction followed by little or no pain, whereas a cramp is more severe in that it is prolonged and painful.

20. An abnormal gait may be a symptom of neurological or muscular disease.

    Rationale: An abnormal gait can indicate a neurological or muscle disorder, so it is imperative to know the different ways this movement can be altered.

Chapter 5. ICD-10-CM: Nervous System

1. The central nervous system includes the brain and the spinal cord. The peripheral nervous system includes the sense organs and the nerves linking the organs, muscles, and glands to the central nervous system.

    Rationale: The nervous system is a complex network of specialized organs, tissues, and cells that coordinate the body's actions and functions. It consists of two main subdivisions: the central nervous system and the peripheral nervous system.

2. The following are all elements of the central nervous system **except**:
    a. Brain
    b. Spinal cord
    c. Connective tissues associated to the brain and spinal cord
    d. Sensory organs

    Rationale: The brain, spinal cord, and associated connective tissues are all elements of the central nervous system.

3. In the central nervous system, the brain and spinal cord receive, integrate, and interpret information, whereas in the peripheral nervous system, the cranial and spinal nerves facilitate communication between the CNS and the rest of the body.

    Rationale: CNS: The brain and spinal cord function as central processing units to receive, integrate, and interpret information, as well as to formulate a response to stimuli. PNS: Consists of cranial nerves and spinal nerves, which serve as communication lines between the CNS and the rest of the body.

4. The peripheral nervous system may be subdivided into the autonomic and the somatic nervous system.

    Rationale: The autonomic nervous system facilitates automatic bodily processes. The somatic (or bodily) nervous system regulates voluntary control over skeletal muscles in response to stimuli.

5. The nervous system works closely with other anatomic systems within the body to maintain homeostatic function.

    Rationale: As an example of how the nervous system works with other body systems, it sends and receives information from the endocrine system to produce and inhibit secretion of hormones to perform a variety of bodily functions, including metabolism.

6. The myelin (e.g., myelin sheath) is a fatty-appearing insulating membrane that covers and protects nerve axons while serving as a conducting mechanism for transmission of electrical signals between nerve cells. An example of a demyelinating disease is multiple sclerosis.

    Rationale: In effect, disorders of the myelin sheath can be loosely equated to problems with electrical wire insulation. These disruptions cause multiple deleterious nervous system effects. For example, multiple sclerosis is a painful demyelinating disease that adversely affects muscle control.

7. Diplacusis is commonly known as being "tone deaf."
    a. True
    b. False

    Rationale: Diplacusis describes a cochlear dysfunction in which the patient hears a single auditory stimulus as two sounds. This condition may be colloquially described as being "tone deaf."

8. Disorders specified as "extrapyramidal" refer to the conditions affecting the areas of the brain that coordinate muscle movement.

   Rationale: Extrapyramidal disorders are so named for the complex pathways and feedback loops that lie outside the tracts of the motor cortex that extend through the pyramid-shaped regions of the medulla. Certain pyramidal pathways innervate motor neurons of the brainstem or spinal cord, whereas the extrapyramidal tracts conduct and modulate motor activity indirectly, transmitting nerve impulses to the spinal cord from the pons and medulla of the brain using motor neurons of the basal ganglia, cerebellum, and thalamus.

9. Transient ischemic attack (TIA) and related syndromes, classified to the circulatory system in ICD-9-CM, have been reclassified to the nervous system in ICD-10-CM.

   Rationale: TIA and related syndromes include basilar and carotid artery syndromes and transient global amnesia. These conditions, although vascular in origin, manifest neurological symptoms and sequelae due to the anatomy involved.

10. High intraocular pressure may be an indication of what disease?
    a. Hypotension
    b. Glaucoma
    c. Oscillopsia
    d. Madarosis

    Rationale: In glaucoma, pseudoexfoliation of the lens capsule is characterized by small, grayish particles deposited on the pupillary margin of the iris, anterior chamber, and lens. This occurs when cells within the eye release dandruff-like flakes. The outer layers of the lens slough off and block normal flow of the aqueous humor. Material deposited on the front surface of the lens in the eye may be partially rubbed off by the pupil moving over the lens. This exfoliation process may occlude the outflow track (trabecular meshwork) and cause intraocular pressure to rise.

11. Codes for ophthalmic manifestations of diabetes mellitus in ICD-9-CM depend on etiology manifestations, whereas in ICD-10-CM, they depend on combination codes.

    Rationale: ICD-10-CM effectively employs combination codes that replace etiology-manifestation coding for diabetic ophthalmic disease. The ICD-10-CM chapter 4 endocrine disease codes (E00–E88) include the causal disease (diabetes mellitus), type of disease, specific ophthalmic manifestation, and associated conditions or complications. An excludes note at the beginning of the chapter informs the coder that those conditions due to endocrine, nutritional, and metabolic diseases (E00–E88), such as diabetes mellitus, are more appropriately classified elsewhere.

12. ICD-10-CM codes have been restructured and refined to accurately reflect disease processes by reflecting advancing medical technologies and study of the patient populations. For example, in the eye and adnexa section, the term senile, which has connotations of dementia, has been replaced with the term age-related. In the ear and mastoid process chapter, central auditory processing disorder, which was classified as a developmental delay in ICD-9-CM, is reclassified as a disorder of the sense organs in ICD-10-CM.

    Rationale: ICD-10-CM code descriptions have been updated to reflect current clinical terminology and to better represent conditions as they are understood by advancing medical technologies and through study of patient populations. For example, chapter 7, "Diseases of the Eye and Adnexa," replaces the term "senile" with "age-related," where appropriate. The term "senile" has been confused with an age-related dementia, cognitive decline, or other degenerative mental health condition beyond that associated with the normal aging process.

Instead, the term "age-related" associates a stated condition only with the natural aging process without implying a change in mental or cognitive status. Chapter 8, "Diseases of the Ear and Mastoid Process," includes central auditory processing disorder (ICD-9-CM 315.32), which was formerly classified as a developmental delay in chapter 5, "Mental Health Disorders." ICD-10-CM reclassified the condition to category H93 as a disorder of the sense organs. This reclassification more appropriately identifies the under-lying physiological causal factors associated with the disorder's manifestations.

13. The entire ear works as a sensory system by which sound waves are collected, amplified, and conducted to the brain for processing of the nervous impulses and to elicit a response. The three parts of the ear (the outer, middle, and inner ear) work together to achieve this goal.

    Rationale: The canals of the outer ear lead to the eardrum (middle ear). The eardrum (tympanic membrane) is attached to the ossicles, which amplify and conduct sound to the structures of the inner ear. The cochlea of the inner ear contains hair cells that vibrate when the eardrum and ossicles conduct a sound to them. The movement of these tiny hair cells transmits electrical impulses down the auditory nerve to the brain, which processes the stimuli as sound and facilitates responsive mechanisms.

14. The following are all types of cataracts ***except***:
    a. Descemet's
    b. Nuclear
    c. Posterior subcapsular
    d. Cuneiform

    Rationale: Nuclear, posterior subcapsular, and cuneiform are all types of cataracts. Descemet's is actually a membrane found within the eye itself. It is the collagenous inner layer of the corneal endothelium.

15. The left side of the brain controls the motor function on the left side of the body and vice versa.
    a. True
    b. False

    Rationale: The left side of the body is controlled by the right side of the brain and vice versa.

Chapter 6. ICD-10-CM: Endocrine System

1. Where are the parathyroid glands located?
   a. Brain
   b. **In the neck behind the thyroid**
   c. On top of each kidney
   d. Abdomen

   Rationale: The parathyroid is located behind the thyroid gland at the front of the neck. There are four glands: a superior pair and an inferior pair.

2. The thymus gland plays a role in which of the following?
   a. Digestion
   b. **Immune defenses**
   c. Insulin production
   d. Sexual and reproductive function

   Rationale: Hormones produced within the thymus are known collectively as thymosins. These play a key role in the development and maintenance of immune defenses by controlling white blood cell maturation.

3. A goiter is an enlargement of what gland?
   a. Pituitary
   b. Parathyroid
   c. Thymus
   d. **Thyroid**

   Rationale: A goiter is described as an abnormal enlargement of the thyroid gland, commonly caused by a deficiency of dietary iodine.

4. Low blood sugar is called:
   a. Hyperglycemia
   b. **Hypoglycemia**
   c. Hyperparathyroidism
   d. Thyroiditis

   Rationale: Hypoglycemia is an abnormally low blood glucose level caused by excessive insulin produced by the pancreas. This is sometimes associated with tumors or an overdose of insulin to treat diabetes.

5. What causes Cushing's disease?
   a. High blood pressure
   b. Obesity
   c. **Benign tumor/hyperplasia**
   d. Malignant tumor

   Rationale: Cushing's disease is specific to one cause of Cushing's syndrome, a benign tumor or hyperplasia in the pituitary gland that produces large amounts of adrenocorticotropic hormone (ACTH), which subsequently elevates cortisol.

6. Hypoparathyroidism is due to an abnormally low amount of what hormone?
   a. Follicle stimulating hormone (FSH)
   b. Parathyroid hormone (PTH)
   c. Growth hormone (GH)
   d. Thyrotropin (TSH)

   Rationale: Hypoparathyroidism is a condition in which one or more of the parathyroid glands secrete an abnormally low amount of the parathyroid hormone (PTH).

7. What part of the eye does a cataract affect?
   a. Retina
   b. Lens
   c. Choroid
   d. Sclera

   Rationale: A cataract is a clouding or opacity of the lens that prevents clear images from forming on the retina, causing vision impairment or blindness.

8. What distinguishes Type 1 diabetes from Type 2?
   a. Insulin injections are always required
   b. Age of patient
   c. Glucose blood level
   d. Hypoglycemia

   Rationale: The primary factor that distinguishes Type 1 diabetes from Type 2 diabetes is the absence of naturally occurring insulin within the body. Type 1 diabetics require insulin injections to survive. Type 2 diabetics may improve their health with insulin injections, and may even come to require insulin, but the administration of insulin has no bearing on code selection for Type 2 diabetes, nor does the age of onset.

9. What two types of glandular tissue is the endocrine system composed of?
   a. Epithelial
   b. Connective
   c. Muscle
   d. Exocrine and endocrine

   Rationale: The endocrine system is composed of hormone-secreting cells and two different types of glandular tissue: exocrine and endocrine.

10. What is the main cause of thiamine deficiency?
    a. Malabsorption
    b. Alcoholism
    c. Diabetes
    d. Hypothyroidism

    Rationale: Alcoholism is the main cause of thiamine (vitamin B1) deficiency in the United States.

Chapter 7. ICD-10-CM: Cardiovascular System

1. In addition to supplying oxygen and nutrients to the body and carrying away carbon dioxide and other waste products, the cardiovascular system is integral to:
    a. Stabilizing body temperature
    b. Maintaining pH balance
    c. Transporting hormones
    d. **All of the above**

   Rationale: The primary functions of the cardiovascular system are to transport oxygen, nutrients, and hormones to the cells of the body, as well as to remove waste products, including carbon dioxide and heat. The cardiovascular system is also instrumental in regulating the body's temperature, maintaining pH balance, and regulating the cells' water content. Protective white blood cells, antibodies, complement proteins, and clotting factors circulate in the cardiovascular system and are carried to the site of an injury to protect the body when needed.

2. The tricuspid valve is found:
    a. Between the atria of the heart
    b. **Between the right atrium and the right ventricle**
    c. Between the ventricles of the heart
    d. Between the left atrium and the left ventricle

   Rationale: Collectively, the bicuspid and the tricuspid valves are referred to as the atrioventricular (AV) valves. The tricuspid valve is found between the right atrium and the right ventricle, and the mitral valve is between the left atrium and the left ventricle.

3. The process whereby carbon dioxide is passed from the blood to the alveoli in the lungs to be exhaled and oxygen from the air is passed from the lungs into the blood is known as:
    a. **Alveolar capillary exchange**
    b. Homeostasis
    c. Reoxygenation
    d. Collateral circulation

   Rationale: The layers of cells that line the alveoli and the surrounding capillaries are very thin and in close proximity to each other. It is here that carbon dioxide is passed from the blood to the alveoli to be exhaled and oxygen from the air is passed from the lungs into the blood, a process known as alveolar capillary exchange.

4. Blood in the right ventricle is:
   a. **Picked up by the pulmonary circulation to be reoxygenated via the pulmonary trunk**
   b. Pumped into the systemic circulation
   c. Pumped to the aorta
   d. Collected in the vena cava

   Rationale: Blood that is deficient in oxygen and laden with carbon dioxide returns to the right atrium of the heart through the superior vena cava and the inferior vena cava. The blood then goes to the right ventricle, where it is picked up by the pulmonary circulation to be reoxygenated. Blood leaves the right ventricle via the pulmonary trunk, which splits into the right and left pulmonary arteries. These branches further divide, becoming successively smaller until they become pulmonary capillaries surrounding the alveoli in the lungs.

5. The microscopic arterioles function to control blood flow into the capillary networks. Changes at this level also affect blood pressure in the following way(s):
   a. Arteriole vasodilatation decreases blood pressure
   b. Arteriole vasoconstriction increases blood pressure
   c. **a and b**
   d. None of the above

   Rationale: Muscular (distributing) arteries are mid-size arteries that are branches of the elastic arteries. Varying in size from the pencil-sized axillary and femoral arteries to the small, string-size arteries that carry blood to organs, the thick walls of these arteries are able to regulate blood flow with vasoconstriction and vasodilatation. Some examples of muscular arteries include the brachial and radial arteries of the arm. Branching into increasingly smaller arteries, the muscular arteries eventually branch out into the microscopic arterioles that function to control blood flow into the capillary networks. Changes at this level can impact blood pressure, with arteriole vasodilatation decreasing blood pressure and arteriole vasoconstriction increasing blood pressure.

6. Blood is supplied to the brain by the:
   a. Subclavian artery
   b. Brachiocephalic branch
   c. Ascending aorta
   d. **Carotid and vertebral arteries**

   Rationale: The carotid and vertebral arteries supply oxygenated blood to the brain. The carotid arteries are easily palpated under the jaw: one on the left and one on the right. At the top of the neck, the carotids bifurcate into the external and internal carotid arteries. The external carotid arteries provide blood and nutrients to the face and scalp, while the internal carotid arteries supply the anterior three-fifths of the cerebrum, with the exception of parts of the temporal and occipital lobes. The vertebral arteries course along the spinal column, joining together to create the single basilar artery (vertebrobasilar arteries) near the brain stem at the skull base. These arteries nourish the posterior two-fifths of the cerebrum, part of the cerebellum, and the brain stem.

7. Rheumatic heart disease primarily affects which area(s) of the heart:
   a. Endocardium
   b. Coronary ostia
   c. Pulmonary vein
   d. **Valves**

   Rationale: Acute rheumatic fever, a complication of strep pharyngitis in children, results in a variety of cardiac conditions in more than a third of patients affected. Depending on the extent of heart inflammation involved, patients with the acute form of the disease may develop heart failure, pericarditis, myocarditis, and endocarditis, which is manifested as insufficiency of the mitral (65 to 70 percent of cases) and aortic valves (25 percent of cases). Chronic disease may result in arrhythmias, ventricular dysfunction, and dilation of the atria. In adults, it is the most common cause of mitral valve stenosis and the leading cause for valvular replacement surgery. Although the mitral valve is most commonly affected, the aortic and tricuspid valves may also be involved.

8. Arteriosclerosis, also referred to as "hardening of the arteries," occurs when the arteries become narrowed due to atherosclerosis, and then become hardened by fibrous tissue and calcification. This condition can affect:
   a. Heart only
   b. Brain only
   c. Extremities only
   d. Every system in the body

   Rationale: As arteriosclerosis continues, it results in a decrease in blood and oxygen supply to the affected organ. Eventually, the plaque may cause severe or complete obstruction of the artery, causing tissue necrosis. Although this process is often associated with the heart, it may occur in any of the organs, including the brain, kidneys, intestines, eyes, and limbs.

9. Other names for unstable angina include all of the following with the exception of:
   a. Acute coronary insufficiency
   b. Prinzmetal's variant angina
   c. Preinfarction angina
   d. Intermediate syndrome

   Rationale: Other names for unstable angina include acute coronary insufficiency, preinfarction angina, and intermediate syndrome. Prinzmetal's (variant) angina is a rare form caused by vasospasm.

10. Once plaque begins to build up in an artery of the leg, the following changes take place:
    a. The flow of blood and oxygen is reduced
    b. The walls of the artery become stiff
    c. Arterial walls become unable to dilate
    d. All of the above

    Rationale: The primary cause of arterial disease of the lower extremities is atherosclerosis. Once the plaque begins to build up in the artery, not only is blood flow reduced, but the arterial walls become stiffer and unable to dilate. This means the leg muscles don't receive adequate blood and oxygen when demand is increased, such as by walking and exercising.

11. Which of the following statements is false concerning aortic dissection?
    a. A dissecting aneurysm occurs when there is deterioration of the middle layer of the artery
    b. Hypertension increases and extends the damage to the damaged aorta
    c. Arteriosclerosis is not related to aortic dissection
    d. Surgery may or may not be required

    Rationale: A dissecting aneurysm occurs when the middle arterial layer (media) deteriorates (medial necrosis). Hypertension and arteriosclerosis play a role in this process, causing further damage until a rupture occurs in the innermost arterial layer, which allows blood to fill the wall of the aorta, causing separation of the layers. When the rupture extends through the outermost wall, fatal hemorrhage occurs. There are two types of aortic dissections. Type A dissection may be treated medically for a period of time with interventional catheterization or using open surgical techniques. Type B is treated medically with regular monitoring and medications that include antihypertensive and cholesterol lowering agents.

12. The single greatest risk factor for superficial venous thrombosis and DVT is:
    a. A past medical history of these conditions
    b. Varicose veins
    c. Stroke
    d. Pregnancy

    Rationale: Although the greatest single risk factor for superficial venous thrombosis and DVT is a past medical history, other risk factors include:
    - Aging
    - Abdominal cancer
    - Blood coagulation disorders
    - Extended bed rest or sitting (e.g., such as on an airplane)
    - Heart failure
    - Intravenous (IV) catheter usage/use of irritating medications in the IV
    - Oral contraceptives
    - Pregnancy
    - Stroke
    - Trauma
    - Varicose veins

13. The difference between the two pressures, the systolic and the diastolic, is referred to as:
    a. Perfusion gradient
    b. Pulse pressure
    c. Ventricular differential
    d. Stroke volume

    Rationale: Blood pressure measures the force exerted against the arterial walls produced by the left ventricle during contraction (systole), and pressure that remains in the arteries when the ventricle relaxes (diastole). Blood pressure readings are measured in millimeters of mercury (mmHg) and expressed as two numbers (e.g., 120/80). Either one or both of these numbers may be too high (hypertension). The difference between the two pressures, the systolic and the diastolic, is referred to as the pulse pressure.

14. Examining the dilated retina is integral to assessing damage sustained due to hypertension because it:
    a. Allows visualization of the inner arterial and venous systems (e.g., arteriole narrowing and vessel sclerosis)
    b. Indicates systemic disease prior to the onset of symptoms
    c. Can indicate malignant and accelerating hypertension
    d. All of the above

    Rationale: Examining the dilated retina is integral to assessing damage sustained due to hypertension. Examining the retinal microvascular allows a view of the inner arterial and venous systems and detects the onset of systemic diseases before symptoms becoming evident. Manifestations of arteriosclerosis include narrowing of the arterioles and sclerosis of the vessels. Cotton wool spots and flame-shaped hemorrhages are often found in hypertensive retinopathy. Edema of the disc indicates malignant hypertension. In many instances, the retinal examination provides the first clue the patient has hypertension. A diagnosis of malignant hypertension includes the presence of papilledema, with swelling of the optic disc in the eye, caused by an increase in intracranial pressure. On the other hand, accelerated hypertension is a recent major increase over the patient's baseline blood pressure, not associated with target organ damage. Fundoscopic examination often reveals flame-shaped hemorrhages or soft exudates, but without papilledema.

15. The precerebral arteries are designated as the:
    a. Left anterior descending, circumflex, and marginal branch
    b. Carotid, subclavian, and cerebral
    c. Basilar, carotid, and vertebral arteries
    d. Vertebral, mesenteric, anterior communicating

    Rationale: The precerebral arteries are designated as the basilar, carotid, and vertebral arteries. The internal-carotid and vertebral arteries converge at the circle of Willis. It is from the circle of Willis that other arteries—the anterior cerebral artery (ACA), the middle cerebral artery (MCA), and the posterior cerebral artery (PCA)—arise and travel to all parts of the brain. The mesenteric artery is in the abdomen, and the left anterior descending, circumflex, and marginal branch are all coronary arteries.

Chapter 8. ICD-10-CM: Blood and Blood-Forming Organs

1. What are the three main functions of blood?
   a. Transportation
   b. Regulation
   c. Protection

   Rationale: Blood serves many purposes that can be divided into three main functions: transportation, regulation, protection.

2. What are the formed elements found in blood?
   a. Red blood cells
   b. White blood cells
   c. Platelets

   Rationale: There are formed elements, consisting of red blood cells, white blood cells, and platelets, and plasma, in which the formed elements "float."

3. The plasma is the liquid that suspends the formed elements.

   Rationale: There are formed elements, consisting of red blood cells, white blood cells, and platelets, and plasma, in which the formed elements "float."

4. Erythrocytes are also known as red blood cells.

   Rationale: Red blood cells, or erythrocytes, make up more than 99 percent of the formed elements.

5. The red blood cells' main function is to carry oxygen to cells and transport some carbon dioxide away.

   Rationale: Red blood cells travel throughout the body delivering oxygen and removing some of the carbon dioxide the cells release.

6. Hemoglobin is the protein responsible for the red color of blood.

   Rationale: The protein molecules, known as **hemoglobin**, are responsible for the blood's color. When the RBCs are carrying oxygen, the blood appears bright red; when the hemoglobin is de-oxygenated, the blood appears blue when viewed through blood vessel walls.

7. What are the four blood types?
   a. A
   b. B
   c. AB
   d. O

   Rationale: The blood type group is determined by identifying up to two antigens on the surface of an erythrocyte. These antigens are known as antigen A and antigen B. The absence or presence of these determine the four blood types:
   - **A:** Antigen A is present.
   - **B:** Antigen B is present.
   - **AB:** Both antigens are present.
   - **O:** Neither antigen is present.

8. Rh-negative means there are negative antigens present on the surface of the red blood cell.

    a. True
    b. False

    Rationale: Also attached to erythrocytes, there are many types of Rh antigens and if any of these are present, the blood is considered Rh-positive. If none are present, Rh-negative.

9. The main function of leukocytes is to fight infection.

    Rationale: Unlike the red blood cells, there is more than one type of white blood cell, but they all share the same basic function, to fight infection.

10. Name the three types of granulocytes.

    a. Neutrophil
    b. Eosinophils
    c. Basophils

    Rationale: There are three types of granulocytes: neutrophils, eosinophils, and basophils.

11. Most lymphocytes are stored in the body's lymphoid tissue.

    Rationale: These types of cells can live for years in the body's lymphoid tissue (e.g., lymph nodes, spleen, etc.), hence the name lymphocyte.

12. Thrombocytes are also called platelets.

    Rationale: Platelets, also known as thrombocytes, are different from the other formed elements found in the blood in that they are not cells in the strict sense, since they lack a nucleus.

13. Plasma helps maintain the pH of the blood.

    a. True
    b. False

    Rationale: The constant adjusting of the different components of the plasma is what maintains an acceptable Ph of blood.

14. Name the three steps in hemostasis.

    a. Vessel spasm
    b. Platelet plug
    c. Coagulation

    Rationale: First, the vessel induces a local spasm of its smooth-muscle lining, constricting the flow of blood to the area to allow more time for the other two responses to occur. At this point, platelets flood the area and form a platelet plug, temporarily sealing it. To form the plug, the normally smooth platelet cells begin to swell and grow spike-like processes in order to stick to other platelets and the exposed collagen fibers of the endothelial lining of the vessel. The last step, referred to as coagulation, takes more than 30 substances, called factors, to complete.

15. Three examples of foods containing vitamin B12 are meat, poultry, and dairy.

    Rationale: Dietary B12 deficiency occurs most commonly in chronic alcoholics and elderly on a "tea and toast" diet; occasionally, this does impact people with strict vegan diets as the majority of dietary B12 comes from the ingestion of meat, poultry, and dairy products.

16. Sickle cell anemia occurs only in patients who also have thalassemia.
    a. True
    b. False

    Rationale: Sickle cell can occur with or without thalassemia, depending on the patient's genetics.

17. Other than acute and chronic, what are the two main types of leukemia?
    a. Lymphocytic
    b. Myeloid

    Rationale: Most leukemias can be classified as myeloid or lymphoid, depending on the malfunctioning stem cell producing the abnormal cells. Lymphocytic leukemia evolves from the lymphoid stem cells and myeloid leukemia the myeloid cells. These can be further divided into acute and chronic types—acute developing suddenly and chronic developing over a period of time.

18. The three phases of leukemia are active, in remission, and in relapse.

    Rationale: An important factor in choosing a code for any type of leukemia in either classification system is whether the cancer is active, in remission, or in relapse. The disease is considered active when it is first discovered and is current and causing signs and symptoms. Once treatment is rendered, usually in the form of chemotherapy or induction therapy, the abnormal blood cells disappear from the blood and the disease disappears. When this occurs, the patient is considered in remission. Relapse occurs when the disease returns after the patient has achieved remission. A patient can relapse multiple times.

Chapter 9. ICD-10-CM: Lymphatic System

1. What lymphatic structure is bean-shaped and encapsulated?
   a. Lymphatic nodules
   b. Spleen
   c. Adenoids
   d. **Lymph nodes**

   Rationale: Lymph nodes are encapsulated, unlike lymphatic nodules. In addition, lymph nodes are bean-shaped, and lymphatic nodules do not have a singular shape.

2. What is the name of the fluid that flows through the lymphatic system?
   a. Interstitial fluid
   b. **Lymph**
   c. B-cells
   d. Microphages

   Rationale: Interstitial fluid enters the lymphatic vessel and becomes lymph. Lymph is the name for the fluid that flows through the lymph vessels and nodes.

3. What is the main purpose of the lymphatic system?
   a. Move fluid though the blood vessels
   b. **Provide immunity to foreign substances**
   c. Aid in development of leukocytes
   d. Provide nourishment to the spleen

   Rationale: The main purpose of the lymphatic system is to provide immunity to foreign substances. Although interstitial fluid enters the lymphatic system, it flows through the lymphatic vessels, not blood vessels. The lymphatic system includes the spleen, whose main purpose is to aid in immunity.

4. Where is interstitial fluid found?
   a. **In the tissues at the cell level**
   b. In the lymphatic trunk
   c. In the thymus vessels
   d. In lymph nodules

   Rationale: Interstitial fluid is found within the tissues at the cell level, and the lymphatic capillaries collect interstitial fluid from the tissues via a one-way structure.

5. What tissues do not contain lymphatic vessels?
   a. Cardiac
   b. **Avascular**
   c. Thymus
   d. Gastrointestinal

   Rationale: Avascular tissues do not have lymphatic vessels. These include cartilage, epidermis, and corneal tissue.

6. What role does the thymus play in immune response?
   a. **T-cells mature within the thymus**
   b. B-cells mature within the thymus
   c. Provides nutrients for the lymph nodes
   d. Both a and b

   Rationale: B-cells are not located in the thymus. T-cells mature in the thymus and learn to identify foreign matter before moving as mature T-cells into the lymph nodes, spleen, and lymphatic tissue.

7. Lymph nodes are found along the lymphatic vessels and may be solitary or in groups.
   a. **True**
   b. False

   Rationale: Lymph nodes are located along the lymphatic vessels and although they may be solitary, they are often grouped together or fairly close together.

8. What are the main categories of lymphatic cancer?
   a. **Hodgkin's lymphoma and all other lymphomas**
   b. Non-Hodgkin's lymphoma and Hodgkin's lymphoma
   c. Hodgkin's lymphoma and sarcoidosis
   d. All lymphomas are terminal

   Rationale: Lymphatic cancer is categorized as Hodgkin's lymphoma and all other lymphomas. Reticulosarcoma, lymphosarcoma, Burkitt's tumor, marginal zone lymphoma, mantle cell, large cell lymphoma, primary central nervous system, anaplastic large cell, and other variants of lymphoma are all included in the other lymphomas category.

9. What is the primary function of microphages?
   a. Ingest and destroy foreign matter
   b. Destroy immune cells
   c. Ingest and destroy dead tissue and cells
   d. **Both a and c**

   Rationale: Microphages are small phagocytes that ingest foreign matter and other small things like dead tissue and cells.

10. What organ contains red and white pulp?
    a. Adenoids
    b. Thymus
    c. **Spleen**
    d. Peyer's patches

    Rationale: The spleen contains red and white pulp. The red pulp consists of splenic cords or tissue that contains microphages, lymphocytes, red blood cells, plasma cells, and granulocytes. The white pulp contains lymphatic tissue with lymphocytes and microphages.

11. What is hyposplenism?
    a. A reduction in the size of the spleen
    b. **A reduction in spleen function**
    c. An increase in spleen function
    d. An increase in the size of the spleen

    Rationale: "Hypo" is the root word meaning low or deficient. In this case, hyposplenism describes a reduction in spleen function.

12. Localized enlarged lymph nodes typically involve 1 area(s) of the body, whereas generalized enlarged lymph nodes typically involve 2 or more area(s) of the body.

    Rationale: Although not official guidelines, these are the common guidelines followed when assigning localized versus generalized lymphadenopathy codes.

13. What additional information do coders need to report infectious mononucleosis in ICD-10-CM?

    a. Type of virus, such as gammaherpesviral mononucleosis or cytomegaloviral mononucleosis
    b. Whether the patient incurred complications
    c. Both a and b
    d. None of the above

    Rationale: In ICD-10-CM, the type of virus and whether the patient incurred complications are both important factors when coding infectious mononucleosis.

14. Match the types of follicular lymphoma grades with the types of cells involved:

    a. Grade I   d   Centrocytes are still present
    b. Grade II   a   < 5 centroblasts per high power field
    c. Grade III   c   > 15 centroblasts per high power field
    d. Grade IIIa   e   Follicles consist almost entirely of centroblasts
    e. Grade IIIb   b   6–15 centroblasts per high power field

    Rationale: Although there is some controversy over the grading system, the World Health Organization recommends the following:

    - Grade I: < 5 centroblasts per high power field
    - Grade II: 6–15 centroblasts per high power field
    - Grade III: > 15 centroblasts per high power field
        - grade IIIa: centrocytes are still present
        - grade IIIb: follicles consist almost entirely of centroblasts

15. Immune reconstitution syndrome is limited to HIV-positive patients.

    a. True
    b. False

    Rationale: Immune reconstitution syndrome can affect any patient who has been immunocompromised.

Chapter 10. ICD-10-CM: Respiratory System

1. What is the function of cilia?
   a. They prompt the sneezing reaction
   b. They have no known function
   c. **They trap particles entering with air and prevent them from entering further into the respiratory system**
   d. They are the first step in the body's immune response system

   Rationale: Within the nose there are hairs, or cilia, that catch germs and other particles inhaled with air. However, cilia do not catch all germs, which is why infections can occur within the bronchial tubes and lungs.

2. Which structure is included in the upper respiratory tract?
   a. Diaphragm
   b. Alveoli
   c. **Pharynx**
   d. Lung

   Rationale: The upper respiratory tract contains the nose, pharynx, and larynx. The lower respiratory tract contains the trachea, bronchial tree, and the lungs.

3. What is the primary function that occurs within the lungs?
   a. **Oxygen and carbon dioxide exchange**
   b. Fluid waste expulsion
   c. Involuntary muscle contraction
   d. Absorption of dust particles

   Rationale: The air moves into the lungs and bronchial tubes, reaching the alveoli, which transport the oxygen to the capillaries where hemoglobin helps it flow into the bloodstream. As the oxygen is absorbed, the carbon dioxide is also extracted from the capillaries into the alveoli to be exhaled as a waste gas. Gas exchange that takes place within the lungs is referred to as external respiration, and exchange taking place within body tissues is referred to as internal respiration.

4. The trachea is commonly referred to as:
   a. Larynx
   b. Pharynx
   c. Esophagus
   d. **Windpipe**

   Rationale: The trachea, or windpipe, begins at the larynx and splits into two bronchi branches within the chest: the left and right primary bronchi. The trachea is 12 centimeters in length and 2½ centimeters wide and is made up of C-shaped rings of cartilage within the smooth muscle.

Comprehensive Anatomy and Physiology for ICD-10-CM and ICD-10-PCS Coding

5. How many bronchial tubes branch off into the lungs?
   a. One
   b. Two
   c. Three
   d. Four

   Rationale: The bronchial tubes are part of the respiratory structure connecting the lungs to the trachea, allowing for air exchange within the lungs. The trachea, or windpipe, begins at the larynx and splits into two bronchi branches within the chest: the left and right primary bronchi. The right bronchus enters the right lung and is shorter and wider than the left. The left bronchus enters the left lung. Once the bronchi enter the lungs, they split into secondary bronchi, one for each lobe within the lung.

6. Where is the carina located?
   a. In the lungs
   b. In the sinuses
   c. In the diaphragm
   d. In the trachea

   Rationale: The carina is the area where the division in the trachea leads to the right and left bronchi and is made up of the last of the tracheal cartilage. The membrane in this area is the most sensitive to foreign matter and primarily responsible for the reflex to expel any irritants.

7. How many lobes are in the left lung?
   a. Two
   b. Three
   c. One
   d. Five

   Rationale: The left lung contains two lobes while the right lung contains three. This is due to the placement of the heart within the thoracic cavity, leaving the left lung somewhat smaller than the right lung. The right lung is thicker and wider than the left lung, but it is shorter than the left since the diaphragm is slightly higher on the right side due to the position of the liver.

8. What is aspergillosis?
   a. A virus
   b. An injury
   c. A genetic disorder
   d. A fungal infection

   Rationale: Aspergillosis is a fungal infection that typically does not affect people with a normal immune system. The fungus grows in stored grain, compost, and other vegetation during the decay process. This condition presents as pneumonia or a fungal growth where there was a previous lung disorder such as tuberculosis or a lung abscess.

Appendix A. **Knowledge Assessment Answers**

9. What physiological changes occur in emphysema?
   a. Deterioration of the bronchioles
   b. A pH imbalance
   c. Fluid accumulation within the lungs
   d. None of the above

   Rationale: Emphysema is considered a factor in chronic obstructive pulmonary disease (COPD). This condition restricts the air flow during exhalation because of gradual deterioration of the bronchioles. This air restriction causes difficulty in breathing. As this condition progresses, the spherical air sacs within the lungs become irregular and contain holes, reducing not only the number of air sacs but also the amount of oxygen that can circulate into the blood from the lungs. As the air sacs deteriorate, the openings collapse, trapping air within the lungs.

10. What structures are responsible for speech?
    a. Vocal cords
    b. Pharynx
    c. Sinuses
    d. All of the above

    Rationale: Ligaments within the vocal cords stretch into the airway, which constricts the glottis. When air hits this area, vibrations produce sound. To create understandable speech, the pharynx, mouth, nasal cavity, and sinuses provide a type of echo chamber.

11. Which body part houses the adenoids?
    a. Sinuses
    b. Nasopharynx
    c. Oropharynx
    d. Mouth

    Rationale: The back wall of the nasopharynx is where the adenoids are positioned. The oropharynx is the middle portion of the pharynx at the back of the mouth, starting at the soft palate and running to the hyoid bone. The palatine and lingual tonsils are within the oropharynx.

12. What is the common name of the disease caused by the *Bordetella pertussis* bacteria?
    a. Strep throat
    b. Asthma
    c. Ascariasis
    d. Whooping cough

    Rationale: Whooping cough is a common symptom/condition associated with pneumonia called pertussis, named after the bacterium *Bordetella pertussis* that is the cause. Before widespread vaccination for these bacteria began in the 1940s, whooping cough killed 5,000 to 10,000 people in the United States every year. With vaccination, that number has dropped to fewer than 30 per year. Parapertussis is similar to whooping cough in etiology and symptoms and can occur at any age, although it typically affects children ages 3 to 5 years. Parapertussis occurs less frequently than pertussis and has a shorter duration as well. Vaccination against whooping cough does not provide immunity to parapertussis, and most people recover completely. Complications due to this infection are extremely rare.

13. What is the cure for pneumoconiosis?
    a. Removal of irritant causing the symptoms
    b. Antibiotics
    c. **There is no cure**
    d. Rest and plenty of fluids

    Rationale: Pneumoconiosis is due to the inhalation of dust particles typically associated with occupations that require regular exposure to mineral dusts. This condition is a form of interstitial lung disease that contributes to the inflammation of the air sacs, causing the lung tissue to harden. There is no cure for this disease, and treatment focuses on managing the patient's symptoms.

14. What is one of the major complications of a pulmonary contusion?
    a. There are none, a contusion is a superficial injury
    b. **Fluid accumulation within the alveoli**
    c. High mortality rate
    d. A life-long, chronic lung condition

    Rationale: A contusion is a superficial injury, often a bruise, resulting from trauma without a break in the skin. However, even this kind of injury can have serious complications when the contusion affects the respiratory system, particularly the lungs. A pulmonary contusion affects the lung tissue itself, leading to fluid and blood accumulation within the alveoli of the lung. About 20 percent of blunt chest injury cases also report pulmonary contusions. In some cases, crackling noises can be heard in the chest through a stethoscope. If the contusion is left undiagnosed, complications such as atelectasis, pneumonia, and respiratory failure may occur. Once diagnosed, most lung contusions resolve in less than a week with fluid restriction and careful observation. Larger contusions may require more extensive treatment like oxygen or mechanical ventilation.

15. How can a physician differentiate a pleural friction rub from a pericardial rub?
    a. By a chest x-ray
    b. Grating sounds within the chest
    c. **Absence of irregular sounds when the patient holds his or her breath**
    d. Indicated by whether or not patient has chest pain

    Rationale: Pleural friction rub causes low, grating sounds heard when pleural surfaces rub against each other. This may be confused with a pericardial rub, so cessation of the sound when the patient holds his or her breath would indicate pleural friction rub. When the lungs are affected by SLE, symptoms include chest pain when breathing deeply, coughing up blood, and shortness of breath. A physician may hear a pleural friction rub when the patient is examined, and a chest x-ray may show pleuritis or pleurisy.

Chapter 11. ICD-10-CM: Digestive System

1. The digestive system consists *only* of the mouth, pharynx, esophagus, small intestine, large intestine, and anus.
   a. True
   b. **False**

   Rationale: The digestive system consists of an alimentary canal and several accessory organs.

2. What are some examples of the digestive system accessory organs?
   a. **Pancreas, liver, gallbladder**
   b. Spleen, tonsils, lymph nodes
   c. Esophagus, stomach, large intestine
   d. All of the above

   Rationale: The accessory organs of the digestive system include teeth, tongue, salivary glands, liver, gallbladder, and pancreas.

3. What are the wave-like movements of a tubular structure, where alternate contraction and relaxation occurs and the contents of the tube are propelled forward, an example of?
   a. Rhythm method
   b. **Peristalsis**
   c. Wave current
   d. Body wave locomotion

   Rationale: Peristalsis is the movement of a tubular structure, characterized by waves of alternate circular contraction and relaxation of the tube by which contents are propelled forward.

4. The secretion of pancreatic juices aid the digestive process by breaking down which substances?
   a. Carbohydrates
   b. Proteins and Fats
   c. Nucleic Acids
   d. **All of the above**

   Rationale: The pancreas plays an important part in digestion by secreting pancreatic juice. Pancreatic juice contains enzymes that digest carbohydrates, fats, proteins, and nucleic acids.

5. The cause of edentulism is no longer significant when selecting the appropriate code in ICD-10-CM.
   a. True
   b. **False**

   Rationale: Coders still need to identify the cause of edentulism when selecting codes in ICD-10-CM.

Comprehensive Anatomy and Physiology for ICD-10-CM and ICD-10-PCS Coding

6. What additional details need to be documented to accurately code sialoadenitis?
   a. The presence of any obstructions
   b. Any additional complications
   c. **Whether the disease is acute, chronic, or recurrent**
   d. None of the above

   Rationale: To code this disease accurately in ICD-10-CM, coders need to know if the disease is acute, acute recurrent, chronic, or unspecified.

7. What condition is now included in codes for alcoholic hepatitis and cirrhosis of the liver?
   a. Abscess
   b. AIDS
   c. **Ascites**
   d. Aggression

   Rationale: In ICD-10-CM, coding for alcoholic hepatitis and cirrhosis has been further specified as occurring with or without ascites.

8. Peliosis hepatitis is one of the several conditions that were included in the code for unspecified hepatitis in ICD-9-CM, but will now have its own code in ICD-10-CM.
   a. True
   b. **False**

   Rationale: Conditions such as toxic liver disease, nonalcoholic steatohepatitis, and peliosis hepatitis have been expanded in ICD-10-CM to have their own code.

9. What are some of the causal conditions of acute/chronic pancreatitis that are now important to know when coding pancreatitis?
   a. **Drug/alcohol-induced pancreatitis**
   b. Iron deficiency pancreatitis
   c. Dysplastic pancreatitis
   d. None of the above

   Rationale: Some of the causal conditions of pancreatitis that are included in the codes for the disease in ICD-10-CM are cytolomegaloviral pancreatitis, idiopathic pancreatitis, biliary pancreatitis, alcohol-induced pancreatitis, and drug-induced pancreatitis.

10. What is the major physiological difference between coding for Barrett's esophagus in ICD-9-CM as opposed to ICD-10-CM?
    a. **Coders need to determine if dysplasia is present and identify the grade**
    b. Coders need to identify the root cause of the condition
    c. Coders need to identify if esophagitis is present
    d. All of the above

    Rationale: In addition to coding the Barrett's esophagus, coders now have to look for details on the presence of dysplasia and understand how the grades of dysplasia will be documented.

11. What clinical concept from ICD-9-CM will no longer be required in ICD-10-CM for proper code selection of the various types of gastric ulcers?
    a. With or without hemorrhage
    b. **With or without obstruction**
    c. With or without perforation
    d. All of the above

    Rationale: Coders no longer need to identify whether an obstruction is present. The only two complications of ulcers included in the code descriptions for ICD-10-CM are hemorrhage and perforation.

12. What new clinical concepts must be considered when coding in ICD-10-CM for diverticular disease?
    a. **With or without abscess/perforation**
    b. With or without hemorrhage
    c. With or without obstruction
    d. All of the above

    Rationale: When coding for diverticular disease in ICD-10-CM, coders need also to look for documentation on whether there is a perforation or abscess. In ICD-9-CM, the only distinguishing factor is whether a hemorrhage is present.

13. What complications of Crohn's disease are identified by the sixth character of the codes?
    a. Rectal bleeding
    b. Intestinal obstruction
    c. Fistula or abscess
    d. **All of the above**

    Rationale: Coding for Crohn's disease and its complications in ICD-10-CM depends on selecting the appropriate fifth and sixth characters. The fifth character Ø (zero) indicates that there are no complications. The fifth character 1 indicates that there are complications—coders need to identify the complications such as rectal bleeding, intestinal obstructions, fistulas, or abscess.

14. The ICD-9-CM code category regional enteritis has been renamed Crohn's disease in ICD-10-CM.
    a. **True**
    b. False

    Rationale: ICD-9-CM category 555 Regional enteritis currently maps to ICD-10-CM category K5Ø Crohn's disease.

15. Why is it important that coders pay close attention to the specific location of the stomal malfunction/complication in ICD-10-CM?
    a. Complications occur only in certain parts of the intestine
    b. The specific part of the intestine determines which codes to use
    c. Colostomy and enterostomy complications are no longer included in the same code category
    d. **Both b and c**

    Rationale: In ICD-9-CM, colostomy and enterostomy complications are grouped together under category 569.6. In ICD-10-CM, these have been split into two separate categories. Coders need to pay close attention to the specific part of the intestine experiencing the complication to determine if it is a colostomy or enterostomy complication.

16. What is an inflammation of the meninges due to *Salmonella typhi* or associated with typhoid fever?

    a. Typhoid pneumonia

    b. Typhoid arthritis

    c. Typhoid osteomyelitis

    d. Typhoid meningitis

    Rationale: Meningitis is an inflammation of the meninges. Inflammation documented as being due to *Salmonella typhi* or with typhoid fever is considered typhoid meningitis.

17. Intestinal trichomoniasis is classified as a protozoal intestinal disease in ICD-10-CM.

    a. True

    b. False

    Rationale: In ICD-10-CM, the condition intestinal trichomoniasis is classified as a protozoal intestinal disease along with other protozoal intestinal diseases like microsporidiosis, sarcocystosis, and sarcosporidiosis.

Chapter 12. ICD-10-CM: Urinary System

1. Name the six organs of the urinary system.
    a. Two kidneys, two ureters, one bladder, and one urethra
    b. Two kidneys, two ureters, and two sphincter muscles
    c. Two kidneys, two sphincter muscles, and two urethras
    d. Two kidneys, two ureters, and two urethras

    Rationale: The urinary system is a collection of various organs, tubes, muscles, and nerves whose function is to create, store, and transport urine out of the body. It comprises two kidneys, two ureters, the bladder, two sphincter muscles, and the urethra.

2. What is the primary function of the urinary system?
    a. Create, store, and transport urine
    b. Promote absorption of nutrients
    c. Regulate blood volume and pH
    d. Excrete hormones

    Rationale: The urinary system, in conjunction with the lungs, skin, and intestines, excretes waste and keeps chemicals and water in the body in balance. Specifically, the urinary system removes urea from the blood. Urea is generated when foods containing proteins (meat, poultry, some vegetables) break down in the body.

3. Approximately how many nephrons does each kidney have?
    a. 100,000
    b. 500,000
    c. 1,000,000
    d. More than 1,000,000

    Rationale: Blood comes into the kidneys by way of arteries that branch within the kidneys into small clusters of looping blood vessels. These clusters are called glomeruli, the tiny units in the kidney where blood is cleaned. Approximately 1 million glomeruli (filters) are in each kidney.

4. What is the functional unit of the kidney?
    a. Medulla
    b. Calices
    c. Nephron
    d. Glomerulus

    Rationale: Every glomerulus and tubule unit combined is called a nephron, or the functional unit of the kidneys.

5. The kidneys:
    a. Help regulate blood volume
    b. Help control blood pressure
    c. Help control pH
    d. All of the above

    Rationale: The kidneys perform other necessary functions, including regulating blood ionic composition, blood pH, blood pressure, and blood glucose level, and aiding in the production of three important hormones (erythropoietin [EPO], renin, and calcitriol).

6. What organ in the urinary system is the reservoir for urine?
   a. Kidneys
   b. **Bladder**
   c. Renal pelvis
   d. Ureters

   Rationale: The urinary bladder is a triangular or pear-shaped, expandable hollow organ located in the pelvic area, held in place by ligaments that bind to the pelvic bones. It is the organ in the urinary system that stores urine and allows urination to be infrequent and voluntary. The urinary bladder muscles relax in order to allow urine to enter from the ureters and contract to excrete urine from the body by way of the urethra. Layers of muscle tissue stretch to house urine with a capacity of 400 to 600 mL being considered normal.

7. What drains urine from the kidneys to the ureters?
   a. Sphincter muscles
   b. Nephrons
   c. Urethra
   d. **Renal pelvis**

   Rationale: Once the urine is formed, it passes through the nephrons and down the renal tubules of the kidney and is subsequently funneled from the renal pelvis, the area at the center of the kidney, into the ureters, which then transport the urine to the bladder.

8. The ureters are tube-shaped structures about _____ to _____ long and connect the kidneys to the bladder.
   a. 24–30 inches
   b. 10–20 inches
   c. 15–24 inches
   d. **8–10 inches**

   Rationale: The ureters are tube-shaped structures approximately 8 to 10 inches long that connect the kidney to the urinary bladder.

9. What is the capacity of an adult bladder?
   a. **400–500 mL**
   b. 100–300 mL
   c. 700–900 mL
   d. Greater than 1,000 mL

   Rationale: In the average healthy adult, approximately two cups, or 400 to 500 mL, of urine can be stored in the bladder for approximately two to five hours.

10. All of the following belong in the urinary system, except:
    a. Bladder
    b. **Prostate**
    c. Ureters
    d. Urethra

    Rationale: The urinary system comprises two kidneys, two ureters, the bladder, two sphincter muscles, and the urethra.

Chapter 13. ICD-10-CM: Reproductive Systems

Male Reproductive System

1. Which organs make up the external male reproductive system?
    a. Penis, prostate, and scrotum
    b. Penis, scrotum, and testicles
    c. Penis, testicles, and vas deferens
    d. Penis, seminal vesicles, and scrotum

    Rationale: Three primary organs make up the external male reproductive system: the penis, scrotum, and testicles (testes).

2. Which is not considered an internal accessory organ of the male reproductive system?
    a. Bulbourethral gland
    b. Ejaculatory duct
    c. Epididymis
    d. Testicle

    Rationale: The male reproductive system consists of internal organs, also referred to as accessory organs, that include the epididymis, vas deferens, ejaculatory ducts, urethra, seminal vesicles, prostate gland, and the bulbourethral glands.

3. What are the three hormones primarily involved in the regulation of the male reproductive system?
    a. FSH, LH, and testosterone
    b. FSH, TSH, and LH
    c. TSH, LH, and testosterone
    d. ADH, LH, and testosterone

    Rationale: Hormones primarily involved in the regulation of the male reproductive system include follicle-stimulating hormone (FSH), luteinizing hormone (LH), and testosterone.

4. How many ejaculatory ducts are in the male reproductive system?
    a. Four
    b. Three
    c. Two
    d. One

    Rationale: There are two ejaculatory ducts, approximately 2 cm in length, formed by the fusing of the vas deferens and the seminal vesicles. The ducts begin at the base of the prostate, running both forward and downward between the middle and lateral lobes, as well as along the sides of the prostatic utricle and ending just within the utricle margins, diminishing in size as they do so.

5. What is phimosis?
    a. Abnormal enlargement of the scrotal veins
    b. Constriction or tightening of the prepuce or foreskin
    c. Urological emergency requiring immediate treatment
    d. Condition that describes a total absence of sperm in the ejaculate fluid

    Rationale: Phimosis is a constriction, or tightening, of the prepuce (foreskin). In this condition, the foreskin contracts and is not able to be retracted or pulled back behind the glans or tip of the penis.

6. What organ in the male reproductive system controls the temperature of the testes to ensure normal sperm development?
   a. Epididymis
   b. Vas deferens
   c. **Scrotum**
   d. Bulbourethral gland

   Rationale: The main function of the scrotum is to control the temperature of the testes to that of slightly lower-than-normal body temperature in order to ensure healthy sperm development. The scrotum wall contains special muscles that contract and relax, thereby allowing the testicles to move closer to the body as necessary for warmth or further away in order to cool the temperature back down.

7. What organ has the task of ejaculating semen upon orgasm?
   a. Ejaculatory duct
   b. Prostate
   c. Seminal vesicle
   d. **Urethra**

   Rationale: As discussed in the urinary chapter, the tube that carries urine from the bladder is called the urethra. In males, the urethra has the additional responsibility of ejaculating semen upon orgasm. During intercourse, the penis is erect and the flow of urine is blocked from the urethra, thereby permitting only the release of semen upon orgasm.

8. Which organ is described as small, pea-sized, and yellow in color?
   a. **Bulbourethral gland**
   b. Seminal vesicle
   c. Vas deferens
   d. Epididymis

   Rationale: Bulbourethral glands, also known as Cowper's glands, are small, pea-sized, yellowish colored, lobular-like bodies located behind and to the sides of the urethra, below the prostate gland.

9. What condition describes a burning or aching type of pain coming from the area of the prostate?
   a. Prostatosis syndrome
   b. Proctalgia
   c. Oligospermia
   d. **Prostatodynia syndrome**

   Rationale: Prostatodynia syndrome describes a deep burning or aching type of pain that appears to originate from the prostate.

10. Which organ makes testosterone and generates sperm?
    a. **Testes**
    b. Prostate
    c. Scrotum
    d. Vas deferens

    Rationale: The last of the external male sex organs are the testicles (testes), which make the primary male sex hormone, testosterone, and generate sperm. Most men have two testes. The testicles are oval in shape and approximately the size of large olives, protected at either end by the spermatic cord.

Female Reproductive System

1. Which organs make up the external female reproductive system?
    a. Labia majora, labia minora, vagina, and clitoris
    b. **Labia majora, labia minor, clitoris, and Bartholin's glands**
    c. Bartholin's glands, clitoris, vagina, and uterus
    d. Vagina, clitoris, ovaries, and labia majora

    Rationale: The female reproductive system comprises external and internal structures. External structures include the labia majora, labia minora, Bartholin's glands, and the clitoris. These organs allow sperm to enter the body, as well as to safeguard the internal genital organs from infection.

2. Which is not an internal organ of the female reproductive system?
    a. Vagina
    b. Ovaries
    c. Fallopian tubes
    d. **Bartholin's glands**

    Rationale: The internal female reproductive organs include the vagina, uterus, ovaries, and fallopian tubes.

3. What are the four hormones involved in the regulation of the female reproductive system?
    a. **FSH, LH, estrogen, and progesterone**
    b. FSH, TSH, LH, and estrogen
    c. TSH, LH, estrogen, and progesterone
    d. TSH, LDH, testosterone, and progesterone

    Rationale: During the follicular phase, two of the four major hormones involved in the menstrual cycle are released, follicle stimulating hormone (FSH) and luteinizing hormone (LH). These two hormones activate the production of estrogen, a third hormone involved in the menstrual cycle. In the third phase of the cycle, after release of the egg, the corpus luteum emits the hormones estrogen and progesterone. As the fourth hormone in the menstrual cycle, progesterone prepares the uterus for the possibility of receiving a fertilized egg to implant. Progesterone and estrogen stimulate the endometrium (lining of the uterus) to thicken, filling it with fluids and nutrients necessary to nourish the fetus.

4. How many lobes are in each female breast?
    a. 5–10
    b. 10–15
    c. **15–20**
    d. Greater than 20

    Rationale: Approximately 15 to 20 lobes are in each breast, emanating from the nipple and areolar area, that appear to be arranged in a wheel-spoke pattern.

5. What is dysplasia?
    a. Twisting of ovarian artery and vein
    b. **Abnormal changes in cells**
    c. A gynecological emergency requiring immediate treatment
    d. Bleeding into the fallopian tubes

    Rationale: Dysplasia describes abnormal changes in the cells found on the surface of the vagina. It is categorized by three stages: mild, moderate, and severe.

6. What organ in the female reproductive system is also referred to as the birth canal?
    a. Uterus
    b. Ovary
    c. Vagina
    d. Cervix

    Rationale: The vagina, often referred to as the birth canal, is a passageway that adjoins the lower part of the uterus, called the cervix, to the outside of the body.

7. Which disorder is considered the fifth most common gynecological emergency condition?
    a. Torsion of the fallopian tube
    b. Moderate dysplasia
    c. Vulvovaginitis
    d. Torsion of the ovary

    Rationale: As the fifth most common gynecologic emergency, torsion, or twisting of the ovary, affects females of all age ranges.

8. Which organ is described as pear-shaped and hollow?
    a. Uterus
    b. Fallopian tube
    c. Vagina
    d. Bartholin's glands

    Rationale: The hollow, pear-shaped organ, which houses the fetus during development, is called the uterus. It has two parts: the cervix or lower portion, and the corpus or main body. Naturally, the corpus is designed to expand to accommodate a developing baby. The cervix contains a channel that permits sperm to enter and menstrual blood to exit when fertilization does not occur.

9. What common condition affecting the female reproductive system causes swelling, itching, and burning in the vagina, as well as an abnormal discharge from bacteria related to a variety of different kinds of germs?
    a. Dysplasia
    b. Acquired atrophy
    c. Acute salpingitis
    d. Vaginitis

    Rationale: Vaginitis is a condition that encompasses symptoms such as swelling, itching, and burning in the vagina, often accompanied by an abnormal discharge that can be caused by several different kinds of germs.

10. Name the phases of the menstrual cycle.
    a. Follicular, ovulation, and luteal
    b. Follicular, luteal, and pregnancy
    c. Ovulation, luteal, and menstruation
    d. Follicular, ovulation, and menstruation

    Rationale: The menstrual cycle is the process by which a woman's body prepares for the possibility of pregnancy. The term "menstru" means monthly; hence the word menstruation describes the monthly shedding of the uterine lining. On average, a menstrual cycle is 28 days long and takes place in three phases: follicular phase, ovulation, and the luteal phase.

Pregnancy, Childbirth, and the Puerperium

1. What does the seventh character for multiple gestations indicate?
    a. The specific fetal anomaly affecting the fetus
    b. **The identity of the affected fetus**
    c. The episode of care
    d. None of the above

    Rationale: A seventh-character extension for multiple gestations in categories that designate maternal care for a fetal anomaly, damage, or other problem is required in order to indicate the affected fetus.

2. What is afibrinogenemia?
    a. A type of spontaneous abortion
    b. A protein required to stop bleeding
    c. An abnormal attachment by the placenta to the uterine wall
    d. **A rare, inherited blood disorder**

    Rationale: Afibrinogenemia is an uncommon, inherited blood disorder that affects the blood's ability to clot by causing a serious deficiency in fibrinogen, a protein produced by the liver. This protein is required to stop bleeding by forming clots.

3. What degree of blood loss is considered a severe postpartum hemorrhage?
    a. **1,000 ml**
    b. 500 ml
    c. 1,500 ml
    d. Between 500 and 1,000 ml

    Rationale: A postpartum hemorrhage is defined as a blood loss of greater than 500 ml after the birth of a baby, and a severe postpartum hemorrhage constitutes blood loss of more than 1,000 ml after delivery.

4. What is the third stage of labor?
    a. The period of time just before delivery
    b. The period of time immediately following delivery
    c. **The period of time between the birth and expulsion of the placenta**
    d. The period of time after expulsion of the placenta

    Rationale: The third stage of labor is the period of time between the birth of the baby and the expulsion of the placenta. It is during this time frame when the uterine muscles contract downward and the placenta begins to separate from the uterine walls.

5. What condition is defined as the premature removal of the products of conception from the uterus?
    a. Placenta increta
    b. **Spontaneous abortion**
    c. Placenta percreta
    d. Legally induced abortion

    Rationale: A spontaneous abortion is defined as the premature expulsion or removal of the products of conception from the uterus.

6. What is disseminated intravascular coagulation (DIC)?
   a. A type of gestational diabetes
   b. A postpartum hemorrhage
   c. **A serious disorder where proteins that control blood clotting become abnormally active**
   d. An uncommon, inherited blood disorder that affects the blood's ability to clot by causing a serious deficiency in fibrinogen, a protein produced by the liver

   Rationale: Disseminated intravascular coagulation (DIC) is a serious disorder in which the proteins that control blood clotting become abnormally active.

7. What condition is defined as the intentional expulsion of the products of conception by a medical professional?
   a. Spontaneous abortion
   b. Placenta percreta
   c. Afibrinogenemia
   d. **Legally induced abortion**

   Rationale: A legally induced abortion is the intentional expulsion of the products of conception from the uterus performed by a medical professional within the boundaries of the law. This often occurs by the patient's choice (elective), through a court order or other mandated action (legal), or for reasons such as the mother's health or life is at risk (therapeutic).

8. What are the three subclassifications under gestational diabetes?
   a. **Diet controlled, insulin controlled, and unspecified**
   b. Pregnancy, childbirth, and the puerperium
   c. First, second, and third trimester
   d. Antepartum, delivered, and postpartum

   Rationale: Codes classified to category O24.4 Gestational diabetes mellitus, have three subcategories: O24.41 Gestational diabetes in pregnancy, O24.42 Gestational diabetes in childbirth, and O24.43 Gestational diabetes in the puerperium. Under each subcategory, there are three subclassifications denoted by characters 0, 4, or 9, indicating whether the gestational diabetes is diet controlled, insulin controlled, or unspecified, respectively.

Chapter 14. ICD-10-PCS Introduction

1. There are 31 body systems in the medical/surgical section (Ø).

2. When coding an amputation, the appropriate root operation value is detachment and is only offered in which two body systems?
   a. Upper and lower bones
   b. Subcutaneous tissue and fascia
   c. Anatomical regions, lower extremities
   d. Anatomical regions, upper extremities

   Rationale: Detachment is the correct root operation for amputation. See the alphabetical index or Appendix D: Optum360's Root Operation Conversion Table. Detachment is only contained in the anatomical upper and lower extremity body systems because these systems encompass into one code all of the layers of the other various body systems (e.g., skin, subcutaneous and fascia, vessels, nerves, and muscle).

3. Label the following arteries as located in the upper or lower artery body system.
   a. Innominate artery Upper
   b. Superior mesenteric artery Lower
   c. Subclavian artery, left Upper
   d. Colic artery, right Lower

   Rationale: Body systems designated as upper or lower contain body parts located above or below the diaphragm, respectively. For assistance in determining which is the correct choice, consult the Character Meaning Tables contained in the beginning of each body system of this book and also located in Optum360's *ICD-10-PCS Complete Official Code Set* coding book.

4. Match the root operations with the correct ICD-10-PCS definitions.

a.	Excision	6	1.	Partially closing off an orifice or the lumen of a tubular body part.
b.	Resection	3	2.	Completely closing an orifice or lumen of a tubular body part.
c.	Bypass	7	3.	Cutting out or off, without replacement, all of a body part.
d.	Drainage	5	4.	Taking or cutting out solid matter from a body part.
e.	Occlusion	2	5.	Taking or letting out fluids and/or gases from a body part.
f.	Restriction	1	6.	Cutting out or off, without replacement, a portion of a body part.
g.	Extirpation	4	7.	Altering the route of passage of the contents of a tubular body part.

5. What PCS body parts do the following terms correspond to?
   a. Abdominal aortic plexus — Use abdominal sympathetic nerve
   b. Biceps femoris muscle — Use upper leg muscle, right/left
   c. Choana — Use nasopharynx
   d. Gastric lymph node — Use lymphatic, aortic
   e. Infundibulopelvic ligament — Use uterine supporting structure
   f. Mitral annulus — Use mitral valve
   g. Pancreatic vein — Use splenic vein
   h. Rima glottidis — Use larynx
   i. Sinus venosus — Use atrium, right
   j. Sweat gland — Use skin

6. What other body terms are included with each of the following PCS body part characters?
   a. Auditory ossicle, right/left — Includes incus, malleus, ossicular chain, stapes
   b. Brain — Includes cerebrum, corpus callosum, encephalon
   c. Esophagus, upper — Includes cervical esophagus
   d. Optic nerve — Includes optic chiasma, second cranial nerve
   e. Tibia, right/left — Includes lateral/medial condyle of tibia, medial malleolus

7. Using the Alphabetical Index of ICD-10-PCS, what appropriate PCS body part does the index lead to for the following specific body part terms?
   a. Anterior crural nerve — Use nerve, femoral
   b. Brachiocephalic artery — Use artery, innominate

   Note: Check the Character Meaning Table to find that the innominate artery is in the upper artery body system.

   c. Hepatic flexure — Use colon, ascending
   d. Jugular body — Use glomus jugulare
   e. Sacral lymph node — Use lymphatic, pelvis

8. Shaving of the cartilage of a joint is coded in the bursae and ligament body system because it supports the joint.
   a. True
   b. False

   Rationale: Cartilage of a joint is considered a joint structure and is coded to the body part in the upper or lower joint body system to which the procedure is being performed.

9. Which root operation *always* needs a device?
   a. Reposition
   b. Restriction
   c. Replacement
   d. Repair

   Rationale: Root operation replacement, in addition to change, insertion, removal, revision, and supplement, can only be coded along with a device.

10. When a laparoscope is used to aid an open procedure, the fifth character assigned for the approach would never be Ø for open.

    a. True
    b. False

    Rationale: Procedures performed using the open approach with percutaneous endoscopic assistance are coded to the approach open.

Chapter 15. ICD-10-PCS: Nervous and Circulatory Systems

1. If a patient has a procedure performed on the third cranial nerve, which body part character in the central nervous system is reported?
    a. **H Oculomotor nerve**
    b. L Abducens nerve
    c. J Trochlear nerve
    d. M Facial nerve

    Rationale: The third cranial nerve is also known as the oculomotor nerve. In the central nervous system table, the oculomotor nerve body part character is H.

2. Which of the following terms is NOT included in the foot artery body part in the lower arteries body system?
    a. Arcuate artery
    b. Lateral tarsal artery
    c. Medial plantar artery
    d. **Fibular artery**

    Rationale: The arcuate artery, lateral tarsal artery, and medial plantar artery are all found in the foot. The fibular artery is found in the lower leg and is part of the peroneal artery body part character (T, U).

3. If a procedure is performed on the tentorium cerebelli, it would likely be assigned to body part character value 2 in the central nervous system section.
    a. **True**
    b. False

    Rationale: The tentorium cerebelli is a horizontal projection of the meningeal dura mater that separates the cerebellum in the posterior cranial fossa from the posterior portion of the cerebral hemispheres. Dura mater is assigned to character value 2 in the central nervous system section.

4. A procedure performed on the pelvic splanchnic nerve would be assigned to which body part character in which section of ICD-10-PCS?
    a. Character K under the peripheral nervous system
    b. **Character M under the peripheral nervous system**
    c. Character Q under the central nervous system
    d. Character R under the central nervous system

    Rationale: The pelvic splanchnic nerve is found within the abdomen and is part of the sympathetic nervous system. It provides parasympathetic innervation to the anterior portions of the abdominal cavity. It is a part of the peripheral nervous system.

5. In the qualifier section (character 7) for the central and peripheral nervous system, the nerves listed detail the site the graft was transferred from.
    a. True
    b. **False**

    Rationale: In the qualifier section, the nerve listed represents the site where the nerves are transferred to.

6. Which procedure is defined as "expanding an orifice or the lumen of a tubular body part"?
    a. Bypass
    b. Insertion
    c. Division
    d. **Dilation**

    Rationale: ICD-10-PCS defines dilation as "expanding an orifice or the lumen of a tubular body part."

7. In the heart and great vessels section, a procedure performed on the right ventricle uses the same body part character as a procedure performed on the left ventricle.
    a. True
    b. **False**

    Rationale: There are two separate body part characters used to report procedures on the right and left ventricles of the heart — K for the right ventricle and L for the left ventricle. Character M is also provided for procedures performed on the ventricular septum.

8. A procedure performed on the posterior communicating artery would likely be assigned to which body part character in the upper arteries body system?
    a. R Face artery
    b. **G Intracranial artery**
    c. K Internal carotid artery
    d. M External carotid artery

    Rationale: The posterior communicating artery is one of the cerebrovascular arteries found within the Circle of Willis. It is assigned to the intracranial artery body part character G.

9. What root operation is defined as "putting in a nonbiological appliance that monitors, assists, performs, or prevents a physiological function but does not physically take the place of a body part"?
    a. **Insertion**
    b. Restriction
    c. Occlusion
    d. Destruction

    Rationale: ICD-10-PCS defines insertion as "putting in a nonbiological appliance that monitors, assists, performs, or prevents a physiological function but does not physically take the place of a body part."

10. A procedure performed on the Scarpa's ganglion would be assigned to body part character N in the central nervous system.
    a. **True**
    b. False

    Rationale: Scarpa's ganglion is a grouping of nerves related to the acoustic nerve, and is assigned to body part character N in the central nervous system section of ICD-10-PCS.

Chapter 16. ICD-10-PCS: Lymphatic, Sense Organ, and Respiratory Systems

1. Which approach is defined as "entry of instrumentation through a natural or artificial external opening to reach the site of the procedure"?

    a. Open

    b. Percutaneous

    c. Via natural or artificial opening

    d. External

    Rationale: An approach via a natural or artificial opening means that the instrumentation enters the body through a natural opening in the body, such as the mouth, or via an artificial opening, such as an ostomy. Examples of these procedures are endotracheal tube insertions or Foley catheter placements.

2. Which root operation is defined as "taking or letting out fluid and/or gases from a body part"?

    a. Extirpation

    b. Release

    c. Change

    d. Drainage

    Rationale: ICD-10-PCS defines drainage as "taking or letting out fluid and/or gases from a body part."

3. What body part character would be assigned for a procedure performed in the lymphatic and hemic systems on the bone marrow of the sternum?

    a. T Bone marrow

    b. Q Bone marrow, sternum

    c. 7 Lymphatic, thorax

    d. S Bone marrow, vertebral

    Rationale: Since additional detail is provided in the example, the higher level body part character can be chosen. Body part character Q Bone marrow, sternum, would be the most appropriate choice.

4. Which procedure is defined as "putting back in or on all or a portion of a separated body part to its normal location or other suitable location"?

    a. Reattachment

    b. Alteration

    c. Revision

    d. Transfer

    Rationale: ICD-10-PCS defines reattachment as "putting back in or on all or a portion of a separated body part to its normal location or other suitable location."

5. A procedure is performed on the antrum of Highmore and is assigned to body part character Q or R in the ear, nose, and sinus body system.

    a. True

    b. False

    Rationale: The antrum of Highmore is another name for the maxillary sinuses. In order to accurately assign the body part character, the coder must know which side of the sinus the procedure was performed on.

6. A patient has a procedure performed on the left side of the diaphragm. Which of the following body part characters would be the most appropriate choice from the respiratory body system?
   a. T Diaphragm
   b. 2 Carina
   c. **S Diaphragm, left**
   d. L Lung, left

   Rationale: When a high level of detail is provided in the documentation, choose the most detailed code. In this example, the most detailed body part character is S Diaphragm, left.

7. The lung pleura is the ridge at the junction of the trachea and the bronchi formed by a projection of the lowest tracheal cartilage separating the openings of the two bronchi.
   a. True
   b. **False**

   Rationale: The carina is the ridge at the junction of the trachea and the bronchi formed by a projection of the lowest tracheal cartilage separating the openings of the two bronchi.

8. Which procedure involves modifying the anatomic structure of a body part without affecting function?
   a. Bypass
   b. **Alteration**
   c. Map
   d. Reposition

   Rationale: ICD-10-PCS defines alteration as "modifying the anatomic structure of a body part without affecting the function of the body part." Alteration procedures are typically performed for cosmetic reasons.

9. If a procedure is performed on the zonule of Zinn on the right side, which body part character from the eye body system would likely be assigned?
   a. **J Lens, right**
   b. E Retina, right
   c. K Lens, left
   d. L Extraocular muscle, right

   Rationale: The zonule of Zinn is a ring of fibrous strands that serves as a ligament to help anchor the lens to the ciliary body.

10. A procedure performed on the optic disc would be assigned to one of the lens body part characters in the eye body system.
    a. True
    b. **False**

    Rationale: The optic disc is part of the retina, not the lens and would be assigned to one of the retina body part characters, based on laterality.

Chapter 17. ICD-10-PCS: Digestive and Endocrine Systems

1. What root operation is defined as "freeing a body part from an abnormal physical constraint by cutting or by use of force"?

    a. Release
    b. Division
    c. Removal
    d. Revision

    Rationale: ICD-10-PCS defines release as "freeing a body part from an abnormal physical constraint by cutting or by use of force."

2. How many codes are necessary to code EGD biopsies of the stomach, including the antrum, cardia, and fundus?

    Three codes:

    ØDB78ZX   Excision of stomach, pylorus, via natural or artificial opening, endoscopic approach, diagnostic

    ØDB48ZX   Excision of esophagogastric junction, via natural or artificial opening, endoscopic approach, diagnostic

    ØDB68ZX   Excision of stomach, via natural or artificial opening, endoscopic approach, diagnostic

    Rationale: Even though all three biopsies are of the stomach, they are performed on different body part values, so three codes are necessary to accurately code this procedure. The cardia can be accessed by the index and body part key referring to esophagogastric junction. The antrum is located in the pylorus area of the stomach. The body part key refers pyloric antrum to stomach, pylorus. The fundus does not have a separate body part value in the key and since it is part of the stomach, it is coded to the body part value of 6 Stomach.

3. The vermillion border is the area around the _____?

    a. Teeth
    b. Lips
    c. Tonsils
    d. Larynx

    Rationale: The vermillion border is found around the edge of the lip.

4. Which procedure involves putting in or on all or a portion of a living body part taken from another individual or animal to physically take the place and/or function of all or a portion of a similar body part?

    a. Transplantation
    b. Transfer
    c. Reposition
    d. Reattachment

    Rationale: ICD-10-PCS defines transplantation as "putting in or on all or a portion of a living body part taken from another individual or animal to physically take the place and/or function of all or a portion of a similar body part."

Appendix A. Knowledge Assessment Answers

5. A procedure performed on the duct of Wirsung would likely be assigned to body part character D in the hepatobiliary system and pancreas body system.

   a. True
   b. False

   Rationale: The duct of Wirsung is another name for the pancreatic duct, which is assigned to body part character D.

6. Inspection of the suprarenal glands bilaterally is assigned to which body part character in the endocrine system table?

   a. S Endocrine gland
   b. 5 Adrenal gland
   c. 4 Adrenal glands, bilateral
   d. 8 Carotid bodies, bilateral

   Rationale: The suprarenal glands are also known as the adrenal glands. In this example, the inspection was performed bilaterally so body part character 4 is the most appropriate code selection.

7. A resection involves cutting out or off, without replacement, a portion of a body part.

   a. True
   b. False

   Rationale: The procedure described above is an excision, defined in ICD-10-PCS as "cutting out or off, without replacement, a portion of a body part."

8. Documentation provides information on a procedure performed on the epiploic foramen. Where is this found in the gastrointestinal system?

   a. Ascending colon
   b. Esophagogastric junction
   c. Rectum
   d. Abdominal cavity, connecting the two layers of peritoneum

   Rationale: The epiploic foramen connects the two layers of peritoneum in the abdominal cavity, serving as a passage between the two.

9. Which procedure involves putting in or on biological or synthetic material that physically takes the place and/or function of all or a portion of a body part?

   a. Change
   b. Replacement
   c. Insertion
   d. Transfer

   Rationale: Replacement is defined by ICD-10-PCS as "putting in or on biological or synthetic material that physically takes the place and/or function of all or a portion of a body part."

10. A procedure performed on the anorectal junction would likely be assigned to body part character R in the gastrointestinal body system.

    a. True
    b. False

    Rationale: The anorectal junction is the junction between the rectum and the anus. Procedures performed on the anorectal junction should be assigned to body part character P Rectum, in the gastrointestinal body system.

Chapter 18. ICD-10-PCS: Skin, Subcutaneous Tissue, and Musculoskeletal Systems

1. A patient has a procedure performed on the right platysma muscle. Which body part character in the muscle system table (K) would be utilized?
   a. C Hand muscle, right
   b. 2 Neck muscle, right
   c. F Trunk muscle, right
   d. V Foot muscle, right

   Rationale: The platysma is found in the region of the neck. The appropriate character assignment is 2 Neck muscle, right.

2. Qualifiers (character 7) in the skin and breast body system are used, when appropriate, to describe grafting procedures, such as specific thickness of the graft or site and type of graft.
   a. True
   b. False

   Rationale: The qualifier character is used for various types of grafting procedures. The information provided in the qualifier character details the thickness of the graft, or perhaps the site and type of graft in the instance of some flap grafts. The grafts in the skin and breast system are typically assigned to root operation characters R Replacement, U Supplement, and X Transfer. For allogenic and autogenic tissue grafts, as well as synthetic grafts of the skin, qualifiers 3 and 4 are used to indicate full thickness and partial thickness grafts. For breast procedures, various qualifiers are used to detail different types of flap grafts.

3. A procedure performed on the galea aponeurotica would be assigned to which body part character in the subcutaneous tissue and fascia body system?
   a. T Subcutaneous tissue and fascia, trunk
   b. 6 Subcutaneous tissue and fascia, chest
   c. 0 Subcutaneous tissue and fascia, scalp
   d. 1 Subcutaneous tissue and fascia, face

   Rationale: The galea aponeurotica is a fibrous membrane that covers the upper part of the cranium, and is assigned to body part character 0 Subcutaneous tissue and fascia, scalp.

4. Which procedure involves restoring, to the extent possible, a body part to its normal anatomic structure and function?
   a. Repair
   b. Reposition
   c. Revision
   d. Supplement

   Rationale: ICD-10-PCS defines repair as "restoring, to the extent possible, a body part to its normal anatomic structure and function."

Appendix A. Knowledge Assessment Answers

5. The quadratus lumborum muscle is found in what part of the body?
    a. Calf
    b. Arm
    c. Thigh
    d. **Back**

    Rationale: The quadratus lumborum muscle is found in the back, and is part of the trunk muscle body part characters F and G in the muscles body system.

6. The scalene muscle is assigned to body part character 1 under the muscle body system.
    a. True
    b. **False**

    Rationale: The scalene muscle is found in the neck, and is assigned to body part character 2 or 3, depending upon which side of the neck the procedure was performed.

7. A repair procedure is performed on the extensor digitorum longus tendon on the left leg. What is the appropriate body part character assignment from the tendons body system table?
    a. W Foot tendon, left
    b. T Ankle tendon, left
    c. **P Lower leg tendon, left**
    d. Y Lower tendon

    Rationale: To determine the accurate body part characters within the tendon table, coders should reference the body part key for muscles. This can assist in finding the most appropriate general grouping and a corresponding PCS character value for tendons. The extensor digitorum longus tendon is found in the lower leg, as is the extensor digitorum longus muscle. From the information provided, it is also indicated that the procedure involved the left side, making character P Lower leg tendon, the most appropriate answer.

8. Which procedure involves joining together portions of an articular body part rendering the articular body part immobile?
    a. Fragmentation
    b. Extirpation
    c. Destruction
    d. **Fusion**

    Rationale: ICD-10-PCS defines fusion as "joining together portions of an articular body part rendering the articular body part immobile."

9. The olecranon process is part of the elbow, but is classified in ICD-10-PCS to the body part character for ulna.
    a. **True**
    b. False

    Rationale: The olecranon process is the end of the ulna that projects beyond the humerus and forms the tip of the elbow.

10. A procedure performed at the calcaneocuboid joint on the left side is assigned to which body part character from the lower joints body system?

    a. C Knee joint, left
    b. J Tarsal joint, left
    c. L Metatarsal-tarsal joint, left
    d. Y Lower joint

    Rationale: The calcaneocuboid joint is one of the many tarsal joints found in the foot, and articulates the joint between the calcaneus (heel bone) and the cuboid (tarsal bone). When a procedure is performed on the left side, the corresponding appropriate body part character is assigned.

Chapter 19. ICD-10-PCS: Genitourinary Systems

1. What root operation is defined as "completely closing an orifice or lumen of a tubular body part"?
   a. Insertion
   b. Restriction
   c. Occlusion
   d. Destruction

   Rationale: ICD-10-PCS defines occlusion as "completely closing an orifice or lumen of a tubular body part."

2. What body part character is reported for a procedure performed on the left oviduct in the female reproductive system?
   a. D Uterus and cervix
   b. 6 Fallopian tube, left
   c. 1 Ovary, left
   d. G Vagina

   Rationale: The oviduct is another term used to describe the fallopian tube. When examining the table for the female reproductive system, the appropriate choice for the left fallopian tube body part character is 6 Fallopian tube, left.

3. What body part character is reported when a procedure is performed on the renal capsule on the left side?
   a. 1 Kidney, left
   b. 2 Kidneys, bilateral
   c. 5 Kidney
   d. 4 Kidney pelvis, left

   Rationale: The renal capsule is the fibrous outer covering of the kidney. The ICD-10-PCS Body Part Key classifies the renal capsule to kidney.

4. A procedure performed on the Cowper's gland is assigned to body part character 9 in the urinary system.
   a. True
   b. False

   Rationale: The bulbourethral or Cowper's gland is found in the male urethral region, and is assigned to body part character D in the urinary system.

5. A procedure performed on the salpinx bilaterally is assigned to which body part character in the female reproductive system?
   a. 3 Ovary
   b. F Cul-de-sac
   c. 2 Ovaries, bilateral
   d. 7 Fallopian tubes, bilateral

   Rationale: Salpinx is another term for fallopian tubes. When performed bilaterally, the appropriate assignment for the body part character is 7 Fallopian tubes, bilateral, in the female reproductive system.

6. Which procedure is defined as "cutting into a body part without draining fluids and/or gases from the body part in order to separate or transect a body part"?
   a. Detachment
   b. **Division**
   c. Occlusion
   d. Resection

   Rationale: ICD-10-PCS defines division as "cutting into a body part without draining fluids and/or gases from the body part in order to separate or transect a body part."

7. A procedure performed on the Bartholin's gland is assigned to which body part character in the female reproductive system?
   a. **L Vestibular gland**
   b. F Cul-de-sac
   c. B Endometrium
   d. V Ova

   Rationale: The Bartholin's gland is classified as one of the vestibular glands. The appropriate body part character assignment is L Vestibular gland.

8. A procedure performed on the renal pelvis is assigned to the body part character for kidney.
   a. True
   b. **False**

   Rationale: ICD-10-PCS provides body part characters for the kidney pelvis, representing both the right and left sides. Assign the appropriate body part character depending upon which side the procedure was performed.

9. Which root operation could be described as "breaking solid matter in a body part into pieces"?
   a. Extirpation
   b. Resection
   c. **Fragmentation**
   d. Removal

   Rationale: ICD-10-PCS defines fragmentation as "breaking solid matter in a body part into pieces."

10. The cul-de-sac is a blind pouch or sac formed by the caudal portion of the parietal peritoneum in the lower abdomen.
    a. **True**
    b. False

    Rationale: The cul-de-sac, also known as the rectouterine pouch, is part of the female reproductive system in ICD-10-PCS. It is found between the rectum and the back wall of the uterus.

Chapter 20. ICD-10-PCS: Anatomical Regions Systems

1. Which root operation is defined as "taking or cutting out solid matter from a body part"?
   a. Excision
   b. **Extirpation**
   c. Extraction
   d. Fragmentation

   Rationale: ICD-10-PCS defines extirpation as "taking or cutting out solid matter from a body part."

2. In the hand, detachment of the complete third ray is defined as an amputation of the middle finger through the carpometacarpal joint.
   a. **True**
   b. False

   Rationale: Based on the table of qualifiers found in chapter 20, a complete third ray amputation is through the carpometacarpal joint of the middle finger. Detachment is the root operation used for amputation.

3. Which procedure is described as "stopping, or attempting to stop, post-procedural bleeding"?
   a. Insertion
   b. Repair
   c. **Control**
   d. Alteration

   Rationale: ICD-10-PCS defines control as "stopping, or attempting to stop, post-procedural bleeding."

4. Which approach involves "entry, by puncture or minor incision, of instrumentation through the skin or mucous membrane and any other body layers necessary to reach and visualize the site of the procedure"?
   a. Percutaneous
   b. External
   c. Open
   d. **Percutaneous endoscopic**

   Rationale: A percutaneous endoscopic approach involves puncture or minor incision as opposed to a major incision. This puncture or minor incision is for placement of instrumentation for visualization of the operative site.

Appendix B. Body Part Key

Body Part Key:
Alphabetic, by specific body site

Anatomical Term	PCS Description
Abdominal aortic plexus	Abdominal Sympathetic Nerve
Abdominal esophagus	Esophagus, Lower
Abductor hallucis muscle	Foot Muscle, Right
	Foot Muscle, Left
Accessory cephalic vein	Cephalic Vein, Right
	Cephalic Vein, Left
Accessory obturator nerve	Lumbar Plexus
Accessory phrenic nerve	Phrenic nerve
Accessory spleen	Spleen
Acetabulofemoral joint	Hip Joint, Left
	Hip Joint, Right
Achilles tendon	Lower Leg Tendon, Right
	Lower Leg Tendon, Left
Acromioclavicular ligament	Shoulder Bursa and Ligament, Right
	Shoulder Bursa and Ligament, Left
Acromion (process)	Scapula, Left
	Scapula, Right
Adductor brevis muscle	Upper Leg Muscle, Right
	Upper Leg Muscle, Left
Adductor hallucis muscle	Foot Muscle, Right
	Foot Muscle, Left
Adductor longus muscle	Upper Leg Muscle, Right
	Upper Leg Muscle, Left
Adductor magnus muscle	Upper Leg Muscle, Right
	Upper Leg Muscle, Left
Adenohypophysis	Pituitary Gland
Alar ligament of axis	Head and Neck Bursa and Ligament
Alveolar process of mandible	Mandible, Left
	Mandible, Right
Alveolar process of maxilla	Maxilla, Left
	Maxilla, Right
Anal orifice	Anus
Anatomical snuffbox	Lower Arm and Wrist Tendon, Right
	Lower Arm and Wrist Tendon, Left
Angular artery	Face Artery
Angular vein	Face Vein, Left
	Face Vein, Right
Annular ligament	Elbow Bursa and Ligament, Right
	Elbow Bursa and Ligament, Left
Anorectal junction	Rectum
Ansa cervicalis	Cervical Plexus

Anatomical Term	PCS Description
Antebrachial fascia	Subcutaneous Tissue and Fascia, Right Lower Arm
	Subcutaneous Tissue and Fascia, Left Lower Arm
Anterior (pectoral) lymph node	Lymphatic, Left Axillary
	Lymphatic, Right Axillary
Anterior cerebral artery	Intracranial Artery
Anterior cerebral vein	Intracranial Vein
Anterior choroidal artery	Intracranial Artery
Anterior circumflex humeral artery	Axillary Artery, Right
	Axillary Artery, Left
Anterior communicating artery	Intracranial Artery
Anterior cruciate ligament (ACL)	Knee Bursa and Ligament, Right
	Knee Bursa and Ligament, Left
Anterior crural nerve	Femoral Nerve
Anterior facial vein	Face Vein, Left
	Face Vein, Right
Anterior intercostal artery	Internal Mammary Artery, Right
	Internal Mammary Artery, Left
Anterior interosseous nerve	Median Nerve
Anterior lateral malleolar artery	Anterior Tibial Artery, Right
	Anterior Tibial Artery, Left
Anterior lingual gland	Minor Salivary Gland
Anterior medial malleolar artery	Anterior Tibial Artery, Right
	Anterior Tibial Artery, Left
Anterior spinal artery	Vertebral Artery, Right
	Vertebral Artery, Left
Anterior tibial recurrent artery	Anterior Tibial Artery, Right
	Anterior Tibial Artery, Left
Anterior ulnar recurrent artery	Ulnar Artery, Right
	Ulnar Artery, Left
Anterior vagal trunk	Vagus Nerve
Anterior vertebral muscle	Neck Muscle, Right
	Neck Muscle, Left
Antihelix	External Ear, Right
	External Ear, Left
	External Ear, Bilateral
Antitragus	External Ear, Right
	External Ear, Left
	External Ear, Bilateral
Antrum of Highmore	Maxillary Sinus, Right
	Maxillary Sinus, Left
Aortic annulus	Aortic Valve

© 2015 Optum360, LLC

Anatomical Term	PCS Description
Aortic arch	Thoracic Aorta
Aortic intercostal artery	Thoracic Aorta
Apical (subclavicular) lymph node	Lymphatic, Left Axillary
	Lymphatic, Right Axillary
Apneustic center	Pons
Aqueduct of Sylvius	Cerebral Ventricle
Aqueous humour	Anterior Chamber, Right
	Anterior Chamber, Left
Arachnoid mater, intracranial	Cerebral Meninges
Arachnoid mater, spinal	Spinal Meninges
Arcuate artery	Foot Artery, Right
	Foot Artery, Left
Areola	Nipple, Left
	Nipple, Right
Arterial canal (duct)	Pulmonary Artery, Left
Aryepiglottic fold	Larynx
Arytenoid cartilage	Larynx
Arytenoid muscle	Neck Muscle, Right
	Neck Muscle, Left
Ascending aorta	Thoracic Aorta
Ascending palatine artery	Face Artery
Ascending pharyngeal artery	External Carotid Artery, Right
	External Carotid Artery, Left
Atlantoaxial joint	Cervical Vertebral Joint
Atrioventricular node	Conduction Mechanism
Atrium dextrum cordis	Atrium, Right
Atrium pulmonale	Atrium, Left
Auditory tube	Eustachian Tube, Right
	Eustachian Tube, Left
Auerbach's (myenteric) plexus	Abdominal Sympathetic Nerve
Auricle	External Ear, Right
	External Ear, Left
	External Ear, Bilateral
Auricularis muscle	Head Muscle
Axillary fascia	Subcutaneous Tissue and Fascia, Right Upper Arm
	Subcutaneous Tissue and Fascia, Left Upper Arm
Axillary nerve	Brachial Plexus
Bartholin's (greater vestibular) gland	Vestibular Gland
Basal (internal) cerebral vein	Intracranial Vein
Basal nuclei	Basal Ganglia
Basilar artery	Intracranial Artery
Basis pontis	Pons

Anatomical Term	PCS Description
Biceps brachii muscle	Upper Arm Muscle, Right
	Upper Arm Muscle, Left
Biceps femoris muscle	Upper Leg Muscle, Right
	Upper Leg Muscle, Left
Bicipital aponeurosis	Subcutaneous Tissue and Fascia, Right Lower Arm
	Subcutaneous Tissue and Fascia, Left Lower Arm
Bicuspid valve	Mitral Valve
Body of femur	Femoral Shaft, Right
	Femoral Shaft, Left
Body of fibula	Fibula, Left
	Fibula, Right
Bony labyrinth	Inner Ear, Left
	Inner Ear, Right
Bony orbit	Orbit, Left
	Orbit, Right
Bony vestibule	Inner Ear, Left
	Inner Ear, Right
Botallo's duct	Pulmonary Artery, Left
Brachial (lateral) lymph node	Lymphatic, Left Axillary
	Lymphatic, Right Axillary
Brachialis muscle	Upper Arm Muscle, Right
	Upper Arm Muscle, Left
Brachiocephalic artery or trunk	Innominate Artery
Brachiocephalic vein	Innominate Vein, Right
	Innominate Vein, Left
Brachioradialis muscle	Lower Arm and Wrist Muscle, Right
	Lower Arm and Wrist Muscle, Left
Broad ligament	Uterine Supporting Structure
Bronchial artery	Thoracic Aorta
Buccal gland	Buccal Mucosa
Buccinator lymph node	Lymphatic, Head
Buccinator muscle	Facial Muscle
Bulbospongiosus muscle	Perineum Muscle
Bulbourethral (Cowper's) gland	Urethra
Bundle of His	Conduction Mechanism
Bundle of Kent	Conduction Mechanism
Calcaneocuboid ligament	Foot Bursa and Ligament, Right
	Foot Bursa and Ligament, Left
Calcaneocuboid joint	Tarsal Joint, Right
	Tarsal Joint, Left
Calcaneofibular ligament	Ankle Bursa and Ligament, Right
	Ankle Bursa and Ligament, Left
Calcaneus	Tarsal, Left
	Tarsal, Right

Appendix B. Body Part Key—Body Part Key: Alphabetic, by specific body site

Anatomical Term	PCS Description
Capitate bone	Carpal, Left
	Carpal, Right
Cardia	Esophagogastric Junction
Cardiac plexus	Thoracic Sympathetic Nerve
Cardioesophageal junction	Esophagogastric Junction
Caroticotympanic artery	Internal Carotid Artery, Right
	Internal Carotid Artery, Left
Carotid glomus	Carotid Bodies, Bilateral
	Carotid Body, Right
	Carotid Body, Left
Carotid sinus nerve	Glossopharyngeal Nerve
Carotid sinus	Internal Carotid Artery, Right
	Internal Carotid Artery, Left
Carpometacarpal (CMC) joint	Metacarpocarpal Joint, Right
	Metacarpocarpal Joint, Left
Carpometacarpal ligament	Hand Bursa and Ligament, Right
	Hand Bursa and Ligament, Left
Cauda equina	Lumbar Spinal Cord
Cavernous plexus	Head and Neck Sympathetic Nerve
Celiac ganglion	Abdominal Sympathetic Nerve
Celiac (solar) plexus	Abdominal Sympathetic Nerve
Celiac lymph node	Lymphatic, Aortic
Celiac trunk	Celiac Artery
Central axillary lymph node	Lymphatic, Left Axillary
	Lymphatic, Right Axillary
Cerebral aqueduct (Sylvius)	Cerebral Ventricle
Cerebrum	Brain
Cervical esophagus	Esophagus, Upper
Cervical facet joint	Cervical Vertebral Joints, 2 or more
	Cervical Vertebral Joint
Cervical ganglion	Head and Neck Sympathetic Nerve
Cervical intertransverse ligament	Head and Neck Bursa and Ligament
Cervical interspinous ligament	Head and Neck Bursa and Ligament
Cervical ligamentum flavum	Head and Neck Bursa and Ligament
Cervical lymph node	Lymphatic, Left Neck
	Lymphatic, Right Neck
Cervicothoracic facet joint	Cervicothoracic Vertebral Joint
Choana	Nasopharynx
Chondroglossus muscle	Tongue, Palate, Pharynx Muscle
Chorda tympani	Facial Nerve
Choroid plexus	Cerebral Ventricle
Ciliary body	Eye, Left
	Eye, Right
Ciliary ganglion	Head and Neck Sympathetic Nerve

Anatomical Term	PCS Description
Circle of Willis	Intracranial Artery
Circumflex illiac artery	Femoral Artery, Right
	Femoral Artery, Left
Claustrum	Basal Ganglia
Coccygeal body	Coccygeal Glomus
Coccygeus muscle	Trunk Muscle, Left
Cochlea	Inner Ear, Left
	Inner Ear, Right
Cochlear nerve	Acoustic Nerve
Columella	Nose
Common digital vein	Foot Vein, Left
	Foot Vein, Right
Common facial vein	Face Vein, Left
	Face Vein, Right
Common fibular nerve	Peroneal Nerve
Common hepatic artery	Hepatic Artery
Common iliac (subaortic) lymph node	Lymphatic, Pelvis
Common interosseous artery	Ulnar Artery, Right
	Ulnar Artery, Left
Common peroneal nerve	Peroneal Nerve
Condyloid process	Mandible, Left
	Mandible, Right
Conus arteriosus	Ventricle, Right
Conus medullaris	Lumbar Spinal Cord
Coracoacromial ligament	Shoulder Bursa and Ligament, Right
	Shoulder Bursa and Ligament, Left
Coracobrachialis muscle	Upper Arm Muscle, Right
	Upper Arm Muscle, Left
Coracoclavicular ligament	Shoulder Bursa and Ligament, Right
	Shoulder Bursa and Ligament, Left
Coracohumeral ligament	Shoulder Bursa and Ligament, Right
	Shoulder Bursa and Ligament, Left
Coracoid process	Scapula, Left
	Scapula, Right
Corniculate cartilage	Larynx
Corpus callosum	Brain
Corpus cavernosum	Penis
Corpus spongiosum	Penis
Corpus striatum	Basal Ganglia
Corrugator supercilii muscle	Facial Muscle
Costocervical trunk	Subclavian Artery, Right
	Subclavian Artery, Left
Costoclavicular ligament	Shoulder Bursa and Ligament, Right
	Shoulder Bursa and Ligament, Left
Costotransverse joint	Thoracic Vertebral Joint

© 2015 Optum360, LLC

Anatomical Term	PCS Description	Anatomical Term	PCS Description
Costotransverse ligament	Thorax Bursa and Ligament, Right	Deep transverse perineal muscle	Perineum Muscle
	Thorax Bursa and Ligament, Left	Deferential artery	Internal Iliac Artery, Right
Costovertebral joint	Thoracic Vertebral Joint		Internal Iliac Artery, Left
Costoxiphoid ligament	Thorax Bursa and Ligament, Right	Deltoid fascia	Subcutaneous Tissue and Fascia, Right Upper Arm
	Thorax Bursa and Ligament, Left		Subcutaneous Tissue and Fascia, Left Upper Arm
Cowper's (bulbourethral) gland	Urethra	Deltoid ligament	Ankle Bursa and Ligament, Right
Cremaster muscle	Perineum Muscle		Ankle Bursa and Ligament, Left
Cribriform plate	Ethmoid Bone, Right	Deltoid muscle	Shoulder Muscle, Right
	Ethmoid Bone, Left		Shoulder Muscle, Left
Cricoid cartilage	Trachea	Deltopectoral (infraclavicular) lymph node	Lymphatic, Left Upper Extremity
Cricothyroid artery	Thyroid Artery, Right		Lymphatic, Right Upper Extremity
	Thyroid Artery, Left	Denticulate (dentate) ligament	Spinal Meninges
Cricothyroid muscle	Neck Muscle, Right	Depressor anguli oris muscle	Facial Muscle
	Neck Muscle, Left	Depressor labii inferioris muscle	Facial Muscle
Crural fascia	Subcutaneous Tissue and Fascia, Right Upper Leg	Depressor septi nasi muscle	Facial Muscle
	Subcutaneous Tissue and Fascia, Left Upper Leg	Depressor supercilii muscle	Facial Muscle
Cubital lymph node	Lymphatic, Left Upper Extremity	Dermis	Skin
	Lymphatic, Right Upper Extremity	Descending genicular artery	Femoral Artery, Right
Cubital nerve	Ulnar Nerve		Femoral Artery, Left
Cuboid bone	Tarsal, Left	Diaphragma sellae	Dura Mater
	Tarsal, Right	Distal humerus	Humeral Shaft, Right
Cuboideonavicular joint	Tarsal Joint, Right		Humeral Shaft, Left
	Tarsal Joint, Left	Distal humerus, involving joint	Elbow Joint, Right
Culmen	Cerebellum		Elbow Joint, Left
Cuneiform cartilage	Larynx	Distal radioulnar joint	Wrist Joint, Right
Cuneonavicular ligament	Foot Bursa and Ligament, Right		Wrist Joint, Left
	Foot Bursa and Ligament, Left	Dorsal digital nerve	Radial Nerve
Cuneonavicular joint	Tarsal Joint, Right	Dorsal metacarpal vein	Hand Vein, Left
	Tarsal Joint, Left		Hand Vein, Right
Cutaneous (transverse) cervical nerve	Cervical Plexus	Dorsal metatarsal artery	Foot Artery, Right
Deep cervical fascia	Subcutaneous Tissue and Fascia, Anterior Neck		Foot Artery, Left
Deep cervical vein	Vertebral Vein, Right	Dorsal metatarsal vein	Foot Vein, Left
	Vertebral Vein, Left		Foot Vein, Right
Deep circumflex iliac artery	External Iliac Artery, Right	Dorsal scapular artery	Subclavian Artery, Right
	External Iliac Artery, Left		Subclavian Artery, Left
Deep facial vein	Face Vein, Left	Dorsal scapular nerve	Brachial Plexus
	Face Vein, Right	Dorsal venous arch	Foot Vein, Left
Deep femoral artery	Femoral Artery, Right		Foot Vein, Right
	Femoral Artery, Left	Dorsalis pedis artery	Anterior Tibial Artery, Right
Deep femoral (profunda femoris) vein	Femoral Vein, Right		Anterior Tibial Artery, Left
	Femoral Vein, Left	Duct of Santorini	Pancreatic Duct, Accessory
Deep palmar arch	Hand Artery, Right	Duct of Wirsung	Pancreatic Duct
	Hand Artery, Left		

Anatomical Term	PCS Description
Ductus deferens	Vas Deferens, Right
	Vas Deferens, Left
	Vas Deferens, Bilateral
	Vas Deferens
Duodenal ampulla	Ampulla of Vater
Duodenojejunal flexure	Jejunum
Dura mater, intracranial	Dura Mater
Dura mater, spinal	Spinal Meninges
Dural venous sinus	Intracranial Vein
Earlobe	External Ear, Right
	External Ear, Left
	External Ear, Bilateral
Eighth cranial nerve	Acoustic Nerve
Ejaculatory duct	Vas Deferens, Right
	Vas Deferens, Left
	Vas Deferens, Bilateral
	Vas Deferens
Eleventh cranial nerve	Accessory Nerve
Encephalon	Brain
Ependyma	Cerebral Ventricle
Epidermis	Skin
Epidural space, intracranial	Epidural Space
Epidural space, spinal	Spinal Canal
Epiploic foramen	Peritoneum
Epithalamus	Thalamus
Epitroclear lymph node	Lymphatic, Left Upper Extremity
	Lymphatic, Right Upper Extremity
Erector spinae muscle	Trunk Muscle, Right
	Trunk Muscle, Left
Esophageal artery	Thoracic Aorta
Esophageal plexus	Thoracic Sympathetic Nerve
Ethmoidal air cell	Ethmoid Sinus, Right
	Ethmoid Sinus, Left
Extensor carpi radialis muscle	Lower Arm and Wrist Muscle, Right, Left
Extensor carpi ulnaris muscle	Lower Arm and Wrist Muscle, Right, Left
Extensor digitorum brevis muscle	Foot Muscle, Right
	Foot Muscle, Left
Extensor digitorum longus muscle	Lower Leg Muscle, Right
	Lower Leg Muscle, Left
Extensor hallucis brevis muscle	Foot Muscle, Right
	Foot Muscle, Left
Extensor hallucis longus muscle	Lower Leg Muscle, Right
	Lower Leg Muscle, Left
External anal sphincter	Anal Sphincter
External auditory meatus	External Auditory Canal, Right
	External Auditory Canal, Left

Anatomical Term	PCS Description
External maxillary artery	Face Artery
External naris	Nose
External oblique aponeurosis	Subcutaneous Tissue and Fascia, Trunk
External oblique muscle	Abdomen Muscle, Right
	Abdomen Muscle, Left
External popliteal nerve	Peroneal Nerve
External pudendal artery	Femoral Artery, Right
	Femoral Artery, Left
External pudendal vein	Greater Saphenous Vein, Right
	Greater Saphenous Vein, Left
External urethral sphincter	Urethra
Extradural space, intracranial	Epidural Space
Extradural space, spinal	Spinal Canal
Facial artery	Face Artery
False vocal cord	Larynx
Falx cerebri	Dura Mater
Fascia lata	Subcutaneous Tissue and Fascia, Right Upper Leg
	Subcutaneous Tissue and Fascia, Left Upper Leg
Femoral head	Upper Femur, Right
	Upper Femur, Left
Femoral lymph node	Lymphatic, Left Lower Extremity
	Lymphatic, Right Lower Extremity
Femoropatellar joint	Knee Joint, Right
	Knee Joint, Left
	Knee Joint, Femoral Surface, Right
	Knee Joint, Femoral Surface, Left
Femorotibial joint	Knee Joint, Right
	Knee Joint, Left
	Knee Joint, Tibial Surface, Right
	Knee Joint, Tibial Surface, Left
Fibular artery	Peroneal Artery, Right
	Peroneal Artery, Left
Fibularis brevis muscle	Lower Leg Muscle, Right
	Lower Leg Muscle, Left
Fibularis longus muscle	Lower Leg Muscle, Right
	Lower Leg Muscle, Left
Fifth cranial nerve	Trigeminal Nerve
First cranial nerve	Olfactory Nerve
First intercostal nerve	Brachial Plexus
Flexor carpi ulnaris muscle	Lower Arm and Wrist Muscle, Left
	Lower Arm and Wrist Muscle, Right
Flexor digitorum brevis muscle	Foot Muscle, Right
	Foot Muscle, Left

Anatomical Term	PCS Description	Anatomical Term	PCS Description
Flexor digitorum longus muscle	Lower Leg Muscle, Right	Glenohumeral joint	Shoulder Joint, Right
	Lower Leg Muscle, Left		Shoulder Joint, Left
Flexor hallucis brevis muscle	Foot Muscle, Right	Glenohumeral ligament	Shoulder Bursa and Ligament, Right
	Foot Muscle, Left		Shoulder Bursa and Ligament, Left
Flexor hallucis longus muscle	Lower Leg Muscle, Right	Glenoid fossa (of scapula)	Glenoid Cavity, Right
	Lower Leg Muscle, Left		Glenoid Cavity, Left
Flexor pollicis longus muscle	Lower Arm and Wrist Muscle, Right	Glenoid ligament (labrum)	Shoulder Joint, Right
	Lower Arm and Wrist Muscle, Left		Shoulder Joint, Left
Foramen magnum	Occipital Bone, Right	Globus pallidus	Basal Ganglia
	Occipital Bone, Left	Glossoepiglottic fold	Epiglottis
Foramen of Monro (intraventricular)	Cerebral Ventricle	Glottis	Larynx
		Gluteal lymph node	Lymphatic, Pelvis
Foreskin	Prepuce	Gluteal vein	Hypogastric Vein, Right
Fossa of Rosenmuller	Nasopharynx		Hypogastric Vein, Left
Fourth cranial nerve	Trochlear Nerve	Gluteus maximus muscle	Hip Muscle, Right
Fourth ventricle	Cerebral Ventricle		Hip Muscle, Left
Fovea	Retina, Left	Gluteus medius muscle	Hip Muscle, Right
	Retina, Right		Hip Muscle, Left
Frenulum labii inferioris	Lower Lip	Gluteus minimus muscle	Hip Muscle, Right
Frenulum labii superioris	Upper Lip		Hip Muscle, Left
Frenulum linguae	Tongue	Gracilis muscle	Upper Leg Muscle, Right
Frontal lobe	Cerebral Hemisphere		Upper Leg Muscle, Left
Frontal vein	Face Vein, Left	Great auricular nerve	Cervical Plexus
	Face Vein, Right	Great cerebral vein	Intracranial Vein
Fundus uteri	Uterus	Great saphenous vein	Greater Saphenous Vein, Right
Galea aponeurotica	Subcutaneous Tissue and Fascia, Scalp		Greater Saphenous Vein, Left
Ganglion impar (ganglion of Walther)	Sacral Sympathetic Nerve	Greater alar cartilage	Nose
		Greater occipital nerve	Cervical Nerve
Gasserian ganglion	Trigeminal Nerve	Greater splanchnic nerve	Thoracic Sympathetic Nerve
Gastric lymph node	Lymphatic, Aortic	Greater superficial petrosal nerve	Facial Nerve
Gastric plexus	Abdominal Sympathetic Nerve		
Gastrocnemius muscle	Lower Leg Muscle, Right	Greater trochanter	Upper Femur, Right
	Lower Leg Muscle, Left		Upper Femur, Left
Gastrocolic ligament	Greater Omentum	Greater tuberosity	Humeral Head, Right
Gastrocolic omentum	Greater Omentum		Humeral Head, Left
Gastroduodenal artery	Hepatic Artery	Greater vestibular (Bartholin's) gland	Vestibular Gland
Gastroesophageal (GE) junction	Esophagogastric Junction		
Gastrohepatic omentum	Lesser Omentum	Greater wing	Sphenoid Bone, Right
Gastrophrenic ligament	Greater Omentum		Sphenoid Bone, Left
Gastrosplenic ligament	Greater Omentum	Hallux	1st Toe, Left
			1st Toe, Right
Gemellus muscle	Hip Muscle, Right	Hamate bone	Carpal, Left
	Hip Muscle, Left		Carpal, Right
Geniculate ganglion	Facial Nerve	Head of fibula	Fibula, Left
Geniculate nucleus	Thalamus		Fibula, Right
Genioglossus muscle	Tongue, Palate, Pharynx Muscle	Helix	External Ear, Right
Genitofemoral nerve	Lumbar Plexus		External Ear, Left
Glans penis	Prepuce		External Ear, Bilateral

Anatomical Term	PCS Description
Hepatic artery proper	Hepatic Artery
Hepatic flexure	Ascending Colon
Hepatic lymph node	Lymphatic, Aortic
Hepatic plexus	Abdominal Sympathetic Nerve
Hepatic portal vein	Portal Vein
Hepatogastric ligament	Lesser Omentum
Hepatopancreatic ampulla	Ampulla of Vater
Humeroradial joint	Elbow Joint, Right
	Elbow Joint, Left
Humeroulnar joint	Elbow Joint, Right
	Elbow Joint, Left
Humerus, distal	Humeral Shaft, Right, Left
Hyoglossus muscle	Tongue, Palate, Pharynx Muscle
Hyoid artery	Thyroid Artery, Right
	Thyroid Artery, Left
Hypogastric artery	Internal Iliac Artery, Right
	Internal Iliac Artery, Left
Hypopharynx	Pharynx
Hypophysis	Pituitary Gland
Hypothenar muscle	Hand Muscle, Right
	Hand Muscle, Left
Ileal artery	Superior Mesenteric Artery
Ileocolic artery	Superior Mesenteric Artery
Ileocolic vein	Colic Vein
Iliac crest	Pelvic Bone, Right
	Pelvic Bone, Left
Iliac fascia	Subcutaneous Tissue and Fascia, Right Upper Leg
	Subcutaneous Tissue and Fascia, Left Upper Leg
Iliac lymph node	Lymphatic, Pelvis
Iliacus muscle	Hip Muscle, Right
	Hip Muscle, Left
Iliofemoral ligament	Hip Bursa and Ligament, Right
	Hip Bursa and Ligament, Left
Iliohypogastric nerve	Lumbar Plexus
Ilioinguinal nerve	Lumbar Plexus
Iliolumbar artery	Internal Iliac Artery, Right
	Internal Iliac Artery, Left
Iliolumbar ligament	Trunk Bursa and Ligament, Right
	Trunk Bursa and Ligament, Left
Iliotibial tract (band)	Subcutaneous Tissue and Fascia, Right Upper Leg
	Subcutaneous Tissue and Fascia, Left Upper Leg
Ilium	Pelvic Bone, Right
	Pelvic Bone, Left

Anatomical Term	PCS Description
Incus	Auditory Ossicle, Right
	Auditory Ossicle, Left
Inferior cardiac nerve	Thoracic Sympathetic Nerve
Inferior cerebellar vein	Intracranial Vein
Inferior cerebral vein	Intracranial Vein
Inferior epigastric artery	External Iliac Artery, Right
	External Iliac Artery, Left
Inferior epigastric lymph node	Lymphatic, Pelvis
Inferior genicular artery	Popliteal Artery, Right
	Popliteal Artery, Left
Inferior gluteal artery	Internal Iliac Artery, Right
	Internal Iliac Artery, Left
Inferior gluteal nerve	Sacral Plexus
Inferior hypogastric plexus	Abdominal Sympathetic Nerve
Inferior labial artery	Face Artery
Inferior longitudinal muscle	Tongue, Palate, Pharynx Muscle
Inferior mesenteric ganglion	Abdominal Sympathetic Nerve
Inferior mesenteric lymph node	Lymphatic, Mesenteric
Inferior mesenteric plexus	Abdominal Sympathetic Nerve
Inferior oblique muscle	Extraocular Muscle, Right
	Extraocular Muscle, Left
Inferior pancreaticoduodenal artery	Superior Mesenteric Artery
Inferior phrenic artery	Abdominal Aorta
Inferior rectus muscle	Extraocular Muscle, Right
	Extraocular Muscle, Left
Inferior suprarenal artery	Renal Artery, Right
	Renal Artery, Left
Inferior tarsal plate	Lower Eyelid, Right
	Lower Eyelid, Left
Inferior thyroid vein	Innominate Vein, Right
	Innominate Vein, Left
Inferior tibiofibular joint	Ankle Joint, Right
	Ankle Joint, Left
Inferior turbinate	Nasal Turbinate
Inferior ulnar collateral artery	Brachial Artery, Right
	Brachial Artery, Left
Inferior vesical artery	Internal Iliac Artery, Right
	Internal Iliac Artery, Left
Infraauricular lymph node	Lymphatic, Head
Infraclavicular (deltopectoral) lymph node	Lymphatic, Left Upper Extremity
	Lymphatic, Right Upper Extremity

Comprehensive Anatomy and Physiology for ICD-10-CM and ICD-10-PCS Coding

Anatomical Term	PCS Description
Infrahyoid muscle	Neck Muscle, Right
	Neck Muscle, Left
Infraparotid lymph node	Lymphatic, Head
Infraspinatus fascia	Subcutaneous Tissue and Fascia, Right Upper Arm
	Subcutaneous Tissue and Fascia, Left Upper Arm
Infraspinatus muscle	Shoulder Muscle, Right
	Shoulder Muscle, Left
Infundibulopelvic ligament	Uterine Supporting Structure
Inguinal canal	Inguinal Region, Right
	Inguinal Region, Left
	Inguinal Region, Bilateral
Inguinal triangle	Inguinal Region, Right
	Inguinal Region, Left
	Inguinal Region, Bilateral
Interatrial septum	Atrial Septum
Intercarpal joint	Carpal Joint, Right
	Carpal Joint, Left
Intercarpal ligament	Hand Bursa and Ligament, Right
	Hand Bursa and Ligament, Left
Interclavicular ligament	Shoulder Bursa and Ligament, Right
	Shoulder Bursa and Ligament, Left
Intercostal lymph node	Lymphatic, Thorax
Intercostal nerve	Thoracic Nerve
Intercostal muscle	Thorax Muscle, Right
	Thorax Muscle, Left
Intercostobrachial nerve	Thoracic Nerve
Intercuneiform joint	Tarsal Joint, Right
	Tarsal Joint, Left
Intercuneiform ligament	Foot Bursa and Ligament, Right
	Foot Bursa and Ligament, Left
Intermediate cuneiform bone	Tarsal, Left
	Tarsal, Right
Internal (basal) cerebral vein	Intracranial Vein
Internal anal sphincter	Anal Sphincter
Internal carotid plexus	Head and Neck Sympathetic Nerve
Internal iliac vein	Hypogastric Vein, Right
	Hypogastric Vein, Left
Internal maxillary artery	External Carotid Artery, Right
	External Carotid Artery, Left
Internal naris	Nose
Internal oblique muscle	Abdomen Muscle, Right
	Abdomen Muscle, Left
Internal pudendal artery	Internal Iliac Artery, Left
	Internal Iliac Artery, Right

Anatomical Term	PCS Description
Internal pudendal vein	Hypogastric Vein, Right
	Hypogastric Vein, Left
Internal thoracic artery	Internal Mammary Artery, Right
	Internal Mammary Artery, Left
	Subclavian Artery, Right
	Subclavian Artery, Left
Internal urethral sphincter	Urethra
Interphalangeal (IP) joint	Finger Phalangeal Joint, Right
	Finger Phalangeal Joint, Left
	Toe Phalangeal Joint, Right
	Toe Phalangeal Joint, Left
Interphalangeal ligament	Foot Bursa and Ligament, Right
	Foot Bursa and Ligament, Left
	Hand Bursa and Ligament, Right
	Hand Bursa and Ligament, Left
Interspinalis muscle	Trunk Muscle, Right
	Trunk Muscle, Left
Interspinous ligament	Head and Neck Bursa and Ligament
	Trunk Bursa and Ligament, Right
	Trunk Bursa and Ligament, Left
Intertransverse ligament	Trunk Bursa and Ligament, Right
	Trunk Bursa and Ligament, Left
Intertransversarius muscle	Trunk Muscle, Right
	Trunk Muscle, Left
Interventricular foramen (Monro)	Cerebral Ventricle
Interventricular septum	Ventricular Septum
Intestinal lymphatic trunk	Cisterna Chyli
Ischiatic nerve	Sciatic Nerve
Ischiocavernosus muscle	Perineum Muscle
Ischiofemoral ligament	Hip Bursa and Ligament, Right
	Hip Bursa and Ligament, Left
Ischium	Pelvic Bone, Right
	Pelvic Bone, Left
Jejunal artery	Superior Mesenteric Artery
Jugular body	Glomus Jugulare
Jugular lymph node	Lymphatic, Left Neck
	Lymphatic, Right Neck
Labia majora	Vulva
Labia minora	Vulva
Labial gland	Upper Lip
	Lower Lip
Lacrimal canaliculus	Lacrimal Duct, Right
	Lacrimal Duct, Left
Lacrimal punctum	Lacrimal Duct, Right
	Lacrimal Duct, Left

Appendix B. Body Part Key—Body Part Key: Alphabetic, by specific body site

Anatomical Term	PCS Description
Lacrimal sac	Lacrimal Duct, Right
	Lacrimal Duct, Left
Laryngopharynx	Pharynx
Lateral (brachial) lymph node	Lymphatic, Left Axillary
	Lymphatic, Right Axillary
Lateral canthus	Upper Eyelid, Right
	Upper Eyelid, Left
Lateral collateral ligament (LCL)	Knee Bursa and Ligament, Right
	Knee Bursa and Ligament, Left
Lateral condyle of femur	Lower Femur, Right
	Lower Femur, Left
Lateral condyle of tibia	Tibia, Left
	Tibia, Right
Lateral cuneiform bone	Tarsal, Left
	Tarsal, Right
Lateral epicondyle of femur	Lower Femur, Right
	Lower Femur, Left
Lateral epicondyle of humerus	Humeral Shaft, Right
	Humeral Shaft, Left
Lateral femoral cutaneous nerve	Lumbar Plexus
Lateral malleolus	Fibula, Left
	Fibula, Right
Lateral meniscus	Knee Joint, Right
	Knee Joint, Left
Lateral nasal cartilage	Nose
Lateral plantar artery	Foot Artery, Right
	Foot Artery, Left
Lateral plantar nerve	Tibial Nerve
Lateral rectus muscle	Extraocular Muscle, Right
	Extraocular Muscle, Left
Lateral sacral artery	Internal Iliac Artery, Right
	Internal Iliac Artery, Left
Lateral sacral vein	Hypogastric Vein, Right
	Hypogastric Vein, Left
Lateral sural cutaneous nerve	Peroneal Nerve
Lateral tarsal artery	Foot Artery, Right
	Foot Artery, Left
Lateral temporomandibular ligament	Head and Neck Bursa and Ligament
Lateral thoracic artery	Axillary Artery, Right
	Axillary Artery, Left
Latissimus dorsi muscle	Trunk Muscle, Right
	Trunk Muscle, Left
Least splanchnic nerve	Thoracic Sympathetic Nerve
Left ascending lumbar vein	Hemiazygos Vein

Anatomical Term	PCS Description
Left atrioventricular valve	Mitral Valve
Left auricular appendix	Atrium, Left
Left colic vein	Colic Vein
Left coronary sulcus	Heart, Left
Left gastric artery	Gastric Artery
Left gastroepiploic artery	Splenic Artery
Left gastroepiploic vein	Splenic Vein
Left inferior phrenic vein	Renal Vein, Left
Left inferior pulmonary vein	Pulmonary Vein, Left
Left jugular trunk	Thoracic Duct
Left lateral ventricle	Cerebral Ventricle
Left ovarian vein	Renal Vein, Left
Left second lumbar vein	Renal Vein, Left
Left subclavian trunk	Thoracic Duct
Left subcostal vein	Hemiazygos Vein
Left superior pulmonary vein	Pulmonary Vein, Left
Left suprarenal vein	Renal Vein, Left
Left testicular vein	Renal Vein, Left
Leptomeninges, intracranial	Cerebral Meninges
Leptomeninges, spinal	Spinal Meninges
Lesser alar cartilage	Nose
Lesser occipital nerve	Cervical Plexus
Lesser splanchnic nerve	Thoracic Sympathetic Nerve
Lesser trochanter	Upper Femur, Right
	Upper Femur, Left
Lesser tuberosity	Humeral Head, Right
	Humeral Head, Left
Lesser wing	Sphenoid Bone, Right
	Sphenoid Bone, Left
Levator anguli oris muscle	Facial Muscle
Levator ani muscle	Trunk Muscle, Left
Levator labii superioris alaeque nasi muscle	Facial Muscle
Levator labii superioris muscle	Facial Muscle
Levator palpebrae superioris muscle	Upper Eyelid, Right
	Upper Eyelid, Left
Levator scapulae muscle	Neck Muscle, Right
	Neck Muscle, Left
Levator veli palatini muscle	Tongue, Palate, Pharynx Muscle
Levatores costarum muscle	Thorax Muscle, Right
	Thorax Muscle, Left
Ligament of head of fibula	Knee Bursa and Ligament, Right
	Knee Bursa and Ligament, Left

Anatomical Term	PCS Description	Anatomical Term	PCS Description
Ligament of the lateral malleolus	Ankle Bursa and Ligament, Right	Medial canthus	Lower Eyelid, Right
	Ankle Bursa and Ligament, Left		Lower Eyelid, Left
Ligamentum flavum	Trunk Bursa and Ligament, Right	Medial collateral ligament (MCL)	Knee Bursa and Ligament, Right
	Trunk Bursa and Ligament, Left		Knee Bursa and Ligament, Left
Lingual artery	External Carotid Artery, Right	Medial condyle of femur	Lower Femur, Right
	External Carotid Artery, Left		Lower Femur, Left
Lingual tonsil	Tongue	Medial condyle of tibia	Tibia, Left
Locus ceruleus	Pons		Tibia, Right
Long thoracic nerve	Brachial Plexus	Medial cuneiform bone	Tarsal, Left
Lumbar artery	Abdominal Aorta		Tarsal, Right
Lumbar facet joint	Lumbar Vertebral Joint	Medial epicondyle of femur	Lower Femur, Right
Lumbar ganglion	Lumbar Sympathetic Nerve		Lower Femur, Left
Lumbar lymph node	Lymphatic, Aortic	Medial epicondyle of humerus	Humeral Shaft, Right
Lumbar lymphatic trunk	Cisterna Chyli		Humeral Shaft, Left
Lumbar splanchnic nerve	Lumbar Sympathetic Nerve	Medial malleolus	Tibia, Left
Lumbosacral facet joint	Lumbosacral Joint		Tibia, Right
Lumbosacral trunk	Lumbar Nerve	Medial meniscus	Knee Joint, Right
Lunate bone	Carpal, Left		Knee Joint, Left
	Carpal, Right	Medial plantar artery	Foot Artery, Right
Lunotriquetral ligament	Hand Bursa and Ligament, Right		Foot Artery, Left
	Hand Bursa and Ligament, Left	Medial plantar nerve	Tibial Nerve
Macula	Retina, Left	Medial popliteal nerve	Tibial Nerve
	Retina, Right	Medial rectus muscle	Extraocular Muscle, Right
Malleus	Auditory Ossicle, Right		Extraocular Muscle, Left
	Auditory Ossicle, Left	Medial sural cutaneous nerve	Tibial Nerve
Mammary duct	Breast, Bilateral	Median antebrachial vein	Basilic Vein, Right
	Breast, Left		Basilic Vein, Left
	Breast, Right	Median cubital vein	Basilic Vein, Right
Mammary gland	Breast, Bilateral		Basilic Vein, Left
	Breast, Left	Median sacral artery	Abdominal Aorta
	Breast, Right	Mediastinal lymph node	Lymphatic, Thorax
Mammillary body	Hypothalamus	Meissner's (submucous) plexus	Abdominal Sympathetic Nerve
Mandibular nerve	Trigeminal Nerve	Membranous urethra	Urethra
Mandibular notch	Mandible, Left	Mental foramen	Mandible, Left
	Mandible, Right		Mandible, Right
Manubrium	Sternum	Mentalis muscle	Facial Muscle
Masseter muscle	Head Muscle	Mesoappendix	Mesentery
Masseteric fascia	Subcutaneous Tissue and Fascia, Face	Mesocolon	Mesentery
Mastoid (postauricular) lymph node	Lymphatic, Left Neck	Metacarpal ligament	Hand Bursa and Ligament, Right
	Lymphatic, Right Neck		Hand Bursa and Ligament, Left
Mastoid air cells	Mastoid Sinus, Right	Metacarpophalangeal ligament	Hand Bursa and Ligament, Right
	Mastoid Sinus, Left		Hand Bursa and Ligament, Left
Mastoid process	Temporal Bone, Right	Metatarsal ligament	Foot Bursa and Ligament, Right
	Temporal Bone, Left		Foot Bursa and Ligament, Left
Maxillary artery	External Carotid Artery, Right	Metatarsophalangeal ligament	Foot Bursa and Ligament, Right
	External Carotid Artery, Left		Foot Bursa and Ligament, Left
Maxillary nerve	Trigeminal Nerve		

Anatomical Term	PCS Description
Metatarsophalangeal (MTP) joint	Metatarsal-Phalangeal Joint, Right
	Metatarsal-Phalangeal Joint, Left
Metathalamus	Thalamus
Midcarpal joint	Carpal Joint, Right
	Carpal Joint, Left
Middle cardiac nerve	Thoracic Sympathetic Nerve
Middle cerebral artery	Intracranial Artery
Middle cerebral vein	Intracranial Vein
Middle colic vein	Colic Vein
Middle genicular artery	Popliteal Artery, Right
	Popliteal Artery, Left
Middle hemorrhoidal vein	Hypogastric Vein, Right
	Hypogastric Vein, Left
Middle rectal artery	Internal Iliac Artery, Right
	Internal Iliac Artery, Left
Middle suprarenal artery	Abdominal Aorta
Middle temporal artery	Temporal Artery, Right
	Temporal Artery, Left
Middle turbinate	Nasal Turbinate
Mitral annulus	Mitral Valve
Molar gland	Buccal Mucosa
Musculocutaneous nerve	Brachial Plexus
Musculophrenic artery	Internal Mammary Artery, Right
	Internal Mammary Artery, Left
Musculospiral nerve	Radial Nerve
Myelencephalon	Medulla Oblongata
Myenteric (Auerbach's) plexus	Abdominal Sympathetic Nerve
Myometrium	Uterus
Nail bed	Finger Nail
	Toe Nail
Nail plate	Finger Nail
	Toe Nail
Nasal cavity	Nose
Nasal concha	Nasal Turbinate
Nasalis muscle	Facial Muscle
Nasolacrimal duct	Lacrimal Duct, Right
	Lacrimal Duct, Left
Navicular bone	Tarsal, Left
	Tarsal, Right
Neck of femur	Upper Femur, Right
	Upper Femur, Left
Neck of humerus (anatomical) (surgical)	Humeral Head, Right
	Humeral Head, Left
Nerve to the stapedius	Facial Nerve
Neurohypophysis	Pituitary Gland
Ninth cranial nerve	Glossopharyngeal Nerve
Nostril	Nose

Anatomical Term	PCS Description
Obturator artery	Internal Iliac Artery, Right
	Internal Iliac Artery, Left
Obturator lymph node	Lymphatic, Pelvis
Obturator muscle	Hip Muscle, Right
	Hip Muscle, Left
Obturator nerve	Lumbar Plexus
Obturator vein	Hypogastric Vein, Right
	Hypogastric Vein, Left
Obtuse margin	Heart, Left
Occipital artery	External Carotid Artery, Right
	External Carotid Artery, Left
Occipital lobe	Cerebral Hemisphere
Occipital lymph node	Lymphatic, Left Neck
	Lymphatic, Right Neck
Occipitofrontalis muscle	Facial Muscle
Olecranon bursa	Elbow Bursa and Ligament, Right
	Elbow Bursa and Ligament, Left
Olecranon process	Ulna, Left
	Ulna, Right
Olfactory bulb	Olfactory Nerve
Ophthalmic artery	Internal Carotid Artery, Right
	Internal Carotid Artery, Left
Ophthalmic nerve	Trigeminal Nerve
Ophthalmic vein	Intracranial Vein
Optic chiasma	Optic Nerve
Optic disc	Retina, Left
	Retina, Right
Optic foramen	Sphenoid Bone, Right
	Sphenoid Bone, Left
Orbicularis oculi muscle	Upper Eyelid, Right
	Upper Eyelid, Left
Orbicularis oris muscle	Facial Muscle
Orbital fascia	Subcutaneous Tissue and Fascia, Face
Orbital portion of ethmoid bone	Orbit, Left
	Orbit, Right
Orbital portion of frontal bone	Orbit, Left
	Orbit, Right
Orbital portion of lacrimal bone	Orbit, Left
	Orbit, Right
Orbital portion of maxilla	Orbit, Left
	Orbit, Right
Orbital portion of palatine bone	Orbit, Left
	Orbit, Right
Orbital portion of sphenoid bone	Orbit, Left
	Orbit, Right
Orbital portion of zygomatic bone	Orbit, Left
	Orbit, Right

© 2015 Optum360, LLC

Anatomical Term	PCS Description
Oropharynx	Pharynx
Ossicular chain	Auditory Ossicle, Right
	Auditory Ossicle, Left
Otic ganglion	Head and Neck Sympathetic Nerve
Oval window	Middle Ear, Left
	Middle Ear, Right
Ovarian artery	Abdominal Aorta
Ovarian ligament	Uterine Supporting Structure
Oviduct	Fallopian Tube, Right
	Fallopian Tube, Left
Palatine gland	Buccal Mucosa
Palatine tonsil	Tonsils
Palatine uvula	Uvula
Palatoglossal muscle	Tongue, Palate, Pharynx Muscle
Palatopharyngeal muscle	Tongue, Palate, Pharynx Muscle
Palmar (volar) metacarpal vein	Hand Vein, Right
	Hand Vein, Left
Palmar (volar) digital vein	Hand Vein, Left
	Hand Vein, Right
Palmar cutaneous nerve	Median Nerve
	Radial Nerve
Palmar fascia (aponeurosis)	Subcutaneous Tissue and Fascia, Right Hand
	Subcutaneous Tissue and Fascia, Left Hand
Palmar interosseous muscle	Hand Muscle, Right
	Hand Muscle, Left
Palmar ulnocarpal ligament	Wrist Bursa and Ligament, Right
	Wrist Bursa and Ligament, Left
Palmaris longus muscle	Lower Arm and Wrist Muscle, Right
	Lower Arm and Wrist Muscle, Left
Pancreatic artery	Splenic Artery
Pancreatic plexus	Abdominal Sympathetic Nerve
Pancreatic vein	Splenic Vein
Pancreaticosplenic lymph node	Lymphatic, Aortic
Paraaortic lymph node	Lymphatic, Aortic
Pararectal lymph node	Lymphatic, Mesenteric
Parasternal lymph node	Lymphatic, Thorax
Paratracheal lymph node	Lymphatic, Thorax
Paraurethral (Skene's) gland	Vestibular Gland
Parietal lobe	Cerebral Hemisphere
Parotid lymph node	Lymphatic, Head
Parotid plexus	Facial Nerve
Pars flaccida	Tympanic Membrane, Right
	Tympanic Membrane, Left
Patellar ligament	Knee Bursa and Ligament, Right
	Knee Bursa and Ligament, Left

Anatomical Term	PCS Description
Patellar tendon	Knee Tendon, Right
	Knee Tendon, Left
Patellofemoral joint	Knee Joint, Right
	Knee Joint, Left
	Knee Joint, Femoral Surface, Right
	Knee Joint, Femoral Surface, Left
Pectineus muscle	Upper Leg Muscle, Right
	Upper Leg Muscle, Left
Pectoral (anterior) lymph node	Lymphatic, Left Axillary
	Lymphatic, Right Axillary
Pectoral fascia	Subcutaneous Tissue and Fascia, Chest
Pectoralis major muscle	Thorax Muscle, Left
	Thorax Muscle, Right
Pectoralis minor muscle	Thorax Muscle, Left
	Thorax Muscle, Right
Pelvic splanchnic nerve	Abdominal Sympathetic Nerve
	Sacral Sympathetic Nerve
Penile urethra	Urethra
Pericardiophrenic artery	Internal Mammary Artery, Right
	Internal Mammary Artery, Left
Perimetrium	Uterus
Peroneus brevis muscle	Lower Leg Muscle, Right
	Lower Leg Muscle, Left
Peroneus longus muscle	Lower Leg Muscle, Right
	Lower Leg Muscle, Left
Petrous part of temporal bone	Temporal Bone, Right
	Temporal Bone, Left
Pharyngeal constrictor muscle	Tongue, Palate, Pharynx Muscle
Pharyngeal plexus	Vagus Nerve
Pharyngeal recess	Nasopharynx
Pharyngeal tonsil	Adenoids
Pharyngotympanic tube	Eustachian Tube, Right
	Eustachian Tube, Left
Pia mater, intracranial	Cerebral Meninges
Pia mater, spinal	Spinal Meninges
Pinna	External Ear, Right
	External Ear, Left
	External Ear, Bilateral
Piriform recess (sinus)	Pharynx
Piriformis muscle	Hip Muscle, Right
	Hip Muscle, Left
Pisiform bone	Carpal, Left
	Carpal, Right
Pisohamate ligament	Hand Bursa and Ligament, Right
	Hand Bursa and Ligament, Left
Pisometacarpal ligament	Hand Bursa and Ligament, Right
	Hand Bursa and Ligament, Left

Appendix B. Body Part Key—Body Part Key: Alphabetic, by specific body site

Anatomical Term	PCS Description
Plantar digital vein	Foot Vein, Left
	Foot Vein, Right
Plantar fascia (aponeurosis)	Subcutaneous Tissue and Fascia, Right Foot
	Subcutaneous Tissue and Fascia, Left Foot
Plantar metatarsal vein	Foot Vein, Left
	Foot Vein, Right
Plantar venous arch	Foot Vein, Left
	Foot Vein, Right
Platysma muscle	Neck Muscle, Right
	Neck Muscle, Left
Plica semilunaris	Conjunctiva, Right
	Conjunctiva, Left
Pneumogastric nerve	Vagus Nerve
Pneumotaxic center	Pons
Pontine tegmentum	Pons
Popliteal ligament	Knee Bursa and Ligament, Right
	Knee Bursa and Ligament, Left
Popliteal lymph node	Lymphatic, Left Lower Extremity
	Lymphatic, Right Lower Extremity
Popliteal vein	Femoral Vein, Right
	Femoral Vein, Left
Popliteus muscle	Lower Leg Muscle, Right
	Lower Leg Muscle, Left
Postauricular (mastoid) lymph node	Lymphatic, Left Neck
	Lymphatic, Right Neck
Postcava	Inferior Vena Cava
Posterior (subscapular) lymph node	Lymphatic, Left Axillary
	Lymphatic, Right Axillary
Posterior auricular artery	External Carotid Artery, Right
	External Carotid Artery, Left
Posterior auricular nerve	Facial Nerve
Posterior auricular vein	External Jugular Vein, Right
	External Jugular Vein, Left
Posterior cerebral artery	Intracranial Artery
Posterior chamber	Eye, Left
	Eye, Right
Posterior circumflex humeral artery	Axillary Artery, Right
	Axillary Artery, Left
Posterior communicating artery	Intracranial Artery
Posterior cruciate ligament (PCL)	Knee Bursa and Ligament, Right
	Knee Bursa and Ligament, Left
Posterior facial (retromandibular) vein	Face Vein, Left
	Face Vein, Right
Posterior femoral cutaneous nerve	Sacral Plexus

Anatomical Term	PCS Description
Posterior inferior cerebellar artery (PICA)	Intracranial Artery
Posterior interosseous nerve	Radial Nerve
Posterior labial nerve	Pudendal Nerve
Posterior scrotal nerve	Pudendal Nerve
Posterior spinal artery	Vertebral Artery, Right
	Vertebral Artery, Left
Posterior tibial recurrent artery	Anterior Tibial Artery, Right
	Anterior Tibial Artery, Left
Posterior ulnar recurrent artery	Ulnar Artery, Right
	Ulnar Artery, Left
Posterior vagal trunk	Vagus Nerve
Preauricular lymph node	Lymphatic, Head
Precava	Superior Vena Cava
Prepatellar bursa	Knee Bursa and Ligament, Right
	Knee Bursa and Ligament, Left
Pretracheal fascia	Subcutaneous Tissue and Fascia, Anterior Neck
Prevertebral fascia	Subcutaneous Tissue and Fascia, Posterior Neck
Princeps pollicis artery	Hand Artery, Right
	Hand Artery, Left
Procerus muscle	Facial Muscle
Profunda brachii	Brachial Artery, Right
	Brachial Artery, Left
Profunda femoris (deep femoral) vein	Femoral Vein, Right
	Femoral Vein, Left
Pronator quadratus muscle	Lower Arm and Wrist Muscle, Right
	Lower Arm and Wrist Muscle, Left
Pronator teres muscle	Lower Arm and Wrist Muscle, Right
	Lower Arm and Wrist Muscle, Left
Prostatic urethra	Urethra
Proximal radioulnar joint	Elbow Joint, Right
	Elbow Joint, Left
Psoas muscle	Hip Muscle, Right
	Hip Muscle, Left
Pterygoid muscle	Head Muscle
Pterygoid process	Sphenoid Bone, Right
	Sphenoid Bone, Left
Pterygopalatine (sphenopalatine) ganglion	Head and Neck Sympathetic Nerve
Pubic ligament	Trunk Bursa and Ligament, Right
	Trunk Bursa and Ligament, Left
Pubis	Pelvic Bone, Right
	Pelvic Bone, Left
Pubofemoral ligament	Hip Bursa and Ligament, Right
	Hip Bursa and Ligament, Left

Anatomical Term	PCS Description	Anatomical Term	PCS Description
Pudendal nerve	Sacral Plexus	Renal calyx	Kidney
Pulmoaortic canal	Pulmonary Artery, Left		Kidney, Left
Pulmonary annulus	Pulmonary Valve		Kidney, Right
Pulmonary plexus	Thoracic Sympathetic Nerve		Kidneys, Bilateral
	Vagus Nerve	Renal capsule	Kidney
Pulmonic valve	Pulmonary Valve		Kidney, Left
Pulvinar	Thalamus		Kidney, Right
Pyloric antrum	Stomach, Pylorus		Kidneys, Bilateral
Pyloric canal	Stomach, Pylorus	Renal cortex	Kidney
Pyloric sphincter	Stomach, Pylorus		Kidney, Left
Pyramidalis muscle	Abdomen Muscle, Right		Kidney, Right
	Abdomen Muscle, Left		Kidneys, Bilateral
Quadrangular cartilage	Nasal Septum	Renal plexus	Abdominal Sympathetic Nerve
Quadrate lobe	Liver	Renal segment	Kidney
Quadratus femoris muscle	Hip Muscle, Right		Kidney, Left
	Hip Muscle, Left		Kidney, Right
Quadratus lumborum muscle	Trunk Muscle, Right		Kidneys, Bilateral
	Trunk Muscle, Left	Renal segmental artery	Renal Artery, Right
Quadratus plantae muscle	Foot Muscle, Right		Renal Artery, Left
	Foot Muscle, Left	Retroperitoneal lymph node	Lymphatic, Aortic
Quadriceps (femoris)	Upper Leg Muscle, Right	Retroperitoneal space	Retroperitoneum
	Upper Leg Muscle, Left	Retropharyngeal lymph node	Lymphatic, Left Neck
Radial collateral ligament	Elbow Bursa and Ligament, Right		Lymphatic, Right Neck
	Elbow Bursa and Ligament, Left	Retropubic space	Pelvic Cavity
Radial collateral carpal ligament	Wrist Bursa and Ligament, Right	Rhinopharynx	Nasopharynx
	Wrist Bursa and Ligament, Left	Rhomboid major muscle	Trunk Muscle, Right
Radial notch	Ulna, Left		Trunk Muscle, Left
	Ulna, Right	Rhomboid minor muscle	Trunk Muscle, Right
Radial recurrent artery	Radial Artery, Right		Trunk Muscle, Left
	Radial Artery, Left	Right ascending lumbar vein	Azygos Vein
Radial vein	Brachial Vein, Right	Right atrioventricular valve	Tricuspid Valve
	Brachial Vein, Left	Right auricular appendix	Atrium, Right
Radialis indicis	Hand Artery, Right	Right colic vein	Colic Vein
	Hand Artery, Left	Right coronary sulcus	Heart, Right
Radiocarpal joint	Wrist Joint, Right	Right gastric artery	Gastric Artery
	Wrist Joint, Left	Right gastroepiploic vein	Superior Mesenteric Vein
Radiocarpal ligament	Wrist Bursa and Ligament, Right	Right inferior phrenic vein	Inferior Vena Cava
	Wrist Bursa and Ligament, Left	Right inferior pulmonary vein	Pulmonary Vein, Right
Rectosigmoid junction	Sigmoid Colon	Right jugular trunk	Lymphatic, Right Neck
Radioulnar ligament	Wrist Bursa and Ligament, Right	Right lateral ventricle	Cerebral Ventricle
	Wrist Bursa and Ligament, Left	Right lymphatic duct	Lymphatic, Right Neck
Rectus abdominis muscle	Abdomen Muscle, Right	Right ovarian vein	Inferior Vena Cava
	Abdomen Muscle, Left	Right second lumbar vein	Inferior Vena Cava
Rectus femoris muscle	Upper Leg Muscle, Right	Right subclavian trunk	Lymphatic, Right Neck
	Upper Leg Muscle, Left		
Recurrent laryngeal nerve	Vagus Nerve		

Appendix B. Body Part Key—Body Part Key: Alphabetic, by specific body site

Anatomical Term	PCS Description
Right subcostal vein	Azygos Vein
Right superior pulmonary vein	Pulmonary Vein, Right
Right suprarenal vein	Inferior Vena Cava
Right testicular vein	Inferior Vena Cava
Rima glottidis	Larynx
Risorius muscle	Facial Muscle
Round ligament of uterus	Uterine Supporting Structure
Round window	Inner Ear, Left
	Inner Ear, Right
Sacral ganglion	Sacral Sympathetic Nerve
Sacral lymph node	Lymphatic, Pelvis
Sacral splanchnic nerve	Sacral Sympathetic Nerve
Sacrococcygeal ligament	Trunk Bursa and Ligament, Right
	Trunk Bursa and Ligament, Left
Sacrococcygeal symphysis	Sacrococcygeal Joint
Sacroiliac ligament	Trunk Bursa and Ligament, Right
	Trunk Bursa and Ligament, Left
Sacrospinous ligament	Trunk Bursa and Ligament, Right
	Trunk Bursa and Ligament, Left
Sacrotuberous ligament	Trunk Bursa and Ligament, Right
	Trunk Bursa and Ligament, Left
Salpingopharyngeus muscle	Tongue, Palate, Pharynx Muscle
Salpinx	Fallopian Tube, Left
	Fallopian Tube, Right
Saphenous nerve	Femoral Nerve
Sartorius muscle	Upper Leg Muscle, Right
	Upper Leg Muscle, Left
Scalene muscle	Neck Muscle, Right
	Neck Muscle, Left
Scaphoid bone	Carpal, Left
	Carpal, Right
Scapholunate ligament	Hand Bursa and Ligament, Right
	Hand Bursa and Ligament, Left
Scaphotrapezium ligament	Hand Bursa and Ligament, Right
	Hand Bursa and Ligament, Left
Scarpa's (vestibular) ganglion	Acoustic Nerve
Sebaceous gland	Skin
Second cranial nerve	Optic Nerve
Sella turcica	Sphenoid Bone, Right
	Sphenoid Bone, Left
Semicircular canal	Inner Ear, Left
	Inner Ear, Right
Semimembranosus muscle	Upper Leg Muscle, Right
	Upper Leg Muscle, Left

Anatomical Term	PCS Description
Semitendinosus muscle	Upper Leg Muscle, Right
	Upper Leg Muscle, Left
Septal cartilage	Nasal Septum
Serratus anterior muscle	Thorax Muscle, Right
	Thorax Muscle, Left
Serratus posterior muscle	Trunk Muscle, Right
	Trunk Muscle, Left
Seventh cranial nerve	Facial Nerve
Short gastric artery	Splenic Artery
Sigmoid artery	Inferior Mesenteric Artery
Sigmoid flexure	Sigmoid Colon
Sigmoid vein	Inferior Mesenteric Vein
Sinoatrial node	Conduction Mechanism
Sinus venosus	Atrium, Right
Sixth cranial nerve	Abducens Nerve
Skene's (paraurethral) gland	Vestibular Gland
Small saphenous vein	Lesser Saphenous Vein, Right
	Lesser Saphenous Vein, Left
Solar (celiac) plexus	Abdominal Sympathetic Nerve
Soleus muscle	Lower Leg Muscle, Right
	Lower Leg Muscle, Left
Sphenomandibular ligament	Head and Neck Bursa and Ligament
Sphenopalatine (pterygopalatine) ganglion	Head and Neck Sympathetic Nerve
Spinal nerve, cervical	Cervical Nerve
Spinal nerve, lumbar	Lumbar Nerve
Spinal nerve, sacral	Sacral Nerve
Spinal nerve, thoracic	Thoracic Nerve
Spinous process	Cervical Vertebra
	Lumbar Vertebra
	Thoracic Vertebra
Spiral ganglion	Acoustic Nerve
Splenic flexure	Transverse Colon
Splenic plexus	Abdominal Sympathetic Nerve
Splenius capitis muscle	Head Muscle
Splenius cervicis muscle	Neck Muscle, Right
	Neck Muscle, Left
Stapes	Auditory Ossicle, Right
	Auditory Ossicle, Left
Stellate ganglion	Head and Neck Sympathetic Nerve
Stensen's duct	Parotid Duct, Right
	Parotid Duct, Left
Sternoclavicular ligament	Shoulder Bursa and Ligament, Right
	Shoulder Bursa and Ligament, Left
Sternocleidomastoid artery	Thyroid Artery, Right
	Thyroid Artery, Left

© 2015 Optum360, LLC

Anatomical Term	PCS Description
Sternocleidomastoid muscle	Neck Muscle, Right
	Neck Muscle, Left
Sternocostal ligament	Thorax Bursa and Ligament, Right
	Thorax Bursa and Ligament, Left
Styloglossus muscle	Tongue, Palate, Pharynx Muscle
Stylomandibular ligament	Head and Neck Bursa and Ligament
Stylopharyngeus muscle	Tongue, Palate, Pharynx Muscle
Subacromial bursa	Shoulder Bursa and Ligament, Right
	Shoulder Bursa and Ligament, Left
Subaortic (common iliac) lymph node	Lymphatic, Pelvis
Subarachnoid space, intracranial	Subarachnoid Space
Subarachnoid space, spinal	Spinal Canal
Subclavicular (apical) lymph node	Lymphatic, Left Axillary
	Lymphatic, Right Axillary
Subclavius muscle	Thorax Muscle, Right
	Thorax Muscle, Left
Subclavius nerve	Brachial Plexus
Subcostal artery	Thoracic Aorta
Subcostal muscle	Thorax Muscle, Right
	Thorax Muscle, Left
Subcostal nerve	Thoracic Nerve
Subdural space, intracranial	Subdural Space
Subdural space, spinal	Spinal Canal
Submandibular ganglion	Facial Nerve
	Head and Neck Sympathetic Nerve
Submandibular gland	Submaxillary Gland, Right
	Submaxillary Gland, Left
Submandibular lymph node	Lymphatic, Head
Submaxillary ganglion	Head and Neck Sympathetic Nerve
Submaxillary lymph node	Lymphatic, Head
Submental artery	Face Artery
Submental lymph node	Lymphatic, Head
Submucous (Meissner's) plexus	Abdominal Sympathetic Nerve
Suboccipital nerve	Cervical Nerve
Suboccipital venous plexus	Vertebral Vein, Right
	Vertebral Vein, Left
Subparotid lymph node	Lymphatic, Head
Subscapular aponeurosis	Subcutaneous Tissue and Fascia, Right Upper Arm
	Subcutaneous Tissue and Fascia, Left Upper Arm
Subscapular artery	Axillary Artery, Right
	Axillary Artery, Left

Anatomical Term	PCS Description
Subscapular (posterior) lymph node	Lymphatic, Left Axillary
	Lymphatic, Right Axillary
Subscapularis muscle	Shoulder Muscle, Right
	Shoulder Muscle, Left
Substantia nigra	Basal Ganglia
Subtalar (talocalcaneal) joint	Tarsal Joint, Right
	Tarsal Joint, Left
Subtalar ligament	Foot Bursa and Ligament, Right
	Foot Bursa and Ligament, Left
Subthalamic nucleus	Basal Ganglia
Superficial epigastric artery	Femoral Artery, Left
	Femoral Artery, Right
Superficial epigastric vein	Greater Saphenous Vein, Left
	Greater Saphenous Vein, Right
Superficial circumflex iliac vein	Greater Saphenous Vein, Left
	Greater Saphenous Vein, Right
Superficial palmar arch	Hand Artery, Right
	Hand Artery, Left
Superficial palmar venous arch	Hand Vein, Left
	Hand Vein, Right
Superficial transverse perineal muscle	Perineum Muscle
Superficial temporal artery	Temporal Artery, Right
	Temporal Artery, Left
Superior cardiac nerve	Thoracic Sympathetic Nerve
Superior cerebellar vein	Intracranial Vein
Superior cerebral vein	Intracranial Vein
Superior clunic (cluneal) nerve	Lumbar Nerve
Superior epigastric artery	Internal Mammary Artery, Right
	Internal Mammary Artery, Left
Superior genicular artery	Popliteal Artery, Right
	Popliteal Artery, Left
Superior gluteal artery	Internal Iliac Artery, Right
	Internal Iliac Artery, Left
Superior gluteal nerve	Lumbar Plexus
Superior hypogastric plexus	Abdominal Sympathetic Nerve
Superior labial artery	Face Artery
Superior laryngeal artery	Thyroid Artery, Right
	Thyroid Artery, Left
Superior laryngeal nerve	Vagus Nerve
Superior longitudinal muscle	Tongue, Palate, Pharynx Muscle
Superior mesenteric ganglion	Abdominal Sympathetic Nerve
Superior mesenteric lymph node	Lymphatic, Mesenteric

Anatomical Term	PCS Description	Anatomical Term	PCS Description
Superior mesenteric plexus	Abdominal Sympathetic Nerve	Sweat gland	Skin
Superior oblique muscle	Extraocular Muscle, Right	Talocalcaneal ligament	Foot Bursa and Ligament, Right
	Extraocular Muscle, Left		Foot Bursa and Ligament, Left
Superior olivary nucleus	Pons	Talocalcaneal (subtalar) joint	Tarsal Joint, Right
Superior rectal artery	Inferior Mesenteric Artery		Tarsal Joint, Left
Superior rectal vein	Inferior Mesenteric Vein	Talocalcaneonavicular joint	Tarsal Joint, Right
Superior rectus muscle	Extraocular Muscle, Right		Tarsal Joint, Left
	Extraocular Muscle, Left	Talocalcaneonavicular ligament	Foot Bursa and Ligament, Right
Superior tarsal plate	Upper Eyelid, Right		Foot Bursa and Ligament, Left
	Upper Eyelid, Left	Talocrural joint	Ankle Joint, Right
Superior thoracic artery	Axillary Artery, Right		Ankle Joint, Left
	Axillary Artery, Left	Talofibular ligament	Ankle Bursa and Ligament, Right
Superior thyroid artery	External Carotid Artery, Right		Ankle Bursa and Ligament, Left
	External Carotid Artery, Left	Talus bone	Tarsal, Left
	Thyroid Artery, Right		Tarsal, Right
	Thyroid Artery, Left	Tarsometatarsal joint	Metatarsal-Tarsal Joint, Right
Superior turbinate	Nasal Turbinate		Metatarsal-Tarsal Joint, Left
Superior ulnar collateral artery	Brachial Artery, Right	Tarsometatarsal ligament	Foot Bursa and Ligament, Right
	Brachial Artery, Left		Foot Bursa and Ligament, Left
Supraclavicular nerve	Cervical Plexus	Temporal lobe	Cerebral Hemisphere
Supraclavicular (Virchow's) lymph node	Lymphatic, Left Neck	Temporalis muscle	Head Muscle
	Lymphatic, Right Neck	Temporoparietalis muscle	Head Muscle
Suprahyoid lymph node	Lymphatic, Head	Tensor fasciae latae muscle	Hip Muscle, Right
Suprahyoid muscle	Neck Muscle, Right		Hip Muscle, Left
	Neck Muscle, Left	Tensor veli palatini muscle	Tongue, Palate, Pharynx Muscle
Suprainguinal lymph node	Lymphatic, Pelvis	Tenth cranial nerve	Vagus Nerve
Supraorbital vein	Face Vein, Left	Tentorium cerebelli	Dura Mater
	Face Vein, Right	Teres major muscle	Shoulder Muscle, Right
Suprarenal gland	Adrenal Glands, Bilateral		Shoulder Muscle, Left
	Adrenal Gland, Right	Teres minor muscle	Shoulder Muscle, Right
	Adrenal Gland, Left		Shoulder Muscle, Left
	Adrenal Gland	Testicular artery	Abdominal Aorta
Suprarenal plexus	Abdominal Sympathetic Nerve	Thenar muscle	Hand Muscle, Right
Suprascapular nerve	Brachial Plexus		Hand Muscle, Left
Supraspinatus fascia	Subcutaneous Tissue and Fascia, Right Upper Arm	Third cranial nerve	Oculomotor Nerve
		Third occipital nerve	Cervical Nerve
	Subcutaneous Tissue and Fascia, Left Upper Arm	Third ventricle	Cerebral Ventricle
		Thoracic aortic plexus	Thoracic Sympathetic Nerve
Supraspinatus muscle	Shoulder Muscle, Right	Thoracic esophagus	Esophagus, Middle
	Shoulder Muscle, Left	Thoracic facet joint	Thoracic Vertebral Joint
Supraspinous ligament	Trunk Bursa and Ligament, Right	Thoracic ganglion	Thoracic Sympathetic Nerve
	Trunk Bursa and Ligament, Left	Thoracoacromial artery	Axillary Artery, Right
Suprasternal notch	Sternum		Axillary Artery, Left
Supratrochlear lymph node	Lymphatic, Left Upper Extremity	Thoracolumbar facet joint	Thoracolumbar Vertebral Joint
	Lymphatic, Right Upper Extremity		
Sural artery	Popliteal Artery, Right	Thymus gland	Thymus
	Popliteal Artery, Left		

Anatomical Term	PCS Description	Anatomical Term	PCS Description
Thyroarytenoid muscle	Neck Muscle, Right	Triquetral bone	Carpal, Left
	Neck Muscle, Left		Carpal, Right
Thyrocervical trunk	Thyroid Artery, Right	Trochanteric bursa	Hip Bursa and Ligament, Right
	Thyroid Artery, Left		Hip Bursa and Ligament, Left
Thyroid cartilage	Larynx	Twelfth cranial nerve	Hypoglossal Nerve
Tibialis anterior muscle	Lower Leg Muscle, Right	Tympanic cavity	Middle Ear, Right
	Lower Leg Muscle, Left		Middle Ear, Left
Tibialis posterior muscle	Lower Leg Muscle, Right	Tympanic nerve	Glossopharyngeal Nerve
	Lower Leg Muscle, Left	Tympanic part of temoporal bone	Temporal Bone, Right
Tibiofemoral joint	Knee Joint, Right		Temporal Bone, Left
	Knee Joint, Left	Ulnar collateral ligament	Elbow Bursa and Ligament, Right
	Knee Joint, Tibial Surface, Right		Elbow Bursa and Ligament, Left
	Knee Joint, Tibial Surface, Left	Ulnar collateral carpal ligament	Wrist Bursa and Ligament, Right
Tracheobronchial lymph node	Lymphatic, Thorax		Wrist Bursa and Ligament, Left
Tragus	External Ear, Right	Ulnar notch	Radius, Left
	External Ear, Left		Radius, Right
	External Ear, Bilateral	Ulnar vein	Brachial Vein, Right
Transversalis fascia	Subcutaneous Tissue and Fascia, Trunk		Brachial Vein, Left
Transverse acetabular ligament	Hip Bursa and Ligament, Left	Umbilical artery	Internal Iliac Artery, Right
	Hip Bursa and Ligament, Right		Internal Iliac Artery, Left
Transverse (cutaneous) cervical nerve	Cervical Plexus	Ureteral orifice	Ureter
			Ureter, Left
Transverse facial artery	Temporal Artery, Right		Ureter, Right
	Temporal Artery, Left		Ureters, Bilateral
Transverse humeral ligament	Shoulder Bursa and Ligament, Right	Ureteropelvic junction (UPJ)	Kidney Pelvis, Right
	Shoulder Bursa and Ligament, Left		Kidney Pelvis, Left
Transverse ligament of atlas	Head and Neck Bursa and Ligament	Ureterovesical orifice	Ureter, Left
			Ureter, Right
Transverse scapular ligament	Shoulder Bursa and Ligament, Right	Uterine artery	Internal Iliac Artery, Right
	Shoulder Bursa and Ligament, Left		Internal Iliac Artery, Left
Transverse thoracis muscle	Thorax Muscle, Right	Uterine cornu	Uterus
	Thorax Muscle, Left	Uterine tube	Fallopian Tube, Right
Transversospinalis muscle	Trunk Muscle, Right		Fallopian Tube, Left
	Trunk Muscle, Left	Uterine vein	Hypogastric Vein, Right
Transversus abdominis muscle	Abdomen Muscle, Right		Hypogastric Vein, Left
	Abdomen Muscle, Left	Vaginal artery	Internal Iliac Artery, Right
Trapezium bone	Carpal, Left		Internal Iliac Artery, Left
	Carpal, Right	Vaginal vein	Hypogastric Vein, Right
Trapezius muscle	Trunk Muscle, Right		Hypogastric Vein, Left
	Trunk Muscle, Left	Vastus intermedius muscle	Upper Leg Muscle, Right
Trapezoid bone	Carpal, Left		Upper Leg Muscle, Left
	Carpal, Right	Vastus lateralis muscle	Upper Leg Muscle, Right
Triceps brachii muscle	Upper Arm Muscle, Right		Upper Leg Muscle, Left
	Upper Arm Muscle, Left	Vastus medialis muscle	Upper Leg Muscle, Right
Tricuspid annulus	Tricuspid Valve		Upper Leg Muscle, Left
Trifacial nerve	Trigeminal Nerve	Ventricular fold	Larynx
Trigone of bladder	Bladder	Vermiform appendix	Appendix

Anatomical Term	PCS Description
Vermilion border	Lower Lip
	Upper Lip
Vertebral arch	Cervical Vertebra
	Lumbar Vertebra
	Thoracic Vertebra
Vertebral canal	Spinal Canal
Vertebral foramen	Cervical Vertebra
	Lumbar Vertebra
	Thoracic Vertebra
Vertebral lamina	Cervical Vertebra
	Lumbar Vertebra
	Thoracic Vertebra
Vertebral pedicle	Cervical Vertebra
	Lumbar Vertebra
	Thoracic Vertebra
Vesical vein	Hypogastric Vein, Right
	Hypogastric Vein, Left
Vestibular (Scarpa's) ganglion	Acoustic Nerve
Vestibular nerve	Acoustic Nerve
Vestibulocochlear nerve	Acoustic Nerve

Anatomical Term	PCS Description
Virchow's (supraclavicular) lymph node	Lymphatic, Left Neck
	Lymphatic, Right Neck
Vitreous body	Vitreous, Left
	Vitreous, Right
Vocal fold	Vocal Cord, Right
	Vocal Cord, Left
Volar (palmar) digital vein	Hand Vein, Left
	Hand Vein, Right
Volar (palmar) metacarpal vein	Hand Vein, Left
	Hand Vein, Right
Vomer bone	Nasal Septum
Vomer of nasal septum	Nasal Bone
Xiphoid process	Sternum
Zonule of Zinn	Lens, Left
	Lens, Right
Zygomatic process of frontal bone	Frontal Bone, Right
	Frontal Bone, Left
Zygomatic process of temporal bone	Temporal Bone, Right
	Temporal Bone, Left
Zygomaticus muscle	Facial Muscle

Appendix C. Body Part Definitions

Body Part Definitions: Alphabetic, by PCS character description

Anatomical Term	PCS Description
1st Toe, Left 1st Toe, Right	Includes: Hallux
Abdomen Muscle, Left Abdomen Muscle, Right	Includes: External oblique muscle Internal oblique muscle Pyramidalis muscle Rectus abdominis muscle Transversus abdominis muscle
Abdominal Aorta	Includes: Inferior phrenic artery Lumbar artery Median sacral artery Middle suprarenal artery Ovarian artery Testicular artery
Abdominal Sympathetic Nerve	Includes: Abdominal aortic plexus Auerbach's (myenteric) plexus Celiac (solar) plexus Celiac ganglion Gastric plexus Hepatic plexus Inferior hypogastric plexus Inferior mesenteric ganglion Inferior mesenteric plexus Meissner's (submucous) plexus Myenteric (Auerbach's) plexus Pancreatic plexus Pelvic splanchnic nerve Renal plexus Solar (celiac) plexus Splenic plexus Submucous (Meissner's) plexus Superior hypogastric plexus Superior mesenteric ganglion Superior mesenteric plexus Suprarenal plexus
Abducens Nerve	Includes: Sixth cranial nerve
Accessory Nerve	Includes: Eleventh cranial nerve
Acoustic Nerve	Includes: Cochlear nerve Eighth cranial nerve Scarpa's (vestibular) ganglion Spiral ganglion Vestibular (Scarpa's) ganglion Vestibular nerve Vestibulocochlear nerve
Adenoids	Includes: Pharyngeal tonsil
Adrenal Gland Adrenal Gland, Left Adrenal Gland, Right Adrenal Glands, Bilateral	Includes: Suprarenal gland
Ampulla of Vater	Includes: Duodenal ampulla Hepatopancreatic ampulla
Anal Sphincter	Includes: External anal sphincter Internal anal sphincter
Ankle Bursa and Ligament, Left Ankle Bursa and Ligament, Right	Includes: Calcaneofibular ligament Deltoid ligament Ligament of the lateral malleolus Talofibular ligament
Ankle Joint, Left Ankle Joint, Right	Includes: Inferior tibiofibular joint Talocrural joint
Anterior Chamber, Left Anterior Chamber, Right	Includes: Aqueous humour
Anterior Tibial Artery, Left Anterior Tibial Artery, Right	Includes: Anterior lateral malleolar artery Anterior medial malleolar artery Anterior tibial recurrent artery Dorsalis pedis artery Posterior tibial recurrent artery
Anus	Includes: Anal orifice
Aortic Valve	Includes: Aortic annulus
Appendix	Includes: Vermiform appendix
Ascending Colon	Includes: Hepatic flexure
Atrial Septum	Includes: Interatrial septum
Atrium, Left	Includes: Atrium pulmonale Left auricular appendix
Atrium, Right	Includes: Atrium dextrum cordis Right auricular appendix Sinus venosus
Auditory Ossicle, Left Auditory Ossicle, Right	Includes: Incus Malleus Ossicular chain Stapes
Axillary Artery, Left Axillary Artery, Right	Includes: Anterior circumflex humeral artery Lateral thoracic artery Posterior circumflex humeral artery Subscapular artery Superior thoracic artery Thoracoacromial artery
Azygos Vein	Includes: Right ascending lumbar vein Right subcostal vein

© 2015 Optum360, LLC

Comprehensive Anatomy and Physiology for ICD-10-CM and ICD-10-PCS Coding

Anatomical Term	PCS Description
Basal Ganglia	**Includes:** Basal nuclei Claustrum Corpus striatum Globus pallidus Substantia nigra Subthalamic nucleus
Basilic Vein, Left **Basilic Vein, Right**	**Includes:** Median antebrachial vein Median cubital vein
Bladder	**Includes:** Trigone of bladder
Brachial Artery, Left **Brachial Artery, Right**	**Includes:** Inferior ulnar collateral artery Profunda brachii Superior ulnar collateral artery
Brachial Plexus	**Includes:** Axillary nerve Dorsal scapular nerve First intercostal nerve Long thoracic nerve Musculocutaneous nerve Subclavius nerve Suprascapular nerve
Brachial Vein, Left **Brachial Vein, Right**	**Includes:** Radial vein Ulnar vein
Brain	**Includes:** Cerebrum Corpus callosum Encephalon
Breast, Bilateral **Breast, Left** **Breast, Right**	**Includes:** Mammary duct Mammary gland
Buccal Mucosa	**Includes:** Buccal gland Molar gland Palatine gland
Carotid Bodies, Bilateral **Carotid Body, Left** **Carotid Body, Right**	**Includes:** Carotid glomus
Carpal Joint, Left **Carpal Joint, Right**	**Includes:** Intercarpal joint Midcarpal joint
Carpal, Left **Carpal, Right**	**Includes:** Capitate bone Hamate bone Lunate bone Pisiform bone Scaphoid bone Trapezium bone Trapezoid bone Triquetral bone
Celiac Artery	**Includes:** Celiac trunk
Cephalic Vein, Left Cephalic Vein, Right	**Includes:** Accessory cephalic vein
Cerebellum	**Includes:** Culmen
Cerebral Hemisphere	**Includes:** Frontal lobe Occipital lobe Parietal lobe Temporal lobe
Cerebral Meninges	**Includes:** Arachnoid mater, intracranial Leptomeninges, intracranial Pia mater, intracranial
Cerebral Ventricle	**Includes:** Aqueduct of Sylvius Cerebral aqueduct (Sylvius) Choroid plexus Ependyma Foramen of Monro (intraventricular) Fourth ventricle Interventricular foramen (Monro) Left lateral ventricle Right lateral ventricle Third ventricle
Cervical Nerve	**Includes:** Greater occipital nerve Spinal nerve, cervical Suboccipital nerve Third occipital nerve
Cervical Plexus	**Includes:** Ansa cervicalis Cutaneous (transverse) cervical nerve Great auricular nerve Lesser occipital nerve Supraclavicular nerve Transverse (cutaneous) cervical nerve
Cervical Vertebra	**Includes:** Spinous process Vertebral arch Vertebral foramen Vertebral lamina Vertebral pedicle
Cervical Vertebral Joint	**Includes:** Atlantoaxial joint Cervical facet joint
Cervical Vertebral Joints, 2 or more	**Includes:** Cervical facet joint
Cervicothoracic Vertebral Joint	**Includes:** Cervicothoracic facet joint
Cisterna Chyli	**Includes:** Intestinal lymphatic trunk Lumbar lymphatic trunk
Coccygeal Glomus	**Includes:** Coccygeal body
Colic Vein	**Includes:** Ileocolic vein Left colic vein Middle colic vein Right colic vein

Appendix C. Body Part Definitions—Body Part Definitions: Alphabetic, by PCS character description

Anatomical Term	PCS Description
Conduction Mechanism	Includes: Atrioventricular node Bundle of His Bundle of Kent Sinoatrial node
Conjunctiva, Left Conjunctiva, Right	Includes: Plica semilunaris
Dura Mater	Includes: Diaphragma sellae Dura mater, intracranial Falx cerebri Tentorium cerebelli
Elbow Bursa and Ligament, Left Elbow Bursa and Ligament, Right	Includes: Annular ligament Olecranon bursa Radial collateral ligament Ulnar collateral ligament
Elbow Joint, Left Elbow Joint, Right	Includes: Distal humerus, involving joint Humeroradial joint Humeroulnar joint Proximal radioulnar joint
Epidural Space	Includes: Epidural space, intracranial Extradural space, intracranial
Epiglottis	Includes: Glossoepiglottic fold
Esophagogastric Junction	Includes: Cardia Cardioesophageal junction Gastroesophageal (GE) junction
Esophagus, Lower	Includes: Abdominal esophagus
Esophagus, Middle	Includes: Thoracic esophagus
Esophagus, Upper	Includes: Cervical esophagus
Ethmoid Bone, Left Ethmoid Bone, Right	Includes: Cribriform plate
Ethmoid Sinus, Left Ethmoid Sinus, Right	Includes: Ethmoidal air cell
Eustachian Tube, Left Eustachian Tube, Right	Includes: Auditory tube Pharyngotympanic tube
External Auditory Canal, Left External Auditory Canal, Right	Includes: External auditory meatus
External Carotid Artery, Left External Carotid Artery, Right	Includes: Ascending pharyngeal artery Internal maxillary artery Lingual artery Maxillary artery Occipital artery Posterior auricular artery Superior thyroid artery

Anatomical Term	PCS Description
External Ear, Bilateral External Ear, Left External Ear, Right	Includes: Antihelix Antitragus Auricle Earlobe Helix Pinna Tragus
External Iliac Artery, Left External Iliac Artery, Right	Includes: Deep circumflex iliac artery Inferior epigastric artery
External Jugular Vein, Left External Jugular Vein, Right	Includes: Posterior auricular vein
Extraocular Muscle, Left Extraocular Muscle, Right	Includes: Inferior oblique muscle Inferior rectus muscle Lateral rectus muscle Medial rectus muscle Superior oblique muscle Superior rectus muscle
Eye, Left Eye, Right	Includes: Ciliary body Posterior chamber
Face Artery	Includes: Angular artery Ascending palatine artery External maxillary artery Facial artery Inferior labial artery Submental artery Superior labial artery
Face Vein, Left Face Vein, Right	Includes: Angular vein Anterior facial vein Common facial vein Deep facial vein Frontal vein Posterior facial (retromandibular) vein Supraorbital vein
Facial Muscle	Includes: Buccinator muscle Corrugator supercilii muscle Depressor anguli oris muscle Depressor labii inferioris muscle Depressor septi nasi muscle Depressor supercilii muscle Levator anguli oris muscle Levator labii superioris alaeque nasi muscle Levator labii superioris muscle Mentalis muscle Nasalis muscle Occipitofrontalis muscle Orbicularis oris muscle Procerus muscle Risorius muscle Zygomaticus muscle

Anatomical Term	PCS Description
Facial Nerve	**Includes:** Chorda tympani Geniculate ganglion Greater superficial petrosal nerve Nerve to the stapedius Parotid plexus Posterior auricular nerve Seventh cranial nerve Submandibular ganglion
Fallopian Tube, Left Fallopian Tube, Right	**Includes:** Oviduct Salpinx Uterine tube
Femoral Artery, Left Femoral Artery, Right	**Includes:** Circumflex iliac artery Deep femoral artery Descending genicular artery External pudendal artery Superficial epigastric artery
Femoral Nerve	**Includes:** Anterior crural nerve Saphenous nerve
Femoral Shaft, Left Femoral Shaft, Right	**Includes:** Body of femur
Femoral Vein, Left Femoral Vein, Right	**Includes:** Deep femoral (profunda femoris) vein Popliteal vein Profunda femoris (deep femoral) vein
Fibula, Left Fibula, Right	**Includes:** Body of fibula Head of fibula Lateral malleolus
Finger Nail	**Includes:** Nail bed Nail plate
Finger Phalangeal Joint, Left Finger Phalangeal Joint, Right	**Includes:** Interphalangeal (IP) joint
Foot Artery, Left Foot Artery, Right	**Includes:** Arcuate artery Dorsal metatarsal artery Lateral plantar artery Lateral tarsal artery Medial plantar artery
Foot Bursa and Ligament, Left Foot Bursa and Ligament, Right	**Includes:** Calcaneocuboid ligament Cuneonavicular ligament Intercuneiform ligament Interphalangeal ligament Metatarsal ligament Metatarsophalangeal ligament Subtalar ligament Talocalcaneal ligament Talocalcaneonavicular ligament Tarsometatarsal ligament

Anatomical Term	PCS Description
Foot Muscle, Left Foot Muscle, Right	**Includes:** Abductor hallucis muscle Adductor hallucis muscle Extensor digitorum brevis muscle Extensor hallucis brevis muscle Flexor digitorum brevis muscle Flexor hallucis brevis muscle Quadratus plantae muscle
Foot Vein, Left Foot Vein, Right	**Includes:** Common digital vein Dorsal metatarsal vein Dorsal venous arch Plantar digital vein Plantar metatarsal vein Plantar venous arch
Frontal Bone, Left Frontal Bone, Right	**Includes:** Zygomatic process of frontal bone
Gastric Artery	**Includes:** Left gastric artery Right gastric artery
Glenoid Cavity, Left Glenoid Cavity, Right	**Includes:** Glenoid fossa (of scapula)
Glomus Jugulare	**Includes:** Jugular body
Glossopharyngeal Nerve	**Includes:** Carotid sinus nerve Ninth cranial nerve Tympanic nerve
Greater Omentum	**Includes:** Gastrocolic ligament Gastrocolic omentum Gastrophrenic ligament Gastrosplenic ligament
Greater Saphenous Vein, Left Greater Saphenous Vein, Right	**Includes:** External pudendal vein Great saphenous vein Superficial circumflex iliac vein Superficial epigastric vein
Hand Artery, Left Hand Artery, Right	**Includes:** Deep palmar arch Princeps pollicis artery Radialis indicis Superficial palmar arch
Hand Bursa and Ligament, Left Hand Bursa and Ligament, Right	**Includes:** Carpometacarpal ligament Intercarpal ligament Interphalangeal ligament Lunotriquetral ligament Metacarpal ligament Metacarpophalangeal ligament Pisohamate ligament Pisometacarpal ligament Scapholunate ligament Scaphotrapezium ligament
Hand Muscle, Left Hand Muscle, Right	**Includes:** Hypothenar muscle Palmar interosseous muscle Thenar muscle

Appendix C. Body Part Definitions—Body Part Definitions: Alphabetic, by PCS character description

Anatomical Term	PCS Description
Hand Vein, Left **Hand Vein, Right**	**Includes:** Dorsal metacarpal vein Palmar (volar) digital vein Palmar (volar) metacarpal vein Superficial palmar venous arch Volar (palmar) digital vein Volar (palmar) metacarpal vein
Head and Neck Bursa and Ligament	**Includes:** Alar ligament of axis Cervical interspinous ligament Cervical intertransverse ligament Cervical ligamentum flavum Interspinous ligament Lateral temporomandibular ligament Sphenomandibular ligament Stylomandibular ligament Transverse ligament of atlas
Head and Neck Sympathetic Nerve	**Includes:** Cavernous plexus Cervical ganglion Ciliary ganglion Internal carotid plexus Otic ganglion Pterygopalatine (sphenopalatine) ganglion Sphenopalatine (pterygopalatine) ganglion Stellate ganglion Submandibular ganglion Submaxillary ganglion
Head Muscle	**Includes:** Auricularis muscle Masseter muscle Pterygoid muscle Splenius capitis muscle Temporalis muscle Temporoparietalis muscle
Heart, Left	**Includes:** Left coronary sulcus Obtuse margin
Heart, Right	Right coronary sulcus
Hemiazygos Vein	**Includes:** Left ascending lumbar vein Left subcostal vein
Hepatic Artery	**Includes:** Common hepatic artery Gastroduodenal artery Hepatic artery proper
Hip Bursa and Ligament, Left **Hip Bursa and Ligament, Right**	**Includes:** Iliofemoral ligament Ischiofemoral ligament Pubofemoral ligament Transverse acetabular ligament Trochanteric bursa
Hip Joint, Left **Hip Joint, Right**	**Includes:** Acetabulofemoral joint

Anatomical Term	PCS Description
Hip Muscle, Left **Hip Muscle, Right**	**Includes:** Gemellus muscle Gluteus maximus muscle Gluteus medius muscle Gluteus minimus muscle Iliacus muscle Obturator muscle Piriformis muscle Psoas muscle Quadratus femoris muscle Tensor fasciae latae muscle
Humeral Head, Left **Humeral Head, Right**	**Includes:** Greater tuberosity Lesser tuberosity Neck of humerus (anatomical)(surgical)
Humeral Shaft, Left **Humeral Shaft, Right**	**Includes:** Distal humerus Humerus, distal Lateral epicondyle of humerus Medial epicondyle of humerus
Hypogastric Vein, Left **Hypogastric Vein, Right**	**Includes:** Gluteal vein Internal iliac vein Internal pudendal vein Lateral sacral vein Middle hemorrhoidal vein Obturator vein Uterine vein Vaginal vein Vesical vein
Hypoglossal Nerve	**Includes:** Twelfth cranial nerve
Hypothalamus	**Includes:** Mammillary body
Inferior Mesenteric Artery	**Includes:** Sigmoid artery Superior rectal artery
Inferior Mesenteric Vein	**Includes:** Sigmoid vein Superior rectal vein
Inferior Vena Cava	**Includes:** Postcava Right inferior phrenic vein Right ovarian vein Right second lumbar vein Right suprarenal vein Right testicular vein
Inguinal Region, Bilateral **Inguinal Region, Left** **Inguinal Region, Right**	**Includes:** Inguinal canal Inguinal triangle
Inner Ear, Left **Inner Ear, Right**	**Includes:** Bony labyrinth Bony vestibule Cochlea Round window Semicircular canal
Innominate Artery	**Includes:** Brachiocephalic artery Brachiocephalic trunk

Comprehensive Anatomy and Physiology for ICD-10-CM and ICD-10-PCS Coding

Anatomical Term	PCS Description
Innominate Vein, Left Innominate Vein, Right	**Includes:** Brachiocephalic vein Inferior thyroid vein
Internal Carotid Artery, Left Internal Carotid Artery, Right	**Includes:** Caroticotympanic artery Carotid sinus Ophthalmic artery
Internal Iliac Artery, Left Internal Iliac Artery, Right	**Includes:** Deferential artery Hypogastric artery Iliolumbar artery Inferior gluteal artery Inferior vesical artery Internal pudendal artery Lateral sacral artery Middle rectal artery Obturator artery Superior gluteal artery Umbilical artery Uterine artery Vaginal artery
Internal Mammary Artery, Left Internal Mammary Artery, Right	**Includes:** Anterior intercostal artery Internal thoracic artery Musculophrenic artery Pericardiophrenic artery Superior epigastric artery
Intracranial Artery	**Includes:** Anterior cerebral artery Anterior choroidal artery Anterior communicating artery Basilar artery Circle of Willis Middle cerebral artery Posterior cerebral artery Posterior communicating artery Posterior inferior cerebellar artery (PICA)
Intracranial Vein	**Includes:** Anterior cerebral vein Basal (internal) cerebral vein Dural venous sinus Great cerebral vein Inferior cerebellar vein Inferior cerebral vein Internal (basal) cerebral vein Middle cerebral vein Ophthalmic vein Superior cerebellar vein Superior cerebral vein
Jejunum	**Includes:** Duodenojejunal flexure
Kidney	**Includes:** Renal calyx Renal capsule Renal cortex Renal segment
Kidney Pelvis, Left Kidney Pelvis, Right	**Includes:** Ureteropelvic junction (UPJ)

Anatomical Term	PCS Description
Kidney, Left Kidney, Right Kidneys, Bilateral	**Includes:** Renal calyx Renal capsule Renal cortex Renal segment
Knee Bursa and Ligament, Left Knee Bursa and Ligament, Right	**Includes:** Anterior cruciate ligament (ACL) Lateral collateral ligament (LCL) Ligament of head of fibula Medial collateral ligament (MCL) Patellar ligament Popliteal ligament Posterior cruciate ligament (PCL) Prepatellar bursa
Knee Joint, Femoral Surface, Left Knee Joint, Femoral Surface, Right	**Includes:** Femoropatellar joint Patellofemoral joint
Knee Joint, Left Knee Joint, Right	**Includes:** Femoropatellar joint Femorotibial joint Lateral meniscus Medial meniscus Patellofemoral joint Tibiofemoral joint
Knee Joint, Tibial Surface, Left Knee Joint, Tibial Surface, Right	**Includes:** Femorotibial joint Tibiofemoral joint
Knee Tendon, Left Knee Tendon, Right	**Includes:** Patellar tendon
Lacrimal Duct, Left Lacrimal Duct, Right	**Includes:** Lacrimal canaliculus Lacrimal punctum Lacrimal sac Nasolacrimal duct
Larynx	**Includes:** Aryepiglottic fold Arytenoid cartilage Corniculate cartilage Cuneiform cartilage False vocal cord Glottis Rima glottidis Thyroid cartilage Ventricular fold
Lens, Left Lens, Right	**Includes:** Zonule of Zinn
Lesser Omentum	**Includes:** Gastrohepatic omentum Hepatogastric ligament
Lesser Saphenous Vein, Left Lesser Saphenous Vein, Right	**Includes:** Small saphenous vein
Liver	**Includes:** Quadrate lobe

Anatomical Term	PCS Description
Lower Arm and Wrist Muscle, Left Lower Arm and Wrist Muscle, Right	Includes: Anatomical snuffbox Brachioradialis muscle Extensor carpi radialis muscle Extensor carpi ulnaris muscle Flexor carpi radialis muscle Flexor carpi ulnaris muscle Flexor pollicis longus muscle Palmaris longus muscle Pronator quadratus muscle Pronator teres muscle
Lower Eyelid, Left Lower Eyelid, Right	Includes: Inferior tarsal plate Medial canthus
Lower Femur, Left Lower Femur, Right	Includes: Lateral condyle of femur Lateral epicondyle of femur Medial condyle of femur Medial epicondyle of femur
Lower Leg Muscle, Left Lower Leg Muscle, Right	Includes: Extensor digitorum longus muscle Extensor hallucis longus muscle Fibularis brevis muscle Fibularis longus muscle Flexor digitorum longus muscle Flexor hallucis longus muscle Gastrocnemius muscle Peroneus brevis muscle Peroneus longus muscle Popliteus muscle Soleus muscle Tibialis anterior muscle Tibialis posterior muscle
Lower Leg Tendon, Left Lower Leg Tendon, Right	Includes: Achilles tendon
Lower Lip	Includes: Frenulum labii inferioris Labial gland Vermilion border
Lumbar Nerve	Includes: Lumbosacral trunk Spinal nerve, lumbar Superior clunic (cluneal) nerve
Lumbar Plexus	Includes: Accessory obturator nerve Genitofemoral nerve Iliohypogastric nerve Ilioinguinal nerve Lateral femoral cutaneous nerve Obturator nerve Superior gluteal nerve
Lumbar Spinal Cord	Includes: Cauda equina Conus medullaris
Lumbar Sympathetic Nerve	Includes: Lumbar ganglion Lumbar splanchnic nerve
Lumbar Vertebra	Includes: Spinous process Vertebral arch Vertebral foramen Vertebral lamina Vertebral pedicle

Anatomical Term	PCS Description
Lumbar Vertebral Joint	Includes: Lumbar facet joint
Lumbosacral Joint	Includes: Lumbosacral facet joint
Lymphatic, Aortic	Includes: Celiac lymph node Gastric lymph node Hepatic lymph node Lumbar lymph node Pancreaticosplenic lymph node Paraaortic lymph node Retroperitoneal lymph node
Lymphatic, Head	Includes: Buccinator lymph node Infraauricular lymph node Infraparotid lymph node Parotid lymph node Preauricular lymph node Submandibular lymph node Submaxillary lymph node Submental lymph node Subparotid lymph node Suprahyoid lymph node
Lymphatic, Left Axillary	Includes: Anterior (pectoral) lymph node Apical (subclavicular) lymph node Brachial (lateral) lymph node Central axillary lymph node Lateral (brachial) lymph node Pectoral (anterior) lymph node Posterior (subscapular) lymph node Subclavicular (apical) lymph node Subscapular (posterior) lymph node
Lymphatic, Left Lower Extremity	Includes: Femoral lymph node Popliteal lymph node
Lymphatic, Left Neck	Includes: Cervical lymph node Jugular lymph node Mastoid (postauricular) lymph node Occipital lymph node Postauricular (mastoid) lymph node Retropharyngeal lymph node Supraclavicular (Virchow's) lymph node Virchow's (supraclavicular) lymph node
Lymphatic, Left Upper Extremity	Includes: Cubital lymph node Deltopectoral (infraclavicular) lymph node Epitrochlear lymph node Infraclavicular (deltopectoral) lymph node Supratrochlear lymph node

Anatomical Term	PCS Description
Lymphatic, Mesenteric	**Includes:** Inferior mesenteric lymph node Pararectal lymph node Superior mesenteric lymph node
Lymphatic, Pelvis	**Includes:** Common iliac (subaortic) lymph node Gluteal lymph node Iliac lymph node Inferior epigastric lymph node Obturator lymph node Sacral lymph node Subaortic (common iliac) lymph node Suprainguinal lymph node
Lymphatic, Right Axillary	**Includes:** Anterior (pectoral) lymph node Apical (subclavicular) lymph node Brachial (lateral) lymph node Central axillary lymph node Lateral (brachial) lymph node Pectoral (anterior) lymph node Posterior (subscapular) lymph node Subclavicular (apical) lymph node Subscapular (posterior) lymph node
Lymphatic, Right Lower Extremity	**Includes:** Femoral lymph node Popliteal lymph node
Lymphatic, Right Neck	**Includes:** Cervical lymph node Jugular lymph node Mastoid (postauricular) lymph node Occipital lymph node Postauricular (mastoid) lymph node Retropharyngeal lymph node Right jugular trunk Right lymphatic duct Right subclavian trunk Supraclavicular (Virchow's) lymph node Virchow's (supraclavicular) lymph node
Lymphatic, Right Upper Extremity	**Includes:** Cubital lymph node Deltopectoral (infraclavicular) lymph node Epitrochlear lymph node Infraclavicular (deltopectoral) lymph node Supratrochlear lymph node
Lymphatic, Thorax	**Includes:** Intercostal lymph node Mediastinal lymph node Parasternal lymph node Paratracheal lymph node Tracheobronchial lymph node

Anatomical Term	PCS Description
Mandible, Left Mandible, Right	**Includes:** Alveolar process of mandible Condyloid process Mandibular notch Mental foramen
Mastoid Sinus, Left Mastoid Sinus, Right	**Includes:** Mastoid air cells
Maxilla, Left Maxilla, Right	**Includes:** Alveolar process of maxilla
Maxillary Sinus, Left Maxillary Sinus, Right	**Includes:** Antrum of Highmore
Median Nerve	**Includes:** Anterior interosseous nerve Palmar cutaneous nerve
Medulla Oblongata	**Includes:** Myelencephalon
Mesentery	**Includes:** Mesoappendix Mesocolon
Metacarpocarpal Joint, Left Metacarpocarpal Joint, Right	**Includes:** Carpometacarpal (CMC) joint
Metatarsal-Phalangeal Joint, Left Metatarsal-Phalangeal Joint, Right	**Includes:** Metatarsophalangeal (MTP) joint
Metatarsal-Tarsal Joint, Left Metatarsal-Tarsal Joint, Right	**Includes:** Tarsometatarsal joint
Middle Ear, Left Middle Ear, Right	**Includes:** Oval window Tympanic cavity
Minor Salivary Gland	**Includes:** Anterior lingual gland
Mitral Valve	**Includes:** Bicuspid valve Left atrioventricular valve Mitral annulus
Nasal Bone	**Includes:** Vomer of nasal septum
Nasal Septum	**Includes:** Quadrangular cartilage Septal cartilage Vomer bone
Nasal Turbinate	**Includes:** Inferior turbinate Middle turbinate Nasal concha Superior turbinate
Nasopharynx	**Includes:** Choana Fossa of Rosenmuller Pharyngeal recess Rhinopharynx

Appendix C. Body Part Definitions—Body Part Definitions: Alphabetic, by PCS character description

Anatomical Term	PCS Description
Neck Muscle, Left Neck Muscle, Right	Includes: Anterior vertebral muscle Arytenoid muscle Cricothyroid muscle Infrahyoid muscle Levator scapulae muscle Platysma muscle Scalene muscle Splenius cervicis muscle Sternocleidomastoid muscle Suprahyoid muscle Thyroarytenoid muscle
Nipple, Left Nipple, Right	Includes: Areola
Nose	Includes: Columella External naris Greater alar cartilage Internal naris Lateral nasal cartilage Lesser alar cartilage Nasal cavity Nostril
Occipital Bone, Left Occipital Bone, Right	Includes: Foramen magnum
Oculomotor Nerve	Includes: Third cranial nerve
Olfactory Nerve	Includes: First cranial nerve Olfactory bulb
Optic Nerve	Includes: Optic chiasma Second cranial nerve
Orbit, Left Orbit, Right	Includes: Bony orbit Orbital portion of ethmoid bone Orbital portion of frontal bone Orbital portion of lacrimal bone Orbital portion of maxilla Orbital portion of palatine bone Orbital portion of sphenoid bone Orbital portion of zygomatic bone
Pancreatic Duct	Includes: Duct of Wirsung
Pancreatic Duct, Accessory	Includes: Duct of Santorini
Parotid Duct, Left Parotid Duct, Right	Includes: Stensen's duct
Pelvic Bone, Left Pelvic Bone, Right	Includes: Iliac crest Ilium Ischium Pubis
Pelvic Cavity	Includes: Retropubic space
Penis	Includes: Corpus cavernosum Corpus spongiosum

Anatomical Term	PCS Description
Perineum Muscle	Includes: Bulbospongiosus muscle Cremaster muscle Deep transverse perineal muscle Ischiocavernosus muscle Superficial transverse perineal muscle
Peritoneum	Includes: Epiploic foramen
Peroneal Artery, Left Peroneal Artery, Right	Includes: Fibular artery
Peroneal Nerve	Includes: Common fibular nerve Common peroneal nerve External popliteal nerve Lateral sural cutaneous nerve
Pharynx	Includes: Hypopharynx Laryngopharynx Oropharynx Piriform recess (sinus)
Phrenic Nerve	Includes: Accessory phrenic nerve
Pituitary Gland	Includes: Adenohypophysis Hypophysis Neurohypophysis
Pons	Includes: Apneustic center Basis pontis Locus ceruleus Pneumotaxic center Pontine tegmentum Superior olivary nucleus
Popliteal Artery, Left Popliteal Artery, Right	Includes: Inferior genicular artery Middle genicular artery Superior genicular artery Sural artery
Portal Vein	Includes: Hepatic portal vein
Prepuce	Includes: Foreskin Glans penis
Pudendal Nerve	Includes: Posterior labial nerve Posterior scrotal nerve
Pulmonary Artery, Left	Includes: Arterial canal (duct) Botallo's duct Pulmoaortic canal
Pulmonary Valve	Includes: Pulmonary annulus Pulmonic valve
Pulmonary Vein, Left	Includes: Left inferior pulmonary vein Left superior pulmonary vein
Pulmonary Vein, Right	Includes: Right inferior pulmonary vein Right superior pulmonary vein

© 2015 Optum360, LLC

Anatomical Term	PCS Description
Radial Artery, Left Radial Artery, Right	Includes: Radial recurrent artery
Radial Nerve	Includes: Dorsal digital nerve Musculospiral nerve Palmar cutaneous nerve Posterior interosseous nerve
Radius, Left Radius, Right	Includes: Ulnar notch
Rectum	Includes: Anorectal junction
Renal Artery, Left Renal Artery, Right	Includes: Inferior suprarenal artery Renal segmental artery
Renal Vein, Left	Includes: Left inferior phrenic vein Left ovarian vein Left second lumbar vein Left suprarenal vein Left testicular vein
Retina, Left Retina, Right	Includes: Fovea Macula Optic disc
Retroperitoneum	Includes: Retroperitoneal space
Sacral Nerve	Includes: Spinal nerve, sacral
Sacral Plexus	Includes: Inferior gluteal nerve Posterior femoral cutaneous nerve Pudendal nerve
Sacral Sympathetic Nerve	Includes: Ganglion impar (ganglion of Walther) Pelvic splanchnic nerve Sacral ganglion Sacral splanchnic nerve
Sacrococcygeal Joint	Includes: Sacrococcygeal symphysis
Scapula, Left Scapula, Right	Includes: Acromion (process) Coracoid process
Sciatic Nerve	Includes: Ischiatic nerve
Shoulder Bursa and Ligament, Left Shoulder Bursa and Ligament, Right	Includes: Acromioclavicular ligament Coracoacromial ligament Coracoclavicular ligament Coracohumeral ligament Costoclavicular ligament Glenohumeral ligament Interclavicular ligament Sternoclavicular ligament Subacromial bursa Transverse humeral ligament Transverse scapular ligament
Shoulder Joint, Left Shoulder Joint, Right	Includes: Glenohumeral joint Glenoid ligament (labrum)

Anatomical Term	PCS Description
Shoulder Muscle, Left Shoulder Muscle, Right	Includes: Deltoid muscle Infraspinatus muscle Subscapularis muscle Supraspinatus muscle Teres major muscle Teres minor muscle
Sigmoid Colon	Includes: Rectosigmoid junction Sigmoid flexure
Skin	Includes: Dermis Epidermis Sebaceous gland Sweat gland
Sphenoid Bone, Left Sphenoid Bone, Right	Includes: Greater wing Lesser wing Optic foramen Pterygoid process Sella turcica
Spinal Canal	Includes: Epidural space, spinal Extradural space, spinal Subarachnoid space, spinal Subdural space, spinal Vertebral canal
Spinal Meninges	Includes: Arachnoid mater, spinal Denticulate (dentate) ligament Dura mater, spinal Leptomeninges, spinal Pia mater, spinal
Spleen	Includes: Accessory spleen
Splenic Artery	Includes: Left gastroepiploic artery Pancreatic artery Short gastric artery
Splenic Vein	Includes: Left gastroepiploic vein Pancreatic vein
Sternum	Includes: Manubrium Suprasternal notch Xiphoid process
Stomach, Pylorus	Includes: Pyloric antrum Pyloric canal Pyloric sphincter
Subarachnoid Space	Includes: Subarachnoid space, intracranial
Subclavian Artery, Left Subclavian Artery, Right	Includes: Costocervical trunk Dorsal scapular artery Internal thoracic artery
Subcutaneous Tissue and Fascia, Scalp	Includes: Galea aponeurotica
Subcutaneous Tissue and Fascia, Face	Includes: Masseteric fascia Orbital fascia

Appendix C. Body Part Definitions—Body Part Definitions: Alphabetic, by PCS character description

Anatomical Term	PCS Description
Subcutaneous Tissue and Fascia, Anterior Neck	Includes: Deep cervical fascia Pretracheal fascia
Subcutaneous Tissue and Fascia, Posterior Neck	Includes: Prevertebral fascia
Subcutaneous Tissue and Fascia, Chest	Includes: Pectoral fascia
Subcutaneous Tissue and Fascia, Right Upper Arm Subcutaneous Tissue and Fascia, Left Upper Arm	Includes: Axillary fascia Deltoid fascia Infraspinatus fascia Subscapular aponeurosis Supraspinatus fascia
Subcutaneous Tissue and Fascia, Right Lower Arm Subcutaneous Tissue and Fascia, Left Lower Arm	Includes: Antebrachial fascia Bicipital aponeurosis
Subcutaneous Tissue and Fascia, Right Hand Subcutaneous Tissue and Fascia, Left Hand	Includes: Palmar fascia (aponeurosis)
Subcutaneous Tissue and Fascia, Right Upper Leg Subcutaneous Tissue and Fascia, Left Upper Leg	Includes: Crural fascia Fascia lata Iliac fascia Iliotibial tract (band)
Subcutaneous Tissue and Fascia, Right Foot Subcutaneous Tissue and Fascia, Left Foot	Includes: Plantar fascia (aponeurosis)
Subcutaneous Tissue and Fascia, Trunk	Includes: External oblique aponeurosis Transversalis fascia
Subdural Space	Includes: Subdural space, intracranial
Submaxillary Gland, Left Submaxillary Gland, Right	Includes: Submandibular gland
Superior Mesenteric Artery	Includes: Ileal artery Ileocolic artery Inferior pancreaticoduodenal artery Jejunal artery
Superior Mesenteric Vein	Includes: Right gastroepiploic vein
Superior Vena Cava	Includes: Precava
Tarsal Joint, Left Tarsal Joint, Right	Includes: Calcaneocuboid joint Cuboideonavicular joint Cuneonavicular joint Intercuneiform joint Subtalar (talocalcaneal) joint Talocalcaneal (subtalar) joint Talocalcaneonavicular joint

Anatomical Term	PCS Description
Tarsal, Left Tarsal, Right	Includes: Calcaneus Cuboid bone Intermediate cuneiform bone Lateral cuneiform bone Medial cuneiform bone Navicular bone Talus bone
Temporal Artery, Left Temporal Artery, Right	Includes: Middle temporal artery Superficial temporal artery Transverse facial artery
Temporal Bone, Left Temporal Bone, Right	Includes: Mastoid process Petrous part of temporal bone Tympanic part of temporal bone Zygomatic process of temporal bone
Thalamus	Includes: Epithalamus Geniculate nucleus Metathalamus Pulvinar
Thoracic Aorta	Includes: Aortic arch Aortic intercostal artery Ascending aorta Bronchial artery Esophageal artery Subcostal artery
Thoracic Duct	Includes: Left jugular trunk Left subclavian trunk
Thoracic Nerve	Includes: Intercostal nerve Intercostobrachial nerve Spinal nerve, thoracic Subcostal nerve
Thoracic Sympathetic Nerve	Includes: Cardiac plexus Esophageal plexus Greater splanchnic nerve Inferior cardiac nerve Least splanchnic nerve Lesser splanchnic nerve Middle cardiac nerve Pulmonary plexus Superior cardiac nerve Thoracic aortic plexus Thoracic ganglion
Thoracic Vertebra	Includes: Spinous process Vertebral arch Vertebral foramen Vertebral lamina Vertebral pedicle
Thoracic Vertebral Joint	Includes: Costotransverse joint Costovertebral joint Thoracic facet joint
Thoracolumbar Vertebral Joint	Includes: Thoracolumbar facet joint

Comprehensive Anatomy and Physiology for ICD-10-CM and ICD-10-PCS Coding

Anatomical Term	PCS Description
Thorax Bursa and Ligament, Left Thorax Bursa and Ligament, Right	**Includes:** Costotransverse ligament Costoxiphoid ligament Sternocostal ligament
Thorax Muscle, Left Thorax Muscle, Right	**Includes:** Intercostal muscle Levatores costarum muscle Pectoralis major muscle Pectoralis minor muscle Serratus anterior muscle Subclavius muscle Subcostal muscle Transverse thoracis muscle
Thymus	**Includes:** Thymus gland
Thyroid Artery, Left Thyroid Artery, Right	**Includes:** Cricothyroid artery Hyoid artery Sternocleidomastoid artery Superior laryngeal artery Superior thyroid artery Thyrocervical trunk
Tibia, Left Tibia, Right	**Includes:** Lateral condyle of tibia Medial condyle of tibia Medial malleolus
Tibial Nerve	**Includes:** Lateral plantar nerve Medial plantar nerve Medial popliteal nerve Medial sural cutaneous nerve
Toe Nail	**Includes:** Nail bed Nail plate
Toe Phalangeal Joint, Left Toe Phalangeal Joint, Right	**Includes:** Interphalangeal (IP) joint
Tongue	**Includes:** Frenulum linguae Lingual tonsil
Tongue, Palate, Pharynx Muscle	**Includes:** Chondroglossus muscle Genioglossus muscle Hyoglossus muscle Inferior longitudinal muscle Levator veli palatini muscle Palatoglossal muscle Palatopharyngeal muscle Pharyngeal constrictor muscle Salpingopharyngeus muscle Styloglossus muscle Stylopharyngeus muscle Superior longitudinal muscle Tensor veli palatini muscle
Tonsils	**Includes:** Palatine tonsil
Trachea	**Includes:** Cricoid cartilage
Transverse Colon	**Includes:** Splenic flexure
Tricuspid Valve	**Includes:** Right atrioventricular valve Tricuspid annulus
Trigeminal Nerve	**Includes:** Fifth cranial nerve Gasserian ganglion Mandibular nerve Maxillary nerve Ophthalmic nerve Trifacial nerve
Trochlear Nerve	**Includes:** Fourth cranial nerve
Trunk Bursa and Ligament, Left Trunk Bursa and Ligament, Right	**Includes:** Iliolumbar ligament Interspinous ligament Intertransverse ligament Ligamentum flavum Pubic ligament Sacrococcygeal ligament Sacroiliac ligament Sacrospinous ligament Sacrotuberous ligament Supraspinous ligament
Trunk Muscle, Left Trunk Muscle, Right	**Includes:** Coccygeus muscle Erector spinae muscle Interspinalis muscle Intertransversarius muscle Latissimus dorsi muscle Levator ani muscle Quadratus lumborum muscle Rhomboid major muscle Rhomboid minor muscle Serratus posterior muscle Transversospinalis muscle Trapezius muscle
Tympanic Membrane, Left Tympanic Membrane, Right	**Includes:** Pars flaccida
Ulna, Left Ulna, Right	**Includes:** Olecranon process Radial notch
Ulnar Artery, Left Ulnar Artery, Right	**Includes:** Anterior ulnar recurrent artery Common interosseous artery Posterior ulnar recurrent artery
Ulnar Nerve	**Includes:** Cubital nerve
Upper Arm Muscle, Left Upper Arm Muscle, Right	**Includes:** Biceps brachii muscle Brachialis muscle Coracobrachialis muscle Triceps brachii muscle
Upper Eyelid, Left Upper Eyelid, Right	**Includes:** Lateral canthus Levator palpebrae superioris muscle Orbicularis oculi muscle Superior tarsal plate
Upper Femur, Left Upper Femur, Right	**Includes:** Femoral head Greater trochanter Lesser trochanter Neck of femur

Anatomical Term	PCS Description
Upper Leg Muscle, Left **Upper Leg Muscle, Right**	**Includes:** Adductor brevis muscle Adductor longus muscle Adductor magnus muscle Biceps femoris muscle Gracilis muscle Pectineus muscle Quadriceps (femoris) Rectus femoris muscle Sartorius muscle Semimembranosus muscle Semitendinosus muscle Vastus intermedius muscle Vastus lateralis muscle Vastus medialis muscle
Upper Lip	**Includes:** Frenulum labii superioris Labial gland Vermilion border
Ureter **Ureter, Left** **Ureter, Right** **Ureters, Bilateral**	**Includes:** Ureteral orifice Ureterovesical orifice
Urethra	**Includes:** Bulbourethral (Cowper's) gland Cowper's (bulbourethral) gland External urethral sphincter Internal urethral sphincter Membranous urethra Penile urethra Prostatic urethra
Uterine Supporting Structure	**Includes:** Broad ligament Infundibulopelvic ligament Ovarian ligament Round ligament of uterus
Uterus	**Includes:** Fundus uteri Myometrium Perimetrium Uterine cornu
Uvula	**Includes:** Palatine uvula
Vagus Nerve	**Includes:** Anterior vagal trunk Pharyngeal plexus Pneumogastric nerve Posterior vagal trunk Pulmonary plexus Recurrent laryngeal nerve Superior laryngeal nerve Tenth cranial nerve

Anatomical Term	PCS Description
Vas Deferens **Vas Deferens, Bilateral** **Vas Deferens, Left** **Vas Deferens, Right**	**Includes:** Ductus deferens Ejaculatory duct
Ventricle, Right	**Includes:** Conus arteriosus
Ventricular Septum	**Includes:** Interventricular septum
Vertebral Artery, Left **Vertebral Artery, Right**	**Includes:** Anterior spinal artery Posterior spinal artery
Vertebral Vein, Left **Vertebral Vein, Right**	**Includes:** Deep cervical vein Suboccipital venous plexus
Vestibular Gland	**Includes:** Bartholin's (greater vestibular) gland Greater vestibular (Bartholin's) gland Paraurethral (Skene's) gland Skene's (paraurethral) gland
Vitreous, Left **Vitreous, Right**	**Includes:** Vitreous body
Vocal Cord, Left **Vocal Cord, Right**	**Includes:** Vocal fold
Vulva	**Includes:** Labia majora Labia minora
Wrist Bursa and Ligament, Left **Wrist Bursa and Ligament, Right**	**Includes:** Palmar ulnocarpal ligament Radial collateral carpal ligament Radiocarpal ligament Radioulnar ligament Ulnar collateral carpal ligament
Wrist Joint, Left **Wrist Joint, Right**	**Includes:** Distal radioulnar joint Radiocarpal joint

Appendix D.
Root Operation Definitions

	0	Medical and Surgical		
0	Alteration	Definition:	Modifying the natural anatomic structure of a body part without affecting the function of the body part
		Explanation:	Principal purpose is to improve appearance
		Examples:	Face lift, breast augmentation
1	Bypass	Definition:	Altering the route of passage of the contents of a tubular body part
		Explanation:	Rerouting contents of a body part to a downstream area of the normal route, to a similar route and body part, or to an abnormal route and dissimilar body part. Includes one or more anastomoses, with or without the use of a device.
		Examples:	Coronary artery bypass, colostomy formation
2	Change	Definition:	Taking out or off a device from a body part and putting back an identical or similar device in or on the same body part without cutting or puncturing the skin or a mucous membrane
		Explanation:	All CHANGE procedures are coded using the approach EXTERNAL
		Example:	Urinary catheter change, gastrostomy tube change
3	Control	Definition:	Stopping, or attempting to stop, postprocedural bleeding
		Explanation:	The site of the bleeding is coded as an anatomical region and not to a specific body part
		Examples:	Control of post-prostatectomy hemorrhage, control of post-tonsillectomy hemorrhage
4	Creation	Definition:	Making a new genital structure that does not take over the function of a body part
		Explanation:	Used only for sex change operations
		Examples:	Creation of vagina in a male, creation of penis in a female
5	Destruction	Definition:	Physical eradication of all or a portion of a body part by the direct use of energy, force, or a destructive agent
		Explanation:	None of the body part is physically taken out
		Examples:	Fulguration of rectal polyp, cautery of skin lesion
6	Detachment	Definition:	Cutting off all or part of the upper or lower extremities
		Explanation:	The body part value is the site of the detachment, with a qualifier if applicable to further specify the level where the extremity was detached
		Examples:	Below knee amputation, disarticulation of shoulder
7	Dilation	Definition:	Expanding an orifice or the lumen of a tubular body part
		Explanation:	The orifice can be a natural orifice or an artificially created orifice. Accomplished by stretching a tubular body part using intraluminal pressure or by cutting part of the orifice or wall of the tubular body part.
		Examples:	Percutaneous transluminal angioplasty, pyloromyotomy
8	Division	Definition:	Cutting into a body part, without draining fluids and/or gases from the body part, in order to separate or transect a body part
		Explanation:	All or a portion of the body part is separated into two or more portions
		Examples:	Spinal cordotomy, osteotomy
9	Drainage	Definition:	Taking or letting out fluids and/or gases from a body part
		Explanation:	The qualifier DIAGNOSTIC is used to identify drainage procedures that are biopsies
		Examples:	Thoracentesis, incision and drainage

Continued on next page

0 — Medical and Surgical (Continued)

B	Excision	Definition:	Cutting out or off, without replacement, a portion of a body part
		Explanation:	The qualifier DIAGNOSTIC is used to identify excision procedures that are biopsies
		Examples:	Partial nephrectomy, liver biopsy
C	Extirpation	Definition:	Taking or cutting out solid matter from a body part
		Explanation:	The solid matter may be an abnormal byproduct of a biological function or a foreign body; it may be imbedded in a body part or in the lumen of a tubular body part. The solid matter may or may not have been previously broken into pieces.
		Examples:	Thrombectomy, choledocholithotomy
D	Extraction	Definition:	Pulling or stripping out or off all or a portion of a body part by the use of force
		Explanation:	The qualifier DIAGNOSTIC is used to identify extractions that are biopsies
		Examples:	Dilation and curettage, vein stripping
F	Fragmentation	Definition:	Breaking solid matter in a body part into pieces
		Explanation:	Physical force (e.g., manual, ultrasonic) applied directly or indirectly is used to break the solid matter into pieces. The solid matter may be an abnormal byproduct of a biological function or a foreign body. The pieces of solid matter are not taken out.
		Examples:	Extracorporeal shockwave lithotripsy, transurethral lithotripsy
G	Fusion	Definition:	Joining together portions of an articular body part, rendering the articular body part immobile
		Explanation:	The body part is joined together by fixation device, bone graft, or other means
		Examples:	Spinal fusion, ankle arthrodesis
H	Insertion	Definition:	Putting in a nonbiological appliance that monitors, assists, performs, or prevents a physiological function but does not physically take the place of a body part
		Explanation:	None
		Examples:	Insertion of radioactive implant, insertion of central venous catheter
J	Inspection	Definition:	Visually and/or manually exploring a body part
		Explanation:	Visual exploration may be performed with or without optical instrumentation. Manual exploration may be performed directly or through intervening body layers.
		Examples:	Diagnostic arthroscopy, exploratory laparotomy
K	Map	Definition:	Locating the route of passage of electrical impulses and/or locating functional areas in a body part
		Explanation:	Applicable only to the cardiac conduction mechanism and the central nervous system
		Examples:	Cardiac mapping, cortical mapping
L	Occlusion	Definition:	Completely closing an orifice or lumen of a tubular body part
		Explanation:	The orifice can be a natural orifice or an artificially created orifice
		Examples:	Fallopian tube ligation, ligation of inferior vena cava
M	Reattachment	Definition:	Putting back in or on all or a portion of a separated body part to its normal location or other suitable location
		Explanation:	Vascular circulation and nervous pathways may or may not be reestablished
		Examples:	Reattachment of hand, reattachment of avulsed kidney
N	Release	Definition:	Freeing a body part from an abnormal physical constraint by cutting or by use of force
		Explanation:	Some of the restraining tissue may be taken out but none of the body part is taken out
		Examples:	Adhesiolysis, carpal tunnel release
P	Removal	Definition:	Taking out or off a device from a body part
		Explanation:	If a device is taken out and a similar device put in without cutting or puncturing the skin or mucous membrane, the procedure is coded to the root operation CHANGE. Otherwise, the procedure for taking out a device is coded to the root operation REMOVAL.
		Examples:	Drainage tube removal, cardiac pacemaker removal

Continued on next page

Appendix D. Root Operation Definitions

	0	**Medical and Surgical**		**(Continued)**
Q	Repair	Definition:	Restoring, to the extent possible, a body part to its normal anatomic structure and function
		Explanation:	Used only when the method to accomplish the repair is not one of the other root operations
		Examples:	Colostomy takedown, herniorrhaphy, suture of laceration
R	Replacement	Definition:	Putting in or on a biological or synthetic material that physically takes the place and/or function of all or a portion of a body part
		Explanation:	The body part may have been taken out or replaced, or may be taken out, physically eradicated, or rendered nonfunctional during the REPLACEMENT procedure. A REMOVAL procedure is coded for taking out the device used in a previous replacement procedure.
		Examples:	Total hip replacement, bone graft, free skin graft
S	Reposition	Definition:	Moving to its normal location, or other suitable location, all or a portion of a body part
		Explanation:	The body part is moved to a new location from an abnormal location, or from a normal location where it is not functioning correctly. The body part may or may not be cut out or off to be moved to the new location.
		Examples:	Reposition of undescended testicle, fracture reduction
T	Resection	Definition:	Cutting out or off, without replacement, all of a body part
		Explanation:	None
		Examples:	Total nephrectomy, total lobectomy of lung
V	Restriction	Definition:	Partially closing an orifice or the lumen of a tubular body part
		Explanation:	The orifice can be a natural orifice or an artificially created orifice
		Examples:	Esophagogastric fundoplication, cervical cerclage
W	Revision	Definition:	Correcting, to the extent possible, a portion of a malfunctioning device or the position of a displaced device
		Explanation:	Revision can include correcting a malfunctioning or displaced device by taking out or putting in components of the device such as a screw or pin
		Examples:	Adjustment of position of pacemaker lead, recementing of hip prosthesis
U	Supplement	Definition:	Putting in or on biological or synthetic material that physically reinforces and/or augments the function of a portion of a body part
		Explanation:	The biological material is non-living, or is living and from the same individual. The body part may have been previously replaced, and the SUPPLEMENT procedure is performed to physically reinforce and/or augment the function of the replaced body part.
		Examples:	Herniorrhaphy using mesh, free nerve graft, mitral valve ring annuloplasty, put a new acetabular liner in a previous hip replacement
X	Transfer	Definition:	Moving, without taking out, all or a portion of a body part to another location to take over the function of all or a portion of a body part
		Explanation:	The body part transferred remains connected to its vascular and nervous supply
		Examples:	Tendon transfer, skin pedicle flap transfer
Y	Transplantation	Definition:	Putting in or on all or a portion of a living body part taken from another individual or animal to physically take the place and/or function of all or a portion of a similar body part
		Explanation:	The native body part may or may not be taken out, and the transplanted body part may take over all or a portion of its function
		Examples:	Kidney transplant, heart transplant

Root Operation Definitions for Other Sections

	1	Obstetrics	
2	Change	Definition:	Taking out or off a device from a body part and putting back an identical or similar device in or on the same body part without cutting or puncturing the skin or a mucous membrane
		Explanation:	All CHANGE procedures are coded using the approach EXTERNAL
		Examples:	Replacement of fetal scalp electrode
9	Drainage	Definition:	Taking or letting out fluids and/or gases from a body part
		Explanation:	The qualifier DIAGNOSTIC is used to identify drainage procedures that are biopsies
		Examples:	Biopsy of amniotic fluid
A	Abortion	Definition:	Artificially terminating a pregnancy
		Explanation:	Subdivided according to whether an additional device such as a laminaria or abortifacient is used, or whether the abortion was performed by mechanical means
		Examples:	Transvaginal abortion using vacuum aspiration technique
D	Extraction	Definition:	Pulling or stripping out or off all or a portion of a body part by the use of force
		Explanation:	The qualifier DIAGNOSTIC is used to identify extraction procedures that are biopsies
		Examples:	Low-transverse C-section
E	Delivery	Definition:	Assisting the passage of the products of conception from the genital canal
		Explanation:	Applies only to manually-assisted, vaginal delivery
		Examples:	Manually-assisted delivery
H	Insertion	Definition:	Putting in a nonbiological appliance that monitors, assists, performs, or prevents a physiological function but does not physically take the place of a body part
		Explanation:	None
		Examples:	Placement of fetal scalp electrode
J	Inspection	Definition:	Visually and/or manually exploring a body part
		Explanation:	Visual exploration may be performed with or without optical instrumentation. Manual exploration may be performed directly or through intervening body layers.
		Examples:	Bimanual pregnancy exam
P	Removal	Definition:	Taking out or off a device from a body part, region or orifice
		Explanation:	If a device is taken out and a similar device put in without cutting or puncturing the skin or mucous membrane, the procedure is coded to the root operation CHANGE. Otherwise, the procedure for taking out a device is coded to the root operation REMOVAL.
		Examples:	Removal of fetal monitoring electrode
Q	Repair	Definition:	Restoring, to the extent possible, a body part to its normal anatomic structure and function
		Explanation:	Used only when the method to accomplish the repair is not one of the other root operations
		Examples:	In utero repair of congenital diaphragmatic hernia
S	Reposition	Definition:	Moving to its normal location, or other suitable location, all or a portion of a body part
		Explanation:	The body part is moved to a new location from an abnormal location, or from a normal location where it is not functioning correctly. The body part may or may not be cut out or off to be moved to the new location.
		Examples:	External version of fetus
T	Resection	Definition:	Cutting out or off, without replacement, all of a body part
		Explanation:	None
		Examples:	Total excision of tubal pregnancy
Y	Transplantation	Definition:	Putting in or on all or a portion of a living body part taken from another individual or animal to physically take the place and/or function of all or a portion of a similar body part
		Explanation:	The native body part may or may not be taken out, and the transplanted body part may take over all or a portion of its function
		Examples:	In utero fetal kidney transplant

2 Placement

0	Change	Definition:	Taking out or off a device from a body region and putting back an identical or similar device in or on the same body region without cutting or puncturing the skin or a mucous membrane
		Explanation:	Procedures performed without making an incision or a puncture
		Examples:	Change of vaginal packing
1	Compression	Definition:	Putting pressure on a body region
		Explanation:	Procedures performed without making an incision or a puncture
		Examples:	Placement of pressure dressing on abdominal wall
2	Dressing	Definition:	Putting material on a body region for protection
		Explanation:	Procedures performed without making an incision or a puncture
		Examples:	Application of sterile dressing to head wound
3	Immobilization	Definition:	Limiting or preventing motion of a body region
		Explanation:	Used in all inpatient settings for splint and brace placement, except in rehabilitation settings
		Examples:	Placement of splint on left finger
4	Packing	Definition:	Putting material in a body region or orifice
		Explanation:	Procedures performed without making an incision or a puncture
		Examples:	Placement of nasal packing
5	Removal	Definition:	Taking out or off a device from a body part
		Explanation:	Procedures performed without making an incision or a puncture
		Examples:	Removal of stereotactic head frame
6	Traction	Definition:	Exerting a pulling force on a body region in a distal direction
		Explanation:	Traction in this section includes only the task performed using a mechanical traction apparatus
		Examples:	Lumbar traction using motorized split-traction table

3 Administration

0	Introduction	Definition:	Putting in or on a therapeutic, diagnostic, nutritional, physiological, or prophylactic substance except blood or blood products
		Explanation:	All other substances administered, such as antineoplastic substance
		Examples:	Nerve block injection to median nerve
1	Irrigation	Definition:	Putting in or on a cleansing substance
		Explanation:	Substance given is a cleansing substance or dialysate
		Examples:	Flushing of eye
2	Transfusion	Definition:	Putting in blood or blood products
		Explanation:	Substance given is a blood product or a stem cell substance
		Examples:	Transfusion of cell saver red cells into central venous line

4 Measurement and Monitoring

0	Measurement	Definition:	Determining the level of a physiological or physical function at a point in time
		Explanation:	Describes a single level taken
		Examples:	External electrocardiogram(EKG), single reading
1	Monitoring	Definition:	Determining the level of a physiological or physical function repetitively over a period of time
		Explanation:	Describes a series of levels obtained at intervals
		Examples:	Urinary pressure monitoring

Comprehensive Anatomy and Physiology for ICD-10-CM and ICD-10-PCS Coding

occuring outside the body (handwritten)

5 — Extracorporeal Assistance and Performance

0	Assistance	Definition:	Taking over a portion of a physiological function by extracorporeal means
		Explanation:	Procedures that support a physiological function but do not take complete control of it
		Examples:	Hyperbaric oxygenation of wound
1	Performance	Definition:	Completely taking over a physiological function by extracorporeal means
		Explanation:	Procedures in which complete control is exercised over a physiological function
		Examples:	Cardiopulmonary bypass in conjunction with CABG
2	Restoration	Definition:	Returning, or attempting to return, a physiological function to its original state by extracorporeal means
		Explanation:	Only external cardioversion and defibrillation procedures. Failed cardioversion procedures are also included in the definition of restoration, and are coded the same as successful procedures.
		Examples:	Attempted cardiac defibrillation, unsuccessful

6 — Extracorporeal Therapies

0	Atmospheric Control	Definition:	Extracorporeal control of atmospheric pressure and composition
		Explanation:	None
		Examples:	Antigen-free air conditioning, series treatment
1	Decompression	Definition:	Extracorporeal elimination of undissolved gas from body fluids
		Explanation:	A single type of procedure—treatment for decompression sickness (the bends) in a hyperbaric chamber
		Examples:	Hyperbaric decompression treatment, single
2	Electromagnetic Therapy	Definition:	Extracorporeal treatment by electromagnetic rays
		Explanation:	None
		Examples:	TMS (transcranial magnetic stimulation), series treatment
3	Hyperthermia	Definition:	Extracorporeal raising of body temperature
		Explanation:	To treat temperature imbalance, and as an adjunct radiation treatment for cancer. When performed to treat temperature imbalance, the procedure is coded to this section. When performed for cancer treatment, whole-body hyperthermia is classified as a modality qualifier in section D, "Radiation Therapy."
		Examples:	None
4	Hypothermia	Definition:	Extracorporeal lowering of body temperature
		Explanation:	None
		Examples:	Whole body hypothermia treatment for temperature imbalances, series
5	Pheresis	Definition:	Extracorporeal separation of blood products
		Explanation:	Used in medical practice for two main purposes: to treat diseases where too much of a blood component is produced, such as leukemia, or to remove a blood product such as platelets from a donor, for transfusion into a patient who needs them
		Examples:	Therapeutic leukopheresis, single treatment
6	Phototherapy	Definition:	Extracorporeal treatment by light rays
		Explanation:	Phototherapy to the circulatory system means exposing the blood to light rays outside the body, using a machine that recirculates the blood and returns it to the body after phototherapy
		Examples:	Phototherapy of circulatory system, series treatment
7	Ultrasound Therapy	Definition:	Extracorporeal treatment by ultrasound
		Explanation:	None
		Examples:	Therapeutic ultrasound of peripheral vessels, single treatment

Continued on next page

Appendix D. Root Operation Definitions

6	Extracorporeal Therapies			(Continued)
8	Ultraviolet Light Therapy	Definition:	Extracorporeal treatment by ultraviolet light	
		Explanation:	None	
		Examples:	Ultraviolet light phototherapy, series treatment	
9	Shock Wave Therapy	Definition:	Extracorporeal treatment by shockwaves	
		Explanation:	None	
		Examples:	Shockwave therapy of plantar fascia, single treatment	

7	Osteopathic		
0	Treatment	Definition:	Manual treatment to eliminate or alleviate somatic dysfunction and related disorders
		Explanation:	None
		Examples:	Fascial release of abdomen, osteopathic treatment

8	Other Procedures		
0	Other Procedures	Definition:	Methodologies which attempt to remediate or cure a disorder or disease
		Explanation:	For nontraditional, whole-body therapies including acupuncture and meditation
		Examples:	Acupuncture, yoga therapy

9	Chiropractic		
B	Manipulation	Definition:	Manual procedure that involves a directed thrust to move a joint past the physiological range of motion, without exceeding the anatomical limit
		Explanation:	None
		Examples:	Chiropractic treatment of cervical spine, short lever specific contact

Note: Sections B-H (Imaging through Substance Abuse Treatment) do not include root operations. The character 3 position represents type of procedure, therefore those definitions are not included in this appendix. See appendix J for definitions of the type (character 3) or type qualifiers (character 5) that provide details of the procedures performed.

Appendix E.
Root Operation Conversion Table

Documented Procedure	PCS Root Operation		Key Objective of Procedure/Comment
Common Suffixes			
-centesis	Drainage	9	
-desis	Fusion	G	
-ectomy	Excision	B	Cutting out or off, without replacement, **a portion of a body part**
	Resection	T	Cutting out or off, without replacement, **all** of a body part
-exeresis	Extraction	D	
-lysis	Release	N	
-oscopy	Inspection	J	
-otomy	Division	8	Cutting into body part **w/o** taking out fluids and/or gases to separate or transect a body part
	Drainage	9	**Taking out fluids and/or gases**
-pexy	Repair	Q	**Restoring to normal anatomy or function**—Used only when no other root operation is applicable
	Reposition	S	**Move** body part to a **new location** (e.g., free flaps)
-plasty	Repair	Q	**Restoring to normal anatomy or function**—Used only when no other root operation is applicable
	Replacement **DVC**	R	Putting in/on biological/synthetic material **to take the place and/or function of a body part**
	Supplement **DVC**	U	Putting in/on biologic/synthetic material **to reinforce and/or augment the function** of a body part
-plication	Restriction	V	
-rraphy	Repair	Q	
-stasis	Control	3	
-tripsy	Fragmentation	F	
Common Procedures			
Adenoidectomy			5th character Approach = **X External**
partial	Excision	B	Coded separately from concomitant tonsillectomy
total	Resection	T	Coded separately from concomitant tonsillectomy
Adhesiolysis	Release	N	4th character Body Part = Body part being freed
Advancement (flap)	Reposition	S	**Move** body part to a **new location** (e.g., free flaps)
	Transfer	X	Move body part to another location **to take over the function,** still **connected to its vascular and nervous supply**
Amniocentesis	Drainage	9	See table 1Ø9.
Amputation (extremity)	Detachment	6	

DVC Root operation for procedures that always involve a device.

Documented Procedure	PCS Root Operation		Key Objective of Procedure/Comment
Anastomosis	Bypass	1	
Aneurysm clipping	Restriction	V	
Angiocardiography (e.g., with cardiac cath)	Fluoroscopy	1	See table B21.
Angioplasty	Dilation	7	**Expanding orifice** or lumen (e.g., PTCA)
	Repair	Q	**Restoring to normal anatomy or function**—Used only when no other root operation is applicable
	Replacement [DVC]	R	Putting in/on biological/synthetic material **to take the place and/or function of a body part**
	Supplement [DVC]	U	Putting in/on biologic/synthetic material **to reinforce and/or augment the function** of a body part
Annuloplasty with ring	Supplement [DVC]	U	Use Synthetic Substitute for ring
Antrostomy	Drainage	9	
Appendectomy	Excision	B	
	Resection	T	
Arthrocentesis	Drainage	9	
Arthroplasty	Repair	Q	**Restoring to normal anatomy or function**—Used only when no other root operation is applicable
	Replacement [DVC]	R	Putting in/on biological/synthetic material **to take the place and/or function of a body part**
	Supplement [DVC]	U	Putting in/on biologic/synthetic material **to reinforce and/or augment the function** of a body part
Arthroscopy	Inspection	J	
Aspiration	Drainage	9	
Banding	Restriction	V	
Biopsy	Drainage	9	Taking out **fluids and/or gases**; 7th character Qualifier = **X Diagnostic**
	Excision	B	**Cutting** out a **portion** of a body part (e.g., punch or wedge); 7th character Qualifier = **X Diagnostic**
	Extraction	D	Pulling out or off, or stripping out by the use of force, some or all of a body part without replacement (e.g., bone marrow, endometrium); 7th character Qualifier = **X Diagnostic**
Blepharoplasty	Repair	Q	**Restoring to normal anatomy or function**—Used only when no other root operation is applicable
	Replacement [DVC]	R	Putting in/on biological/synthetic material **to take the place and/or function of a body part**
	Reposition	S	**Move** a body part to a new location retaining normal function
	Supplement [DVC]	U	Putting in/on biologic/synthetic material **to reinforce and/or augment the function** of a body part
Bone marrow, biopsy	Extraction	D	
Bone marrow, transplant	Administration/ Transfusion	2	See table 302.
Bunionectomy	Excision	B	4th character Body Part = **N or P Metatarsal, Right or Left**
Calculus removal	Extirpation	C	

[DVC] Root operation for procedures that always involve a device.

Appendix E. Root Operation Conversion Table

Documented Procedure	PCS Root Operation		Key Objective of Procedure/Comment
Capsulorrhaphy, joint	Repair	Q	
Cardiac catheterization, diagnostic	Measurement	Ø	See table 4AØ.
Carpal tunnel repair	Release	N	4th character Body Part = **5 Median Nerve**
Caesarean section	Extraction	D	4th character Body Part = **Ø Products of Conception**
Cauterization	Destruction	5	**Physical eradication by the direct use of energy, force or a destructive agent**
	Repair	Q	**Restoring to normal anatomy or function**—Used only when no other root operation is applicable
Chemoembolization	Introduction	Ø	See table 3EØ.
Chemotherapy infusion	Introduction	Ø	See table 3EØ.
Clamping	Occlusion	L	
Clipping (e.g., aneurysm)	Restriction	V	
Closure	Occlusion	L	**Completely closing** an orifice or the lumen
	Repair	Q	**Restoring to normal anatomy or function**—Used only when no other root operation is applicable
Coagulation	Destruction	5	
Colonoscopy, diagnostic	Inspection	J	4th character Body Part = **D Lower Intestinal Tract**
Colostomy	Bypass, Colon	1	**Altering route** of passage of contents of a **tubular** body part; Body System GI
	Drainage	9	**Taking out fluids and/or gases**
Compression	Restriction	V	
Craniotomy	Drainage, CNS	9	
	Division, Head and Facial Bones	8	
	Drainage, Head and Facial Bones	9	
Crushing, nerve	Destruction	5	
Cryoablation	Destruction	5	
Cryotherapy	Destruction	5	
Curettage	Excision	B	**Cutting out or off**, without replacement, a portion of a body part
	Extraction	D	**Pulling** or stripping out by the use of force
Cystocele repair	Repair	Q	2nd character = **J Subcutaneous Tissue & Fascia**; 4th character Body Part = **C Pelvic Region**
Cystoscopy (diagnostic)	Inspection	J	
Debridement			
excisional	Excision	B	
nonexcisional	Extraction	D	
Denervation	Destruction	5	
Dilation & Curettage	Extraction	D	
Disarticulation	Detachment	6	
Discectomy, diskectomy	Excision	B	Cutting out or off, without replacement, a **portion** of a body part
	Resection	T	Cutting out or off, without replacement, **all** of a body part

DVC Root operation for procedures that always involve a device.

Comprehensive Anatomy and Physiology for ICD-10-CM and ICD-10-PCS Coding

Documented Procedure	PCS Root Operation		Key Objective of Procedure/Comment
Diversion	Bypass	1	4th character Body Part = **From** – 7th character Qualifier = **To** (except in coronary artery bypass—the body part identifies the number of coronary artery sites bypassed **To**, with qualifier specifying the vessel bypassed **From**)
Diverticulectomy	Excision	B	2nd character Body System = **D Gastrointestinal System**
Elevation, bone fragments, skull	Reposition	S	
Embolectomy	Extirpation	C	
Embolization	Occlusion	L	
Endarterectomy	Extirpation	C	2nd character Body System = **3 or 4, Upper or Lower Arteries**
Endometrial biopsy	Extraction	D	
Enucleation, eyeball, w/o implant	Resection	T	
w/ implant	Replacement [DVC]	R	
Episiotomy	Division	8	2nd character Body System = **W Anatomical Regions, General**
ERCP	Fluoroscopy	1	See table BF1.
ESWL	Fragmentation	F	
Evacuation			
hematoma	Extirpation	C	
other fluid	Drainage	9	
Evisceration, eyeball, w/o implant	Resection	T	
w/ implant	Replacement [DVC]	R	
Examination	Inspection	J	
Exchange, device	Change [DVC]	2	
Exploration	Inspection	J	
Fasciotomy	Division	8	Cutting into body part **w/o** taking out fluids and/or gases **to separate or transect a body part**; Body System **J** Subcutaneous Tissue & Fascia
	Drainage	9	**Taking out fluids and/or gases**; Body System = **J Subcutaneous Tissue & Fascia**
Feeding tube placement	Insertion [DVC]	H	
Fistulization	Bypass	1	**Altering route** of passage of **contents** of a **tubular** body part
	Drainage	9	**Taking out fluids and/or gases**
	Repair	Q	**Restoring to normal anatomy or function**—Used only when no other root operation is applicable
Fixation, bone			
w/ fracture reduction	Reposition	S	
w/o fracture reduction	Insertion [DVC]	H	
Flap closure	Transfer	X	
Foley catheter placement	Drainage	9	
Foreign body removal	Extirpation	C	
Fulguration	Destruction	5	
Full-thickness skin grafting	Replacement [DVC]	R	

[DVC] Root operation for procedures that always involve a device.

Appendix E. Root Operation Conversion Table

Documented Procedure	PCS Root Operation		Key Objective of Procedure/Comment
Fundoplication, GI	Restriction	V	
Gastroscopy	Inspection	J	
Gastrostomy	Bypass	1	**Altering route** of passage of **contents** of a **tubular** body part
	Drainage	9	**Taking out fluids and/or gases**
Graft	Replacement [DVC]	R	Putting in/on biological/synthetic material **to take the place and/or function of a body part**
	Supplement [DVC]	U	Putting in/on biologic/synthetic material **to reinforce and/or augment the function** of a body part
Hemicolectomy	Resection	T	
Hemilaminectomy	Excision	B	2nd character Body System = **P or Q Upper or Lower Bones**
Hernia repair			
w/mesh	Supplement [DVC]	U	
w/o mesh	Repair	Q	
Hysterectomy (lap-assisted total vaginal)	Resection	T	
Implantation	Insertion [DVC]	H	Putting in **appliance** that **monitors, assists, performs or prevents** a physiological function
	Replacement [DVC]	R	Putting in/on biological/synthetic material **to take the place and/or function of a body part**
Incisional procedures (no tissue removed)	Division	8	(e.g., osteotomy, neurotomy, spinal cordotomy)
for drainage	Drainage	9	**Taking out fluids and/or gases** (e.g., I&D abscess or cyst, bursotomy, laparotomy, oophorotomy)
Induction of labor			
AROM	Drainage, Pregnancy	9	
Oxytocin	Introduction, Hormone		See table 3E0; 6th character Substance = **V Hormone**
Infusion	Introduction		See table 3E0.
Injection	Introduction		See table 3E0.
Instillation	Introduction		See table 3E0.
Insufflation	Introduction		See table 3E0.
Interruption	Occlusion	L	
Intrathecal infusion pump placement	Insertion [DVC]	H	In most cases, the 2nd character Body System = **J Subcutaneous Tissue & Fascia**
Intubation			
airway, trachea	Insertion [DVC]	H	
airway, mouth & throat	Insertion [DVC]	H	
airway, esophagus	Insertion [DVC]	H	
drainage device	Drainage	9	
feeding device	Insertion [DVC]	H	
Iridotomy	Drainage	9	
Jejunostomy	Bypass	1	
	Drainage	9	

[DVC] Root operation for procedures that always involve a device.

Documented Procedure	PCS Root Operation		Key Objective of Procedure/Comment
Keratoplasty	Repair	Q	**Restoring to normal anatomy or function**—Used only when no other root operation is applicable
	Replacement **DVC**	R	Putting in/on biological/synthetic material **to take the place and/or function of a body part**
	Supplement **DVC**	U	Putting in/on biologic/synthetic material **to reinforce and/or augment the function** of a body part
Laceration suturing	Repair	Q	
Laminectomy	Excision	B	2nd character Body System = **P or Q Upper or Lower Bones**
Laparoscopy	Inspection	J	
Laparotomy			
for drainage	Drainage	9	2nd character Body System = **W Cavity, Peritoneal**
exploratory	Inspection	J	2nd character Body System = **W Cavity, Peritoneal**
Lavage	Irrigation		See table 3E1.
diagnostic bronchial alveolar	Drainage	9	2nd character Body System = **B Respiratory**
Lengthening			
bone, with device	Insertion **DVC**	H	6th character Qualifier = **8 External Fixation Device, Limb Lengthening**
muscle, by incision	Division	8	
tendon, by incision	Division	8	
Ligation	Occlusion	L	
Liposuction			5th character Approach = **3 Percutaneous**
for medical reasons	Extraction	D	
for cosmetic reasons	Alteration	Ø	
Lithotripsy	Fragmentation	F	
w/ removal of fragments	Extirpation	C	
Lobectomy lung			
total	Resection	T	
partial	Excision	B	
Lobotomy	Division	8	
Lumbar puncture (spinal tap)	Drainage, spinal canal	9	
Lymphadenectomy			
partial	Excision	B	
total, entire chain	Resection	T	
Lysis	Release	N	4th character Body Part = Body part being freed
Mammoplasty	Alteration	Ø	**Modifying natural anatomic structure** w/o affecting the function for **cosmetic** purpose
	Repair	Q	**Restoring to normal anatomy or function**—Used only when no other root operation is applicable
	Replacement **DVC**	R	Putting in/on biological/synthetic material **to take the place and/or function of a body part**
	Supplement **DVC**	U	Putting in/on biologic/synthetic material **to reinforce and/or augment the function** of a body part
Manipulation, adhesions	Release	N	4th character Body Part = Body part being freed

DVC Root operation for procedures that always involve a device.

Appendix E. Root Operation Conversion Table

Documented Procedure	PCS Root Operation		Key Objective of Procedure/Comment
Mastectomy			
partial or lumpectomy	Excision	B	
total w/ implants or flap reconstruction	Replacement **DVC**	R	
total w/o implants	Resection	T	
Mastoidectomy			
partial	Excision	B	
total	Resection	T	
Mechanical ventilation	Performance, respiratory		See table 5A1.
Meniscectomy			
partial	Excision	B	
total	Resection	T	
Myringoplasty	Repair	Q	2nd character Body System = **9 Ear, Nose, Sinus**
	Replacement **DVC**	R	2nd character Body System = **9 Ear, Nose, Sinus**
	Supplement **DVC**	U	2nd character Body System = **9 Ear, Nose, Sinus**
Myringotomy	Drainage	9	2nd character Body System = **9 Ear, Nose, Sinus**
Nephrectomy			
partial	Excision	B	
total	Resection	T	
Nephrolithotomy	Extirpation	C	
Nephrostomy	Bypass	1	**Altering route** of passage of **contents** of a **tubular** body part
	Drainage	9	**Taking out fluids and/or gases**
Nephrotomy	Drainage	9	**Taking out fluids and/or gases**
	Division	8	**Cutting into** a body part w/o draining fluids and/or gases **to separate or transect** a body part
Neurolysis	Release	N	**Freeing** a body part from **abnormal physical constraint**; 4th character Body Part = Body part being freed
Neuroplasty	Repair	Q	**Restoring to normal anatomy or function**—Used only when no other root operation is applicable; 2nd character Body System = **Ø or 1 Central or Peripheral Nervous System**
	Supplement **DVC**	U	Putting in/on biologic/synthetic material **to reinforce and/or augment the function** of a body part; 2nd character Body System = **Ø or 1 Central or Peripheral Nervous System**
Neurorrhaphy	Repair	Q	
Obliteration	Destruction	5	
Omentectomy	Excision	B	Cutting out or off, without replacement, **a portion** of a body part; 2nd character Body System = **D Gastrointestinal System**
	Resection	T	Cutting out or off, without replacement, **all** of a body part; 2nd character Body System = **D Gastrointestinal System**

DVC Root operation for procedures that always involve a device.

Comprehensive Anatomy and Physiology for ICD-10-CM and ICD-10-PCS Coding

Documented Procedure	PCS Root Operation			Key Objective of Procedure/Comment
Oophorectomy				2nd character Body System = **U Female Reproductive System**
partial	Excision		B	
total	Resection		T	
Orchiectomy				2nd character Body System = **V Male Reproductive System**
partial	Excision		B	
total	Resection		T	
Orchiopexy	Repair		Q	Body System = **V Male Reproductive System**
	Reposition		S	Body System = **V Male Reproductive System**
Osteotomy	Division		8	**Cutting into** a body part w/o draining fluids and/or gases **to separate or transect** a body part
	Drainage		9	**Taking out fluids and/or gases**
Otoplasty	Repair		Q	**Restoring to normal anatomy or function**—Used only when no other root operation is applicable
	Replacement	DVC	R	Putting in/on biological/synthetic material **to take the place and/or function of a body part**
	Supplement	DVC	U	Putting in/on biologic/synthetic material **to reinforce and/or augment the function** of a body part
Paracentesis (abdominal)	Drainage		9	2nd character Body System = **W Anatomical Regions, General**
Parathyroidectomy				2nd character Body System = **G Endocrine System**
partial	Excision		B	
total	Resection		T	
PEG (percutaneous endoscopic gastrostomy)	Insertion	DVC	H	6th character Device = **U Feeding Device**
PEJ (percutaneous endoscopic jejunostomy)	Insertion	DVC	H	6th character Device = **U Feeding Device**
Pericardiocentesis	Drainage		9	2nd character Body System = **W Anatomical Regions, General**
Photocoagulation	Destruction		5	
	Repair		Q	
Pleurocentesis	Drainage		9	2nd character Body System = **W Anatomical Regions, General**
Pleurodesis				
chemical	Introduction			See table 3E0; 4th character Body Part = **L Pleural Cavity**
mechanical (surgical)	Destruction		5	See table 0B5.
Plication	Restriction		V	
Pneumonectomy	Resection		T	2nd character Body System = **B Respiratory System**
Polypectomy	Excision		B	
Proctectomy				
partial	Excision		B	
total	Resection		T	

DVC Root operation for procedures that always involve a device.

Appendix E. Root Operation Conversion Table

Documented Procedure	PCS Root Operation		Key Objective of Procedure/Comment
Proctopexy	Repair	Q	**Restoring to normal anatomy or function**—Used only when no other root operation is applicable
	Reposition	S	**Move** body part to a new location retaining normal function
Proctoplasty	Repair	Q	**Restoring to normal anatomy or function**—Used only when no other root operation is applicable
	Supplement [DVC]	U	Putting in/on biologic/synthetic material **to reinforce and/or augment the function** of a body part
Proctostomy	Drainage	9	
Prostatectomy			
partial (by lobe)	Excision	B	
total	Resection	T	
PTCA	Dilation	7	
Pull-through, rectal	Resection	T	
Punch biopsy	Excision	B	7th character Qualifier = **X Diagnostic**
Puncture	Drainage	9	
Pyelostomy	Drainage	9	Taking out fluids and/or gases; 2nd character Body System = **T Urinary System**
	Bypass	1	**Altering route** of passage of **contents** of a **tubular** body part; 2nd character Body System = **T Urinary System**
Pyelotomy	Drainage	9	2nd character Body System = **T Urinary System**
Pyloroplasty	Repair	Q	**Restoring to normal anatomy or function**—Used only when no other root operation is applicable
	Supplement [DVC]	U	Putting in/on biologic/synthetic material **to reinforce and/or augment the function** of a body part
Recession	Repair	Q	**Restoring to normal anatomy or function**—Used only when no other root operation is applicable
	Reposition	S	**Move** body part to a new location retaining normal function
Reconstruction	Repair	Q	**Restoring to normal anatomy or function**—Used only when no other root operation is applicable
	Replacement [DVC]	R	Putting in/on biological/synthetic material **to take the place and/or function of a body part**
	Supplement [DVC]	U	Putting in/on biologic/synthetic material **to reinforce and/or augment the function** of a body part
Rectopexy	Repair	Q	**Restoring to normal anatomy or function**—Used only when no other root operation is applicable
	Reposition	S	**Move** body part to a new location retaining normal function
Rectoplasty	Repair	Q	**Restoring to normal anatomy or function**—Used only when no other root operation is applicable; 2nd character Body System = **D Gastrointestinal System**
	Supplement [DVC]	U	Putting in/on biologic/synthetic material **to reinforce and/or augment the function** of a body part

[DVC] Root operation for procedures that always involve a device.

© 2015 Optum360, LLC

Comprehensive Anatomy and Physiology for ICD-10-CM and ICD-10-PCS Coding

Documented Procedure	PCS Root Operation		Key Objective of Procedure/Comment
Reduction			
dislocation	Reposition	S	
fracture	Reposition	S	
intussusception, intestinal	Reposition	S	
mammoplasty	Excision	B	
prolapse	Reposition	S	
torsion	Reposition	S	
volvulus, GI	Reposition	S	
Reimplantation	Reposition	S	**Move** body part to a new location retaining normal function
	Transfer	X	Move to another location **to take over the function** still **connected to its vascular and nervous supply**
	Reattachment	M	**Putting back in or on a separated** body part to its **normal location** or other suitable location
Reinforcement	Repair	Q	**Restoring to normal anatomy or function**—Used only when no other root operation is applicable
	Supplement DVC	U	Putting in/on biologic/synthetic material **to reinforce and/or augment the function** of a body part
Relaxation, scar tissue	Release	N	4th character Body Part = Body part being freed
Reopening, operative site			
control of bleeding	Control	3	
examination only	Inspection	J	
Rhinoplasty	Alteration	Ø	**Modifying natural anatomic structure** w/o affecting the function for **cosmetic** purpose
	Repair	Q	**Restoring to normal anatomy or function**—Used only when no other root operation is applicable
	Replacement DVC	R	Putting in/on **biological/synthetic material to take the place and/or function of a body part**
	Supplement DVC	U	Putting in/on biologic/synthetic material **to reinforce and/or augment the function** of a body part
Rhytidectomy	Alteration	Ø	
Roux-en-Y operation	Bypass	1	2nd character Body System = **D Gastrointestinal System or F Hepatobiliary System and Pancreas**
Salpingectomy			
partial	Excision	B	
total	Resection	T	
Scleral buckling w/implant	Supplement DVC	U	
Sclerotherapy, mechanical	Destruction	5	
Septoplasty	Repair	Q	**Restoring to normal anatomy or function**—Used only when no other root operation is applicable
	Replacement DVC	R	Putting in/on biological/synthetic material **to take the place and/or function of a body part**
	Reposition	S	**Move** body part to a **new location retaining normal function**
	Supplement DVC	U	Putting in/on biologic/synthetic material **to reinforce and/or augment the function** of a body part

DVC Root operation for procedures that always involve a device.

Appendix E. Root Operation Conversion Table

Documented Procedure	PCS Root Operation		Key Objective of Procedure/Comment
Shunt creation	Bypass	1	
Sigmoidectomy			
partial	Excision	B	
total	Resection	T	
Sphincterotomy	Drainage	9	Taking out fluids and/or gases
	Division	8	**Cutting into** a body part w/o draining fluids and/or gases **to separate or transect** a body part
Stone removal	Extirpation	C	
Stripping	Extraction	D	
Suction	Drainage	9	
Suction curettage (D&C)			
nonobstetric	Extraction	D	4th character Body Part = **B Endometrium** (see table 0UD)
obstetric post-delivery	Extraction	D	4th character Body Part = **1 Products of Conception, Retained** (see table 10D)
Suspension	Reposition	S	
Suture			
laceration repair	Repair	Q	
ligation	Occlusion	L	
Swan-Ganz placement	Insertion [DVC]	H	4th character Body Part = **Pulmonary Artery**; 6th character Device = **Monitoring Device**
Synovectomy	Excision	B	
Takedown			
shunt	Removal [DVC]	P	
shunt (with replacement)	Bypass	1	
stoma	Repair	Q	
Tarsorrhaphy	Repair	Q	
Tendolysis	Release	N	
Thoracentesis	Drainage	9	2nd character Body System = **W Anatomical Regions, General**
Thoracotomy	Drainage	9	2nd character Body System = **W Anatomical Regions, General**
Thrombectomy	Extirpation	C	
Thyroidectomy			
partial	Excision	B	
total	Resection	T	
Tonsillectomy			5th character Approach = **X External**
partial	Excision	B	Coded separately from concomitant adenoidectomy
total	Resection	T	Coded separately from concomitant adenoidectomy
Tracheostomy formation	Bypass	1	
Transection	Division	8	

[DVC] Root operation for procedures that always involve a device.

Documented Procedure	PCS Root Operation		Key Objective of Procedure/Comment
Transposition	Reposition	S	**Move** body part to a new location retaining normal function
	Transfer	X	Move to another location **to take over the function** still **connected to its vascular and nervous supply**
Turbinectomy			
partial	Excision	B	
total	Resection	T	
TURP (transurethral resection of prostate)	Excision	B	
Tympanoplasty	Repair	Q	**Restoring to normal anatomy or function**—Used only when no other root operation is applicable
	Replacement DVC	R	Putting in/on biological/synthetic material **to take the place and/or function of a body part**
	Supplement DVC	U	Putting in/on biologic/synthetic material **to reinforce and/or augment the function** of a body part
Ureterolithotomy	Extirpation	C	
Ureteroscopy	Inspection	J	
Urethral catheterization, indwelling	Drainage	9	
Urethrolithotomy	Extirpation	C	
Urinary diversion	Bypass	1	4th character Body Part = **From** – 7th character Qualifier = **To**
Valvuloplasty	Repair	Q	**Restoring to normal anatomy or function**—Used only when no other root operation is applicable
	Replacement DVC	R	Putting in/on biological/synthetic material **to take the place and/or function of a body part**
	Supplement DVC	U	Putting in/on biologic/synthetic material **to reinforce and/or augment the function** of a body part
Vasectomy	Excision	B	
Vein stripping	Extraction	D	
Ventilation (mechanical)	Performance		See table 5A1.
Ventriculostomy			4th character Body Part = **6 Cerebral Ventricle**
external drainage	Drainage	9	
internal shunt	Bypass	1	
Vitrectomy			
partial	Excision	B	
total	Resection	T	
Washing	Irrigation	1	Administration section
Wedge resection, pulmonary	Excision	B	
Window	Drainage	9	
Z-plasty, skin for scar contracture	Release	N	4th character Body Part = Body part being freed

DVC   Root operation for procedures that always involve a device.